# Mental Health Concepts and Techniques for the Occupational Therapy Assistant

FOURTH EDITION

# Mental Health Concepts and Techniques for the Occupational Therapy Assistant

FOURTH EDITION


Mary Beth Early, M.S., OTR
Professor
Occupational Therapy Assistant Program
LaGuardia Community College
City University of New York
New York, New York



Wolters Kluwer Health | Lippincott Williams & Wilkins
Philadelphia • Baltimore • New York • London
Buenos Aires • Hong Kong • Sydney • Tokyo

*Acquisitions Editor:* Emily J. Lupash
*Managing Editor:* Matthew J. Hauber, Elizabeth Connolly
*Marketing Manager:* Missi Carmen
*Production Editor:* Paula C. Williams
*Designer:* Doug Smock
*Compositor:* International Typesetting and Composition

Fourth Edition



351 West Camden Street
Baltimore, MD 21201

530 Walnut Street
Philadelphia, PA 19106

Printed in China



9 8

**Library of Congress Cataloging-in-Publication Data**

Early, Mary Beth.
Mental health concepts and techniques for the occupational therapy assistant / Mary Beth Early.—4th ed.
p. ; cm.
Includes bibliographical references and index.
ISBN-13: 978-0-7817-7839-8
ISBN-10: 0-7817-7839-5
1. Occupational therapy. 2. Mentally ill—Rehabilitation. 3. Occupational therapy assistants. I. Title.
[DNLM: 1. Occupational Therapy—methods. 2. Allied Health Personnel. 3. Mental Disorders—rehabilitation. WM 450.5.O2 E12m 2009]
RC437.E3 2009
616.89'165—dc22

2007040191

## DISCLAIMER

Care has been taken to confirm the accuracy of the information present and to describe generally accepted practices. However, the authors, editors, and publisher are not responsible for errors or omissions or for any consequences from application of the information in this book and make no warranty, expressed or implied, with respect to the currency, completeness, or accuracy of the contents of the publication. Application of this information in a particular situation remains the professional responsibility of the practitioner; the clinical treatments described and recommended may not be considered absolute and universal recommendations.

The authors, editors, and publisher have exerted every effort to ensure that drug selection and dosage set forth in this text are in accordance with the current recommendations and practice at the time of publication. However, in view of ongoing research, changes in government regulations, and the constant flow of information relating to drug therapy and drug reactions, the reader is urged to check the package insert for each drug for any change in indications and dosage and for added warnings and precautions. This is particularly important when the recommended agent is a new or infrequently employed drug.

Some drugs and medical devices presented in this publication have Food and Drug Administration (FDA) clearance for limited use in restricted research settings. It is the responsibility of the health care provider to ascertain the FDA status of each drug or device planned for use in their clinical practice.

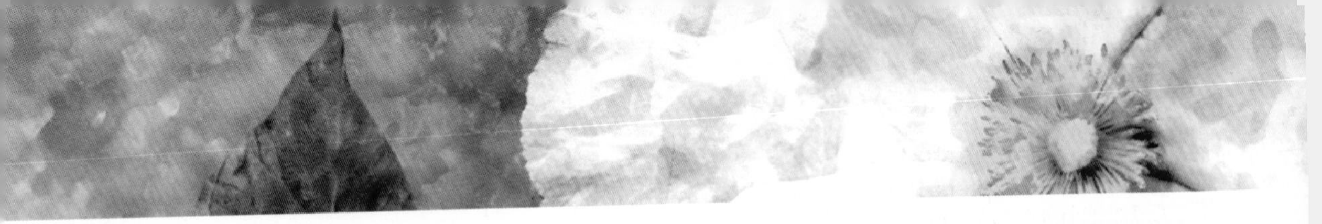

# Preface

Like its predecessors, the fourth edition of *Mental Health Concepts and Techniques* aims to provide the occupational therapy assistant (OTA) student with a comprehensive foundation for the practice of occupational therapy for persons with mental health problems. In addition, the book may be useful to experienced occupational therapy assistants who wish to enter or reenter psychiatric practice. The text may serve as a resource for occupational therapists with supervisory and administrative roles in mental health settings who have an interest in exploring the delineation and relationships between the professional and technical levels of responsibility. It is assumed that readers of this text have prior education in human growth and development, group process, and activities used in occupational therapy.

Much has changed in mental health practice since the first edition. Psychopharmacology has provided medications that better target specific disorders, enabling improved functioning and reducing unwanted side effects. People with psychiatric disorders are increasingly politicized—assertive about their rights, alert and proactive as consumers of services. The terms used to refer to "recipients of services" in the fourth edition reflect current usage. Box 7-1 lists and discusses some of the names given to the recipient of occupational therapy services in psychiatric settings: patient, client, consumer, member, inmate, resident, survivor, and so on. The student and reader are encouraged to tolerate the ambiguity of these terms, to learn to intuit which is the correct name for a specific situation, and to develop an empathic feel for the stigma that attaches to such labels.

The content is arranged into six sections. Section I (Chapters 1 to 5) establishes a framework, discussing the historical origins of psychiatric occupational therapy and the past and current theoretical foundations on which mental health practice is based. Case examples are included to illustrate how each theory can be applied. Information on occupational therapy practice models and theories has been updated and combined into one chapter. A new chapter on *The Occupational Therapy Practice Framework (OTPF)* has been added.

Section II (Chapters 6 to 9) addresses the context of the occupational therapy intervention process and includes chapters on psychiatric diagnosis *(DSM-IV)*, treatment settings, medications, and special groups of consumers. Content on practice with children, adolescents, families, victims of domestic violence, and other groups has been increased. The purpose of gathering such disparate topics under the heading *context* is to draw attention to the effects of these aspects on the occupational therapy process.

Section III (Chapters 10 to 13) focuses on relationships with patients/clients/consumers. There are two reasons this material is placed here: First, the therapeutic relationship with the mental health worker is a primary force in restoring the patient's motivation and ability to function and logically should precede any discipline-specific content. In addition, past students have expressed a need to know what to *do* with the clients whom they meet on level I fieldwork, which may run concurrently with the mental health coursework in some curricula. A chapter on safety is included in this section. The chapter on groups also comes in this section.

Section IV (Chapters 14 to 17) describes the occupational therapy process, beginning with an overview and proceeding to individual chapters on data gathering and evaluation and intervention and documentation. The chapters in this sections correspond to the terminology and concepts of the *OTPF.*

Occupational therapy methods and activities are the focus of Section V (Chapters 18 to 23). These chapters detail specific activities in the areas of daily living skills, education and work, leisure and social participation, management of emotional needs, and cognitive and sensory and motor factors. The final chapter in this section explains how to analyze and adapt activities to fit the needs of individual clients and groups.

Section VI (Chapters 24 and 25) addresses the professional self. Chapter 24, on supervision, provides a perspective on the purpose and use of supervision; it is recommended that this chapter be assigned at the beginning of level I fieldwork. The final chapter, on being organized, is intended to help students and new graduates structure their work time and work environments more efficiently and effectively.

Appendix A contains several case examples, some of which are referred to in the text. Additional case examples are included in Chapters 2 through 6. Appendix B gives several sample group protocols to supplement the material in Chapter 13. The end papers list abbreviations that students and practitioners may encounter in psychiatric settings and medical records.

Those familiar with the prior editions will note an enhanced art program along with some new text features. Chapter objectives help direct readers (especially student readers) to the learning goals for the chapter, and chapter review questions test the readers' comprehension. Point-of-view boxes have also been added to selected chapters to show a different perspective on the topic at hand. This edition continues to employ features from the previous edition as well: Concepts Summary and Vocabulary Review (found throughout selected chapters in Section I) reinforce important concepts and provide definitions for key terms, and Case Examples (also in selected chapters in Section I) provide a practical application of the material.

With each edition we try to move more perfectly toward gender-neutral language. Unfortunately, the third person plural is not always appropriate and in such cases masculine or feminine names or pronouns have been employed.

# Acknowledgments

I am indebted to all those who have helped in direct and indirect ways, over the 27 years that I have worked on the four editions of this text and its predecessor manuals. I remain deeply grateful to Professor JoAnn Romeo Anderson, Dean Irwin Feifer, and former Dean of Faculty Martin Moed for their encouragement and mentorship during the T.A.R. project at LaGuardia Community College in 1980 and 1981; participation in that project enabled me to develop the course manual from which the first edition evolved. I am grateful to LaGuardia Community College, President Gail Mellow, and the City University of New York for providing me with sabbatical leave to work on the fourth edition.

I am most appreciative of the careful suggestions and collegial encouragement of the reviewers of the various editions over the years: Claudia Allen, Linda Barnes, Jody Bortone, Terry Brittell, Leita Chalfin, Phyllis Clements, Carol Endebrock-Lee, Edith Fenton, Yvette Hachtel, Florence Hannes, Diane Harlowe, Noel Hepler, Lorna Jean King, Tom Lawton, Siri Marken, Maureen Matthews, Ann Neville-Jan, Elizabeth Nyberg, Gertrude Pinto, Anne Hiller Scott, Esther Simon, Scott Trudeau, Susan Voorhies, and Marla Wonser.

Contributions, suggestions, and encouragement for the various editions were offered by many including Carlotta Kip and Alfred Blake, Sherrell Powell and Naomi Greenberg, Diane Harlowe and Gloria Graham. Susan Voorhies, COTA, CAODAC, and her supervisor, Anne Brown, OTR, MS, provided group protocols, case examples, and other treatment information for substance abuse for the second edition that have been retained for the fourth. I appreciate the help of Kathleen Kannenberg of AOTA's practice division for information on total quality management (second edition), and Charlotte Lazaro, COTA, during her days as an occupational therapy assistant student, for research on medications and their side effects. Hermine D. Plotnick, MA, OTR, and Margaret D. Rerek, MA, OTR, created the case study for the chapter on psychiatric diagnosis. All of these contributions were significant.

For the fourth edition, I am particularly grateful to Gary Kielhofner and Jessica Marvelle Kramer of the Model of Human Occupation Clearinghouse for granting permission to reproduce pages from the MOHO instruments, to Gloria Furst for sharing the ACTRE, and to Haven Smink of AOTA and to Ina Elfant Asher for sharing the contents of the third edition of *Occupational Therapy Assessment Tools: An Annotated Index* prior to its publication. Jody Bertrand of S&S Worldwide provided photos that help illustrate activities, as did Donna Costa, and the Iyengar Yoga Association of Greater New York.

I thank also the staff at Raven Press and at Lippincott Williams & Wilkins for their editorial and other support over the years. Vickie Thaw was especially encouraging in her stewardship of the project during the development of the second edition. For the third edition, Margaret Biblis, Linda Napora, Amy Amico, Lisa Franko and Mario Fernandez created wonderful text features and a beautiful design, which have been retained for the new edition. For the fourth edition, Elizabeth Connolly provided careful and thoughtful guidance as managing editor. I am also indebted to Kim Battista (artist) and Jennifer Clements (art director) for enhancing the look of the book and the images within it. Also important to making this book possible were the production team, especially Paula Williams, and the acquisitions editor, Emily Lupash. I thank also Arushi Chawla (of International Typesetting and Composition, Noida, India) who was a responsive and responsible contact during the page proof stage.

My family gave unceasingly of devotion and care. In particular I thank my husband, Bob, for consistently and lovingly reminding me that I would manage to complete this edition just as I have completed others, for listening to me when I was working out ideas, and for nourishing me with tasty new dishes and irresistible desserts. Our son, Jeffrey, put up with a great deal of preoccupation and unintentional ignoring while I was immersed in this work; I admire and appreciate his cheerful and accepting attitude and constant good nature. Thanks, guys!

# Contents

## APPENDIX A: CASE EXAMPLES



## APPENDIX B: SAMPLE GROUP PROTOCOLS

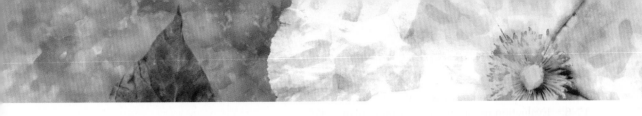

# List of Figures

# List of Tables

# List of Boxes

SECTION I

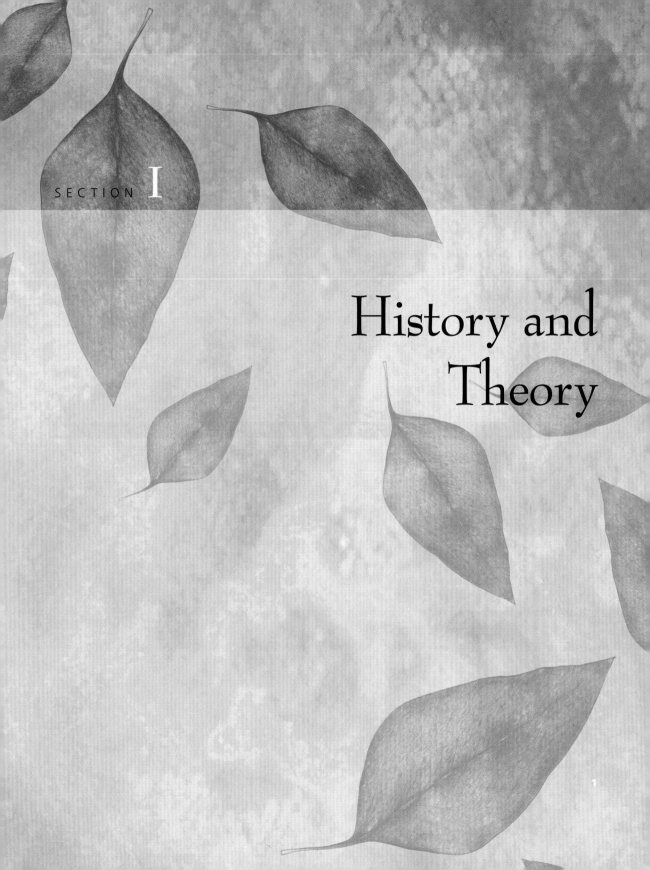

# History and Theory

CHAPTER 1

# History and Basic Concepts

*Occupational therapy has a great deal to learn from its history. The profession was founded on the visionary idea that human beings need, and are nurtured by, their activity as by food and drink and that every human being possesses potential that can be achieved through engagement in occupation.*

ELIZABETH YERXA (48)

## CHAPTER OBJECTIVES

After studying this chapter, the reader will be able to:

1. Contrast *mental health* and *mental illness* and discuss the relationship of occupational functioning to mental health and illness.
2. Explain the unique value of occupational therapy in addressing the occupational needs of persons with mental disorders.
3. Recognize key events in the history of psychiatry.
4. Identify and describe key events in the history of occupational therapy in mental health.
5. List and discuss historical events and figures in occupational therapy practice in mental health.
6. Identify possible future trends for occupational therapy practice in mental health.
7. Describe the roles of the occupational therapy assistant in mental health practice.

We all seem to understand that people with mental health problems have trouble controlling their feelings, thoughts, and behavior. What is less obvious is that people with mental disorders also have trouble doing everyday activities, things the rest of us take for granted. Occupational therapy practitioners address this part of human life—how people carry out the tasks that are important to them, how well they do these tasks, and how satisfied they feel about them. Occupation has been defined as "man's goal-directed use of time, interest, energy, and attention" (5). Occupation is activity with a purpose, with a meaning unique to the person performing it (6). Occupational therapy views engagement in occupation as essential to both physical and mental health. Occupational therapy practitioners evaluate occupational functioning; work with consumers (patients, clients, families) to identify goals; and intervene to help troubled individuals, families, and communities learn new skills, maintain successful and adaptive habits and routines, explore their feelings and interests, and control their lives and destinies.

## MENTAL HEALTH AND MENTAL ILLNESS

Before we look at how occupational therapy approaches the evaluation and treatment of persons with mental health problems, it is useful to consider the terms *mental health* and *mental illness*. The American Psychiatric Association has defined *mental health* as follows: "a state of being, relative rather than absolute. The best indices of mental health are simultaneous success at working, loving, and creating with the capacity for mature and flexible resolution of conflicts between instincts, conscience, important other people, and reality" (19, p. 127).

This definition views mental health in terms of reasonably successful functioning within a framework of daily life activities (working), relationships (loving), and exploration and growth (creating). The ability to resolve conflicts in a mature, not childish or impulsive, fashion is part of successful functioning. The mentally healthy person has a balanced and satisfying life with energies divided among work, leisure, self-care, and care of others. He or she can manage the conflicting demands of instincts (such as drives for sex and self-preservation), conscience (internalized moral rules and standards of behavior), significant other people, and the real external world. What is described here is not a state of absolute or perfect mental health but rather a condition or quality of being able to manage one's daily affairs and respond constructively and creatively to the changing demands and opportunities of real life.

If mental health is relative, defined in relation to changing life conditions, at what point can we say that someone has mental health problems? Throughout recorded history, mental illness has been defined and redefined, reflecting increases in knowledge and understanding and changes in cultural beliefs and values. The American Psychiatric Association has defined *mental disorder* as follows:

> A behavioral or psychological syndrome that causes significant distress (a painful symptom) or disability (impairment in one or more important areas of functioning), or a significantly increased risk of suffering death, pain, or an important loss of freedom. The syndrome is considered to be a manifestation of some behavioral, psychological, or biological dysfunction in the person (and in some cases it is clearly secondary to or due to a general medical condition) (19, p. 127).

We can see from the definition that mental disorder causes considerable discomfort (extreme sadness or rage, for example) and/or impairment in the ability to function, such as to hold a job, and/or a risk to oneself, such as the risk of being imprisoned. Most important for occupational therapy is the emphasis on impairment in "important areas of functioning"—that is, in the abilities to care for oneself, to work or be productive, to engage in effective or productive relationships with others, and to pursue valued leisure activities. Reading further, we learn that the causes of the disorder may be behavioral, psychological, or biological, but these terms are undefined, so we are not sure what this sentence means except that medical disorders can bring on mental disorders.

Crucial for occupational therapy is this definition's emphasis on impaired functioning; difficulty in carrying out daily life activities is cited as one of the major symptoms of mental disorder. Occupational therapy is a most appropriate intervention for such problems because performance in human occupation and daily life activities is its main concern. Also, because occupational therapy uses occupation as its primary treatment tool, patients must act and perform and thus prove to themselves and to others that indeed they *can* function.

## RELATION OF OCCUPATION TO MENTAL HEALTH

The notion that involvement in occupation can improve mental health is hardly new; it appears in records of ancient civilizations from China to Rome. It is such an excellent idea that it is continually rediscovered and acclaimed. At the 1961 annual conference of the American Occupational Therapy Association, Mary Reilly expressed it this way: "That man, through the use of his hands as they are energized by mind and will, can influence the state of his own health" (40, p. 1).

Every person is born with a drive to act on the environment, to change things, to produce things, to work, to use hands and mind. The satisfaction of having an effect and the challenge and pleasure of solving problems give life meaning and purpose. We know that both the unemployed and those employed in routine jobs suffer from stress and mental disorders because they lack the stimulation of challenging activity. Their drive to act is frustrated and weakened. We know too that many of the mentally ill suffer because they cannot do what they once did; disease and social stigma have impaired their capacity to act. Unhappiness and inactivity reinforce each other; those who fail to act become less able to do so.

Occupational therapy uses occupation to reverse the negative cycle of inactivity and disease. Occupation requires attention and energy; it has a unique meaning to the person performing it (26). Activity that engages the entire human being—heart, mind, and body—is powerful therapy. Not every activity is therapeutic, only those that ignite the person's interest and empower the will. Helping the client explore, discover, master, and manage the occupations that give that individual's life purpose and direction is the essence of psychiatric occupational therapy.

## HISTORICAL UNDERSTANDING

The history of the occupational therapy profession is intertwined with that of psychiatry. It is useful to look back and consider the important threads that tie the two professions together. Furthermore, reviewing the history of occupational therapy in mental health can reveal the core values and interests of the profession—values and interests that are still strong today. The moral treatment movement, discussed in the next section, fueled the growth of both professions.

### The Moral Treatment Era

Moral treatment was a pivotal stage in the development of psychiatry as a separate medical discipline. It was based on ideas developed in France by Pinel and in England by Tukes and was first practiced in the United States at McLean Hospital in Massachusetts and at Frankford Asylum in Pennsylvania in the early 19th century (10).

The philosophy of moral treatment included respect for the individual and a belief that the mentally ill would benefit most from a regular daily routine and the opportunity to contribute productively to their own care and to the welfare of society in general through involvement in occupation. Before the advent of moral treatment, the mentally ill were housed in large asylums where they were neglected; observers noted that they were ill-fed, unclothed, and often found lying in their own body wastes. It was not unusual for mentally ill persons to be subjected to restraint and torture.

In contrast, early moral treatment hospitals provided a prescribed routine of daily hygiene, regular meals sometimes prepared by the inmates from crops grown on the hospital grounds, and craft work and recreation. Efforts were made to engage as many inmates as possible in regular employment or occupation, such as kitchen, laundry, general cleaning, grounds work, or building repair within the hospital. The effect of such employment was described by Adolph Meyer, a physician and one of the founders of occupational therapy:

> It had long been interesting to see how groups of a few excited patients can be seated in a corner in a small circle of two or three settees and kept wonderfully contented picking the hair of mattresses, or doing simple tasks not too readily arousing the desire for big movements and uncontrollable excitement and yet not too taxing to their patience. Groups of patients with raffia and basket work, or with various kinds of handwork and weaving and bookbinding and metal and leather work, took the place of the bored wall flowers and of mischief-makers. A pleasure in achievement, a real pleasure in the use and activity of one's hands and muscles and a happy appreciation of time began to be used as incentives in the management of our patients, instead of abstract exhortations to cheer up and to behave according to abstract or repressive rules (36, p. 81).

Occupational therapy arose out of the moral treatment movement. Early occupational therapy practitioners based their work on moral treatment methods and used a variety of occupations, such as arts and crafts, classroom instruction, manual labor, games, sports, social activities, and self-care activities. These were designed to provide a balanced daily program that incorporated work, rest, and leisure. Occupations were planned and graded for the needs and abilities of individuals. Formation of habits and the development of skills and attention were emphasized. The personality of the occupational therapist was important; kindliness, modeling of correct habits, and the ability to analyze and adjust occupations to suit the interests and capacities of patients were valued traits (34).

Ever since the beginning of occupational therapy in mental health, the profession has been greatly influenced and restrained by physician referral and the practice of psychiatry. For this reason, we will look at the history of American psychiatry before returning to the development of occupational therapy later in the chapter.

## Psychiatry in the 20th and 21st Centuries

The medical specialty of psychiatry has evolved greatly in its techniques and interests since the time of moral treatment. Early in the 20th century, the theories of Sigmund Freud (see Chapter 2) and other psychoanalytic theoreticians dominated the field. But, for the severely mentally ill, psychoanalysis, which relies on talking, was not practical. Patients were simply too ill and symptomatic. A number of pseudoscientific methods were used to try to limit the effects of psychotic symptoms. Some of these methods, such as ice water baths and confinement in wooden restraints, were efforts to compel patients to submit to the rules of the institutions in which they were housed.

Through the 1940s, physicians' treatments of major mental disorders aimed at changing the brain by changing the biology of the body. Some treatments included the following:

- Prefrontal lobotomy (a kind of brain surgery, often crudely executed)
- Insulin shock treatment (inducement of coma by lowering blood sugar with injections of insulin)
- Electroconvulsive (shock) therapy (ECT)

A critical development during the 1950s was the discovery and introduction of the major tranquilizers. Finally, a way had been found to control and diminish the psychotic symptoms and extreme behaviors of the seriously mentally ill. The discovery and use of the tranquilizing drugs led indirectly to the passage in 1963 of the Community Mental Health Act (also known as the Community Mental Health Centers Construction Act) (Public Law 88-164), which was designed to establish community-based treatment facilities and to move the mentally ill from institutional settings to community living. Unfortunately, inadequate planning and funding resulted in large numbers of deinstitutionalized mental patients being released into communities lacking resources to meet their needs.

Historians later suggested that persons with chronic psychiatric disorders were not really *de*institutionalized by the 1963 legislation but rather were *trans*institutionalized. In other words, they were moved from one kind of institution (psychiatric hospitals) into other kinds of institutions (jails, prisons, and nursing homes) and not into the community at all (45). Furthermore, the enactment of Medicaid and Medicare legislation in 1965 changed the incentives for the states. Mental health care had been, up to 1965, a state responsibility, but the new legislation made it possible to shift responsibility for funding the care of the seriously mentally ill to the federal government once patients were discharged from the state hospitals (45).

The social and political climate of the 1960s and 1970s generated increased interest in and funding for mental health research, but much of this was directed toward the milder problems of "normal" people who were having difficulty managing stress and away from the seriously mentally ill. As a consequence of the increased attention to those with less serious mental health problems, several new theories (gestalt therapy, milieu therapy, behavioral therapy, and family therapy) were applied by mental health professionals, including occupational therapists, during those years.

The 1960s and 1970s also brought an explosion of interest in and knowledge about the biological foundations of mental disorders. There had long been an interest in the genetics of the major brain disorders (schizophrenia, depression, manic depression. Continued research on diagnosed individuals and their families and the study of the human genome have enabled a better understanding of the link between genetics and the development of mental disorders. The consensus at present is that a genetic predisposition results in disease in vulnerable individuals, but that environmental factors, possibly viruses, are also involved.

At present, the medical specialty of psychiatry is oriented strongly toward biological and biochemical research and pharmacological interventions. Imaging studies, conducted since the 1990s using positron emission tomography (PET), computed tomography (CT), and magnetic resonance imaging (MRI), increasingly show changes in the cerebral cortex, ventricles, and other brain structures and activity of persons with major mental disorders. Pharmaceutical companies fund major research to demonstrate the effectiveness of competing drugs aimed at the considerable market represented by people with psychiatric disorders. Furthermore, drug companies advertise and market directly to consumers. The volume of studies published requires physicians to review results constantly and to adjust their interventions according to the newest best evidence.

Other than medications, the most prevalent form of intervention for persons with mental disorders is associated with the *psychiatric rehabilitation* movement (8). Psychiatric rehabilitation shows strong research evidence of effectiveness and has introduced rehabilitation counselors, social workers, and many allied health paraprofessionals to methods of intervention that are very similar to the traditional methods of occupational therapy. Psychiatric rehabilitation has been adopted by some states, including New York, as the model for treatment within all units of the state mental health system, under the name *intensive psychiatric rehabilitation treatment* (IPRT). Psychiatric rehabilitation, discussed further in Chapter 2, defines its goal as helping persons with mental disorders to function at their best in the environments of their choice. Methods include teaching skills and providing resources.

## Consumers, Families, and Mental Health Parity

One of the most important forces at work on behalf of persons with mental illness is the combined political effort of consumers (persons with mental disorders) and their families. Represented most prominently by the National Alliance on Mental Illness (NAMI), founded in 1979, the consumer movement has helped reduce stigma associated with mental illness and improve the quality of life for persons with mental disorders. Consumers see themselves not as outcasts but rather as members of the community with a voice and with a vision for their future. With NAMI and similar organizations, consumers, families, and professionals together advocate for appropriate housing, community care, supported employment, and other services. In addition, families and consumers provide peer and family support and education (37).

An important focus of the consumer vision is *mental health parity*, a proposed public policy that would require insurance companies to reimburse for mental health care to the same extent as for physical health care. Consumers and families are explored in Chapter 9.

## Occupational Therapy in Mental Health: History and Trends

Returning to the early history of occupational therapy, we see immediately that the profession was very dependent on physicians. From 1917 to the 1950s psychiatric occupational therapists provided comprehensive programs of occupation based loosely on principles of moral treatment within institutional settings. The physician prescribed occupational therapy, often ordering specific activities for patients, and the occupational therapist carried out the treatment. After World War II, interest in rehabilitating veterans led to an emphasis on workmanship and vocational readiness (22).

During the 1940s and 1950s occupational therapy was attacked by the medical profession for failing to have a "scientific basis" (30, 43). In response to that criticism, occupational therapy adopted the vocabulary and concepts of psychoanalysis, the prevailing psychiatric theory. Although occupational therapists continued to work under the prescription of physicians, Gail Fidler, Jay Fidler, and others began to use activities to evaluate their patients' psychodynamics (emotions and psychological defenses). They analyzed activities for their capacity to meet patients' unconscious needs. Activities were matched symbolically to psychic content—for example, clay looks like feces and may symbolize anal-stage concerns (see "Theory of Object Relations" in Chapter 2). This psychoanalytical application of occupational therapy in mental health followed the trend of using occupation to enhance medical outcomes (22) after World War II.

With the introduction of the major tranquilizers in the 1950s, occupational therapists were able to work with patients whose behavior without medication had been so psychotic and bizarre that treatment was difficult or impossible. At first, the main emphasis continued to be psychoanalytical. The theories developed by other disciplines, primarily psychology, during the 1960s and 1970s did not always include a focus on occupation. Of these new therapies, the behavioral approach was the one most used by occupational therapists. Occupational therapists applied the techniques of *behavioral therapy* in their work with the mentally ill and the mentally retarded to diminish acting out and to promote healthy behaviors. By reinforcing desired behavior through carefully selected rewards and by enforcing limits on undesirable behavior, therapists thought they could improve their patients' functioning. Behavioral approaches are discussed in detail in Chapters 2 and 3.

During the 1970s, occupational therapist Lorna Jean King applied *sensory integration* theory and methods developed by A. Jean Ayres, also an occupational therapist, to the treatment of patients with chronic psychiatric disorders. King proposed that poor functioning and grossly abnormal posture in chronic schizophrenia could be attributed to errors in sensory processing, which might be corrected or at least ameliorated by carefully designed sensorimotor programs. Sensory integration is rarely used today for this population but may be employed for treatment of severe behavioral disorders (see Chapter 3).

During the 1980s Claudia Allen outlined and developed her theory of *cognitive disabilities*. Allen proposed that a person's performance in a task indicates the quality of his or her thought. She identified six levels of cognitive functioning, which can be evaluated through performance of unfamiliar small crafts, such as leather lacing or mosaics. The six levels were later elaborated and expanded. Diagnosis of cognitive level can contribute to the psychiatric diagnosis and can be used to predict future functioning and to identify the interventions most likely to be effective (1). Allen's theory is described further in Chapter 3.

Sensory integration and cognitive disabilities attribute the problems in functioning to defects of the structure or function of the nervous system in persons with severe and persistent mental illness. The questions for therapists are to what extent can these defects be corrected or remediated and to what extent can the person learn to work around the defects. Defects that cannot be remediated must be compensated for if the person is to function. King's approach is remedial; Allen's is more compensatory.

Both King's and Allen's theories emphasize activity or occupation as a focus for evaluation and intervention. However, most theories of the 1950s and 1960s were criticized for the absence of this focus and for being *reductionistic* (reducing the patient's problems to isolated elements such as insight or behavior). During the 1960s and 1970s Mary Reilly (40) and others attacked these approaches, arguing for a more comprehensive theory of occupational therapy practice that would focus primarily on the occupational nature of human beings. Kielhofner (31), Kielhofner and Burke (32), and others built on Reilly's work with the *model of human occupation*. This model organized research findings and traditional occupational therapy beliefs to create a comprehensive theory for use in all practice areas, including among others physical medicine, developmental disabilities, and psychiatry. The model proposes that human response to the environment is formed from an interaction among three systems: *(a)* volition (motivation), *(b)* habituation (roles and habits), and *(c)* performance (skills of the mind, brain, and body). The interactions among the three are dynamic, each affecting the other two. The model of human occupation is discussed in Chapter 3.

Some occupational therapists during the 1980s began to apply cognitive behavioral principles (28). This approach, discussed in Chapter 2, investigates the feelings and thoughts that drive behavior. The patient is taught to challenge erroneous ideas. Once the ideas are proven false, there is an opportunity to change the behavior. Cognitive-behavioral therapy and dialectical behavioral therapy, which is derived from it, show strong research evidence of effectiveness.

Since the 1980s Florence Clark and others (14, 27) have been developing a new scientific discipline, *occupational science,* for systematic study of the occupational nature of humans. Research in occupational science is beginning to generate data that help us understand the nature of occupation and that validate the effectiveness of occupational therapy.

Another exciting development for mental health occupational therapy is study of sensory processing by Catana Brown and colleagues (12, 13). Brown has provided an evaluation instrument to help identify sensory sensitivities and differences and has also provided strategies to compensate for these. This is important for persons with serious mental disorders, some of whom are acutely sensitive to environmental factors such as noise or odors. Others may be very insensitive and unaware of sensations from the environment, which causes them to miss cues from other people.

The consumer movement has fueled an interest in exploring the phenomenology of illness, or how the person views what is happening. The telling of a personal story and the appreciation of this story by the therapist are the focus of *narrative reasoning.* Narrative reasoning is a way to study how people understand and tell the stories of their lives; it has enriched our appreciation and analysis of occupation and its relation to individuals (35).

While occupational therapists have been striving to clarify the theoretical understanding of occupation and refine their assessment and intervention techniques, they have also been increasingly concerned about the rapid proliferation and growth of other activity-oriented mental health therapies, all of which share to some extent occupational therapy techniques and theories. Vocational rehabilitation counseling and dance, art, music, and poetry therapies focus on activities that once concerned only occupational therapists. Increasingly, nursing, social work, psychology, and physical therapy are addressing the daily life activities and occupational functioning of persons with mental illness. This sounds so similar to occupational therapy that it can be hard for the uninformed to see the difference. Occupational therapy practitioners employed in psychiatric rehabilitation programs have a unique skill base, activity analysis (discussed in Chapter 23), not shared by the other team members.

The passage of the Americans with Disabilities Act of 1990 (ADA) (Public Law 101–336) has opened new opportunities for practice in mental health occupational therapy, working with consumers trying to gain access to employment and other situations. This law mandates that qualified persons not be excluded from employment and work activities because of disability owing to physical or mental impairments. Occupational therapists and assistants can help prepare persons with mental disabilities for the world of work through training in work, self-advocacy, and attitudinal skills and by collaborating with employers to analyze job functions and to determine reasonable accommodations (16). Whether the potential of the ADA to provide increased participation in employment for disabled persons will ever be realized depends on how the law is implemented, how much it costs the public, and how the benefits of the law are perceived (21, 38). Occupational therapy practitioners have the training and background to assist employers and disabled persons to interpret and apply the law in a cost-effective and reasonable fashion.

The future of occupational therapy in psychiatry is not clear; some even question whether it will maintain a presence in mental health service delivery during the 21st century (39, 46). Continuing shortages of therapists in mental health have been attributed to lower salaries and lower perceived status than in other practice areas, such as physical medicine and pediatrics. The therapist shortage has led to a decline in available fieldwork placements in mental health (29). Practice acts in some states, such as New York, restrict the practice of occupational therapy to physician referrals, obstructing the profession from moving independently into community positions outside the medical model. New York therapists have joined with consumers of mental health services to combine resources (44). In other states, including Wisconsin and California, occupational therapy practitioners have developed innovative community programs and have secured recognition for the profession by advocating with consumers for improved service delivery (18, 41).

Leaders in occupational therapy mental health practice remind us, however, that the coming years will test the profession with bottom-line economics and frequent reengineering of staff configurations in mental health practice (20). Hospital-based practice has declined because of decreased length of stay, staff shortages, and reduced reimbursement. Managed care has limited hospital stays and has capped benefits for mental health care. Occupational therapy practitioners are advised to develop and maintain awareness of political change in regard to mental health parity and to help advocate on behalf of consumers (23).

Despite reduced reimbursement and the movement away from hospital practice, the mentally ill will continue to need and benefit from occupational therapy. We increasingly see these consumers in their homes, workplaces, and communities. The occupational therapist (OT) frequently serves as consultant or manager rather than as provider of direct service. Practitioners teach consumers and families to manage symptoms and maximize occupational functioning. Opportunities for the occupational therapy assistant (OTA) are likely to expand. These opportunities have been and will continue to be found, primarily in the community. The reader is encouraged to consider ideas such as:

- Wellness and health promotion for persons with mental disorders and also for the general population (4)
- Direct interventions and prevention programs to address the occupational problems of victims of domestic violence (25)
- Interventions in the schools and in community after-school programs for school-aged children with mental health problems (9)
- Services for people with mental disorders who have become inmates and parolees of the prison system (42)
- Life coaching and motivational services on a fee-for-service basis (33)
- Outreach and community integration for the homeless (24)

Occupational therapy's greatest challenges are to maintain its professional visibility, claim its unique expertise in occupation (17, 47), and communicate effectively to make patients, insurance companies, and federal agencies aware of its special skills in evaluating and intervening effectively to address the problems of the mentally ill. Figure 1-1 gives a view of the parallel histories of psychiatry and occupational therapy.

## THE ROLE OF THE OCCUPATIONAL THERAPY ASSISTANT

Occupational therapy assistant students sometimes question how the occupational therapist differs from the OTA because they appear at first glance to perform similar job tasks. Comments such as "Why are OTs paid more? They do the same things we do" and "The OT only does paperwork and doesn't even treat patients" are typical. Some professional-level occupational therapy students and therapists also express confusion about the difference between the professional and the technical levels. Understanding the difference is essential for both if they are to work together effectively.

Since 1958, when the American Occupational Therapy Association (AOTA) began to plan for OTAs, their role in mental health treatment has

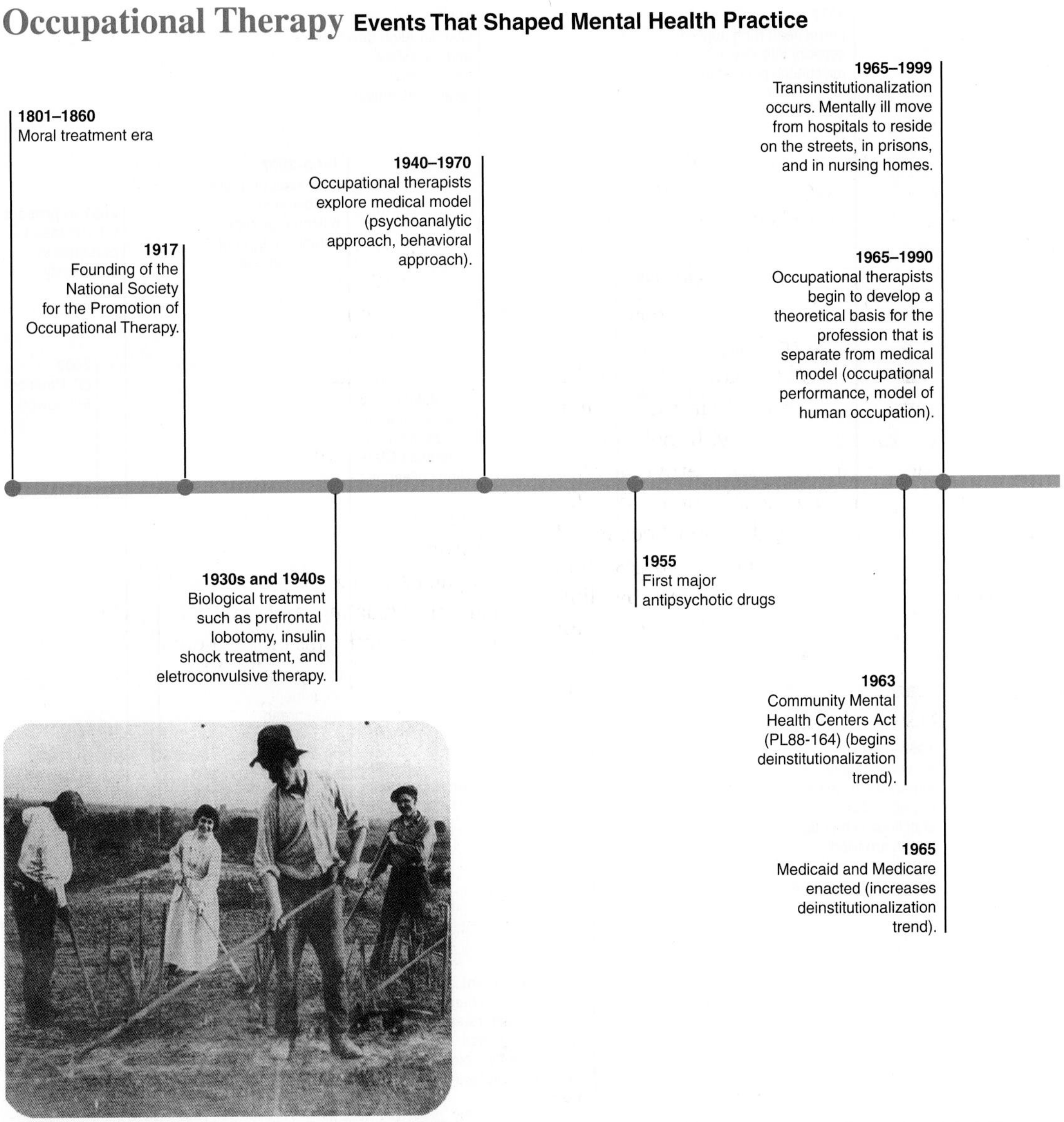
Occupational Therapy Events That Shaped Mental Health Practice
1801–1860
Moral treatment era
1917
Founding of the National Society for the Promotion of Occupational Therapy.
1930s and 1940s
Biological treatment such as prefrontal lobotomy, insulin shock treatment, and eletroconvulsive therapy.
1940–1970
Occupational therapists explore medical model (psychoanalytic approach, behavioral approach).
1955
First major antipsychotic drugs
1963
Community Mental Health Centers Act (PL88-164) (begins deinstitutionalization trend).
1965
Medicaid and Medicare enacted (increases deinstitutionalization trend).
1965–1990
Occupational therapists begin to develop a theoretical basis for the profession that is separate from medical model (occupational performance, model of human occupation).
1965–1999
Transinstitutionalization occurs. Mentally ill move from hospitals to reside on the streets, in prisons, and in nursing homes.

**Figure 1-1. Timeline.** Selected key events in the history of psychiatry, medicine, law, and occupational therapy in mental health.

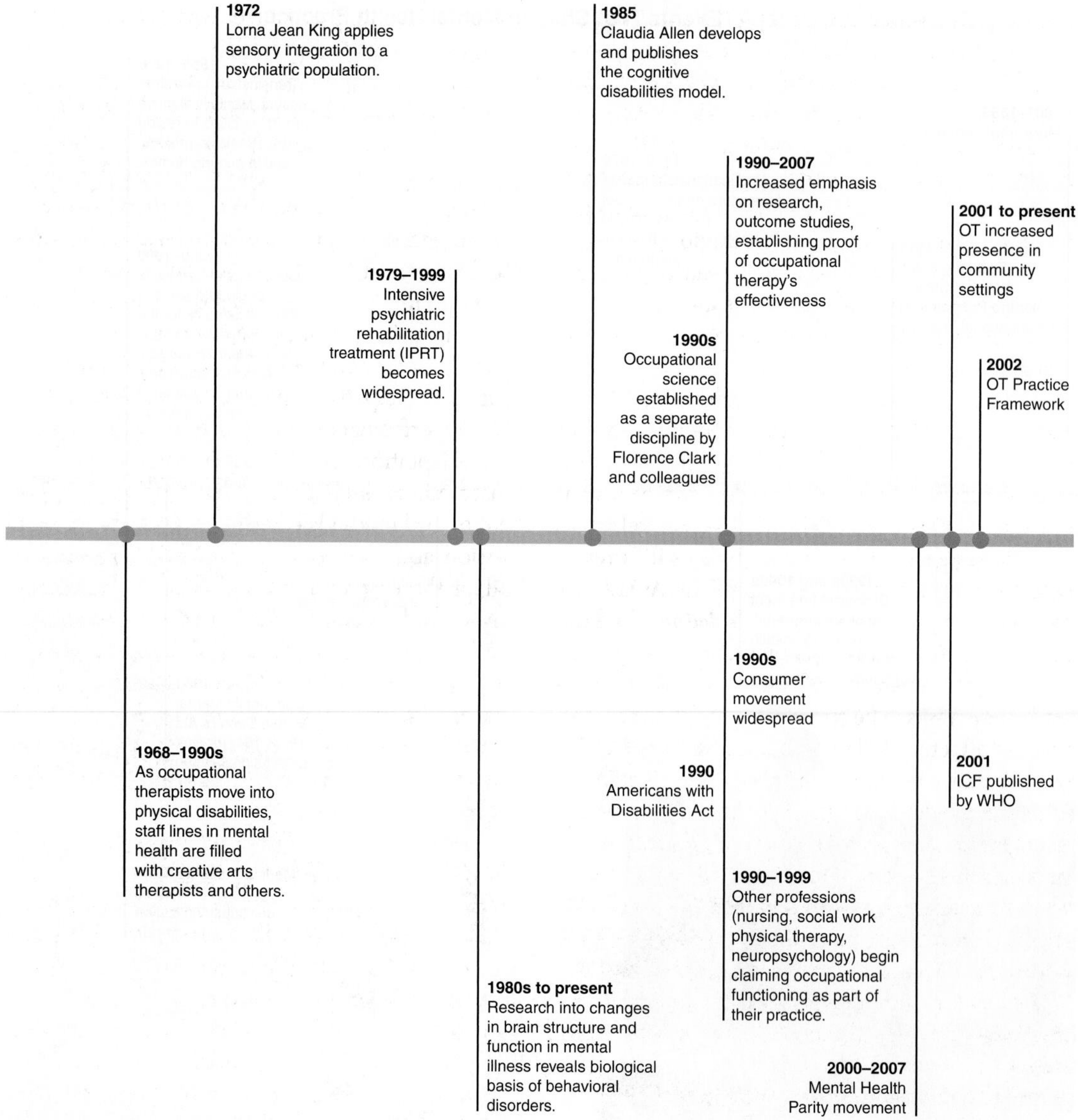


**Figure 1-1.** ***(Continued)***

expanded tremendously. Among the many factors affecting the role of the OTA in the 21st century are the official educational standards and role descriptions provided by the AOTA (2); the licensing and certification guidelines of the various states; and the local market availability of OTs, baccalaureate-level activities therapists, and other mental health practitioners. In addition, the regulations and needs within mental health treatment facilities and community agencies and the experience and skills of individual occupational therapy assistants influence their roles.

To clarify the role of the OTA, the AOTA has in the past conducted several projects on *role delineation.* The purpose of these projects was to outline precisely, or to delineate, the roles of entry-level OTAs and OTs. *Entry-level* refers to new graduates of training programs as differentiated from experienced therapists. The AOTA has consequently published *role guidelines* to help practitioners structure job tasks in a way that reflects the preparation of the OT or OTA to perform these tasks. The most recent of the role documents affecting OTAs was approved by AOTA's representative assembly in 2004 (3). The *Standards for an Accredited Program for the Occupational Therapist and Occupational Therapy Assistant* are periodically reviewed and revised, the most recent version having been adopted in 2006 (2). In 2005 the AOTA's representative assembly redefined the *Standards of Practice for Occupational Therapy* (7). These documents provide a framework for discussing the role of the OTA in a mental health setting.

First it is important to understand that the entry-level OTA is trained to collaborate with a supervising OT to provide occupational therapy services. The OT and the OTA are prepared to perform complementary job functions. Both are involved in all stages of the intervention process from screening and evaluation to discharge planning, but their roles and the areas for which each is responsible are distinct, with the OT taking the leadership role. Differing educational experiences prepare the OTA and the OT.

To be certified by the National Board for Certification in Occupational Therapy (NBCOT), the OTA must successfully complete an assistant-level program in a college or postsecondary institution. The required content includes communication and interpersonal skills; basic biological and behavioral sciences; diseases and conditions treated by occupational therapy; human development; areas of occupation (work, play, leisure, activities of daily living, education, social participation); performance skills and patterns; performance contexts; client factors; analysis, adaptation, and gradation of activities; and instructional techniques. Also included are principles and methods of occupational therapy evaluation and intervention. The assistant learns to adapt the environment and is trained in various structured evaluation and treatment techniques and in basic management and supervision of occupational therapy. At the completion of the program and the required minimum of the equivalent of 16 weeks of full-time related fieldwork, the graduate is eligible to sit for the NBCOT certifying examination (2).

In contrast, to be eligible for registration by the NBCOT, the OT must complete a course of instruction in a university or college that grants degrees at the master's (MA or MS) level. To enter a master's program, applicants must have a baccalaureate degree and must have taken courses in anatomy, psychology, statistics, other social sciences, and sometimes physics or chemistry. The required content at the occupational therapist level includes advanced courses in biological and medical and health sciences, including detailed and rigorous courses in anatomy; physiology; kinesiology; neuroanatomy; neurophysiology; and medical, surgical, neurological, psychiatric, orthopedic, congenital, and developmental disorders. Occupational therapy courses emphasize the exploration and comparison of theories that analyze normal and therapeutic use of activities and the application of these theories at each stage of the treatment process. Unstructured as well as structured evaluation and intervention methods are included along with adaptation and environmental modification of activities, advanced management and supervision concepts and skills, theory building, research methods and statistics, program evaluation and development, social and public policy, and quality assurance methods. The equivalent of 24 weeks of full-time fieldwork is required. After completing the coursework and fieldwork, graduates are eligible to take an examination to be registered and certified by the NBCOT (2).

The training of the OTA and the OT prepares them to work in a complementary fashion, as the following situation illustrates:

**CASE EXAMPLE**

The setting is a community day-treatment center. The clients range in age from 25 to 65 years. Many are inactive and would like to spend their days sitting unoccupied in the lounge. Two OTAs work at the center, leading a variety of groups such as lunch preparation, horticulture, exercise, diet management, and crafts. The supervising OT, who works 8 hours per week at this facility, has a strong interest in supported employment and has recently persuaded the director of the agency to fund the development of a program to help clients prepare for some level of work in the community. One of the OTAs has an interest in this area and has persuaded two community businesses, a fast-food restaurant and a health aids store, to hire clients part-time.

According to evaluations done by the OT, with parts administered by the OTA, the OT and OTA have identified six clients who may be ready for this program. The OTA now runs a job skills group 5 days a week for 40 minutes, geared to prepare clients to begin the specific available jobs. The group employs a psychoeducational approach, focusing on social interaction in situations members may encounter on the job (e.g., responding to a request for assistance). Other topics include proper dress and hygiene, expectations, and responsibilities (to be on time, to work the arranged hours, to ask questions when one needs help) in the world of work. The OTA meets with the OT once a week to review clients' progress. The OTA is concerned that clients may need a staff member with them on the job, at least for the first few days. The OT agrees and has helped the OTA lay out a schedule to phase the clients into the jobs one at a time, with the OTA attending work with the clients initially as a job coach.

The collaboration between OT and OTA in this situation makes use of their different skills. The OT and the OTA have evaluated the clients, the OTA performing parts of the evaluation as instructed by the OT supervisor. From the evaluation results, the OT has matched clients' capabilities and interests with the requirements of the job program. The OTA is carrying out a psychoeducational training regimen designed by both the OT and the OTA. The OTA makes good use of supervision to explore questions related to client progress. The specifics reported by the OTA are useful to the OT when conferring with the director about the need for more occupational therapy lines (e.g., to provide side-by-side coaching). This sort of complementary relationship is only one example of the ways in which OTA and OT work together.

By education, the OTA's area of greatest expertise is performance in areas of occupation. These include work, play, leisure, activities of daily living and instrumental activities of daily living, education, and social participation. Although the OT is educated in these areas, the professional level of education is oriented more toward assessment and evaluation and interventions in client factors and specific performance skills. The OTA is trained in some of the routine and structured techniques used to evaluate and address problems in performance skills and patterns. The OTA is thus able to carry out large segments of the occupational therapy program with supervision from the OT, who is better prepared to design the overall program and to evaluate and plan treatment for complex problems involving a combination of performance skill deficits and problems in client factors.

What the OTA working in a mental health setting actually does on a day-to-day basis varies widely, depending on the experience of the OTA, state law, and the treatment facility and its reimbursement structure. Hypothetically, the OTA could plan and carry out a complete program of independent living skills, grooming and hygiene, cooking and food management skills, money management, use of public and private transportation, shopping, care and selection of clothing, use of telephone and postal services, homemaking, child care, work skills, and play and leisure skills. The OTA may teach coping skills and self-identity skills or may assist the OT in assessing and providing interventions for performance skills such as communication and interaction or cognitive processes. Consider another example of a OTA in mental health practice:

**CASE EXAMPLE**

The setting is a large community service agency. The consumers who attend its programs have serious and persistent mental illnesses such as schizophrenia and bipolar disorder. Many have substance abuse histories as well. Among the many programs provided here are a psychosocial clubhouse, a supported employment program, and a transitional employment program. One OT serves as consultant to the agency 6 hours per week.

An experienced OTA has recently been hired for the psychosocial clubhouse program. This is a new position; the four OTAs working in the employment programs have not had the time to provide any services in the clubhouse. The new OTA began by sitting down with members of the club and formulating a plan; the OT sat in on the first meeting as an observer. In accordance with suggestions from the members, the OTA helps the member leader with the lunch program 5 days a week, providing information and education on nutrition and smart shopping. Another major responsibility is helping set up the photography darkroom; members expressed a strong interest in learning to develop and print photographs with the possible goal of having a photography show. The OTA also meets with individual members to address specific needs such as selecting and caring for clothes appropriate for work, finding leisure opportunities for interests such as weight training, looking up new medications on the Internet, and locating 12-step groups near members' residences. One day a week the OTA accompanies members on a trip to a community resource, such as the YWCA, to learn what additional programs are available. The OTA meets with the OT once a week to review progress, discuss concerns, and prepare for the Level I OTA fieldwork student who will start the next month. Just the past week, the OT commented that the OTA had such a full program it was hard to believe that the position didn't even exist 6 months ago.

This OTA is far more independent than the one in the previous example. This is appropriate for someone with several years of experience and established service competency. Professional development and continuing education amplify the possibilities (15). The OT continues to provide guidance and general supervision and to direct the overall program.

## SUMMARY

The histories of psychiatry and occupational therapy share a common origin in the moral treatment era. Throughout the 20th century, occupational therapy mental health practitioners worked mainly in medical settings and consequently were greatly influenced by events in medicine and psychiatry.

Even as occupational therapy has reembraced its unique professional scope of practice, the profession continues to respond to developments in psychiatry and medicine. Thus OTs and OTAs monitor effects of medication, provide interventions to improve cognitive functioning, and in many states must obtain a physician referral to provide services to a person with mental health problems. However, with the increased political activity of mental health consumers and their families, many occupational therapists and assistants have responded by moving their practices to community settings, providing consumer-focused services. Outside of the medical model, however, these services may not be identified as occupational therapy.

The relationship between the OT and OTA in mental health practice provides greater opportunities for the OTA than in some other practice areas. The OTA carries out major portions of the total occupational therapy program, usually under the supervision of an OT. Chapter 24 addresses the topic of supervision. How much supervision is required depends on state regulations and on administrative patterns within treatment facilities. For example, in New York State, the licensing law for occupational therapists provides specific direction on how the OT and the OTA shall work together. According to this law, a practicing OTA must be under the direct supervision of an OT or a licensed physician. *Direct supervision* is defined variously to mean anything from full-time on-site supervision to monthly cosignature of notes. Other states are less restrictive. Occupational therapy assistants are cautioned to stay current with state regulations and their most recent interpretations.

In each situation the need for supervision varies with the skills and experience of OTA and OT (3). Experienced OTAs may need only general supervision and may be asked to help supervise OT students, as suggested by the three levels of OTAs (generalist, skilled clinician, and master clinician) outlined by Terry Brittell (11). When patients' conditions are complex or change rapidly, the OTA is likely to require and want more supervision. The need for supervision, the number of hours needed, and the depth of supervision can be determined only after considering guidelines and the characteristics of the particular situation.

The future of occupational therapy in providing quality services to persons with mental health problems depends on the ability of OTs and OTAs to work together and to develop staffing patterns that provide quality services at a reasonable cost. Shortages of qualified applicants for OT-level positions in mental health settings were reported across the country for many years; the majority of these positions were released to be filled by other activities therapists. However, OTAs are ideally suited to work with the mental health population, especially those in chronic care settings. The OT who has never worked with a OTA and who has limited understanding of the OTA's training and role may be uncertain of what the OTA can do. By openly and optimistically discussing the possibilities for a complementary and supportive role, OTAs can do much to create and nurture their own future. With increasing emphasis on OTA and OT roles in occupational therapy educational programs, future graduates from professional-level programs should be appropriately prepared to appreciate and employ the skills and contributions of the OTA (2).

## REVIEW QUESTIONS AND ACTIVITIES

1. Differentiate *mental health* and *mental illness;* highlight the differences between these two states.
2. What effect(s) might involvement in occupation have on mental health?
3. What effect(s) might having a mental disorder have on occupational functioning?
4. Describe how occupational therapy can help the occupational functioning of persons with mental disorders.
5. Discuss the following events/eras in the history of psychiatry: moral treatment, discovery of major tranquilizers, deinstitutionalization, consumer movement, brain imaging, human genome, biological and pharmacological orientation.
6. List five people who were important historically for mental health occupational therapy and describe the contributions of each.
7. Name and discuss three major events in the history of occupational therapy in mental health practice.
8. List five areas related to mental health in which occupational therapy might have a role in the future.
9. Describe the role(s) of the occupational therapy assistant in mental health practice.

## REFERENCES


1. Allen C. Occupational Therapy for Psychiatric Diseases: Measurement and Management of Cognitive Disabilities. Boston: Little, Brown, 1985.
2. American Occupational Therapy Association. Accreditation Council for Occupational Therapy Education (ACOTE) Standards and Interpretative Guidelines August 2006. Available at:www.aota.org. Accessed Sept 2006.
3. American Occupational Therapy Association. Guidelines for supervision, roles, and responsibilities during the delivery of occupational therapy services. Am J Occup Ther 2004;58:663–667.
4. American Occupational Therapy Association. Occupational therapy in the promotion of health and the prevention of disease and disability statement. Am J Occup Ther 2001; 55:656–660.
5. American Occupational Therapy Association. Occupational Therapy: Its Definition and Functions. Rockville, MD: AOTA, 1972.
6. American Occupational Therapy Association. Occupational therapy practice framework: Domain and process. Am J Occup Ther 2002;56:609–639.
7. American Occupational Therapy Association. Standards of practice for occupational therapy. Am J Occup Ther 2005;59:663–665.
8. Anthony WA, Cohen M, Farkas M. Psychiatric Rehabilitation. Boston: Center for Psychiatric Rehabilitation, Boston University, Sargent College of Allied Health Professions, 1990.
9. Barnes KJ, Beck AJ, Vogel KA, et al. Perceptions regarding school-based occupational therapy for children with emotional disturbances. Am J Occup Ther 2003;57:337–341.
10. Bockoven JS. Legacy of moral treatment: 1880's to 1910. Am J Occup Ther 1971;5:223–225.
11. Brittell T. Future concepts of the COTA role, Part 2. Am Occup Ther Assoc Ment Health Special Sect Q Newslett 1981;4:1–4.
12. Brown C. What is the best environment for me? A sensory processing perspective. Occup Ther Ment Health 2001;17(3–4):115–125.
13. Brown C, Tollefson N, Dunn W, et al. The adult sensory profile: Measuring patterns of sensory processing. Am J Occup Ther 2001;55:75–82.
14. Clark FA, Parham D, Carlson ME, et al. Occupational science: Academic innovation in the service of occupational therapy's future. Am J Occup Ther 1991;45:300–310.
15. Cottrell RF. COTA education and professional development: An historical review. Am J Occup Ther 2000;54:407–412.
16. Crist PAH, Stoffel VC. The Americans with Disabilities Act of 1990 and employees with mental impairments: Personal efficacy and the environment. Am J Occup Ther 1992;46:434–443.
17. Darnell JL, Heater SL. The Issue Is: Occupational therapist or activity therapist—Which do you choose to be? Am J Occup Ther 1994;48:467–468.
18. Dressler J, MacRae A. Advocacy, partnerships and client centered practice in California. In: Scott AH, ed. New Frontiers in Mental Health. Binghamton, NY: Haworth Press, 1999.
19. Edgerton JE, ed. American Psychiatric Glossary. 7th ed. Washington: American Psychiatric Press, 1994.
20. Fine SB. Surviving the health care revolution: Rediscovering the meaning of "good work." In: Scott AH, ed. New Frontiers in Mental Health. Binghamton, NY: Haworth Press, 1999.
21. Frieden L. The Issue Is: The Americans with Disabilities Act of 1990: Will it work? (pro). Am J Occup Ther 1992;46:468–469.
22. Friedland J. Occupational therapy and rehabilitation: An awkward alliance. Am J Occup Ther 1998;52:372–380.
23. Gallew HA, Haltiwanger E, Sowers J, van den Heever N. Political action and critical analysis: Mental health parity. Occup Ther Ment Health 2004;20(1):1–25.
24. Griner KR. Helping the homeless: An occupational therapy perspective. Occup Ther Ment Health 2006;22(1): 49–61.
25. Helfrich CA, Lafata MJ, MacDonald SL, et al. Domestic abuse across the lifespan: Definitions, identification and risk factors for occupational therapists. Am J Occup Ther Ment Health 2001;16(3–4):5–34.
26. Hinojosa J, Sabari J, Pedretti L. Position Paper: Purposeful activity. Am J Occup Ther 1993;47:1081–1082.
27. Jackson J, Carlson M, Mandel D, et al. Occupation in lifestyle redesign: The well elderly study occupational therapy program. Am J Occup Ther 1998;52:326–336.
28. Johnson MT. Occupational therapists and the teaching of cognitive behavioral skills. Occup Ther Ment Health 1987;7(3):69–81.
29. Kautzmann LN. Alternatives to psychosocial fieldwork: Part of the solution or part of the problem? Am J Occup Ther 1995;49:266–268.
30. Kielhofner G. A model of human occupation: Theory and application. Baltimore: Williams & Wilkins, 1985.
31. Kielhofner G. Conceptual foundations of occupational therapy. Philadelphia: Davis, 1992.
32. Kielhofner G, Burke J. A model of human occupation. Part 1: Conceptual framework and content. Am J Occup Ther 1980;34:572–581.
33. Klippel L. A horse of a different color: Mental health occupational therapy and coaching. Am Occup Ther Assoc Ment Health Special Sect Q Newslett 2006;29:1–4.

34. Licht S. The early history of occupational therapy: An outline. Occup Ther Ment Health 1983;3:1:67–88.
35. Mallinson T, Kielhofner G, Mattingly C. Metaphor and meaning in a clinical interview. Am J Occup Ther 1996; 50:338–346.
36. Meyer A. The philosophy of occupational therapy. Occup Ther Ment Health 1982;2:3:79–86.
37. National Alliance on Mental Illness. Home page. Available at: www.nami.org. Accessed Nov 2006.
38. Nosek MA. The Issue Is: The Americans with Disabilities Act of 1990: Will it work? (con). Am J Occup Ther 1992;46:466–467.
39. O'Neill EH. Health Professions Education for the Future: Schools in Service to the Nation. San Francisco: Pew Health Professions Commission, 1993.
40. Reilly M. The 1961 Eleanor Clarke Slagle Lecture: Occupational therapy can be one of the great ideas of 20th century medicine. Am J Occup Ther 1962;16:1.
41. Samuels L. Responsive changes in mental health in Wisconsin. In: Scott AH, ed. New Frontiers in Mental Health. Binghamton, NY: Haworth Press, 1999.
42. Schindler VP. Occupational therapy in forensic psychiatry: Role development and schizophrenia. Occup Ther Ment Health 2005;20(3–4):1–171.
43. Serrett KD. Another look at occupational therapy's history. Occup Ther Ment Health 1985;5(3):1–31.
44. Tewfik D, Precin P. The New York experience: The remodeling of mental health practice. In: Scott AH, ed. New Frontiers in Mental Health. Binghamton, NY: Haworth Press, 1999.
45. Torrey EF. Out of the Shadows. New York: Wiley, 1997.
46. Walens D, Wittman P, Dickie VA, et al. Current and future education and practice: Issues for occupational therapy practitioners in mental health settings. In: Scott AH, ed. New Frontiers in Mental Health. Binghamton, NY: Haworth Press, 1999.
47. Wood W. Legitimizing occupational therapy's knowledge. Am J Occup Ther 1996;50:626–634.
48. Yerxa EJ. Some implications of occupational therapy's history for its epistemology, values, and relation to medicine. Am J Occup Ther 1992;46:79–83.

## SUGGESTED READINGS

American Occupational Therapy Association. Occupational therapy in the promotion of health and the prevention of disease and disability statement. Am J Occup Ther 2001;55:656–660.

American Occupational Therapy Association. Psychosocial aspects of occupational therapy. Am J Occup Ther 2004;58:669–672.

Bonder BR. Occupational therapy in mental health: Crisis or opportunity? Am J Occup Ther 1987;41:495–499.

Cottrell RF. COTA education and professional development: An historical review. Am J Occup Ther 2000;54:407–412.

Fidler GS. The challenge of change to occupational therapy practice. Occup Ther Ment Health 1991;11(1):1–11.

Fine SB. Working the system: A perspective for managing change. Am J Occup Ther 1988;42:417–419.

Hemphill-Pearson BJ, Hunter M. Holism in mental health practice. Occup Ther Ment Health 1997;13(2):35–49.

Kleinman BL. The challenge of providing occupational therapy in mental health. Am J Occup Ther 1992;46:555–557.

Peloquin SM. Moral treatment: how a caring practice lost its rationale. Am J Occup Ther 1994;48:167–173.

CHAPTER 2

# Medical and Psychological Models of Mental Health and Illness

*For every perceivable phenomenon, devise at least six explanations that indeed explain the phenomenon. There are probably sixty, but if you devise six, this will sensitize you to the complexity of the Universe, the variability of perception. It will prevent you from fixing on the first plausible explanation as The Truth.*

PAULA UNDERWOOD (53, P. 13)

## CHAPTER OBJECTIVES

After studying this chapter, the reader will be able to:

1. Explain why theories are used in mental health practice.
2. Identify and briefly describe seven theories or models used in mental health practice.
3. Define terms associated with each of these theories.
4. State major concepts associated with these theories.

Theories attempt to explain how mental health problems develop and how a therapist may help someone deal with them. Many of the theories occupational therapists have used in mental health practice were originally developed by psychologists or psychiatrists.[1] Although many of these theories are used less widely today, practitioners frequently use techniques based on them. Also occupational therapists (OTs) and occupational therapy assistants (OTAs) often work in treatment settings in which some of the staff use one or more of the theories discussed in this chapter. Chapter 3 explores other theories developed specifically for use in occupational therapy practice.

First, however, why use a theory at all? One very good reason is that a theory provides ideas about what to do in a situation with a patient. Imagine the following scenario:

**CASE EXAMPLE**

Your supervisor on level 1 fieldwork has asked you to cover her cooking group while she goes to a meeting. Because you are comfortable with cooking, you agree to do it. Everything seems to be going fine. All eight members are busy on their tasks. Suddenly one teenage girl starts drawing a knife across her wrist. She isn't actually cutting herself, but just dragging the knife across her skin.

What would you do? Are you finding it hard to think of an answer? Maybe you would like to think about it for a while; but in a real situation, you would not have much time. You would have to respond quickly, and it might help if you had a theory to give you some ideas.

A theory is one way of looking at something, and because there are many ways of looking at how the mind works, we have many theories about it. A theory provides a set of principles that can be used to organize, explain, and predict observable phenomena—in this case, behavior and other aspects of mental health. A theory is one explanation, but there is not yet any one "correct" theory that explains all we want to know about the human mind. Consequently, many theories try to explain the same thing. As an occupational therapy assistant, you will use techniques based on these theories; therefore, you need to know something about them. Techniques are methods or approaches for working with patients or clients.

Six major medical and psychological theories used in mental health treatment are covered in this chapter. You will learn about the main ideas, special vocabulary, and some of the basic techniques of each theory. A seventh popular model for mental health treatment is *atheoretical* (without theory); this model (psychiatric rehabilitation) is also presented in this chapter.

## THEORY OF OBJECT RELATIONS

The theory of object relations is a psychoanalytic theory based on the work of Sigmund Freud and his followers, who believed that mental health and mental illness are determined by our relations with objects in our environment. These objects may be physical (nonhuman) or human. Our abilities to love and respond to other people and to take interest in the things in our environment are seen as expressions of object relations. The way a person relates to things and people gives clues about his or her lifelong pattern of object relations, which is believed to develop through relationships in very early childhood.

According to object relations theory, the infant develops relationships with objects in the environment to satisfy needs, such as hunger and thirst. Humans have inborn tendencies, or *drives,* to try actively to satisfy needs. It is believed that humans are born with drives for self-preservation, pleasure,

[1] Much of the material in this chapter derives from Early (25).

and exploration and that these inborn drives originate in the most primitive part of the self, the *id.* The id is not concerned about other people's feelings but only with satisfying its own needs. At birth, the personality is dominated by the id. It is only through experiences of and relationships with human and nonhuman objects that other parts of the personality develop.

As an example, when very young infants are hungry, they cry. This is their way of expressing their drive for food and their terrible frustration at not being fed. As children develop, they are expected to express their needs in ways that are more socially acceptable. They are put under pressure to adapt to the rules of society. For instance, they must learn to talk about their feelings instead of just striking out. If they cry, they may be sent to their rooms. In the beginning, children's parents make them follow the rules of society, but gradually these rules become part of the children's personalities. Freud called this the *superego.* The superego acts as the conscience or moralizer and tells the person what is right and wrong.

As you might imagine, the id and the superego are often in conflict. For example, a woman who is dieting may pass a bakery window and see a chocolate cake. Her id wants her to eat that chocolate cake. The superego says, in effect, "You shouldn't do that." The conflict between what the id wants and what the superego will allow can generate anxiety. The woman may feel confused and tense, not knowing what to do. Fortunately, a third part of the personality, the *ego,* controls anxiety by compromising between the warring id and superego.

The word *ego,* as it is used in object relations theory, refers to something quite different from the everyday meaning ("He has a big ego."). The ego, the third main part of the personality, performs many mental functions that deal with reality and with the conflicting desires of id and superego. Memory and perception are two important functions of the ego. Another is *reality testing,* or the ability to tell the difference between reality and fantasy and to share the same general ideas about reality that most people do. For example, a student may say that a particular teacher doesn't like her, citing as evidence that the teacher frowns. Is it true that the teacher dislikes the student? Reality testing is needed; the student may gather evidence from other incidents or from feedback from fellow students. Willingness to consider other points of view (e.g., that the teacher keeps saying he can't hear her when the student speaks so softly or that the teacher said he had a headache) indicates good reality testing. Persistence in beliefs despite evidence to the contrary indicates denial of reality and suggests poor reality testing. The business of learning about reality and comparing or testing assumptions about reality consumes much of the ego's time and attention.

The ego also helps control impulses and organize actions. In addition, the ego makes use of many *defense mechanisms,* which compromise among the id, the superego, and the demands of reality. Defense mechanisms ward off or defend against anxiety and other uncomfortable feelings.

One defense mechanism is *displacement,* or the transfer of the id drive to another object. In the case of the woman looking in the bakery window, the ego might substitute another object, so that the woman finds herself thinking of a bathing suit she saw the other day. All of this happens without the woman being aware of it because *all defense mechanisms operate unconsciously.* Some other defense mechanisms are listed in Table 2-1. Understanding the various defense mechanisms helps the occupational therapy assistant speculate on why someone is behaving in a certain way and then helps provide an effective response.

Most mental operations, like defense mechanisms, operate unconsciously. Even so, they may dominate behavior. The conflicting demands of the id and superego create anxiety, which the ego attempts to control, usually by unconscious defense mechanisms. Sometimes the ego consciously tries to control the anxiety through *suppression,* but

**TABLE 2-1 SELECTED DEFENSE MECHANISMS[a]**

| DEFENSE MECHANISM | DEFINITION | EXAMPLE |
|---|---|---|
| Denial | Refusing to believe something that causes anxiety | A mother plans for her child who is mentally retarded to be a doctor. |
| Projection | Believing that an unacceptable feeling of one's own belongs to someone else | A self-isolating patient in a work group says that other patients won't talk to him. |
| Rationalization | Making excuses for unacceptable behavior or feelings | A teenager says he didn't do his homework because he didn't have the right kind of paper. |
| Conversion | Conflicts turned into real physical symptoms | A girl with poor coordination gets a migraine headache when it is time for volleyball. |
| Regression | Functioning at a more primitive developmental level than previously; going back to an immature pattern of behavior | A 7-year-old child who is hospitalized for major surgery begins to walk on tiptoes and suck his thumb. |
| Undoing | Trying to reverse the effects of what one has done by doing the opposite | A patient accuses the therapist of trying to run his life. Later he brings her flowers. |
| Idealization | Overestimating someone or valuing him or her more than the real personality and person seem to merit | A woman says that the group leader is the most handsome and kindest man in the world. |
| Identification | Adopting the habits or characteristics of another person | A teenage girl begins to wear her hair just like her therapist does. |
| Sublimation | Unacceptable wishes channeled into socially acceptable activities | A child who wants to cut things up to see how they work grows up to become a surgeon. |
| Substitution | A realistic goal or object substituted for one that cannot be achieved | A young man fails the examination for the police department, then takes a job as a security guard. |
| Compensation | Efforts to make up for personal deficits; this can also be a conscious effort | A woman, blind from birth, learns to travel without a cane or any other aid. |

[a]All defense mechanisms operate unconsciously and should not be confused with other mental mechanisms, such as suppression, that are conscious.

whether conscious or unconscious defenses are used, occasionally the ego is overwhelmed and unable to resolve the conflict. According to object relations theory, the extreme anxiety that results can cause a breakdown of ego functions—in other words, mental illness. *Mental illness occurs when the ego is unable to achieve a successful compromise among the id, the superego, and the demands of reality.* In mental illness a person's behavior is dominated by tremendous anxiety and by unconscious processes that are out of control.

The supposition that mental illness is caused by unconscious processes creates problems for therapists. How do you help someone deal with something he or she is unaware of? Object relations theory says that to change a person's mental illness, the therapist must bring unconscious conflicts to consciousness and make the person aware of them. Freud discovered that the *analysis of symbols* in patients' dreams provided clues to their unconscious feelings and that by talking with patients about their dreams he could sometimes make them conscious of these feelings. Freud believed that once this consciousness was achieved, the symptoms would be relieved.

Analysis of symbols relies on the fact that many symbols are shared by most people, at least within a particular culture. A symbol is something that stands for something else. Some examples of symbols in American culture are the Statue of Liberty, which symbolizes freedom, and the color red, which symbolizes passion or anger. Red in Chinese culture, however, symbolizes weddings and celebrations, and white (which in Western culture symbolizes purity and is used for weddings) is associated with death. Some symbols seem universal across cultures; the circle, for example, symbolizes unity.

In object relations theory many symbols are used as keys to the meaning of unconscious conflicts. For example, food symbolizes the relationship with the mother, who is the first object to satisfy the hunger need. Thus in our minds food is often associated with love and trust. Most of us occasionally overeat, even when we are not hungry. Because food symbolizes comfort and mother love, overeating may be a symbolic way to meet unconscious needs for love and comfort.

Occupational therapists who follow object relations theory use symbols in arts, crafts, and everyday activities (26, 30, 31). As an example, ceramics can provide an opportunity to explore issues of self-control versus control by others. Because wet clay is so similar to feces in color and texture, it can symbolize the anal period, during which the child learns to control the bowels and to cooperate with his or her parents through self-control. People have widely varying reactions to ceramics. Some cannot wait to handle the clay; others shrink back and may try to avoid it altogether, as the following situation illustrates:

**CASE EXAMPLE**

The occupational therapist is working alone with a 35-year-old woman, Paula, in the ceramics shop. Paula is rolling out small beads, measuring each against the others. She avoids touching the clay with her hands, using tools and plastic gloves instead. When she finishes with each bead, she places it neatly in line with the others.

The therapist comments, "The beads are very neat and precise."

Paula answers, "They have to match."

"Why is that?"

"It would look like a mess if they didn't."

The therapist thinks for a few seconds and then responds, "I have seen some necklaces with beads of all different sizes."

"People who wear those are slobs."

"Oh?"

"They don't care about doing things right."

As this brief dialogue illustrates, there are many ways in which someone can relate to a symbol.

A patient's behavior toward an activity may reveal his or her attitudes and feelings about issues that that activity symbolizes. Because people have their own personal histories, they may also have individual or *idiosyncratic* symbols that are theirs alone. For example, beads may mean something to Paula because of some previous experience of hers; and although clay is a powerful symbol of anal issues, it may not mean this to everyone, and it has many other uses in occupational therapy.

Therapists who employ the object relations approach successfully must understand the theories behind it. This requires years of study and communication with a supervisor who knows the theory well. By focusing on the unconscious meaning of symbols in activities, object relations theory suggests that patients do not need to develop conscious real-life skills. Many occupational therapists think the theory has limited usefulness for this reason. In addition, because this approach attempts to analyze and change unconscious processes, it can take a very long time to achieve results. Consequently, it has been used most often in long-term settings, where patients are expected to remain in treatment for many years. Insurance companies often do not reimburse for this kind of treatment, and few modern inpatient clinics use this theory exclusively.

Another criticism frequently leveled at object relations theory is that it was developed by men and is based on a gender-specific view. In other words, it does not adequately address the psychosexual and psychosocial development of women. Writers Carol Tavris and Carol Gilligan, among others, have summarized and elaborated some theories and principles more applicable to women and girls.

Kielhofner (35) argues that object relations theory is inadequate as a basis for practice in psychiatric occupational therapy, because it ignores the essential therapeutic value of individually chosen productive activity and instead exploits the symbolic elements of activities that are not linked to functional participation in real life. Furthermore, object relations theory does not address the neurological impairments seen in schizophrenia and other major mental disorders. Despite these

## CONCEPTS SUMMARY

1. Humans are born with drives for self-preservation and pleasure. These drives reside in the id, the most primitive and childish part of the personality.
2. Children develop control over the id drives by learning the moral standards of society from their parents. These standards become the superego, a second part of the personality.
3. The id and the superego often conflict because they desire different things: The id wants to satisfy its own needs, and the superego wants to follow the rules. Beyond this, reality may not permit either desire to be satisfied, adding to the conflict.
4. The ego, a third part of the personality, attempts to resolve the conflicting demands of the id, the superego, and reality. It does this through ego functions such as memory, perception, reality testing, and defense mechanisms.
5. The id, ego, and superego operate unconsciously. We are not normally aware of their functioning.
6. When the ego cannot resolve unconscious conflict, anxiety becomes overwhelming and the ego cannot operate normally. This breakdown of ego functions is recognized as mental illness.
7. Ego functions can be strengthened or restored if the person can become conscious of the unconscious conflict that is causing the anxiety.
8. One method of identifying unconscious processes is by the analysis of symbols.

defects, object relations theory provides a structure for thinking about how the mind works. Though not the dominant theory it once was, object relations theory continues to be studied and used today by other professionals working with people who have psychiatric problems; and for this reason, it should be known by OTAs working in mental health.

### VOCABULARY REVIEW

**id** The part of the personality that contains the drives to self-preservation and pleasure. The id is present from birth or before and operates unconsciously.

**object** Anything toward which the id directs its energies to satisfy a drive. Objects may be human (people) or nonhuman (animals and things).

**superego** The part of the personality that contains standards for behavior. The superego is thought to be a representation of rules learned from parents and other authorities. It operates unconsciously.

**ego** The part of the personality that regulates behavior by compromising among the demands of the id, the superego, and reality. The ego contains many functions, such as memory, perception, reality testing, and defense mechanisms. These work together in a continuous process of adapting to reality. Many ego functions operate unconsciously.

**reality testing** The ability to tell the difference between reality and fantasy and to share the same general ideas about reality as everyone else. Reality testing is an ego function.

**defense mechanism** Any of several methods used by the ego to control anxiety and conflict. All defense mechanisms operate unconsciously (Table 2-1).

**conscious** Mental functions of which we are aware. Suppression is one example.

**unconscious** Mental functions of which we normally are not aware. These include the id, the superego, and the defense mechanisms.

**conflict** Opposition between simultaneous demands, such as those of the id and the superego or the self and reality.

**anxiety** An uncomfortable feeling of tension that may arise from unconscious conflict.

**symbol** Something that represents something else. Symbols may be universal, cultural, or idiosyncratic.

**analysis of symbols** One of the methods used in object relations therapy. The therapist analyzes symbols in the patient's dreams or artwork to discover their unconscious meanings.

**suppression** An attempt to control anxiety and conflict by *consciously* controlling or denying it. Suppression is conscious, unlike the defense mechanisms, but it may serve the same purpose in regard to anxiety.

## DEVELOPMENTAL THEORY

There are several versions of developmental theory. The best known are those of Erikson, Piaget, and Gesell. This section outlines the main concepts common to all developmental theories and then explores Erikson's theory of psychosocial development.

The first developmental concept is that *a person matures through a series of stages that occur in a fixed sequence.* At each stage the person encounters specific *developmental tasks* that, when mastered, provide a foundation for later development. For example, a child learns to stand before learning to walk. The standing stage must come before the walking stage. Physical, social, and intellectual growth all occur simultaneously but in a fixed sequence in each area. In other words, children can develop social skills as they are learning to walk, but they cannot walk before they stand. In the normal growth process, development is gradual and spontaneous and eventually produces a mature and functional adult.

However, many factors can interrupt the growth process. Physical disease, poverty, malnutrition, trauma, or emotional or social deprivation can keep a person from mastering the developmental tasks of a particular stage. When this happens, a *developmental lag* may result. A developmental lag is a discrepancy (difference) between a person's behavior and the behavior one would expect of a person of that age. In other words, a person who has a developmental lag has fallen behind in development and is not as mature as his or her peers. Take, for example, the case of David:

## CASE EXAMPLE

David is a 29-year-old man who has attended several colleges, majoring in a variety of subjects but never graduating. He has had a succession of jobs that seem unrelated: dishwasher, produce clerk, busboy, crewman on a sailboat, handyman, horse groom, waiter, messenger, house painter. David has acquired a lot of skills over the years but doesn't stick to anything, and he doesn't know what to do about it. He sees that friends his own age are establishing themselves in careers and settling down with marriage and family life. David feels increasingly distant from his friends. He is extremely depressed and has twice attempted suicide.

A therapist using Erikson's theory of psychosocial development would first analyze where David was lagging in development. According to Erikson, around 3 years of age the child enters a developmental stage termed *initiative versus guilt*. In this stage the developmental task is for the child to establish a sense of purpose and direction (initiative) in activities. The child feels pleasure and power at the ability to affect the world around him or her. This stage lays a foundation for setting goals and working to accomplish them in later life, but this can happen only if the child is permitted to follow his or her own direction.

However, the child's direction may be unacceptable to the parents, who may have their own ideas about what the child should be doing. For example, David's history revealed that his parents pushed him to read at an early age and constantly compared him with his older brother, who could read before he was age 3. David was an active child and good at sports and games, but his parents discouraged these interests and stressed reading as the preferred activity.

Because David was not permitted to pursue his own interests as a child, his sense of purpose (initiative) remained confused and vague. During adolescence, this confusion was reactivated when he attempted to choose a career. Because he had little previous experience in setting his own direction and following it through to success, he was unsure of himself and uncertain of his direction and of how to proceed. This pattern repeated itself over the years. For example, David felt guilty when he enjoyed crewing on the sailboat; he thought he should be doing something "more important" with his life and went back to college but dropped out after one semester.

According to Erikson's theory, mental health problems occur when developmental tasks are not successfully mastered. Failure at one stage of development does not prevent the person from continuing to develop, but problems may result because the foundation is weak. To help a person who has problems because of a developmental lag, the therapist designs situations that will facilitate growth in the deficient area. In other words, if a person has failed to develop adequately in a given area, the therapist can make it easier for the development to occur by creating conditions that encourage growth. For example, in David's case an occupational therapist might expose him to a variety of activities that fit his skills and interests, helping him choose and get involved in an activity that needs fairly consistent effort over a fairly long time (for example, woodworking). The therapist would encourage David when he became disheartened and would try to sustain his interest in the activity by showing him new challenges or problems to solve. The therapist might help him find new ways to use his skills by producing objects for sale or by having him instruct others. The therapist would be careful not to push him too hard; after all, it is *David's* sense of purpose that has to be developed, not the therapist's.

This example focuses on one of the eight stages of psychosocial development proposed in Erikson's theory. The word *psychosocial* refers to the interaction between the self (*psyche*) and society, an interaction that Erikson believed was the core of successful human functioning. Table 2-2 defines and explains the eight stages. Erikson suggested that each stage is organized around a central crisis that has two possible but totally opposite resolutions. For example, the crisis of purpose and self-direction can be resolved as either *initiative* or *guilt.* Erikson argued that there is a continuum of resolutions between these two extremes at any stage and cautioned students not to think of the outcome in good–bad, either–or terms. He also noted that human development is continuous and that anyone facing a problem in the present must rely on the interconnected matrix or network of feelings about earlier developmental events. When a new crisis arises, a person may regress and reexperience the conflicts of earlier developmental stages.

Erikson's and other developmental theories are consistent with many of the basic ideas of occupational therapy. The concept of gradation, of learning through successively more challenging and complex stages, and the focus on solving problems and acquiring skills make developmental theory an appealing choice for working with persons who have poor social relationships and inadequate skills (61). Similarly, occupational therapists have long attempted to meet the patient at his or her own level, matching tasks to abilities and interests.

There are three major difficulties with this approach. The first is that some persons with major mental illnesses (e.g., those diagnosed in childhood or early adolescence) appear to lag in the earliest stage of psychosocial development; they have always had problems trusting others, as their histories show. To change fundamental and life-long mistrust is a serious challenge. Second, like approaches based on object relations theory, which itself has a developmental orientation,[2] application of developmental theory to treatment is possible only over the long term because developmental change is a gradual process. Third, human development involves many complex and interrelated issues that can be understood only through rigorous study, and therapists must be exceptionally well trained to use developmental theory well. One model used in psychiatric occupational therapy that is related to developmental theory is *development of adaptive skills.* This practice model is described in Chapter 3.

## CONCEPTS SUMMARY

1. Human beings mature through a series of stages that occur in a fixed sequence. Specific developmental tasks arise at each stage; the person's experience with these tasks provides a foundation for later development.
2. Problems occur when developmental tasks are not mastered sufficiently well. This causes a lag in development that can interfere with a person's attempts to master other developmental tasks in future stages.
3. A developmental lag can be corrected by exposing the person to a situation that will encourage growth in the deficient area. If the proper conditions are created and the therapist provides corrective guidance, the developmental task can be mastered.

[2]The alert reader may have noticed that Erikson's developmental theory is in some respects similar to object relations theory. Erikson's training and background were psychoanalytic; therefore, much of his work is based on the writings of Freud. Freud's work focused on psychosexual rather than psychosocial development.

## TABLE 2-2 ERIKSON'S EIGHT STAGES OF PSYCHOSOCIAL DEVELOPMENT

| APPROXIMATE AGE | PSYCHOSOCIAL STAGE | EXPLANATION |
|---|---|---|
| Birth–18 months | *Basic Trust* versus *Mistrust* | Infants need nurturance from the mother. If they perceive her as reliable, they develop the capacity to trust others. If not, they tend to mistrust others, feel anxious about others' willingness to meet their needs, and so on. |
| 2–4 years | *Autonomy* versus *Shame and Doubt* | During this period children learn to control their bowel and bladder and become more independent in exploring the environment. Their sense of motivation and will are shaped by the parents' attitudes toward bodily functions and their willingness to allow their children to control themselves. |
| 3–5 years | *Initiative* versus *Guilt* | Preschool and kindergarten children begin to combine skills and plan activities to accomplish goals. They begin to imitate adult roles, try out new ways of doing things, and develop a sense of self-direction. |
| 6–12 years | *Industry* versus *Inferiority* | During elementary school, children acquire skills and work habits. They compare themselves with their peers. Attitudes of parents, teachers, and other children contribute to their sense of competence. |
| Adolescence | *Identity* versus *Role Confusion* | Adolescents experiment with a variety of adult roles. Key issues include vocational choice and gender identification. Rebellion against parents is common, as teenagers try to assert a separate identity. |
| Young adulthood | *Intimacy* versus *Isolation* | The central concern of this period is to find a suitable partner with whom to share life. |
| Middle adulthood | *Generativity* versus *Stagnation* | Adults look toward the future and try to make a contribution to it through work, community leadership, child rearing, and so on. |
| Old age | *Ego Integrity* versus *Despair* | Faced with the prospect of death, older adults review and evaluate their life's choices to see whether they have done what they meant to do. |

### VOCABULARY REVIEW

**development** A process of maturation occurring throughout life.

**developmental stage** A specific level of development, generally believed to occur at a specific time in a human being's life. Various developmental psychologists postulate different theories, each containing a number of developmental stages. Erikson proposed eight stages of psychosocial development. Piaget proposed four stages of cognitive development. Regardless of the particular theory, the stages always occur in a fixed sequence.

**developmental task** A problem or crisis that arises during a developmental stage. Solving the problem shows mastery of the task. An example is choosing a career, traditionally a developmental task of adolescence.

**developmental lag** A delay in development demonstrated by failure to master a developmental task.

**psychosocial development** The ongoing process in which the person resolves conflicts between personal needs and what society demands and permits.

## BEHAVIORAL THEORIES

The behavioral theories are derived from the work of Pavlov, a Russian physiologist who experimented with dogs, and Skinner, an American psychologist who studied how animals responded to stimulation. The central concept of these theories is that all behavior is learned. *Behaviors that have pleasurable results tend to be repeated.* For example:

### CASE EXAMPLE

You are in a new class. The professor says something you do not understand, so you ask a question. He says he is glad you asked that question and gives you an answer that helps you understand. The next time you have a question, you raise your hand.

It seems almost common sense that people repeat actions that result in pleasure or rewards. Imagine what might happen if the professor had given a confusing answer or had in some way made you feel embarrassed for asking the question. You might feel that you should never ask another question. This illustrates a complementary concept: *Actions that have negative or unpleasant consequences tend not to be repeated.*

According to behavioral theories, each person develops through a process of learning from the results of his or her behavior. If adaptive behaviors are rewarded and maladaptive behaviors punished or ignored, the result should be a mature and responsible human being. Sometimes, however, the wrong behaviors are learned. Mental illness, in this theory, is defined as abnormal behavior that results because normal or adaptive behavior was not rewarded or did not have pleasurable consequences. In some cases, abnormal behavior occurs because maladaptive behavior was reinforced.

As an example, take the case of a 2-year-old boy who screams and cries when his mother goes out for an evening. Every time he cries, the babysitter gives him a piece of candy. The undesirable behavior (screaming) has had a pleasurable consequence (candy). Very quickly the child learns that screaming is an effective way of getting candy. In later life, he may carry on the pattern, screaming at other people to get what he wants.

Occupational therapists use a variety of techniques based on behavioral theory. Sometimes this is called an *action–consequence* approach because the therapist tries to change the person's behavior (action) by changing the consequences of the behavior. The therapist may reward new adaptive behaviors or ignore or punish the maladaptive behavior. Some therapists use both methods.

An example is the case of Eric, who repeatedly interrupts while the therapist is working with other patients. He constantly asks for her opinion of his project. Using the action–consequence approach, the therapist tells him to work on his own for 5 minutes, and then she will talk to him. During the 5-minute work period she ignores his disruptive behavior, but after this she will "reward" him with some time and attention.

*Identification of terminal behavior* is the first step in a behavioral treatment program. Terminal behavior is the normal or adaptive behavior that the therapist wants the person to perform. In the case of Eric, this might be working on his own for half an hour. Once the terminal behavior has been identified, the therapist determines a baseline by counting and recording the person's behavior. For example, she might count how often Eric tries to interrupt her during a half-hour period. The *baseline* is a known standard or record of how the person behaved before the treatment was started. Records of the patient's behavior after treatment can be compared with this baseline to determine to what extent the treatment was effective.

Next the therapist selects a reinforcement. Reinforcement is the name given to the therapist's response (consequence) to the client's performance of the desired behavior (action). In Eric's case, the therapist already knows that attention from her will be a good reinforcement. The therapist then decides how often the reinforcement will be given (this is called the *schedule*). The therapist may decide to reward Eric every time he works for 5 minutes without interrupting her. This would be a continuous schedule of reinforcement, because a reward is given every time the action is performed. Usually *continuous schedules* are used at the beginning of treatment, when the therapist is trying to get the person to do the desired action. Later, when the behavior is established, the reinforcement might be scheduled intermittently, not every time the action is performed but only now and then. *Intermittent schedules* are believed to be more effective than continuous schedules once the behavior has been learned.

Often the terminal behavior seems very far from the way the person is acting now. For example, for Eric to sit still and work by himself for half an hour seems like a distant goal. To help Eric reach it, the therapist might use *shaping*. Shaping is a method of working toward a terminal behavior through successive approximations, or small steps. In Eric's case, the therapist might start by expecting him to work on his own for 5 minutes, at the end of which time she talks to him. Once the 5-minute period of independent work has been established, it can be extended to 10 minutes. Then Eric would have to work for 10 minutes to be rewarded. Gradually the half-hour goal would be reached through a series of steps or approximations, each one closer to the goal than the one before.

When the terminal behavior involves learning a complicated routine with several steps, the technique of *chaining* can be used. Chaining is teaching a multistep activity one step at a time. The person does the steps he or she knows, and the therapist does the rest. Gradually the person learns the whole activity. Chaining can begin with the first step (*forward chaining*) or the last step (*backward chaining*). An example of backward chaining is having a person fold the laundry (last step) that someone else has washed. After learning to fold, the person learns how to use the dryer. Gradually, by working backward in this way, he or she learns the entire sequence of washing clothes. Mentally retarded adults appear to learn faster with backward chaining than with forward chaining (56), and this approach can also be effective with other learners who have cognitive disabilities or who lack experience or confidence in a task.

Occupational therapists have used behavioral techniques to treat hyperactive (17) children, severely mentally retarded (57) children, and children with autism and related developmental disorders (55). Unlike therapies based on object relations or developmental concepts, behavioral therapies give quick results, as the following example of a hyperactive child described by Cermak et al. illustrates:

**CASE EXAMPLE**

Tom . . . spent a great deal of time lying on the floor kicking his legs and thrashing around. His behavior was disruptive to the group. In the classroom this conduct disturbed the other children and made it difficult for Tom to sit long enough to finish his schoolwork. The therapists decided to give him the attention he wanted. When he was sitting on the bench, the leader or another member of the group sat next to him and put their arm around him. Surprisingly, after one play session of being on the floor 30 times, Tom was on the floor only twice the next session (17, p. 315).

Like most human efforts, a behavior modification program is only as effective as the thinking and planning behind it, and the consistency of its implementation (41). Table 2-3 shows the steps in designing a behavioral treatment program in occupational therapy as identified by Sieg (46) and gives examples. Sieg's model is strictly behavioral. Occupational therapy treatment approaches based on modified behavioral concepts include Mosey's (40) *activities therapy* and the use of social skills training (14). Because these approaches are so widely used today, they will be discussed in more detail in "Roll Acquisition and Social Skills Training" in Chapter 3.

Behavior therapies have been criticized for treating people like machines; for using unhealthful reinforcers, such as candy, coffee, and cigarettes; and for using aversive reinforcement (punishment). Although the idea that people will respond the way a therapist "programs" them to is

**TABLE 2-3 STEPS IN A BEHAVIORAL TREATMENT PROGRAM[a]**

| STEP | EXAMPLE |
|---|---|
| 1. Identify the terminal behavior. | The therapist and patient select the treatment goal: Jim will initiate conversation with another patient at least twice in each 4-hour work session. |
| 2. Determine the baseline by counting the frequency of the behavior. | Before the beginning of treatment, the therapist records how often Jim starts a conversation with another patient during the group. Baseline data are collected over several sessions. |
| 3. Select a method of counting and recording the behavior. | The therapist notes each time Jim starts a conversation and writes it on a chart. Jim checks the chart each day to verify that it is correct. |
| 4. Select a reinforcer that is meaningful to the patient. | Jim likes to sit in the hospital coffee shop and drink coffee. The therapist decides that he will be given tokens to use for the coffee shop. |
| 5. Determine a schedule of reinforcement. | A continuous schedule helps Jim develop the new behavior quickly. The therapist gives him a token every day he shows the desired behavior. |

[a]Adapted with permission from Sieg KW. Applying the behavioral model to the occupational therapy model. Am J Occup Ther 1974;28:421–428. Copyright © 1974 by the American Occupational Therapy Association, Inc.

repugnant, it is also unrealistic. Therapists who set goals with, rather than for, their patients and who explain the treatment program to them can hardly be accused of treating patients like machines. Although therapists at times use unhealthful reinforcers to get clients to respond; other rewards, such as weekend passes and other privileges, are selected wherever possible. Finally, therapists do not use punishment unless there is no other way to stop patients from harming themselves.

In summary, behavioral theories consist of a group of approaches that have in common the idea that people learn from the consequences of their behavior. Understanding how people learn is important to occupational therapy practitioners who want to help people get rid of maladaptive behaviors and acquire new skills.

## CONCEPTS SUMMARY

1. All behavior is learned.
2. Actions that have had pleasurable consequences tend to be repeated.
3. Normal behavior is learned if adaptive behaviors are rewarded and maladaptive behaviors are punished or ignored.
4. Abnormal behavior is learned if adaptive behavior is not rewarded or maladaptive behavior is reinforced.
5. Abnormal behavior can be changed if the therapist changes the consequences of the behavior.

## VOCABULARY REVIEW

**behavior** Any observable action.

**reinforcement** Consequences of behavior that either encourage or discourage the repetition of the behavior.

**terminal behavior** The treatment goal, the behavior the person will show at the end of a successful treatment program.

**shaping** A method of approaching the terminal behavior gradually, using a series of steps (successive approximations) that lead to the goal.

**chaining** A method of teaching a complex activity a step at a time, starting with either the first or the last step. The therapist performs the remaining steps until the person masters the entire sequence.

**backward chaining** Chaining that starts with the last step. It is believed to be more effective than forward chaining.

**forward chaining** Chaining that starts with the first step.

**schedule of reinforcement** The timing of reinforcement. Schedules may be continuous (reinforcement follows every performance of the desired behavior) or intermittent (reinforcement is given only occasionally).

**extinction** Discouraging an undesired behavior by removing any reinforcement. An example might be a therapist's ignoring a child's temper tantrum instead of responding to it. This is called planned ignoring.

## COGNITIVE-BEHAVIORAL THERAPY

Cognitive-behavioral treatment is based on the work of the psychiatrist Aaron Beck (9–11) and others (8, 27, 59). The many variations on cognitive-behavioral theories all share an underlying assumption: Human behavior is based on what we think and believe. To put this another way, what we think (cognition) determines how we act (behavior). This theory proposes that people with mental health problems have maladaptive patterns of thinking (*cognitions*) that lead to unsuccessful behaviors. Cognitive-behavioral therapy helps the person understand and change negative cognitions, and this process brings about a change in behavior.

Negative cognitions include *automatic thoughts* that occur without the person recognizing them or challenging their logic. For example, someone who says hello to a neighbor and gets little or no response may think, "She doesn't like me. Nobody likes me. I'm just not someone that people like." The negative thought triggers negative feelings (anxiety or depression) and maladaptive behaviors (avoidance of social situations, poor eye contact, and dysfunctional interactions with others).

Cognitive-behavioral approaches link a precipitating event to a person's thoughts about the event and then to the feelings these thoughts evoke. Events are in themselves neutral; they receive their value from our thoughts about them. When an event occurs, a person has thoughts about it, although these thoughts may occur below the level of conscious awareness. These thoughts are evaluative, attaching an *attribution* or meaning to the event. For example, a raise in pay to most people is a positive event. When informed of a raise in pay, most people think, "That means they think I'm doing a good job." However, some attach a negative evaluation to a pay raise; a person might think "Uh oh, now they're going to expect me to work even harder. I'll never be able to meet their expectations."

Thoughts lead to feelings. In the first example, interpreting the raise to mean that others think one is doing a good job can lead to feelings of positive self-evaluation ("I feel really competent and successful"), contentment, excitement, and increased motivation. Ultimately these feelings stimulate associated behaviors, such as confident posture, efforts to solve problems on the job, and pleasant and assertive interactions with co-workers.

In the second example, thinking that a raise indicates unreachable expectations can provoke feelings of anxiety, negative self-evaluation, and hopelessness. The person may elaborate and ruminate on the negative thoughts and associated negative feelings ("Once they find out I can't really handle it, they'll fire me for sure"), and then act on these feelings—for example, by failing to concentrate because of ruminations, procrastinating or avoiding assignments, or coming in late. Again, thoughts provoke feelings that affect the person's behavior, in this case adversely.

Cognitive-behavioral treatment focuses on both cognition and behavior and on the relationship between them. Cognitive techniques involve challenging and modifying negative automatic thoughts and their underlying assumptions. Behavioral techniques focus on identifying behaviors, investigating their consequences, and evaluating their effectiveness. Traditional behavioral techniques such as systematic desensitization are also used.

Of all cognitive-behavioral approaches, Beck's variation is the most widely recognized and practiced. The therapist (any psychotherapist trained in this approach) works one on one with the person to identify negative or distorted thoughts and examine their validity. Therapist and patient also monitor the patient's behavior and evaluate its effectiveness. Homework assignments are designed by the therapist with input from the patient, are carried out by the patient, and are reported to the therapist. Beck discusses this approach as a sort of joint scientific effort of collecting data and testing hypotheses. Homework assignments in this approach include bibliotherapy (assigned reading), graded task assignments, and activity scheduling (9). These are familiar to occupational therapy practitioners, as they have been traditional occupational therapy techniques since the beginnings of our profession.

Other techniques used by Beck include cognitive rehearsal, self-monitoring, and reattribution. *Cognitive rehearsal* is used with patients who have difficulty carrying out tasks, even when they know them well. The person is asked to imagine carrying out each successive step in the task. This helps the person attend to details that might otherwise escape attention and lead to task failure (e.g., forgetting to bring exercise clothing to the gym). *Self-monitoring* requires that the patient notice and record negative cognitions and their associated events with an aim to discovering the frequency of the problem and understanding the chain of events, thoughts, feelings, and behaviors. The person may use a diary, a structured record sheet, a tape recorder, a portable computer, or even a wrist counter to collect data. *Reattribution* is used to challenge the patient's belief that his or her personal shortcomings are responsible for negative external events. This is particularly helpful with depressed persons, who may think that they are responsible for things that are clearly outside their control.

The following is an example of Beck's treatment of a woman who was afraid of being in crowded places. This example shows the use of self-monitoring and desensitization.[3]

**CASE EXAMPLE**

Therapist: What are you afraid of when you're in a crowded place?

Patient: I'm afraid I won't be able to catch my breath. . . .

Therapist: And?

Patient: . . . I'll pass out.

Therapist: Just pass out?

Patient: All right, I know it sounds silly but I'm afraid I will just stop breathing . . . and die.

Therapist: Right now, what do you think are the probabilities that you will suffocate and die?

Patient: Right now, it seems like one chance in a thousand.

Beck asked this patient to visit a crowded store and to write down her estimates of the probability of dying at various steps on the way to the store. The patient's notations and consequent interactions with the therapist were as follows:[4]

**CASE EXAMPLE (*Continued*)**

1. Leaving my house—chances of dying in store: 1 in 1,000
2. Driving into town—chances of dying in store: 1 in 100
3. Parking car in lot—chances of dying in store: 1 in 50
4. Walking to store—chances of dying in store: 1 in 10
5. Entering store—chances of dying in store: 2 to 1
6. In middle of crowd—chances of dying in store: 10 to 1

Therapist: So when you were in the crowd you thought you had a 10 to 1 chance of dying.

Patient: It was crowded and stuffy and I couldn't catch my breath. I felt I was passing out. I really panicked and got out of there.

Therapist: What do you think—right now—were the actual probabilities that you would have died if you stayed in the store?

Patient: Probably one in a million.

With continued treatment the patient learned to remind herself that she had already thought about this rationally and that she was as safe in the store as she was elsewhere. Eventually she was able to visit stores and crowded places with only minimal discomfort.

In addition to Beck, other leaders in the development of cognitive-behavioral treatment include

[3]From Beck (9, p. 253). Used with permission of International Universities Press.

[4]From Beck (9, pp. 253–254). Used with permission of International Universities Press.

Albert Ellis and Albert Bandura. Ellis (27) is the founder of rational-emotive therapy (RET), which works with the ABCs of human experience. An activating event (A) has cognitive, emotional, and behavioral consequences (C). People view or experience A in terms of their beliefs (B). The focus of therapy is on the beliefs (B), which Ellis divides into rational and irrational beliefs. Rational beliefs express personal desires or preferences ("I would like people to like me.") in contrast with irrational beliefs ("People *must* like me or I will not be able to go on."). Irrational beliefs typically begin with the words *should, ought, must,* and so on. Ellis linked these irrational beliefs to cognitive distortions such as all-or-none thinking, personalizing, fortune telling, and overgeneralization.

The aim of RET is for the patient to realize that we create our world through the way we interpret experience. Thus one's own psychological experience is self-created and can be changed. The RET therapist helps the patient to dispute (D) the irrational beliefs to bring about a corrective emotional (E) experience (Table 2-4). The therapist using this approach directly challenges the person's spoken or even unspoken irrational beliefs. The aim is to dispute this thinking and replace it with more rational ideas. Ellis encouraged therapists following his technique to use an active, highly directive, and confrontational approach. Indeed, transcripts of Ellis' therapy sessions reveal techniques that may seem brutal, such as poking fun at the patient and using profanity and insults. According to Ellis, such methods are necessary to challenge and disrupt irrational thinking.

Bandura (8) investigated the effects of social modeling, which uses a skilled model to teach behavior. The model, which may be a person, a video, or a cartoon, demonstrates the behavior, which is copied by the subject. Learning occurs through imitation. This training method is more effective for humans than is trial-and-error learning with external reinforcement (rewards and punishments). Originally Bandura was trying to show that modeling is a more powerful training method than trial and error or operant conditioning (behavioral techniques). Bandura's work explained why children imitate adults even when the behavior they are copying is not appropriate for their age. He also argued convincingly that television violence, even with symbolic models such as cartoon characters, is a potent teacher of violent behavior. He attacked the cathartic (release of emotion) methods used in psychoanalytic approaches, stating that it made no sense to encourage angry people to act out their anger because this increases rather than decreases their anger. Bandura's work is especially relevant to

**TABLE 2-4 COGNITIVE-BEHAVIORAL MODEL BASED ON RATIONAL-EMOTIVE THERAPY OF ELLIS**

| | | |
|---|---|---|
| A | Activating event | Student is assigned to present a speech to a class of 50. |
| B | Belief | "I can't do this. I'll make a fool of myself." |
| C | Consequence | Frightened student stammers, forgets speech, performs poorly. |
| D | Disputation | "What do you mean by 'I can't'?" "You are always well prepared." "You can rehearse this in front of friends." "Have you considered learning some relaxation techniques?" "Have you thought about using cue cards or other memory aids?" |
| E | Corrective emotional experience | Student brings cue cards, uses deep breathing and visualization to relax. Performance is excellent. Everyone applauds loudly. |

occupational therapy because modeling techniques are used extensively in teaching skills to patients (see "Role Acquisition and Social Skills Training" and "Psychoeducation" in Chapter 3).

Cognitive-behavioral therapy has been applied in occupational therapy by Johnston (34) and Taylor (50) and others (42, 51, 60). Johnston described the teaching of communication skills, assertive training, problem solving, and feeling management in a day treatment setting. These skills were taught in groups and individually. Interventions included role-playing; teaching of behaviors; and monitoring of beliefs, assumptions, and self-talk (automatic thoughts).

Taylor's work (50) focused on anger intervention. From a cognitive-behavioral perspective, the link between anger and aggression is learned. One can be angry and act aggressively—or not. Anger intervention teaches nonaggressive management of anger. The major techniques used are *(a)* monitoring physiological arousal, *(b)* practice in arousal control methods, *(c)* monitoring escalating self-talk (angry automatic thoughts), *(d)* promotion of neutral or calming self-talk via humor and diversional activities, *(e)* identification of anger-arousing stimuli, and *(f)* learning strategies to avoid these conditions.

In Taylor's approach the client first learns to identify and contain arousal. Only after arousal has been controlled to some extent are the cognitions behind the arousal addressed. Clients are exposed to activities that induce high and low states of arousal (e.g., physical exercise versus listening to soothing music). Clients are taught to use both high- and low-arousal activities for reducing anger. Although Taylor uses crafts and other traditional activities in her approach, she molds them to the goals of cognitive-behavioral therapy. For example, if physical exercise or wedging clay is used, the client is cautioned not to dwell on angry thoughts because these will perpetuate and accelerate angry arousal. The therapist teaches more appropriate self-talk so that the client can learn to use the activity to promote a calm state.

Once arousal has been controlled, the client explores the cognitive components of anger and learns to change anger-producing cognitions. The emphasis is on problem solving, stress management, and positive and neutral self-talk.

Babiss (7) reported her work using cognitive-behavioral methods and dialectical behavior therapy (DBT). The DBT approach, developed by Marsha Linehan for borderline personality disorder patients (37), helps the patient acknowledge and tolerate unpleasant thoughts and self-destructive impulses and not act on the impulse, even though it may be strong. Controlled studies demonstrate that DBT may be more effective than other approaches (22). In the group described by Babiss, an emotion is the focus of a particular session. Participants identify precipitating events that may bring on that emotion; they then list the behaviors that they use to respond to that emotion. The group helps participants identify constructive or neutral ways of behaving (taking a walk, calling a friend), to substitute for negative and self-destructive ways (drinking, shouting, cutting self).

## CONCEPTS SUMMARY

1. Thinking and behavior are linked.
2. Automatic thoughts and their associated feelings generate behavior.
3. Identifying automatic thoughts and challenging their validity allows us to consider and learn alternative patterns of thinking and behavior.
4. We create our own experience of the world and can change it by becoming aware of how we think and feel.
5. Social models (parents, peers, the media) are powerful teachers of what we think, believe, and feel.

## VOCABULARY REVIEW

**assumptions** The unarticulated rules by which a person orders and organizes experience. These assumptions are arbitrary and are learned or acquired during development. Assumptions may be adaptive, maladaptive, depressogenic (leading to depression), and so on.

**attribution** The meaning attached by the person to an event. Attributions may be either positive or negative.

**automatic thoughts** Thoughts that occur involuntarily and that are provoked by specific events and situations. For persons with psychiatric disorders, these thoughts are often negative and based on faulty assumptions or errors in reasoning.

**cognitions** Thoughts, both rational and irrational.

**cognitive distortions** or **cognitive errors** Errors in reasoning such as overgeneralization, all-or-nothing thinking, and personalization.

**self-talk** One's personal cognitions or internal thoughts. See also *automatic thoughts.* One of the goals of cognitive-behavior therapy is to identify negative, maladaptive self-talk and replace it with positive, adaptive self-talk.

**activity schedule** Used to describe a written self-report of how the person is spending time. Alternatively, a planned or projected schedule the person is assigned to follow as *homework.*

**bibliotherapy** A homework assignment to read books and articles that reinforce material covered in therapy sessions.

**cognitive rehearsal** The technique of carrying out a task in one's imagination.

**graded task assignment** A stepwise series of tasks graded from simple to complex, the purpose of which is to promote engagement in activities, realistic self-assessment, and positive self-evaluation of ability to reach a goal.

**homework** Assignment for the person to work on between therapy contacts. Ideally, homework is designed collaboratively by patient and therapist. Homework is most effective when the therapist shows a genuine interest and reviews it regularly.

**reattribution** A technique used by Beck to challenge the self-blaming thoughts of depressed persons. The purpose is to show that events perceived as negative may not be the person's fault.

**self-monitoring** Noting and recording negative cognitions and the events that precede them.

## CLIENT-CENTERED THERAPY

One of several humanistic therapies, client-centered therapy was developed by psychologist Carl Rogers. Humanistic therapies are concerned with the individual's view of life and with helping people find satisfaction in whatever way makes most sense for them. Rogers used the word *client* to convey a greater sense of self-determination than does the word *patient,* which suggests a dependent role in a medical relationship. He believed that the client's personal development is best fostered by a relationship with a warm, nondirective therapist who accepts the client as the client wishes to be accepted.

A central concept of client-centered therapy is that human beings possess the potential for directing their own growth and development. No matter how psychotic or disorganized the behavior may appear, the client is capable of self-understanding and ultimately of changing behavior.

Another concept is that people direct their own lives. The therapist does not tell the client what to do; the client must determine what action to take. By being *nondirective,* the therapist allows the client to take an individual direction. The therapist does help the client, however, by making the client more aware of feelings and by helping explore the possible consequences of contemplated action. Rogers believes that only when clients are aware of how they feel and of what is likely to happen are they truly free to choose what to do (44).

For example, a high school student, Karen, may plan to go to college because that is what her family expects her to do, even though she is confused and not particularly interested in college. She has suppressed these feelings and is not really aware of them. A client-centered therapist would listen to her and reflect back the hidden feelings that he or she hears. The student, now aware of the feelings, would be more free to choose not to go to college or at least to explore other possibilities.

A third and related concept is that mental health problems occur when a person is not aware of feelings and of the available choices. In other words, people who do not know how they feel about the people and events in their lives are likely to act in disorganized, confused, or maladaptive ways.

A fourth concept is that a person can become more aware of feelings and choices by experiencing them in a relationship with a therapist who genuinely accepts himself or herself and the client. Therapists must be aware of their own feelings and attitudes and be comfortable expressing them. They must be able to provide *unconditional positive regard*—that is, they must continue to like the client no matter what the client does. By accepting the client as is, no matter how bizarre the attitudes or behaviors, the therapist helps the client accept himself or herself. Gradually, the client's self-perception changes, and his or her behavior becomes more organized and more consistent with feelings. The client adapts better to new situations; in short, his or her mental health improves.

The client's relationship with a warm, empathic therapist is the key to the client-centered approach. *Accurate empathy* involves constantly being in the moment so that one can "feel with" the client, sensitively tuning in to the client's feelings and thoughts (18). Client-centered therapists use several techniques that facilitate clients' awareness and expression of feelings. Because occupational therapists use some of these techniques when interviewing and conversing with clients or patients, five are discussed here (32).

One technique is the *open invitation to talk.* This invitation to talk is conveyed through the use of *open questions.* Open questions are designed to require more than a one-word answer. They encourage the client to talk freely and at length. Two examples are "What were your feelings when that happened?" and "Tell me about your family."

The opposite is *closed questions,* such as "Are you married?" and "Were you angry when that happened?" Closed questions require only one- or two-word answers and limit self-expression because the person is likely to stop after that; they are not a client-centered technique. Sometimes closed questions are the quickest way to get specific details from a client, but they have little therapeutic value beyond that.

A second technique used by client-centered therapists is the *minimal response,* which shows that the therapist is listening to the client and that the client should go on talking. Some examples are nodding the head, or saying "Uh-huh" or "Go on." These responses let the client know that the therapist is tuned in to what he or she is saying.

A third technique is *reflection of feeling.* Through this technique, the therapist puts the client's feelings into words and helps him or her experience the emotional content. For example:

**CASE EXAMPLE**

Client: My husband doesn't mean anything by it, by the things he does that, well, you know. [Client looks down at her hands and sighs deeply.] It's just that I feel a certain way that he just can't see. Maybe he doesn't want to. But he's really too busy with his work and everything. He works so hard.

Therapist: You're sad that your husband is too busy to see how you feel. You feel that maybe he works so hard so that he doesn't have to see.

Just as reflection of feeling focuses on the emotional aspect of the client's words, a fourth technique focuses on the narrative content or story. Using *paraphrasing*, the therapist restates in different words what the client has said. This lets the client know that the therapist has been listening and helps the therapist check out whether he or she understood what the client meant. As an example:

**CASE EXAMPLE *(Continued)***

Client: So then Jack said he would take care of it, but he never did. You'd think he would do what he said, but no. So I had to take time off from work to go to Con Edison and pay the bill.

Therapist: Because Jack was so unreliable, you had to lose time from work.

Paraphrasing can help the therapist sort out what the client has been saying, which is particularly valuable when the client speaks for a long time or in a disorganized fashion.

A fifth technique is *withholding judgment.* The therapist refrains from giving an opinion about the client's remarks or behaviors. Clients often look to the therapist for advice, praise, approval, or rejection. The following is an example:

**CASE EXAMPLE *(Continued)***

Client: My mother says I dress too sexy, that's why I have so much trouble. It's none of her business. My clothes are okay, don't you think?

Therapist: What do you think?

Here the therapist is not only withholding judgment but is also encouraging the client to evaluate the situation herself. If the therapist had said, "Your clothes are okay," or "You dress nicely," or "Maybe your mother has a point there," the client might react to the comment instead of thinking out the problem on her own. The therapist is letting her know that she has to decide for herself.

All five of these techniques are derived from similar techniques used in object relations therapy. Like object relations therapy, client-centered therapy requires many sessions and is most practical in long-term treatment. Client-centered therapy, because it relies on clients' ability to direct themselves, seems inappropriate for persons with severe mental disabilities, who may not use words and may seem incapable of making even simple decisions. This issue is at the heart of the persistent debate over the use of the word *client* in occupational therapy practice and literature. Sharrott and Yerxa (47) argue that a client would be capable of choosing and securing occupational therapy services; in contrast, many of the persons served by occupational therapy are so disabled that they are incapable of acting in their own best interests and for that reason should be called patients. On the other hand, since the 1990s, persons with mental health problems have organized politically and prefer (when living in the community) to be called consumers.

Despite these concerns, although it is unusual for an occupational therapist to embrace the entirety of client-centered therapy, psychiatric occupational therapy practitioners continue to use client-centered techniques, which are effective for getting people with mental health problems to express themselves and for establishing a solid therapeutic relationship. They are often combined with other approaches, such as behavioral techniques, which may give faster results in changing a person's behavior (24).

Chapter 10, "Therapeutic Use of Self," describes and illustrates further how Rogers' techniques can be applied by the OTA.

## CONCEPTS SUMMARY

1. Each human being has the potential to direct his or her own growth and development.
2. Each person is free to choose his or her own course of action.
3. Mental health problems can occur when a person is not aware of his or her own feelings and of the available choices.
4. A person can become more aware of feelings and choices by exploring them in a relationship with a warm, empathic therapist who genuinely accepts himself or herself and the client.

## VOCABULARY REVIEW

**accurate empathy** Understanding the feelings and actions of another person, staying attuned to the person's thoughts and feelings. This is contrasted with sympathy, which includes a sense of *feeling* what the other feels.

**warmth** A sense conveyed by the therapist that the therapist feels concerned about the patient's well-being.

**genuineness** A sense conveyed by the therapist that the therapist is really the way he or she appears and is not just putting on an act for the patient's benefit.

**unconditional positive regard** A sense conveyed by the therapist that he or she accepts, likes, and respects the patient regardless of the patient's feelings or actions.

**nondirective behavior** A behavior of the therapist in which he or she refrains from giving an opinion on anything the patient says or does.

**open invitation to talk** An interviewing technique in which questions are worded to require a response longer than one or two words. This encourages the client to talk.

**minimal response** A brief verbal or nonverbal action of the therapist that gives the message that he or she is listening and wants the client to keep talking. Examples are nodding, saying "Go on," and leaning forward in the chair.

**reflection of feeling** The therapist's restatement of the *feeling* conveyed by the client's words or nonverbal expression.

**paraphrasing** The therapist's restatement of the *story* or narrative content conveyed by the client's words.

**withholding judgment** The therapist's deliberate abstinence from giving opinions on the client's behavior, feelings, or intention.

## NEUROSCIENCE THEORIES

*Neuroscience* refers to the entire body of information about the nervous system—how it is organized, what it looks like, and how it operates.

Use of neuroscience theories to plan treatment requires significant knowledge of the anatomy and physiology of the nervous system, content not covered in depth in occupational therapy assistant programs. However, a basic understanding of neuroscience theory is helpful to the occupational therapy assistant. Much of current medical practice in psychiatry is based on neuroscience; the physician may determine the diagnosis and choose medications based on brain imaging studies of the patient or on blood tests. And some occupational therapy practice models in mental health reflect a neuroscience foundation.

How much of our mental and emotional experience results from physical, biological, and chemical events in the brain? Freud himself explored this possibility during his earliest years in medicine, when he worked on the neuroanatomy of the medulla (58). Research since that time has demonstrated many associations between behavior and brain activity. The central concept of the neuroscience theories is that the phenomena we think of as mind and emotion are explained by biochemical and electrical activity in the brain.

Neuroscience theories are based on the assumption that normal human functioning requires a brain that is anatomically normal, with normal neurophysiology and brain chemicals in the proper proportions. Neuroscientists are finding that many kinds of mental illness are associated with variations from these normal conditions. This is particularly obvious in the case of schizophrenia and other severe and persistent mental disorders. Ventricular enlargement is consistently found in the brains of persons with schizophrenia, and abnormalities of brain anatomy and neurotransmitter mechanisms are suspected of contributing to the symptoms of the disease (3, 12, 20). Brain imaging techniques such as computed tomography (CT), positron emission tomography (PET), single-proton emission computed tomography (SPECT), and magnetic resonance imaging (MRI) provide views of deep brain structures in sufficient detail to show atrophy and reduced blood flow in the brains of persons with Alzheimer's disease (39, 62). The research evidence has been so plentiful and convincing that some leading research psychiatrists propose regrouping the major mental illnesses with other disorders of the central nervous system (e.g., multiple sclerosis, Parkinson disease)—in other words, redesignating these conditions as medical problems rather than problems of mental health (52). The National Alliance for the Mentally Ill (NAMI, now the National Alliance on Mental Illness) designated the 1990s as the decade of the brain, but research since then has been so active, productive, and promising that perhaps the 21st century will be the century of the brain. The next (the fifth) edition of the *Diagnostic and Statistical Manual of Mental Disorders* (*DSM-V*), will carry increased information derived from neuroscience research (45).

Because neuroscience assumes that mental illness is caused by a brain defect, logic tells us that treatment must be directed at the brain itself. Treatment of mental illness, according to the neuroscience model, involves changing the abnormal *somatic* (bodily) conditions through somatic intervention. These interventions include chemotherapy (drugs), psychosurgery, and electroconvulsive therapy (ECT). Despite their negative side effects, drugs have been useful in controlling psychotic and affective (mood) symptoms that might otherwise prevent people from participating in rehabilitation. Psychosurgery (stereotactic and laser surgery on the brain) has been used successfully to stop abnormal rage in persons with temporal lobe epilepsy. In addition, ECT (sometimes incorrectly called "shock treatment") is effective in reversing extreme suicidal depressions that fail to respond to drugs. All of these treatments were discovered serendipitously (by accident) and were used for years with little understanding of how they worked; one of the major contributions of recent neuroscience is to demonstrate some of the mechanisms behind them (33). More recently, psychiatrists have begun to stimulate brain centers using technology such as transcranial magnetic stimulation (TMS), vagus nerve stimulation (VNS), and deep brain stimulation (21, 38, 54).

Only physicians can prescribe drugs, surgery, and brain stimulation. The traditional role of occupational therapy in the neuroscience approach is to monitor the effects on functional performance of the somatic treatments prescribed by the physician. By observing how the person performs in activities, the OT or OTA can collect information to help the doctor determine or verify the diagnosis and later decide whether the treatment is working and whether it should be increased, decreased, or modified. Occupational therapy personnel also help patients adjust their approach to activities to cope with the side effects of drugs and ECT (48). This topic is discussed in Chapter 8.

Among the exciting new hypotheses in neuroscience are those relating to *neuroimmunomodulation* (28) and *psychoneuroimmunology* (PNI) (13, 49). Research indicates an interaction between the central nervous system and the immune system; it is this interaction that regulates the immune response of the body. Depression as a diagnosis often occurs with diagnosed medical illnesses such as cardiovascular disease (49). Farber (28) suggests that occupational therapy may strengthen the immune response by reducing helplessness and hopelessness and helping the person establish positive attitudes. Stress management training is one aspect of this.

Three occupational therapy treatment approaches have ties to neuroscience theory. One is Lorna-Jean King's sensory integration approach to the treatment of schizophrenia. King (36) showed that games and postural exercises can bring about changes in the sensorimotor functioning of persons with certain types of chronic schizophrenia. She argued that these activities stimulate the part of the central nervous system that processes and organizes sensory information.

A second occupational therapy approach related to neuroscience was developed by Allen (1), who proposed that the problems psychiatric patients have functioning in daily life originate in physical and chemical abnormalities of the brain. She argued that the role of occupational therapy should be to define the person's functional level very precisely and to modify the environment to help the person function as well as possible. She believes that occupational therapy cannot change the patient's level of function and should instead work on adapting the environment to the disability.

More recently, Brown and co-workers (15, 16), building on the work of Dunn and Westman (23), developed an evaluation of sensory processing for adults and adolescents. She offers strategies for modifying the environment and one's behavior to compensate for sensory differences. Two key notions for this approach are *neurological threshold* and *behavioral response.* The neurological threshold may be high or low and is a measure of how easily a person registers sensation from the environment. The person with a low threshold notices sensations very easily, and someone with a high threshold does not notice sensations that are very obvious to almost everyone else.

The behavioral response is the kind of action taken in regard to sensory information. For example, one person may be very sensitive to odors (low threshold) and another quite insensitive (high threshold). The behavioral response for the person with low threshold may take the form of avoiding department store perfume and cosmetic counters. The person with high threshold may not be aware of his or her own bodily odors or of the need to bathe regularly, with a behavioral response of low registration, or not noticing unpleasant odors. Although olfactory sensation (smell) is the example here, Brown also addresses other sensory systems (vision, taste, hearing, touch).

Both King's and Allen's approaches are discussed further in Chapter 3. The reader who is interested in Brown's ideas is encouraged to consult the references at the end of the chapter.

## CONCEPTS SUMMARY

1. All mental processes, including behavior and emotion, originate in biochemical and electrical activity in the brain.
2. Abnormal behavior and abnormal emotional states (mental illness) are caused by defects either in the anatomy or in the level of chemicals in the brain.
3. Abnormal mental conditions can be controlled by changing either the anatomy or the chemical and electrical activity of the brain. Treatments include surgery, drugs, and ECT.

## VOCABULARY REVIEW

**neurotransmitter** A chemical that transmits nerve impulses from one neuron to another within the central nervous system. Examples are serotonin, dopamine, norepinephrine, and acetylcholine.

**organic** Referring to the structure (anatomy) of the brain, the organ of mind and emotion.

**electroconvulsive therapy (ECT)** A treatment in which an electrical current applied to the brain causes a brief seizure. ECT is most often used to treat severe depression.

**chemotherapy** A treatment in which chemical substances (drugs) are introduced into the body in an effort to cure a disease or control its symptoms.

**psychosurgery** Surgery on the brain in which nerve fibers are cut or destroyed to control abnormal behavior or mood disturbances.

**neuroimmunomodulation** The proposed interactive regulation of immune responses through the combined actions of the neurological, endocrine, and immune systems.

**psychoneuroimmunology** The study of the interaction of the immune system and the central nervous system.

**neurological threshold** The degree to which the person's nervous system registers sensation from the environment.

**behavioral response** Action taken by a person in reaction to sensory information.

## PSYCHIATRIC REHABILITATION

Psychiatric rehabilitation (PsyR) is an approach documented by William Anthony and others (4–6) and Farkas and others (29) at the Sargent College of Allied Health Professions, Boston University. It combines principles and concepts from the fields of physical rehabilitation, client-centered therapy, behavioral psychology, and psychosocial rehabilitation (5, 43). Unlike the other models described in this chapter, PsyR is *eclectic* (drawing on many sources for techniques). As such, it is *atheoretical* (without theory), although it uses techniques associated with several theories. It is not a *treatment theory* and does not attempt to explain why or how mental illness occurs. Rather, it is a *rehabilitation approach* that focuses on how best to help the person with mental illness function optimally in his or her life situation.

PsyR is uncannily similar to occupational therapy in that it is oriented to the present and future, focuses on the development of skills and resources, and uses activities and environmental adaptations as a base for intervention. For decades, occupational therapists had an approach that was highly effective but also undocumented and unpublished; it is not surprising that during the 1970s and 1980s other mental health professionals noticed this and took the opportunity to publish and to develop it further. Pratt and colleagues (43) note that many PsyR techniques have been stolen (from other people), adopted, and improved on. Ironically, a recent position paper from the American Occupational Therapy Association states: "Occupational therapists and occupational therapy assistants working with [occupationally impaired] individuals use psychiatric rehabilitation principles and techniques to help them set and achieve personally meaningful occupational goals" (2, p. 670).

PsyR is included in this text because it has become a popular model for design of programs, because it has a developing research base, and because the occupational therapy practitioner is quite likely to encounter the model in settings that serve persons with mental health problems. Some states in the United States have adopted PsyR as the model for mental health service delivery statewide (4).

Because PsyR is not allied with or based on any theory, we cannot examine its theoretical underpinnings so will instead look at goals, values, and guiding principles (43). Instead of addressing how the clients came to be ill, PsyR focuses on aiding them in achieving a better quality of life, in recovering and integrating themselves in their communities. The *goals* are recovery, community integration, and quality of life (43). The *values* of PsyR are strongly oriented toward client self-direction (self-determination, dignity, and hope). The *guiding principles* include the following:

- Client-centered, individual approach
- Services that emphasize normal functioning in the community
- Focus on the strengths of the client
- Assessment based on the clients' situations
- Coordination of services accessible to clients
- Focus on work
- Focus on skills development
- Environmental modifications and supports
- Family involvement
- Research and outcome orientation

Competencies are achieved by two methods: developing the client's skills and/or improving environmental supports and resources. Many intervention techniques, including psychotropic medication, are considered compatible with this approach; but techniques must be individualized. The client is expected to participate actively in his or her own rehabilitation, with appropriate support from the mental health system and the environment. Because work is a significant organizing theme of adult life, the client's participation and satisfaction in a vocational role are targeted for major intervention.

PsyR is conducted in a three-stage process of *rehabilitation diagnosis, rehabilitation planning,* and *rehabilitation intervention.* The rehabilitation diagnosis is a statement of the environment in which the client—say, Phil—would like to function and the resources and skills he will need for this environment. The rehabilitation diagnosis disregards the symptoms and pathology of disease and thus differs from a medical or psychiatric diagnosis. It is situation specific and individualized.

In the rehabilitation diagnosis stage, on first meeting the client, the psychiatric rehabilitation practitioner sets the stage for collaboration by explaining to the client how he or she can participate in evaluation and planning. The first step in a PsyR diagnosis is setting the *overall rehabilitation goal* (ORG), a statement of the environment and role in which the client would like to live, work, study, and so on. An example is, "Phil would like to live at Livingston Arms, a supported residence." The therapist and the client jointly determine the ORG.

Once the ORG is chosen, the focus shifts to evaluating the client's functional skills. The question to be answered in this phase is, Which of the skills needed in this environment can the client perform and which can he not perform? Practitioner and client work together to list specific skills that correspond to the behavioral requirements of the chosen role and environment. One example might be speaking in turn at community meetings. Client and practitioner can then assess

Phil's skill level and evaluate the level needed in the supportive living environment. If Phil has the needed level of skill, this is listed as a strength. If he lacks it or does not perform it with sufficient frequency or accuracy, it is listed as a deficit.

Because community supports are needed for successful functioning in any environment, a resource assessment is also performed. Again, client and practitioner together list the elements needed for the client to function successfully in the chosen environment. These might include things (spending money, clothing, medication), people (sponsor, buddy, home group), and activities (day treatment, evening leisure program). Again, resources that are available at the required level are listed as strengths and those that are less than adequate are listed as deficits. Thus the rehabilitation diagnosis yields a list of skill strengths and deficits and resource strengths and deficits in relation to an overall rehabilitation goal.

The next stage is the formulation of the rehabilitation plan. The typical diagnosis yields many deficit areas; here the practitioner and client must determine which ones are to be the priorities for intervention. They might select, for example, "Phil will say what he thinks in community meeting" and "Phil will wait until his turn to speak at community meetings." Practitioner and client then discuss and select appropriate interventions, such as direct skills teaching.

The third stage, rehabilitation intervention, is the enactment of the plan. Here the client may, for example, attend a class or individual session to learn a new skill and do homework or other assignments to practice or reinforce the skill. The client may enter a new environment and practice using a skill that he or she understands but does not consistently use. The practitioner works on resource development with the client in this stage, which may mean helping the client find an exercise class in the community, secure spending money from parents, or obtain food stamps.

One of the most important concepts of PsyR is that evaluation and intervention make sense only in relation to the environment in which the client is functioning or intends to be functioning. A client may be "lacking in social skills," but the only social skills that matter are those that are relevant to the particular environment in which he or she interacts. Defining the environment establishes a context in which further evaluation of the client's skills and resources makes sense.

The two main areas of intervention in PsyR are *(a)* developing the client's functional skills and *(b)* modifying the environment to maximize functional use of skills (4). These interventions occur

**BOX 2-1**

**SIX DIMENSIONS OF REHABILITATION READINESS**

The consumer will . . .

1. Perceive a need for rehabilitation
2. View change as desirable
3. Be open to establishing relationships
4. Have sufficient self-understanding
5. Be aware of and able to interact meaningfully with the environment
6. Have significant others who support his or her participation in rehabilitation

Adapted with permission from Cohen MR, Anthony WA, Farkas MD. Assessing and developing readiness for psychiatric rehabilitation. Psychiatr Serv 1997;48:644–646.

after assessment and are targeted at moving the client toward the established ORG. PsyR practitioners also assess the client's *rehabilitation readiness*, defined as "a reflection of consumers' interest in rehabilitation and their self-confidence, not of their capacity to complete a rehabilitation program" (19). The six dimensions of rehabilitation readiness are shown in Box 2-1.

Although PsyR is atheoretical, it does make certain identifiable assumptions. The first is *functioning adequately in the environment of one's choice is possible for everyone.* By analogy with physical rehabilitation, the bilateral upper extremity (BUE) amputee can live in the community, can hold a job, and can enjoy leisure activities.

The second is *to function successfully one must possess the needed skills and resources.* Again, by analogy with physical rehabilitation, to dress oneself, the BUE amputee must learn a new motor pattern (skill) and may need certain adaptive equipment and the assistance of another person (resources) to don the prostheses and the harness that supports them. To live in a supported living situation, the person with a psychiatric disability may have to learn when and how to care for his or her clothing (skill); will need money to purchase laundry products, services, and dry-cleaning; and may need support and reminders from a case manager (resources).

The third is *skills that are lacking can be developed through training, and skills that are present but that are weak can be strengthened through practice.* For skills to make sense, they should be learned and practiced in the environment in which they will be used or one as similar to it as possible. For example, to learn to speak in turn in a group meeting, the client should attend such meetings and practice the skill while there.

The fourth is *environmental supports and resources enable and facilitate successful functioning.* Just as grab bars and a tub-transfer seat make bathing easier for a person with physical weakness and limited standing tolerance, so too can environmental supports make things easier for the person with a psychiatric disability. For example, the support of a case manager can make it easier for the client to avoid relapse and rehospitalization by enabling the client to obtain a prescription for medication or by assisting the client to join a self-help group. In addition to providing supports, the case manager can help the client learn to use them. The client who can recognize that he or she is at risk for a relapse and who knows how to obtain medication or to reach out to a support network is better able to function in the community.

The fifth assumption is *belief in and hope for the future facilitate rehabilitation outcomes.* In other words, a sense of motivation and personal investment are necessary; the client must have a positive expectation that he or she can indeed function.

As stated previously, occupational therapy has a natural fit with PsyR, which is a multidisciplinary approach. Regardless of professional credentials or certification, all practitioners provide similar services. Anthony and colleagues (4) indicate, however, that an activities-oriented background is desirable. As a PsyR practitioner, the OTA would work with the client to develop the rehabilitation diagnosis and rehabilitation plan. Occupational therapy assistants may provide many different rehabilitation interventions, including skills instruction and training, general programming, and development and adaptation of environment supports.

## CONCEPTS SUMMARY

1. Functioning adequately in the environment of one's choice is possible for everyone.
2. To function successfully one must possess both the skills and the resources needed to do so. The selection of skills and resources is highly individual, depending on the person and the immediate context. Persons with chronic psychiatric disorders often lack the necessary skills and resources for functioning in their chosen environments.

3. Skills that are lacking can be developed through training. Skills that are present but weak can be strengthened through practice. Both practice and training make sense only in the environment of choice.
4. Environmental supports and resources enable and facilitate successful functioning. Persons with psychiatric illness can function better when such supports are available and they know how to use them.
5. Belief in and hope for the future facilitate rehabilitation outcomes.

## VOCABULARY REVIEW

**overall rehabilitation goal (ORG)** An agreement between the client and practitioner about the environment and roles the client would like to occupy (where the client intends to live, learn, or work).

**rehabilitation diagnosis** A process to identify the client's ORG. The ORG becomes the basis for evaluating the client's skills (functional assessment), resource strengths, and deficits (resource assessment), in relation to this goal.

**rehabilitation planning** A process that identifies and prescribes high-priority skill and resource goals, the interventions for achieving them, and the personnel responsible.

**rehabilitation intervention** Processes for developing client skills and environmental resources specified in the client's rehabilitation plan. This may include direct skills teaching, skill refinement and practice, coordination and linking of existing resources, and development of new resources.

**rehabilitation readiness** "a reflection of consumers' interest in rehabilitation and their self-confidence, not of their capacity to complete a rehabilitation program" (19).

## SUMMARY

Seven models have been presented in this chapter. Six are based on theory: object relations, developmental, behavioral, cognitive-behavioral, client-centered, and neuroscience. The seventh model, psychiatric rehabilitation, is atheoretical, based on established traditions of intervention from occupational therapy and other rehabilitation professions. The student and OTA may expect to encounter most of these models in some form in mental health settings. The reader is encouraged to observe other occupational therapy practitioners and other mental health professionals, to study their techniques and approaches, and to discuss with them the theories and models they use. This will help clarify the differences among the different models. Comparative research data and outcome studies provide the reader with an appreciation for which approaches are most likely to be effective with particular clients.

Now, consider again the scenario from the beginning of the chapter. How would you respond to the girl in the cooking group? Using each of the seven models in turn, determine what response each model would suggest. What response would be the most successful in your view? Or do you feel that none is quite right? Of course, none of these models, except psychiatric rehabilitation, is particularly relevant to occupational therapy. Chapter 3 explores models developed by occupational therapists specifically for occupational therapy.

## REVIEW QUESTIONS AND ACTIVITIES

1. Why are theories used in practice? Of what value are they?
2. Read the quote from Paula Underwood at the beginning of the chapter. Why do you think this quote was chosen? What does it have to do with theories of mental health?
3. Briefly describe each of the following theories or models of practice and discuss how they differ from each other: object relations, developmental, behavioral, cognitive-behavioral, client-centered, neuroscience, psychiatric rehabilitation
4. Review the vocabulary from each section of the chapter. Test yourself on your ability to write definitions for the terms.
5. Review the concepts for each theory. Then, for each theory, write a brief paragraph explaining the major concepts.
6. Using the material from this chapter, write 10 multiple-choice questions, each with four possible answers. Make the questions reasonably difficult, so that someone who has not read and studied the chapter would not be able to select the correct answer. Share your questions with your instructor and your classmates. Some ideas for questions are: identify techniques or concepts that match a model; given a concise case description, choose the response that matches a particular model; select term that matches a definition given.
7. Choose two theories that seem different from each other. Write an essay contrasting them.
8. Select one of the case vignettes that illustrate theories within the chapter and describe how one would approach the case using a *different* theory or model.

## REFERENCES


1. Allen CK. Occupational Therapy for Psychiatric Disorders: Measurement and Management of Cognitive Disabilities. Boston: Little, Brown, 1985.
2. American Occupational Therapy Association. Psychosocial aspects of occupational therapy. Am J Occup Ther 2004;58:669–672.
3. Andreason NC. Cognitive dysmetria as an integrative theory of schizophrenia: A dysfunction in cortical-subcortical-cerebellar circuitry? Schizophr Bull 1998;24:203–218.
4. Anthony W. Explaining psychiatric rehabilitation by analogy to physical rehabilitation. Psychosoc Rehab J 1982; 5(1):61–65.
5. Anthony W, Cohen M, Farkas M. Psychiatric Rehabilitation. Boston: Center for Psychiatric Rehabilitation, Boston University, 1990.
6. Anthony W, Cohen M, Farkas M. A psychiatric rehabilitation treatment program: Can I recognize one if I see one? Commun Ment Health J 1982;18(2):83–96.
7. Babiss F. An ethnographic study of mental health treatment and outcomes: Doing what works. Occup Ther Ment Health 2002;18(3–4):1–146.
8. Bandura A. Behavioral modifications through modeling procedures In: Krasner L, Ullmann LP, eds. Research in Behavior Modification: New Developments and Implications. New York: Holt, Rinehart & Winston, 1965.
9. Beck AT. Cognitive Therapy and the Emotional Disorders. New York: Meridian, 1976.
10. Beck AT. Love Is Never Enough. New York: Harper & Row, 1988.
11. Beck AT, Rush JA, Shaw BF, Emery G. Cognitive Therapy of Depression. New York: Guilford, 1979.
12. Benes FM. Model generation and testing to probe neural circuitry in the cingulate cortex of postmortem schizophrenic brain. Schizophr Bull 1998;24:219–230.
13. Black PH. Psychoneuroimmunology: Brain and immunity. Scientific American, Nov–Dec 1995:16–25.
14. Brady JP. Social skills training for psychiatric patients. 1: Concepts, methods, and clinical results. Occup Ther Ment Health 1984;4(4):51–68.
15. Brown C. What is the best environment for me? A sensory processing perspective. Occup Ther Ment Health 2001;17(3–4):115–125.
16. Brown C, Tollefson N, Dunn W, et al. The adult sensory profile: Measuring patterns of sensory processing. Am J Occup Ther 2001;55:75–82.
17. Cermak S, Stein F, Abelson C. Hyperactive children and an activity group therapy model. Am J Occup Ther 1973;27:311–315.
18. Client-centered therapy. Harv Ment Health Lett 2006;22(7):1–3.
19. Cohen MR, Antony WA, Farkas MD. Assessing and developing readiness for psychiatric rehabilitation. Psychiatr Serv 1997;48:644–646.
20. Csernansky JG, Grace AA. New models of the pathophysiology of schizophrenia. Schizophr Bull 1998;24:185–188.
21. Deep brain stimulation. Harv Ment Health Lett 2006; 22(10):3–4.
22. Dialectical behavior therapy. Harv Ment Health Lett 2002;19(2):1–3.
23. Dunn W, Westman K. The sensory profile: The performance of a national sample of children without disabilities. Am J Occup Ther 1997;51:25–34.
24. Dunning RE. The occupational therapist as counselor. Am J Occup Ther 1973;27:473–476.
25. Early MB. T.A.R. Introductory Course Workbook. Occupational Therapy: Psychosocial Dysfunction. Long Island City, NY: LaGuardia Community College, 1981.
26. Eklund M. Applying object relations theory to psychosocial occupational therapy: Empirical and theoretical considerations. Occ Ther Ment Health 2000;15(1):1–26.
27. Ellis A. Reason and Emotion in Psychotherapy. New York: Birch Lane, 1994.
28. Farber SD. Neuroscience and occupational therapy: Vital connections [1989 Eleanor Clarke Slagle Lecture]. Am J Occup Ther 1989;43:637–646.
29. Farkas MD, Cohen MR, Nemec PB. Psychiatric rehabilitation programs: Putting concepts into practice? Commun Ment Health J 1988;24(1):7–22.
30. Fidler G, Fidler J. Occupational Therapy: A Communication Process in Psychiatry. New York: Macmillan, 1963.
31. Fidler GS, Velde BP. Activities: Reality and Symbol. Thorofare, NJ: Slack, 1999.
32. Hays JS, Larson K. Interacting with Patients. New York: Macmillan, 1963.
33. Hedaya RJ. Understanding Biological Psychiatry. New York: Norton, 1995.
34. Johnston MT. Occupational therapists and the teaching of cognitive-behavioral skills. Occup Ther Ment Health 1987;7(3):69–81.
35. Kielhofner G. Conceptual foundations of occupational therapy. Philadelphia: Davis, 1992.
36. King L-J. A sensory-integrative approach to schizophrenia. Am J Occup Ther 1974;28:529–536.
37. Linehan M. The cognitive-behavioral treatment of borderline personality disorder. New York: Guilford Press, 1993.
38. Magnetic stimulation of the brain: An update. Harv Ment Health Lett 2005;22(2):4–6.
39. McNeil C. Alzheimer's Disease: Unraveling the Mystery. Washington, DC: National Institutes of Health, 1995.
40. Mosey AC. Activities Therapy. New York: Raven, 1973.
41. Norman CW. Behavior modification: A perspective. Am J Occup Ther 1976;30:491–497.

42. Phillips ME, Bruehl S, Harden RN. Work-related post traumatic stress disorder: Use of exposure therapy in work simulation activities. Am J Occup Ther 1997;51:696–700.
43. Pratt CW, Gill KJ, Barrett NM, Roberts MM. Psychiatric Rehabilitation. 2nd ed. Burlington, MA: Elsevier Academic, 2007.
44. Rogers C. On Becoming a Person: A Therapist's View of Psychotherapy. Boston: Houghton Mifflin, 1961.
45. Rosenbaum JF, Pollock R. DSM V—Plans and Perspectives. Available at: www.medscape.com/viewarticle/436403. Accessed November 2006.
46. Sieg KW. Applying the behavioral model to the occupational therapy model. Am J Occup Ther 1974;28:421–428.
47. Sharrott GW, Yerxa EJ. The Issue Is: Promises to keep: Implications of the referent "patient" versus "client" for those served by occupational therapy. Am J Occup Ther 1985;39:401–405.
48. Smith DA. Effects of psychotropic drugs on the occupational therapy process. Am Occup Ther Assoc Ment Health Special Sect Q Newslett 1981;4(1):1–3.
49. Spollen JJ, Gutman DA. The interaction of depression and medical illness. Available at: www.medscape.com/viewarticle/457165. Accessed Nov 2006.
50. Taylor E. Anger intervention. Am J Occup Ther 1988;42:147–155.
51. Toal-Sullivan D, Henderson PR. Client-oriented role evaluation (CORE): The development of a clinical rehabilitation instrument to assess role change associated with disability. Am J Occup Ther 2004;58:211–220.
52. Torrey EF. Out of the Shadows. New York: Wiley, 1997.
53. Underwood P. Three Strands in the Braid: A Guide for Enablers of Learning. San Anselmo, CA: Tribe of Two, 1991.
54. Vagus nerve stimulation. Harv Ment Health Lett 2002;19(6):3–4.
55. Watling R, Schwartz IS. Understanding and implementing positive reinforcement as an intervention strategy for children with disabilities. Am J Occup Ther 2004;58:113–116.
56. Weber NJ. Chaining strategies for teaching sequenced motor tasks to mentally retarded adults. Am J Occup Ther 1978;32:385–389.
57. Wehman P, Marchant J. Improving the free play skills of severely retarded children. Am J Occup Ther 1978;32: 100–104.
58. Winson J. Brain and Psyche. Garden City, NY: Anchor Doubleday, 1985.
59. Wright JH, Beck AT. Cognitive therapy. In: Hales RE, Yudofsky SE, Talbott JA, eds. American Psychiatric Press Textbook of Psychiatry. 2nd ed. Washington: APA, 1995.
60. Yakobina S, Yakobina S, Tallant BK. I came, I thought, I conquered: Cognitive behaviour approach applied in occupational therapy for the treatment of depressed (dysthymic) females. Occup Ther Ment Health 1997;13(4): 59–73.
61. Zemke R, Gratz RR. The role of theory: Erikson and occupational therapy. Occup Ther Ment Health 1982;2(3): 45–64.
62. Zubenko GZ. Molecular neurobiology of Alzheimer's disease (syndrome?). Harv Rev Psychiatry 1997;5:177–213.

## SUGGESTED READINGS

Cognitive behavioral therapy for schizophrenia. Harv Ment Health Lett 2003;20(4):5–6.

Dialectical behavior therapy. Harvd Ment Health Lett 2002;19(2):1–3.

Giroux Bruce MA, Borg B. Psychosocial Frames of Reference Core for Occupation-Based Practice. 3rd ed. Thorofare, NJ: Slack, 2002.

Pratt CW, Gill KJ, Barrett NM, Roberts MM. Psychiatric Rehabilitation. 2nd ed. Burlington, MA: Elsevier Academic, 2007.

Watling R, Schwartz IS. Understanding and implementing positive reinforcement as an intervention strategy for children with disabilities. Am J Occup Ther 2004;58:113–116.

CHAPTER 3

# Some Practice Models for Occupational Therapy in Mental Health

***There are no whole truths; all truths are half truths. It is trying to treat them as whole truths that plays the devil.***

ALFRED NORTH WHITEHEAD (68)

## CHAPTER OBJECTIVES

After studying this chapter, the reader will be able to:

1. Name and describe six practice models used in psychosocial occupational therapy.
2. Identify medical or psychological theories or models that are compatible with each occupational therapy practice model.
3. Recognize concepts associated with each model.
4. Define terms associated with each model.
5. Discuss, in general terms, which practice model might best address the needs of a particular client and situation.

Chapter 2 presented some of the many theories of how the mind works. Each theory gives us one way of looking at mental health and mental illness—one way to organize, explain, predict, and intervene in behavior. We can think of theories as being similar to eyeglasses with a variety of colored lenses. The world looks different through each color, and we respond differently to what we see when we wear them. Theories are like this; when we look at a client or patient through the lens of a particular theory, we pay attention to the things that that theory says are important and we ignore everything else, just as red lenses make green things prominent and make red things fade away. It can be fascinating to try on these different points of view, but we must ultimately decide which one gives us the most useful view of the person and his or her problems and how to address them through occupational therapy. As service providers, we must consider which one is most consistent with what we know of the individual and his or her goals and problems and which one is best supported by research. At the same time, we must appreciate that no one theory is sufficient, that each forces us to ignore some aspects that might be important.

Because performance of occupation is the chief concern of occupational therapy, any theory useful to occupational therapy practitioners must explain how people's occupation affects their mental health and how their mental health affects their occupation. None of the theories discussed in Chapter 2 does a very good job of this. Object relations theory focuses on the symbolic content of activities as a mirror of unconscious processes. Sharrott (63) and others have criticized this approach for disregarding the person's conscious motivation to choose and participate in the activities of human life. Also, this approach works best with those who have good insight and good verbal skills—only a small fraction of the clients seen in psychiatric occupational therapy.[1] Finally, object relations and psychoanalytic theory have been criticized for being overly subjective (not providing observable results), sexist, and unproved through research (9, 11, 16).

As an occupational therapy approach, client-centered therapy has been criticized for being a talking therapy, not a doing therapy and for lacking the activity core on which occupational therapy is based. Similar to and derived from psychoanalytic therapy, client-centered therapy also works best with those who are articulate and whose cognitive functions are not greatly disturbed. Thus it can be applied effectively to only a few of the clients seen in occupational therapy mental health practice (9, 16).

Like client-centered therapy, developmental theories, such as Erikson's, used in mental health are derived from psychoanalytic foundations. They emphasize social and sexual development. Because some of these theories address the development of the motivation, skills, habits, and attitudes that enable full participation in occupation and activity, occupational therapy practitioners have used developmental concepts in their practice. Later in this chapter, we look at this more closely, with Mosey's model for development of adaptive skills.

Although the behavioral approach has been used in occupational therapy with the developmentally disabled and cognitively impaired, it focuses on learning as a consequence of external rewards. In this, behaviorism conflicts with one of the central values of occupational therapy—the internal reward implicit in the intrinsic motivation for activity. Behaviorism has also been criticized for being superficial and for failing to establish permanent changes in behavior (9, 11). Nonetheless, many of the techniques used in behavioral approaches (role modeling, shaping, chaining) have been applied successfully by occupational therapists (OTs) and occupational therapy assistants (OTAs). We consider these later in the chapter, when we look at social skills training and Mosey's role acquisition

[1].For further discussion of this point, see Bruce MAG, Borg B. Frames of Reference in Psychosocial Occupational Therapy. Thorofare, NJ: Slack, 1987:79.

model, which include concepts and techniques aligned with behavioral and cognitive-behavioral theory.

Neuroscience theories focus on brain anatomy and chemistry. There is much to be learned about the effects of the brain's structure and metabolism on participation and performance of human activity. Because OTs and OTAs are not trained to perform surgery or prescribe drugs, our contribution to this theory is our skill in observing and describing the patient's functional behavior as it may be affected by neurosurgical or neurochemical interventions. Another aspect of neuroscience theory proposed by occupational therapy leaders since the time of Adolph Meyer is that participation in activity may affect brain metabolism, changing the patient's behavior and emotion. We look at both of these aspects later in this chapter, with Allen's theory of cognitive disabilities and King's application of sensory integration with chronic schizophrenics.

Although none of the theories considered in Chapter 2 focuses on the relationship of activity to mental health, some of them have been adapted by occupational therapy practitioners for use in psychiatry. (As we know, the psychiatric rehabilitation model, which does not have a specific theory base, closely resembles traditional occupational therapy.) This chapter describes six occupational therapy practice models that have been used successfully with persons with psychiatric disorders. These practice models are

- The *development of adaptive skills* (also called recapitulation of ontogenesis), based on developmental concepts
- *Role acquisition,* based on developmental and behavioral concepts used together with *social skills training*, which is based primarily on behavioral concepts
- *Psychoeducation,* based on educational principles and techniques
- *Sensory integration,* based on neuroscience foundations
- *Cognitive disabilities*, also based on neuroscience foundations
- *The model of human occupation*, based on occupational behavior theory

Each of these models uses occupation or activity as a treatment medium, and each considers functional performance in daily life activities to be important to mental health. However, all of these models have features that limit their application to only some of the clients seen in mental health settings.

We call these practice models rather than theories because they are ways to organize our thinking about problems in clinical practice, just as a cardboard or plastic model helps architects organize their thoughts about the design of a physical space. As OTAs, you will need to know the evaluation (while not responsible for evaluation, the OTA is often asked to administer assessments) and treatment techniques, or what to do with the client under each practice model. A brief discussion of treatment principles and a case example is given for each model. Because the primary role of the OTA in psychiatry is to carry out treatment, detailed description of clinical techniques will follow in Chapters 10 through 23. Although the technical aspects of treatment are most important to the OTA, I hope that you will also appreciate the power of each practice model as a lens giving a unique view of the patient.

## DEVELOPMENT OF ADAPTIVE SKILLS

The *development of adaptive skills* model, which was conceived by Anne Cronin Mosey (45, 46), and is also called recapitulation of ontogenesis, means the stage-by-stage repeating of development. Mosey (45) identifies six areas of adaptive skills and lists stages of development within each skill. The skills are as follows:[2]

[2] These skills are paraphrased from Mosey (46). Mosey's earlier work included a seventh skill, drive-object skill. For a discussion of this skill see Mosey AC. Three Frames of Reference for Mental Health. Thorofare, NJ: Slack, 1970.

- *Sensory integration skill.* The ability to receive, select, combine, and use information from the balance (vestibular), touch (tactile), and position (proprioceptive) senses to perform functional activities
- *Cognitive skill.* The ability to perceive, represent, and organize sensory information for thinking and problem solving
- *Dyadic interaction skill.* The ability to participate in a variety of relationships involving one other person
- *Group interaction skill.* The ability to participate successfully in a variety of groups; generally this means being able to act as a productive member of the group
- *Self-identity skill.* The ability to recognize one's own assets and limitations and to perceive the self as worthwhile, self-directed, consistent, and reliable
- *Sexual identity skill.* The ability to accept one's sexual nature as natural and pleasurable and to participate in a relatively long-term sexual relationship that considers the needs of both partners

Each of these skills is acquired in a series of stages that follows a developmental sequence. In normal development and in therapy, stages are encountered and mastered in order, and no stage can be skipped.

Table 3-1 gives the breakdown of stages for Mosey's developmental skills. Mosey gives much detail on cognitive skills. However, her terms and descriptions differ from those in the American Occupational Therapy Association's (AOTA's) *Occupational Therapy Practice Framework* (OTPF) (6) and for this reason are likely to be unfamiliar to technical-level students. A key to some terms used by Mosey is provided in Table 3-1.

According to Mosey, development of adaptive skills is a suitable practice model for clients who have not mastered all of the stages of development appropriate for their chronological age. Mosey specifically states, however, that this model does not directly address performance in occupation. The focus is instead on the general skills and behaviors needed to negotiate one's environment successfully (45); these skills in turn support performance in occupation. The aim of this model is to help the person master, step by step, occupation-supporting skills not yet acquired. Four basic concepts guide the use of this model:[3]

1. *The therapist must provide an environment that facilitates growth.* The details and features of the environment depend on the particular subskill. For example, if the subskill of perceiving the self as self-directed is the focus, the clients must be given freedom to make their own decisions and to explore a variety of options. This is best practiced outside the treatment setting, where the options of real life can be found in ample supply. A simulated experience, such as an arts and crafts group, is less likely to develop this skill, regardless of the variety of crafts available.
2. *The subskills are mastered in order.* This follows from item 1; unless clients have already come to recognize and appreciate their assets and limitations, they have great difficulty making choices in an unstructured environment. One cannot begin to attempt to develop a sense of self-direction until one understands one's own capacities and limitations.
3. *Subskills from different areas may be addressed at the same time, provided they are normally acquired at the same chronological age.* Thus the person needing to develop a sense of his or her own assets and limitations might also work on cooperative group skills but not as easily on mature group skills, which depend on learning both self-assessment and cooperative skills.
4. *The patient's intrinsic motivation or desire for mastery of the subskills must be engaged.* Mosey cautions therapists to be exquisitely sensitive to evidence of the client's motivation or lack thereof. For example, anxiety and frustration may suggest that the environment and activities

[3] Mosey lists these as three concepts, combining the second and third into one.

## TABLE 3-1 STAGES IN DEVELOPMENT OF SELECTED ADAPTIVE SKILLS

| ADAPTIVE SKILL | AGE OF MASTERY |
|---|---|
| **Sensory integration** | |
| 1. Ability to integrate tactile subsystems | 0–3 months |
| 2. Ability to integrate primitive postural reflexes | 3–9 months |
| 3. Maturation of righting and equilibrium reactions | 9–12 months |
| 4. Ability to integrate two sides of body, be aware of body parts and their relationship, and plan gross motor movements | 1–2 years |
| 5. Ability to plan fine motor movements | 2–3 years |
| **Cognition** | |
| 1. Ability to use inherent behavioral patterns for environmental interaction | 0–1 months |
| 2. Ability to interrelate visual, manual, auditory, and oral responses | 1–4 months |
| 3. Ability to attend to the environmental consequence of actions with interest, to represent objects in an exoceptual manner, to experience objects, to act on basis of egocentric causality, and to seriate events in which self is involved | 4–9 months |
| 4. Ability to establish a goal and carry out means, to recognize independent existence of objects, to interpret signs, to imitate new behavior, to apprehend influence of space, to perceive other objects as partially causal | 9–12 months |
| 5. Ability to use trial-and-error problem solving, to use tools, to perceive variation in spatial positions, to seriate events in which self is not involved, and to perceive causality of other objects | 12–18 months |
| 6. Ability to represent objects in an image manner, to make believe, to infer a cause given its effect, to act on the basis of combined spatial relations, to attribute omnipotence to others, and to perceive objects as permanent in time and space | 18 months–2 yr |
| 7. Ability to represent objects in a endoceptual manner, to differentiate between thought and action, and to recognize the need for causal sources | 2–5 years |
| 8. Ability to represent objects in a denotative manner, to perceive viewpoint of others, and to decenter | 6–7 years |
| 9. Ability to represent objects in a connotative manner, to use formal logic, and to work in realm of hypothetical | 11–13 years |
| **Dyadic interaction** | |
| 1. Ability to enter into trusting familial relationships | 8–10 months |
| 2. Ability to enter into association relationships | 3–5 years |
| 3. Ability to interact in an authority relationship | 5–7 years |
| 4. Ability to interact in a chum relationship | 10–14 years |
| 5. Ability to enter into a peer, authority relationship | 15–17 years |
| 6. Ability to enter into an intimate relationship | 18–25 years |
| 7. Ability to engage in a nurturing relationship | 20–30 years |
| **Group interaction** | |
| 1. Ability to participate in a parallel group | 18–24 months |
| 2. Ability to participate in a project group | 2–4 years |

**TABLE 3-1 STAGES IN DEVELOPMENT OF SELECTED ADAPTIVE SKILLS *(Continued)***

| ADAPTIVE SKILL | AGE OF MASTERY |
|---|---|
| 3. Ability to participate in an egocentric-cooperative group | 5–7 years |
| 4. Ability to participate in a cooperative group | 9–12 years |
| 5. Ability to participate in a mature group | 15–18 years |
| **Self-identity** | |
| 1. Ability to perceive self as worthy | 9–12 months |
| 2. Ability to perceive assets and limitations of self | 11–15 years |
| 3. Ability to perceive self as self-directed | 20–25 years |
| 4. Ability to perceive self as a productive, contributing member of a social system | 30–35 years |
| 5. Ability to perceive self as having an autonomous identity | 35–50 years |
| 6. Ability to perceive one's own aging process and ultimate death as part of life cycle | 45–60 years |
| **Sexual identity** | |
| 1. Ability to accept and act according to one's pregenital sexual nature | 4–5 years |
| 2. Ability to accept sexual maturation as positive growth | 12–16 years |
| 3. Ability to give and receive sexual gratification | 18–25 years |
| 4. Ability to enter into a sustained sexual relationship characterized by the mutual satisfaction of sexual needs | 20–30 years |
| 5. Ability to accept the sex-related physiological changes that occur as a natural part of the aging process | 35–50 years |

*Exoceptual representation,* memory of stimuli as an action or motor response; *egocentric causality,* belief that one's own actions are completely responsible for object response; *endoceptual representation,* memory of stimuli in terms of felt experience; *denotative representation*, memory of stimuli in terms of words that stand for or name objects; *connotative representation,* memory of stimuli in terms of a more complex set of associations that are associated with an object; *decenter:* distinguish several features or characteristics of an object (be flexible enough to see it from several perspectives). Adapted with permission from Mosey AC. Psychosocial Components of Occupational Therapy. New York: Raven, 1987:416–431.

are not motivating or suitable for the person at this time. When the proper environment, activities, and subskill behaviors are present, the person appears engaged, involved, and interested.

## CASE EXAMPLE

### Judi

Judi has been a client at a suburban community day treatment center for 2 months. She is a 27-year-old unemployed high school graduate who has taken some courses at a local community college but has not declared a major. She has worked in the past, but never for more than a few weeks at a time, and has held many kinds of jobs—shop clerk, supermarket checker, lifeguard, assembly line worker, and office clerk. She has been hospitalized twice for suicide attempts and has attended several different outpatient programs. She lives at home with her widowed mother; they are financially comfortable with the pension and life insurance income from Judi's father, who was a business executive.

Judi's physical appearance is clean but not very attractive. Her hair is well brushed but not attractively cut. Her clothing is new and stylish but not well coordinated, and the colors do not flatter her. Judi appears to relate well to other clients in social situations but often says that she feels left out and that others dislike her. She reports alternately that she feels superior to everyone else and totally inadequate. She has had problems relating to staff members also. Often she seems to agree with a staff suggestion but fails to follow through. At other times she argues with staff over every detail and has several times left the center very abruptly and angrily.

After interviewing Judi and her mother, reviewing her record, and administering a task skills evaluation (done by the OTA), the OT summarizes the findings on the Adaptive Skills Developmental Chart (45). The following subskills are targeted for development in occupational therapy:

- *Dyadic interaction skill.* Subskill 3, the ability to interact in an authority relationship
- *Group interaction skill.* Subskill 3, the ability to participate in an egocentric-cooperative group
- *Self-identity skill.* Subskill 2, the ability to perceive the assets and limitations of the self

Because the first two of these are normally learned at the same chronological age, 5 to 7 years, they were the first to be addressed. Judi was placed in the jewelry production group, an egocentric-cooperative group that meets three afternoons a week for 2.5 hours each time. She was also to meet weekly with Paulette, the OTA, to review progress in the group and to discuss expectations and goals. She was expected to sign in each day in Paulette's office on her arrival at the treatment center.

The activity purpose of the jewelry group was to produce items for sale in the treatment center gift shop. The goal was to help the members develop egocentric-cooperative skills. Design and production decisions were delegated to the group members, who needed some assistance to get started. Evelyn, an OTA assigned to lead this group, provided suggestions and guided the group in making their decisions and generating new ideas. Because group members lacked experience in estimating needs, ordering supplies, and pricing items for sale, Evelyn shared resources and experiences with them. As the group became more confident and as members learned more skills, Evelyn began to step back from the group and let them work things out by themselves. As needed, she intervened in a nonauthoritarian way to help group members recognize each other's needs for approval and for respect from other group members. For example, when Judi complained that she never got a chance to participate in design work, Evelyn helped her problem solve and practice how to ask for it from the group. Judi was surprised and pleased when they agreed to give her a turn.

In her weekly sessions with Judi, Paulette's first goal was to have Judi trust her and want to be with her. Accordingly, Judi was allowed to take candy from a dish on the desk when she signed in each morning, and Paulette was careful to stop what she was doing and pass a few pleasantries with Judi each day. When Judi wore something becoming, Paulette was sure to compliment her. Judi was often late, both for individual sessions and for attendance at the center, but Paulette made little mention of this at first. Once Judi seemed genuinely to look forward to her meetings with Paulette, Paulette introduced the expectation that Judi be more punctual. Initially resentful, Judi gradually accepted this and other demands placed on her. She asked to be placed in a second group, the clerical production group, so that she could work on computer and office skills. Paulette considered it reasonable for Judi at the time and thought it would give her the experience of working with another authority figure. She recommended it to the OT.

The case example of Judi shows how the development of adaptive skills model can be applied by the OTA both in individual meetings and in group activities to promote development of adaptive skills. The example takes place in a long-term community setting, where a client could comfortably receive treatment for many months and even years. This lengthy period is necessary for the development of these adaptive skills, which are ideally learned over quite a long period in the child's life. Therefore, this developmental approach may not be as effective in short-term treatment.

In settings using the development of adaptive skills model, the OTA can be highly instrumental in helping clients progress. Assistants wishing to apply this practice model should obtain regular supervision and would benefit from further study of Mosey's work (45–47).

## CONCEPTS SUMMARY

1. The therapists must provide an environment that facilitates growth as defined by the subskill or subskills to be developed.
2. Subskills are mastered in order.
3. Subskills from different areas may be addressed at the same time, provided they are normally acquired at the same chronological age.
4. The patient's intrinsic motivation, or desire for mastery of the subskills, must be engaged.

## VOCABULARY REVIEW

**recapitulation of ontogenesis** Mosey's title for this practice model; refers to the return to or review of early stages of development.

**sensory integration skill** The ability to receive, select, combine, and use information from the balance (vestibular), touch (tactile), and position (proprioceptive) senses to perform functional activities.

**cognitive skill** The ability to perceive, represent, and organize sensory information for thinking and solving problems.

**dyadic interaction skill** The ability to participate in a variety of relationships involving one other person.

**group interaction skill** The ability to participate successfully in a variety of groups; generally, this means being able to act as a productive member of the group.[4]

**self-identity skill** The ability to recognize one's own assets and limitations and to perceive the self as worthwhile, self-directed, consistent, and reliable.

**sexual identity skill** The ability to accept one's sexual nature as natural and pleasurable and to participate in a relatively long-term sexual relationship that considers the needs of both partners.

## ROLE ACQUISITION AND SOCIAL SKILLS TRAINING

Role acquisition, a term coined by Mosey (45–47), is the learning of all daily life, work, and leisure skills that enable one to participate in a social and productive roles. Roles are student, worker, family member, leisure participant, and many others.

Success in roles depends to some extent on social skills. Social skills training refers to the teaching of interpersonal skills needed to relate to other people effectively in situations as varied as dating and applying for a job (10). Role acquisition and social skills training focus on here-and-now behaviors—how the person is functioning in the present. For example, Mark, a 52-year-old man, has been in institutions for much of his life. In institutions, his needs for food, clothing, and shelter are taken care of by the staff. To live in the community successfully, Mark must acquire daily living skills, such as doing the laundry and shopping for food, and social skills, such as how to talk to shopkeepers and neighbors.

[4] Mosey's levels of group interaction are further explained in Chapter 13.

Because both role acquisition and social skills training use techniques derived from behavioral and especially from cognitive-behavioral theory, the reader may find it helpful to review those sections of Chapter 2 before proceeding further. Role acquisition and social skills training view behavior as motivated from within. The client's needs, wants, and goals are seen as a starting point for clinical intervention. Role acquisition also relies on developmental concepts to explain the sequence and method by which skills that support role behaviors are acquired (45).

## Role Acquisition

The aim of treatment under the role acquisition model is to help the person gain the specific skills needed to function in the occupational and social roles he or she has chosen. Clients need also to develop an awareness of what they are doing and why. This awareness must extend to the environmental context, with an understanding of what is expected and appropriate for that context. To continue with the example of Mark, although he needs to learn ways to care for his clothing, he also has to develop a sense that caring for his clothing will affect how other people see him as a neighbor and member of the community. What Mark believes and understands about what he is doing is just as important as his physical actions. (The reader may note here a similarity to cognitive-behavioral theory.)

Role acquisition is based at least in part on the idea that all behavior is learned. By extension, what has been learned can be unlearned, and new behaviors can be learned to take their place. What has not been learned previously can be learned for the first time. Occupational therapists have long been concerned with how best to help people learn and with discovering under what circumstances learning is most likely to occur. Their collected experience and wisdom can be translated into the following set of 10 principles for planning and providing treatment (8, 46, 55).

### Principle 1: Client Participation

*The person should participate in identifying problems and goals for treatment and in evaluating his or her own progress* (8, 46). This conveys the idea that clients are ultimately responsible for themselves and that their ideas about what they need are important. Not all clients can participate equally in this. Some can tell the therapist exactly what their problems and goals are and spontaneously evaluate their own progress during treatment, but this is rare. Others have such limited awareness of their own deficiencies and needs that developing this awareness itself is a goal of treatment. An example is a severely psychotic patient with chronic schizophrenia who has been living on the street and who has adopted a bizarre costume of twisted and knotted rags held together with duct tape. Persuading this person to give up the costume can be quite difficult. Improving basic hygiene and grooming is a goal the therapist chooses because the patient is incapable of understanding this need. Even so, the therapist should try to explain it.

Involving clients in identifying problems and setting goals can be structured into the first meetings with them. From the start, the assistant should try to learn the client's view of the situation and what he or she wants out of the treatment. Checklists and questionnaires that the client can complete and score independently are useful. Also, the therapist or assistant can present the results of the evaluation to the client and incorporate the client's responses into the intervention plan. An example is sharing the results of an unemployed man's vocational interest evaluation with him and discussing the need for further evaluation of skills and aptitudes before a training program is selected. If the client wants to try a training program before the evaluation is finished, a compromise plan can be arranged.

Some clients have a general view of what they want to achieve but little sense of the steps they must take to get there. An example is a mildly mentally retarded woman in her early 20s who wants to have a boyfriend. Although she can identify this goal, she needs the OTA to help her understand that some intermediate steps might include learning to dress appropriately and make conversation. Once she appreciates how these skills are connected to her goal of having a boyfriend, she may be more interested in learning them.

Some clients are preoccupied with an idealized role. An example is the harried mother of three preschool children who wants to have a picture-perfect home, picture-perfect children, a trim athletic figure, and dinner on the table at exactly 6:30 every evening. Nothing less will satisfy her image of what a mother should be; consequently, she is frequently tense and depressed. In this situation, the therapist or assistant helps the client examine her goals and reason through their implications, perhaps in a discussion group with other members.

Occasionally, a person is too apathetic and unmotivated to identify any goals at all or chooses ones that present no challenge. An example is a 34-year-old man who wants to live with his parents and collect public assistance rather than return to his own apartment and his job as a clerk in a law office. If the person cannot think of suitable goals, the therapist must. Furthermore, the therapist may have to cajole and persuade such a person to become involved in activities at all. Helping clients take the first steps toward involvement in occupation when they feel hopeless and incompetent can dramatically improve the quality of the person's life and his or her motivation for rehabilitation. It is important that occupational therapy practitioners recognize this responsibility and be willing to be assertive with the client in such a situation.

Getting clients to assess their own progress or lack thereof is equally important. For decades the treating professional was seen as all-powerful and the patient as a passive receiver of treatment; although this view has gradually shifted and given way to a more consumer-driven health care model, older clients and those with cognitive disabilities may still depend on the psychiatric system to make their decisions for them. In occupational therapy the client, by engaging in occupation, is carrying out his or her own treatment. The therapist is responsible for making sure clients know what they are supposed to be doing and why. But clients need to learn to pay attention to their performance and their feelings about the activities in which they participate. Being able to assess one's own reaction, to reflect on how an activity feels, how competent one feels doing it, and whether it achieves what one set out to do are skills that help one maintain a balanced, flexible, and satisfying life.

## Principle 2: Personalized Goals

*Choose goals and activities that reflect the client's interests, personal and cultural values, and present and future life roles* (8, 46). No two people are alike, and the OTA or OT must not assume that he or she can predict what is best for the client. Information about the client's interests and values can be obtained through interview or evaluation (such as the Interest Checklist) and sometimes from the medical record or from family members.

Clients' values may be shaped in part by their ethnicity, social class, and culture. Ethnicity refers to race and national origin, for example, Native American, Uzbek, Polish, Jamaican, Korean, Mexican, and Brazilian. Social class refers to the person's rank or status within the larger society. This rank is based in part on educational level and family background and in part on occupation and personal wealth. For example, those whose earnings fall below the poverty level are generally considered to be in the lowest social class, but a Harvard-educated farm worker from a wealthy family would be considered upper class even though his earnings fall in the poverty range.

Culture is a complex and constantly changing concept that includes the customs, beliefs, and objects associated with specific groups of people (39). Each ethnic group has many cultural variations, because family traditions and new customs acquired from association with members of other cultural groups are often quite individual. Consider, for example, the situation of American Jews, who may be Orthodox, Conservative, or Reform in their religious practices; some are so distant from Jewish tradition that they have a Christmas tree in their homes, exchange Christmas gifts, and go to work on Jewish holidays such as Yom Kippur. Likewise, black men from the West Indies have expectations of their wives that are different from those of black men born in the United States.

In addition to the specific cultural group to which the client belongs, the values and trends of the larger culture have to be considered. The best contemporary occupational therapy practice reflects this by involving clients in occupations that are meaningful today and in particular that are meaningful to that person. Media such as weaving, basketry, and copper enameling were adopted by occupational therapists when the practice of these crafts by artisans was diminishing and when home use of crafts was advocated to keep the crafts from dying out. Arts and crafts have risen and fallen in popularity over the years and should not be the primary modality for most clients. Instead, the occupational therapy practitioner must identify and help the client engage in occupations that are meaningful to that specific person, whether it be gardening, using a computer, or managing time and a schedule.

The person's present and future life roles also influence the choice of activity. Activities used in occupational therapy should be geared to helping clients acquire needed skills and making them competent at something they need to do in real life. The best activities are those that will enable the person to handle the everyday demands of life. For example, a high school student hospitalized for a brief period will probably benefit most from keeping up with schoolwork and learning better note-taking and study skills.

## Principle 3: Ability-Based Goals

*Choose goals and activities that provide a realistic challenge but are consistent with the client's present level of ability* (8, 46). Many people who have psychiatric disorders are unable to perform their usual occupations as effectively as they once did. Their thinking may be slow or confused; they may hallucinate (see or hear things that are not there); they may have to make a conscious effort to perform simple motions; and they may have incorrect ideas (delusions) and be so preoccupied with their own concerns that they have trouble attending to what is going on around them. Nonetheless, they may expect themselves to accomplish tasks that are beyond their capability at the moment; they may see less-demanding tasks presented by the OTA as a sign that others think very little of them. The assistant should express absolute conviction that the person will recover and will be able to accomplish more in the future; at the same time, he or she should explain the purpose of the activity and its relation to the client's condition and goals.

Activities should require some effort from clients; otherwise they may just go through the motions without becoming involved. The activities should not be so simple and routine that clients do not have to pay attention to what they are doing. On the other hand, they should not require such intense effort that the person quickly becomes tired or frustrated.

## Principle 4: Increasing Challenges

*Increase challenges and demands as the person's capacity increases.* At the beginning, many clients can work for only short periods or at only simple activities. Positive support from the therapist or assistant may be needed to encourage their first efforts. After a person feels comfortable and reasonably successful, he or she generally is willing and ready to try more difficult tasks. Some improve only slowly, whereas others improve so rapidly that they get bored or tune out unless given new challenges.

## Principle 5: Natural Progression

*Present skills in their natural developmental sequence* (8). All skills are developed in a predictable direction from simple to complex. This is true of motor skills, which begin as gross, generalized motions and progress gradually to finely coordinated movements. Similarly, the ability to interact in a group starts with being able to tolerate other people and only gradually develops into a varied repertoire of ways of actually relating to those people. In both cases there are many steps along the way to full mastery of the skill. It is important to keep this principle in mind when teaching skills to clients. Moving from simple to complex and following a natural, step-by-step sequence strengthens learning because the skills are built on a solidly developed foundation.

## Principle 6: Client Knowledge

*Clients should always know what they are supposed to be learning and why.* The assistant should orient the person to each new activity, never assuming that the person sees the connection between the immediate activity and the treatment goal. Orientation should include an explanation of why the activity is being done, what steps are involved, how long the activity will take, and what is required for successful performance. Someone who has never had a job and who is placed in a prevocational setting may have little idea of what behaviors are expected on the job. Unless the importance of being on time for work is explained, the person may assume that the assistant's emphasis on punctuality is a personal preference. Similarly, if asked to perform unfamiliar tasks, such as filing papers, the person must be told exactly how to go about it.

## Principle 7: Client Awareness

*Clients should be made aware of the effects of their actions* (8). Many clients lack the skill or perspective necessary to evaluate their own performance; if so, the therapist or assistant must do so for them. As Mosey (46) states, "The consequence of an action is important." You can appreciate this yourself just by thinking of how eagerly you await the results of tests, especially those in which you are uncertain of your performance. Similarly, clients need to know whether they have achieved, to what extent, and how they can improve. If the person seems at loose ends about what to do next and does not comment on his or her own success or failure, the assistant has ample evidence that the client needs feedback and guidance from someone else.

Severely disabled persons often make slow progress, and improvements may be so slight as to be barely perceptible. Here the assistant must be especially alert to small changes in behavior so that they can be rewarded immediately. Consider, for example, the person whose social skills are so impaired that he or she keeps eyes downcast and fails to make eye contact with others. To increase this person's eye contact the assistant should respond positively to even the briefest and most glancing look.

There are many ways of responding to a client's efforts and giving feedback. One is through the systematic use of reinforcers, as discussed in Chapter 2. Occupational therapy practitioners need to be aware of their emotional reaction to the client and of the verbal and nonverbal responses they communicate. There is no overestimating the value of tolerance, acceptance, positive support, and a sense of humor in motivating people. However, the assistant must remain in control of the situation and not allow the client to abuse the relationship. Because of the powerful effects of the assistant's reaction on the client's motivation and future behavior, it will be discussed separately in Chapter 10.

## Principle 8: Practice Makes Perfect

*Skills must be practiced repeatedly and then applied to new situations* (8, 46). There is truth to the old saying, Practice makes perfect; and although we do not expect our clients to achieve perfection in everything they attempt, we do want to make sure they know a skill well enough to use it in the future. To ensure this, the assistant must provide opportunities for clients to practice until they are comfortable. A single correct performance cannot be taken as evidence that someone has learned a skill; if Mark does the laundry correctly today, this does not guarantee that he can do so next week. Performing a skill repeatedly strengthens learning and helps transform skills into habits.

Once a skill or habit is well established through practice, variations and shortcuts can be attempted. It is crucial that the client be encouraged to practice new skills and habits in his or her own environment and that someone monitor the efforts there. When, for example, Mark attempts to do the laundry at home, he may discover that the machines in his local coin laundry business operate differently from the one on which he learned. If Mark, like many people with psychiatric disorders, has trouble asking others for help and is unable to solve problems on his own, he may give up on doing his laundry altogether.

Practicing a skill in a variety of situations helps the client see that what works in one situation can work in others. This is called generalization. For example, assembling the necessary supplies before beginning an activity is a skill that works just as well in studying for a test as in doing the laundry. People can be helped to apply learning from one situation to another similar situation by being involved in varied activities and environments. In addition, this variety can help the person learn that a given behavior or skill does not work in all situations. This ability to recognize what behavior is appropriate or not for a given situation is called *discrimination*. An example is knowing that sneakers and sweats should be worn for athletic activities and not for a job interview.

## Principle 9: Parts of the Whole

*If a task is too complex or time consuming to learn all at one time, teach one part at a time, but always do or show the whole activity.* Many tasks that clients need to learn are long, complicated multistep operations. Doing the laundry is an example. The major steps are sorting the clothes by color and type of fabric, assembling laundry supplies (including knowing which laundry products to use and in which order) and money, getting to the laundry shop, loading the clothes in the washer, inserting the coins, adding the detergent and perhaps bleach, running the machine, unloading the washer, loading the dryer, inserting the correct change and turning on the dryer, removing the dry clothes, and folding and/or ironing them. Further refinements include using spot removers and fabric softeners, using net bags for lingerie, adjusting water and dryer temperature, and using special cycles on the washer. The client must also learn which clothes can be machine washed and which must be dry-cleaned or washed by hand.

The most effective way to help someone learn a complex task like this is to go through the entire process with the person many times. However, because of other demands on an assistant's time, this is not often possible, and a complex task can seem overwhelming if presented all at once. The recommended approach is to teach only what can be learned in a given time—for example, folding clothes immediately after removing them from the dryer. Taught in isolation, this step may not make much sense to the client, but connecting this step to the rest of the activity will demonstrate why it is important. This may be done in a variety of ways.

One method for showing how a step or subskill relates to the larger complex activity of which it is a part is to talk it through. In this example, it would necessitate a brief verbal overview of the whole process of doing the laundry, emphasizing why, when, and how the clothes should be folded.

It is important to keep the overview brief and to the point to maintain the person's interest and attention. Because some people have trouble following spoken descriptions and directions, other learning aids such as posters, printed handouts, samples of how a project looks at various stages, photos, or videotapes can also be used. Chaining, as described in Chapter 2, can be incorporated with these techniques.

Another technique is to simplify the activity by removing all but the most basic steps. For example, starting with a load of mixed-color wash-and-wear items in a washer with only one temperature setting, using only detergent (omitting all other laundry products), and using a dryer with a single temperature setting focuses attention on the essential key steps of the activity and reduces confusion.

Activities make most sense when they are presented in context. Barris et al. (8) give the example that a makeup class for adolescent girls becomes more motivating if it is followed by a dance or other activity for which makeup is appropriate. Similarly, an actual trip to a real destination enhances learning how to use the subway or bus, and doing the laundry when the client's clothes are dirty makes more sense than just washing things to show how it is done.

### Principle 10: Imitation

*People learn how to do things by imitating others.* It is easy to see this in small children, who mimic their parents' actions, words, and even intonations. The tendency to learn through imitation continues throughout life; watching how someone does something and then trying to do the same thing is familiar to all of us. This is no less true for people with psychiatric disorders, but with an important difference: Their experience may have included few good role models. Consider the case of a woman who was abused by her parents when she was a child; this the only behavior she is familiar with, and she is likely to repeat it when she has children herself. To learn other ways of managing her children, she has to be exposed to better role models. In a child-care skills group she can learn how to manage her own feelings, reduce stress, and communicate effectively by watching other mothers and imitating what they do.

Clients often look to staff for role models. Being a good role model can be hard work. It requires that the assistant or therapist actually embody the qualities he or she is trying to get the client to develop. A tense therapist cannot help someone relax, and a shy therapist is likely to have trouble developing assertiveness in her clients because she lacks it herself. This is discussed further in Chapter 10.

Fellow clients can also serve as models for imitation. Encouraging a person to observe and copy the behavior of another client reaps a double reward because it increases the confidence of the one being imitated. Clients can also be taught to imitate role models from their past. For example, a childhood teacher or a favorite uncle may possess characteristics useful in the present; in that case, the assistant helps the person remember and focus on the model while attempting the activity.

## Social Skills Training

As mentioned previously, social skills training refers to the teaching of interpersonal skills needed to relate effectively to other people. Many persons with psychiatric disorders have problems in this area. They may fail to make eye contact or to respond to questions asked of them, or they may speak too loudly or stand too close or say bizarre things. Such behavior is a serious handicap when applying for (and keeping) a job, asking someone for a date, meeting new people, or just shopping for food or clothing. Figure 3-1 illustrates someone who strongly desires relationships with others but does not understand the rules of social conduct that lead to mutually positive interactions.

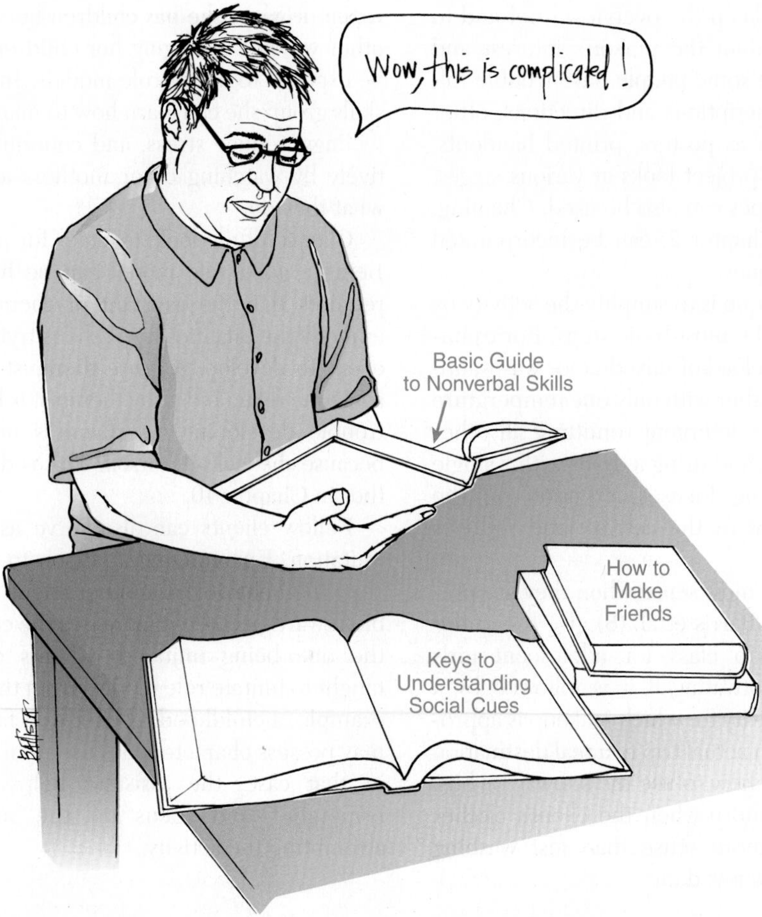


**Figure 3-1. Some people find social behavior very hard to understand.**

Kelly (27) defines social skills as "those identifiable, learned behaviors that individuals use in interpersonal situations to obtain or to maintain reinforcement from their environment." In other words, social skills help us get what we want from others. Others respond to the way we act, and the more awareness and control a person has over his or her social behavior, the more success he or she is likely to have in dealing with other people.

Social skills have been classified in many ways. One way is to group the behaviors that are needed in a given situation. For example, in a job interview the necessary skills include eye contact, emotional expression appropriate to the situation, clear speech at an appropriate volume, listening, responding, sticking to the topic under discussion, stating one's qualifications positively, showing interest, and asking relevant questions.

Another way of grouping skills is by content or purpose. This approach recognizes that the same social skills may apply in a variety of situations; showing interest is important in friendship and dating as well as on the job. Generically, social skills can be classified into four groups (65): self-expressive skills, other-enhancing skills, assertive skills, and communication skills. Among the many self-expressive skills are stating feelings and opinions, stating positive things about oneself, and stating one's values and beliefs. Other-enhancing skills include giving compliments, smiling and expressing interest, and giving support and encouragement. Assertive skills are varied. Making requests, disagreeing with another's opinion or statement of fact, refusing requests, questioning another's behavior, and setting limits on another's aggressiveness are examples. Communication skills include controlling the tone and quality of one's voice, articulating words clearly, and choosing the proper words for a situation. There are many skills in each category besides those listed.

The OTA is unlikely to be involved in the evaluation of clients' social skills; this task is usually performed by the therapist, a social worker, or a psychologist. However, the assistant has many opportunities to observe the client and can contribute these observations to a discussion of the person's social skills. The OTA may also be asked to participate in social skills training (treatment to remedy social skills deficits) and so should know the methods and techniques.

A social skills training session usually consists of four distinct phases: motivation, demonstration, practice, and feedback. These phases are probably already quite familiar to occupational therapy assistant students, as they are similar to those used in the traditional occupational therapy method of instructing a patient in an activity (64). *Motivation* consists of identifying the behavior to be learned and explaining why it is important. The therapist should give examples of the desired behavior and discuss why it is relevant to the person's goals. If the patient can state reasons it is important, so much the better.

In the *demonstration* phase the therapist shows the person how the behavior is performed. Among the many methods that can be used are modeling by the therapist, role-playing by the therapist and another person, and film or videotape models. Regardless of the method, during this phase the patient watches and observes but does not attempt the behavior himself or herself until the practice phase.

*Practice* can be structured to improve learning. One way is to ask the person to rehearse the desired behavior by talking it through. This can reduce anxiety before the actual performance. For example, if the target behavior is asking relevant questions on a job interview, the person would be asked to list some questions first in a discussion with the therapist. Then he or she might try them out in role-playing with another client.

*Feedback* is given at the end of the treatment session to summarize what the person has learned and focus attention on what is to be learned next. However, throughout the session the therapist should also provide immediate feedback on the client's performance. It is important that the feedback be immediate and specific, emphasizing positive aspects of the person's performance and providing concrete details about how to improve it. To illustrate, following the client's role-playing of interviewing for a job, the therapist might say, "Good. You looked me right in the eye while you were talking. Your answers to the questions were brief and to the point. Now let's work on showing more enthusiasm. How much do you want this job? Convince me."

Training in social skills should involve not only learning the appropriate behaviors but learning to perceive when and where they are appropriate (11). Social perception requires reading subtle variations in others' behavior and in the immediate environment. For example, if two people are seated in a room conversing with each other and a third person comes in, several things can happen, depending on the situation and who is involved. One of the seated people might look at the entering person, stand up, and greet him. This would be good manners in many situations, especially if the entering person has authority (e.g., is the boss or an older person). However, if the scene is a student lounge and all three people are students who know each other well and have spent all day together, it may be rude or strange for one person to stand up, in effect ending the conversation.

To summarize, social skills training is a structured approach for teaching interpersonal behaviors. It fits within the general framework of role acquisition and uses behavioral concepts and techniques. Both role acquisition and social skills training can be used as treatment approaches within the model of human occupation; both approaches recognize that the therapist must first motivate the client and that skills and habits are acquired through learning within a social environment. Both approaches assume that if the input from the environment is changed, the client's behavior will change. The case example of Howard illustrates the application of both role acquisition and social skills training.

**CASE EXAMPLE**

## Howard

Howard is a 45-year-old single man who lives with his widowed mother in a two-bedroom apartment in a rundown neighborhood of a large city. Howard was first hospitalized at age 14 and has been in and out of the hospital many times in the intervening years. He has received a dual diagnosis of chronic schizophrenia and mild mental retardation.

Until 3 weeks ago Howard was employed for 25 years by a messenger service. His job was to pick up and deliver packages via the subway and bus system. He got this job following successful vocational rehabilitation during one of his hospitalizations. Recently, however, the old manager, who was fond of Howard, retired, and his replacement found Howard's hygiene "unbearable." This was given as the reason for dismissal. After being fired, Howard began to hallucinate and became afraid to leave his apartment. His mother took him to the emergency room; and after an overnight stay, he was referred to the outpatient day hospital program.

On meeting Howard, the OTA, Gloria, immediately observed that his hygiene was quite poor. His clothes fit badly, his pants were buttoned but unzipped, he had several days' growth of beard, and his hair was uncombed. He wore a dirty yarmulke, which was lopsided despite three bobby pins. He had noticeable body odor and visible food particles stuck in his teeth. He walked with a shuffling gait and kept his eyes downcast. He did answer Gloria's questions, although his answers were often long, rambling, and difficult to follow. At the end of the interview, Howard followed Gloria to the door and continued talking and asking her questions even though she had three times told him the interview was over.

During the evaluation of daily living skills it became evident that Howard knew how to perform basic hygiene and grooming routines but did not always remember to do them and had trouble keeping his attention on what he was doing. He was easily distracted by the presence of other people and would interrupt whatever he was doing to talk to them. An evaluation of task skills revealed similar patterns: Once instructed, Howard was able to perform simple tasks, such as stuffing envelopes, but often stopped in the middle to talk to others and had to be reminded to return to his task. The content of his speech was egocentric and tangential; he talked mostly about himself, TV shows he had seen, and things he had done. He frequently sought approval of his task performance from staff members.

After receiving written permission from Howard to do so, Ben, Gloria's supervisor, interviewed by telephone both Howard's mother and his former employer. The employer said that he felt bad about firing Howard but didn't know how to deal with his poor hygiene and incessant talking. He agreed to take Howard back on a trial basis if these problems were solved. He also stated that the company's insurance policy, under which Howard was still covered, provided for 14 days annually of inpatient psychiatric hospitalization and up to 6 months of outpatient treatment. No new information was obtained from Howard's mother.

Ben evaluated Howard's social skills during a social skills group, using structured role-playing in which other clients played the parts of Howard's employer and various customers. The following problem behaviors were noted: interrupting others who are speaking, failing to make eye contact, introducing inappropriate topics, and failing to perceive and act on the other's desire to end the interaction.

Ben and Gloria discussed the evaluation results with Howard. Howard was most interested in returning to work and agreed to the following goals:

- To perform daily hygiene and grooming routines
- To learn conversational skills appropriate for a job situation

Because social contact was so important to Howard, one-on-one meetings with Gloria were selected as the main reinforcer. Gloria also thought this would provide opportunities for her to explore other aspects of Howard's social behavior in various environments, such as the hospital coffee shop and local stores and parks.

Specific training included a day-long job skills group run by Marlene, another OTA, and a daily morning hygiene group run by Gloria and Paul, a nurse's aide. Howard was also scheduled for evening recreation groups. All staff were directed to give Howard feedback on incorrect behaviors and to praise and support any improvements.

The first target behavior in the job skills group was learning not to interrupt others. Marlene explained this to Howard, giving several examples and indicating other clients who had already mastered this skill and whom Howard could watch as role models. During discussion periods at the end of each day's work, Howard reviewed and assessed his behavior that day and listened to feedback from Marlene and the group members. Other behaviors were taught in the same fashion.

In the daily hygiene skills group Howard practiced his hygiene and grooming under supervision. He gradually relearned the entire sequence of brushing his teeth, showering, shaving, using deodorant, and combing his hair. After Howard had practiced the routine daily for several weeks, he no longer needed reminders.

Howard was able to return to his job after a month, first 2 days per week, gradually increasing to 5 days per week. Gloria visited him twice at work to observe and give him feedback on his behavior at the job. She also coached Howard's employer on how to give constructive feedback. On discharge from day hospital, Howard was enrolled in the evening aftercare program, which he continued to attend for 3 months, at which point he made a successful transition to an evening psychosocial club program near his home.

Throughout his treatment, Howard participated in selecting his own goals and evaluating his own progress. Because his role as a worker was so important to him, this became the focus of the treatment plan. New skills and behaviors were taught sequentially, allowing Howard to succeed first at easy tasks before attempting more difficult ones. Each task was explained to Howard and role models were provided. Finally, the newly acquired skills were carried over to the job, with staff support and supervision.

This example also shows how various levels of occupational therapy staff can work together and with nursing staff to carry out a treatment plan. Both role acquisition and social skills training are approaches well suited to team effort because the goals and methods are easily understood and carried out by all levels of staff.

Social skills training has been criticized as having limited effectiveness. It appears that behavioral change transfers best to environments similar to those used for training (18, 20). Therefore, skills should be taught either in the environment in which they will be used or in an environment carefully designed to mimic the final environment of action.

Schindler (60) has provided extensive guidelines for *role development,* a model based on role acquisition. Schindler applied the role development model for clients with schizophrenia in forensics (prison settings). Schindler's specific examples and explanations of methods may be helpful to practitioners using the models discussed in this section.

## CONCEPTS SUMMARY

1. The person should be involved in selecting problems and goals for treatment and in evaluating his or her own progress.
2. Choose goals and activities that reflect the client's interests, personal and cultural values, and present and future life roles.
3. Choose goals and activities that provide a realistic challenge but are consistent with the client's present level of ability.
4. Increase challenges and demands as the person's capacity increases.
5. Present skills in their natural developmental sequence.
6. Clients should always know what they are supposed to be learning and why.
7. Clients should be made aware of the effects of their actions.
8. Skills should be practiced repeatedly and then applied to new situations.
9. If a task is too complex or time consuming to learn all at one time, one part should be taught at a time, always doing or showing the whole activity.
10. People learn to do things by imitating other people.
11. Skills should be taught in a four-stage process consisting of motivation, demonstration, practice, and feedback.
12. Feedback should be given throughout the learning process and should be immediate, specific, positive, concrete, and directive.

## VOCABULARY REVIEW

**behavior** Defined in "Behavioral Theories" in Chapter 2.

**chaining** Defined in "Behavioral Theories" in Chapter 2.

**reinforcement** Defined in "Behavioral Theories" in Chapter 2.

**extinction** Defined in "Behavioral Theories" in Chapter 2.

**shaping** Defined in "Behavioral Theories" in Chapter 2.

**skills** Basic action patterns that can be combined into a variety of more complex actions.

**social skills** Skills used to relate to other people in a variety of situations.

**generalization** The ability to apply a skill or behavior to new situations that are similar to the one in which it was learned.

**discrimination** The ability to recognize differences in situations that call for a change in behavior.

**imitation** A method of learning by copying or mimicking the behavior of another person.

**target behavior** The new behavior to be learned in the immediate treatment situation.

The target behavior is a short-term goal, which is distinguished from the long-term goal known as the terminal behavior, a desired behavior that will be mastered by the completion of the treatment program.

**motivation** The first stage in the cycle of skills training, in which the target behavior is identified and its importance explained.

**demonstration** The second stage in the cycle of skills training, in which the target behavior is demonstrated to the person via role play, videotape, or other example.

**practice** The third stage in the cycle of skills training, in which the person attempts the target behavior and repeats it until he or she becomes comfortable.

**feedback** This word has several meanings. In the cycle of skills training it is the fourth stage, in which the person's performance of the target behavior is reviewed and summarized. More generally, however, feedback means information from the environment about the effects of one's action. When given by a person, feedback is most effective when it occurs immediately after the behavior is performed, includes positive aspects of the performance, and gives specific information on what can be done to improve it.

## PSYCHOEDUCATION

Psychoeducation is not, strictly speaking, an occupational therapy practice model. Rather, it is an educational approach used by many service providers to improve the skills of persons with mental disorders. The psychiatric rehabilitation (PsyR) model (53) regularly employs psychoeducation. PsyR and psychoeducation both affirm that problem behaviors shown by persons with chronic mental disorders reflect deficient living skills. Psychoeducation assumes that such skill deficits can be remedied by direct teaching and training. The therapist acts as an educator, providing lessons similar to classroom courses, with objectives, learning activities, and homework. Behavioral techniques such as reinforcement are also sometimes used.

Bruce and Borg (11) suggest that psychoeducational approaches exemplify cognitive-behavioral theory. This may appear so because homework and educational assignments are used in both. Psychoeducation, however, focuses primarily on training and development of skills, on functional performance of everyday activities, and to a much lesser degree on faulty cognitions. Psychoeducation draws on the social learning theories of Bandura (see "Cognitive-Behavioral Theory" in Chapter 2), but the techniques and general form of psychoeducation come more directly from educational theory. Psychoeducation also shares an emphasis with role acquisition and social skills training, in that it has similar goals. The difference in psychoeducation is in the emphasis on the *educational* nature of the behavioral change.

A psychoeducation setting is viewed as an educational environment, a place for learning; it is not a clinic or a place for healing or treatment. For a psychoeducation course, the therapy practitioner typically prepares a syllabus containing the course description, rationale, goals, objectives, methods, daily lesson plans, homework assignments, and evaluation or assessment methods (38). The students, as clients are termed to encourage them to adopt this role, take notes in notebooks, keep and use handouts, and do homework. Students who would benefit from increased concentration on a given topic may be directed to use an individualized study method.

Lillie and Armstrong (38) were among the first to apply the psychoeducational model in occupational therapy in their Life Skills Program (LSP). They used a hierarchical model of skill development adapted from Hewett (23). Educational goals increase at each level, reflecting that skill development at earlier levels must be achieved

| *Directions:* Circle number in appropriate column and add for total. | Rarely / Sometimes / Often | Circle rater/student familiarity - 1 2 3 4 5 + | Rarely / Sometimes / Often | NAME ____ RATER ____ DATE ____ | Rarely / Sometimes / Often |
|---|---|---|---|---|---|
| **I. ENTRY LEVEL** | | **IV. RELATIONSHIP LEVEL** | | **VII. ACHIEVEMENT LEVEL** | |
| States desire to attend | 0 1 (2) | Seeks approval | 0 1 (2) | Assumes self-responsibility | 0 1 (2) |
| Stays through classes | 0 1 (2) | Accepts feedback | 0 1 (2) | Completes tasks | 0 1 (2) |
| Hallucinates/delusional | (2) 1 0 | Is outgoing and friendly | 0 1 (2) | Manages stress | (0) 1 2 |
| Is easily distracted | (2) 1 0 | Interacts with peers | 0 1 (2) | Is able to abstract | 0 1 (2) |
| Stays on topic/coherent | 0 1 (2) | Seeks reinforcement | 0 1 (2) | Is self-motivated | 0 1 (2) |
| Is disruptive/combative | (2) 1 0 | Works productively 1-1 | 0 1 (2) | Generalizes | 0 1 (2) |
| Speaks & acts at normal pace | 0 1 (2) | Gives compliments | 0 1 (2) | Competent in ADL skills | 0 (1) 2 |
| Observes limits | 0 1 (2) | Receives compliments | 0 (1) 2 | Makes discharge plans | 0 (1) 2 |
| Affect is appropriate | 0 1 (2) | Uses staff appropriately | 0 1 (2) | Seeks independence | (0) 1 2 |
| Threatens suicide | (2) 1 0 | Shares feelings with others | 0 1 (2) | Generates + self-statements | (0) 1 2 |
| TOTAL | 20 | TOTAL | 19 | TOTAL | 10 |
| **II. ACCEPTANCE LEVEL** | | **V. EXPLORATORY LEVEL** | | | |
| Attentive | 0 1 (2) | Asks questions | 0 1 (2) | | |
| Suspicious, guarded | (2) 1 0 | Seeks new situations | 0 (1) 2 | | |
| Answers questions | 0 1 (2) | Makes suggestions | 0 1 (2) | | |
| Engages others | 0 1 (2) | Tries new behaviors | 0 (1) 2 | | |
| Is rude or indifferent | (2) 1 0 | Requests feedback | 0 1 (2) | | |
| Keeps appointments | 0 1 (2) | Initiates activities | 0 1 (2) | | |
| Withdraws/lacks trust | (2) 1 0 | Reveals feelings | 0 1 (2) | | |
| Refuses feedback | (2) 1 0 | Considers goals | 0 1 (2) | | |
| Denies problems | (2) 1 0 | Role plays | 0 1 (2) | | |
| Accepts contacts with staff | 0 1 (2) | Expresses concern for others | 0 1 (2) | | |
| TOTAL | 20 | TOTAL | 18 | | |
| **III. ORDER LEVEL** | | **VI. MASTERY LEVEL** | | | |
| Appears neat and orderly | 0 1 (2) | Makes decisions | 0 (1) 2 | | |
| Follows rules | 0 1 (2) | Problem solves | 0 (1) 2 | | |
| Adheres to schedule | 0 1 (2) | Exercises good judgment | 0 (1) 2 | | |
| Acts impulsively | (2) 1 0 | Sets treatment goals | 0 1 (2) | | |
| Organizes tasks | 0 1 (2) | Self-reinforces | 0 (1) 2 | | |
| Is rigid or compulsive | (2) 1 0 | Generates alternatives | 0 (1) 2 | | |
| Follows directions | 0 1 (2) | Verbalizes spontaneously | 0 1 (2) | | |
| Complies with treatment | 0 1 (2) | Is able to relax | 0 (1) 2 | | |
| Is punctual | 0 1 (2) | Exerts self-control | 0 1 (2) | | |
| Attends regularly | 0 1 (2) | Takes notes/completes assignments | 0 1 (2) | | |
| TOTAL | 20 | TOTAL | 14 | | |

**SUMMARY GRAPH**

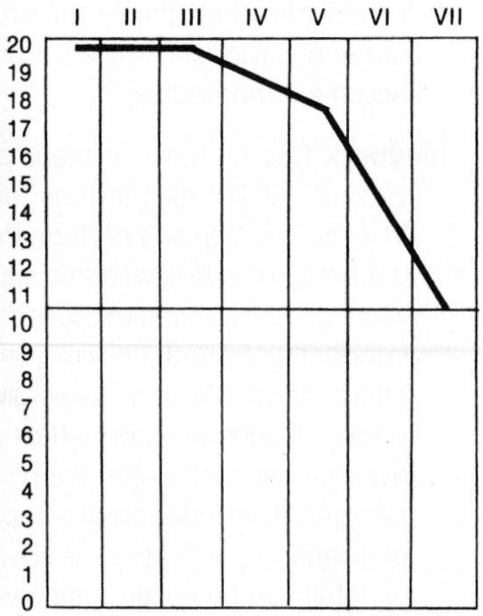

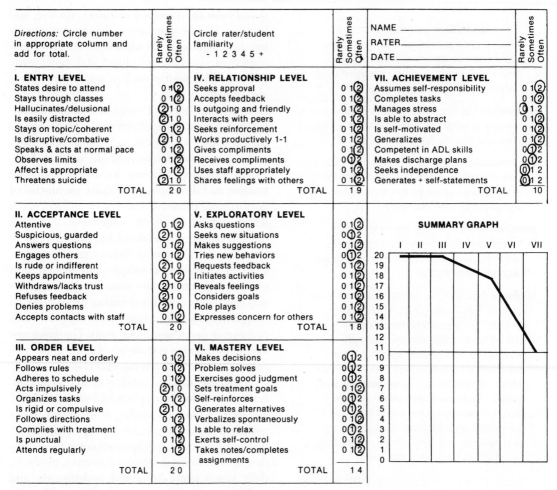

**Figure 3-2. Task checklist.** This example has been completed for a 55-year-old divorced mother of six in her first psychiatric hospitalization for bipolar disease. (Reprinted with permission from Lillie MD, Armstrong HE. Contributions to the development of psychoeducational approaches to mental health service. Am J Occup Ther 1982;36:441. Used with permission of the American Occupational Therapy Association.)

before success can occur at higher levels. A task checklist (TCL) highlights the key behaviors pertaining to each level. Figure 3-2 shows a TCL for a middle-aged woman in her first psychiatric hospitalization for bipolar disorder. The client, who previously functioned normally in the community, felt unsure of herself. It was difficult for her to explore new situations and make decisions. The therapist enrolled her in the exploring community course, which required her to call businesses and bus companies for information, arrange an outing to an unfamiliar site, and so on. This and other psychoeducation experiences increased her confidence to the point that she eventually obtained a volunteer job and moved into her own apartment.

Evaluation of outcome is important in psychoeducation. To what extent do clients actually learn new skills; and, more important, to what extent do they generalize or carry them over into other environments and situations? Hayes and Halford (19), in a review of the literature, noted that many of the techniques (e.g., homework assignments) used in psychoeducation are useful for generalization. However, generalization is usually not stated as a goal and is rarely evaluated. Any psychoeducation program should, therefore, include a post-program assessment *(post-test)* to measure the extent to which students actually learn and apply in their everyday environments the skills taught in the psychoeducation course.

The psychoeducational model has been applied in the rehabilitation of multiply handicapped adults. Courses have focused on functional life skills (cooking, shopping) and appropriate role acquisition (self-advocacy, participation in community recreation). Classroom teaching, homework assignments, and quizzes and examinations involved the clients in their roles as students. Praise and other social reinforcers were used in responses by classroom teachers and in feedback on homework. Outcome was evaluated by pretest and post-test scores and by successful placements in community living.

Occupational therapists have also used the psychoeducation approach to improve skills of persons with codependency problems (49), to teach life skills to persons with chronic psychiatric disorders in a university setting (13), and to instruct psychiatric patients in a maximum-security forensic hospital about human immunodeficiency virus (HIV) and high-risk behaviors (61).

The psychoeducation setting is typically multidisciplinary. Working in a role similar to that of other professionals but using unique occupational therapy skills and perspectives, the occupational therapy practitioner may serve as case manager or as educator. As case manager, the OT or OTA is responsible for assisting the learner in planning a program of study. This includes evaluation, identification of goals, selection of learning opportunities, and measurement of outcomes. The case manager acts as liaison to other services, for example to the physician or social worker, and helps with community transitions and bureaucratic issues. The case manager may serve functions similar to those of homeroom teacher and guidance counselor. The case manager must have service competencies beyond entry level for the OTA.

As educator, the OT or OTA may teach individuals or groups. Padilla (50) describes three teaching approaches that may be used (executive, therapist, and liberationist). Teaching may involve lecturing; guiding role-playing, discussions, and other in-class activities; one-on-one instruction; social modeling; designing and responding to homework assignments; and creating, administering, and evaluating various outcome measures such as pretests and post-tests. Pretests and post-tests, which document the effects of interventions, therefore may be used in outcome studies and would be helpful in research.

The focus of evaluation is identification of deficient areas and of goals that are important to the student. The student is seen as a consumer of an educational service and is expected to participate in self-evaluation and goal setting. The following are some of the methods that have been used for evaluation:

- *Semistructured interview.* With a focus on occupational performance, this identifies areas in which therapist and student may jointly establish goals (49).
- *Task checklist.* Developed by Lillie and Armstrong (38), this is a checklist for assessing student competencies and setting treatment goals.
- *Kohlman Evaluation of Living Skills.* This instrument, which takes only a short time to

administer, measures basic skills in literacy, money management, self-care, and other areas (66).
- *Pretest and post-test.* These may be used to assess the student's mastery of the content of various learning modules both before and after instruction.

In this approach, goals for intervention are identified by the case manager and the student-client jointly (43). Goals should focus on specific behavioral objectives or outcomes. The primary environment used with psychoeducation is educational courses or modules about various life skills. These may include activities of daily living (medication management, shopping, cooking), recreation and leisure, school- and work-related activities, coping skills and management of feelings, relapse prevention and symptom management, decision making and problem solving, and community exploration. Methods of instruction include classroom lectures, guest lectures by experts, films, role-playing and group exercises, videotaping and video feedback, assigned reading, homework assignments, and individual study. Social modeling by the therapist-educator or a peer is often used. Separate one-on-one instruction may focus on needs of individuals.

Psychoeducation makes use of both *in vivo* or naturalistic (real-life) and *simulated* training environments. Students may take a trip to a museum or shopping mall (*in vivo*). Alternatively, they may simulate a community environment using props in the classroom, where they can role-play experiences and interactions before risking themselves *in vivo*.

**CASE EXAMPLE**

## Eloise

Eloise, a 31-year-old single woman who lives alone, is employed as a legal secretary. She began to abuse alcohol at age 11 but decided to stop drinking 5 months ago at the suggestion of her therapist, whom she had begun seeing because of feelings of emptiness and loneliness. A month ago she attempted suicide and was admitted to the hospital, medicated with fluvoxamine maleate (Luvox), and discharged 6 days later to the continuing day treatment program. She is worried about being out of work but is afraid that she will become suicidal again if she returns to her job too soon. Her diagnoses are major depressive episode and dependent personality disorder.

History in the chart revealed that Eloise's parents both abused alcohol; her father is deceased and her relationship with her mother, who continues to drink heavily, is poor. Eloise has had many sexual relationships, most recently with her boss, who is married. According to psychological testing, Eloise possesses exceptional verbal intelligence.

Deshawn, the OT, interviewed Eloise with the Occupational Case Analysis Interview and Rating Scale (OCAIRS) (26). Eloise said that she worked long hours at her job, staying late because she wanted to "be there" for her boss. At home she had few leisure interests, attended AA meetings daily in the mornings before work, and talked with her mother on the phone every night. The phone conversations were invariably argumentative and abusive and left Eloise feeling terrible about herself. Eloise could not identify any friends; women from AA would invite her to have coffee or go to a movie, but she did not accept, fearing rejection. At work she felt she did a very good job but sometimes became paralyzed with not knowing what to do if a problem arose. Eloise was a good student in school, worked hard, and earned high grades. She completed 2 years of college but, at her mother's insistence that she become financially independent, went to work rather than continue. Eloise identified the following goals for herself: *(a)* to return to work, *(b)* to go back to school to get a better job, and *(c)* to have friends.

Based on observations from Eloise's 1st week in the program, Deshawn and Anita, the OTA, independently completed the TCL (Fig. 3-2). They thought perhaps their ratings might change as they came to know Eloise better but estimated that although Eloise had mastered some subskills at the exploratory level, she needed to learn many of the skills at this level (e.g., seeking new situations and trying new behaviors, revealing feelings, initiating activities) and at the two higher levels.

Eloise was placed in the following psychoeducational classes: managing leisure time, women's sexuality, exploring careers, and assertiveness training. Before attending the classes, she completed the pretest for each curriculum of instruction. In addition to group instruction, Eloise was scheduled for one-on-one practice sessions with Anita to reinforce learned skills and to provide feedback privately, which Eloise found less threatening. Within 2 weeks, as Eloise became more comfortable with her classmates, the one-on-one sessions were discontinued. In the assertiveness training class, with Anita's encouragement, Eloise role-played saying no to her boss and carried out simulated conversations with her mother. She completed many worksheet activities and in-class and homework exercises for the other classes. She kept a diary to monitor her thoughts and actions when interacting with male staff, fellow students, and community members.

A month later Eloise returned to work, having requested and obtained a transfer to the rotating pool of secretaries. At Anita's encouragement, she contacted her women AA acquaintances and set up weekly movie dates with them. Post-tests indicated significant learning in all four educational areas. Eloise's TCL ratings showed consistent performance of exploratory-level subskills (score of 20) and development of many mastery-level skills (score of 17). At the exit interview Eloise said, "I see now that I have been afraid of people and would do anything to earn their approval. I don't have to sleep with guys to make them like me. My job now is to figure out who I am and who I want to be. I'm still scared but not as much as before." Eloise was discharged to the evening and weekend program to continue with vocational exploration.

This case example illustrates how deficient interpersonal and intrapersonal skills (in this case from growing up in an abusive alcoholic family) can undermine a person's adult life. Prior to treatment Eloise was unable to say no to her mother or to men, and she evaluated her own worth primarily by how others responded to her. Consequently, she felt depressed and empty. Initially, she had difficulty participating in the classes and discussions, but the one-on-one sessions with the OTA helped her become more comfortable. In her classes in assertiveness training she learned to say no and to ask for what she wanted. She was able to practice these skills with her classmates. She was encouraged to generalize these skills to life situations (*in vivo*). She developed a strategy of ending phone conversations with her mother as soon as they turned abusive. She was able to ask for a transfer at work, which extricated her from the abusive relationship with her boss. And she identified and began to work toward the goal of returning to college.

## CONCEPTS SUMMARY

1. Many of the problems of people with psychiatric disorders are caused by deficits in skills needed for living.
2. These skill deficits represent faulty learning or failure to learn appropriate and successful strategies.
3. Deficits can be remedied and skills taught via an educational program that includes instruction and opportunity to practice skills.
4. Adoption of a classroom setting and an educational framework encourages clients to adopt the role of student, a valued and functional social role.

5. While instruction may occur in groups, each student has an individualized educational plan and objectives.
6. Practice *in vivo* is used to promote generalization.
7. Measurement of outcomes through post-tests reinforces the standards of an educational environment and allows assessment of the student's progress.

## VOCABULARY REVIEW

**generalization** Defined in "Role Acquisition and Social Skills Training" in this chapter.

**social modeling** Defined in "Cognitive-Behavioral Therapy" in Chapter 2.

**syllabus** A written plan for a course of study, typically including a description, a list of learning objectives, reading and homework assignments, evaluation plan, and a calendar or schedule of instructional events.

**lesson plan** A plan for a session of instruction.

**social reinforcer** Behaviors shown by one person to another that tend to promote the frequency of the desired behavior. Praise is one example.

**behavioral objective** A statement in highly specific and objective terms of the actions that will be seen when a given competency is achieved: "For 3 weeks the student will take her medication as scheduled and will independently arrange for refill of prescriptions."

**pretest** An instrument (quiz or test) used to evaluate a student's level of mastery of specific material before instruction is given.

**post-test** An instrument (quiz or test) used to evaluate a student's level of mastery of specific material following instruction.

## SENSORY INTEGRATION

Sensory integration is a theory and practice model initially developed by the occupational therapist A. Jean Ayres (7) for the treatment of learning disorders in children. It was later applied by Lorna Jean King (36), another occupational therapist, to the treatment of adult patients with chronic schizophrenia. Sensory integration theory is based on neuroscience studies of how the brain operates. Although the underlying neuroanatomy and neurophysiology would be difficult for the entry-level assistant to understand without more knowledge of these fields, the basic concepts and assumptions of sensory integration theory are easy to grasp.

*Sensory integration* is the smooth working together of all of the senses to provide information needed for accurate perception and motor action. We will explore this concept one step at a time. First, the senses include not only the five that are commonly recognized (sight, hearing, taste, smell, and touch) but also proprioception, kinesthesia, and vestibular awareness.

*Proprioception* is the sense that helps us identify where parts of our bodies are even if we cannot see them. For example, you don't have to look under your desk to know where your feet are; you have a built-in sense, proprioception, that keeps you informed of their location and position.

*Kinesthesia,* a related sense, gives us information about movement and position of the body as it changes with muscular effort. To illustrate, when you walk through the snow (or, more pleasantly, through shallow water) your brain is aware of the work involved, which muscles are working, and how to compensate for the changes in resistance. This is something that happens automatically; you do not have to think about it.

*Vestibular awareness* is the sense that detects motion and the pull of gravity during movement. For instance, when you fall while learning to roller skate or ride a bicycle, you know that you have gotten off balance and you have a feeling for what speed you are going and in what direction you are likely to fall. You get this information from your vestibular system, which coordinates sensations of balance, velocity, and acceleration.

Sensory integration combines all of the information from the five basic senses and from kinesthesia, proprioception, and vestibular awareness so that you can accurately interpret what is going on around you and act on it. For example, suppose you are about to cross a busy street. You see the traffic and the lights; hear the cars, trucks, and perhaps sirens; smell the fumes. In addition, you feel the pressure of your feet on the concrete and sense where your body weight is centered. You have a sense of how fast you are moving forward and of whether the surface under your feet is level and smooth. To cross the street safely, you have to receive all of this information, interpret it correctly, and act on it accordingly. If a siren gets louder, you must look for the source of it to learn whether you can cross safely when the light is with you.

We do not usually give much thought to the complex neurological, sensory, and perceptual processing that supports everyday actions like this. This is not the case, however, with learning-disabled children and some persons with schizophrenia. King (36) hypothesized that persons diagnosed as having the chronic type of schizophrenia suffer from a proprioceptive deficit, a disturbance in the sense of where the body is in space. She further suggested that this proprioceptive disturbance causes other observable symptoms, such as difficulties in perception, problems with body image, and motor incoordination.

Before discussing the physical signs and symptoms of this proprioceptive defect, one must appreciate some of the difficulties faced by the person with chronic schizophrenia. Corbett (12) vividly describes how he imagines the chronic schizophrenic experiences the world when he talks about a patient who walked hunched over with his hands holding his head because he believed the ceiling was only 2 inches away.

Imagine for yourself, then, what it would be like to live in a world where sensation and perception are unreliable. All of a sudden things feel very strange. Your clothing hurts. The sidewalk seems to be rising up at you. Ordinary smells seem overpowering. Your fork feels like it's made of some spongy material, and it gets bigger and bigger when you bring it to your mouth. Your tongue feels so large you can't believe it fits inside your mouth. The world moves up and down with every step you take. Memories and ideas come charging at you and feel more real than what is going on around you. When you try to study, the words on the page turn squiggly and you can't make sense of them. Not only that but the sound of the air-conditioner is as loud as a jet plane and you become fascinated by the texture of the paint on the walls and can't concentrate on anything else. You can see that this would be very unpleasant, and it's easy to understand why schizophrenia may interfere with even simple activities.[5]

In addition to these hallucinations and perceptual inconsistencies, persons in a psychotic episode may have problems moving about in the environment, partly because they cannot tell where things are but also because they have to plan every movement consciously. Nothing seems to happen automatically; every action requires conscious effort. For instance, to climb a flight of stairs the person may have to lift each knee deliberately to raise the foot for each step. This phenomenon is known as decomposition of movement, because previously automatic motor behaviors become decomposed, or broken up out of their pattern. General slowing of movement, known as psychomotor retardation, is also common.

King (36) speculated that some persons with schizophrenia have defects in their reception or processing of proprioceptive and vestibular information and that these sensory integrative deficits contribute to or perhaps even cause their psychotic symptoms. On the basis of several research studies demonstrating poor vestibular reactions in

---

[5] Based on descriptions given by Corbett (12).

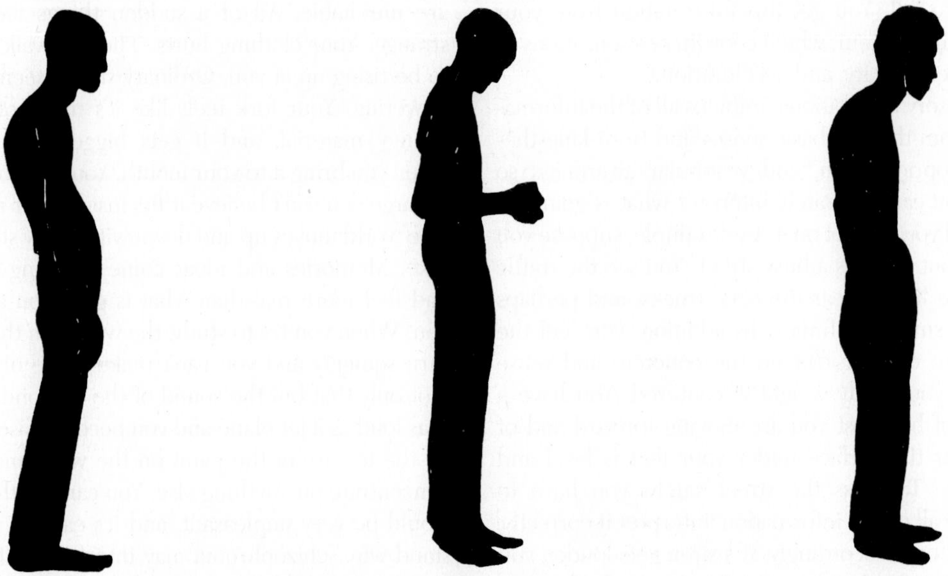

**Figure 3-3. Process schizophrenic postures.** (Reprinted with permission from King LJ. A sensory-integrative approach to schizophrenia. Am J Occup Ther 1974:28:529–536.)

persons with schizophrenia, she hypothesized that a defect in the vestibular or balance system might be the cause of hallucinations and perceptual disturbances. King identified six postural and movement patterns commonly observed in chronic schizophrenia after many years of illness (Fig. 3-3).

- An S-curve posture, in which the head and neck are flexed, the shoulders rounded, the abdomen protruding, and the pelvis tipped forward.
- A shuffling gait, a style of walking with the feet constantly in flat contact with the floor.
- Difficulty raising the arms above the head.
- Inflexibility of the neck and shoulder joints, which prevents the head from rotating or tipping back.
- A resting posture in which the shoulders and hips are flexed, adducted, and internally rotated.
- Various changes in the hand, including weakness of grip, ulnar deviation, and loss of tone and bulk in the muscles acting on the thumb.

King attributed these features to an underlying problem in the central nervous system and demonstrated that a treatment program of gross motor activities could improve mobility. At the same time, she noted that the patients receiving the treatment also spoke more often and more freely, expressed emotion more spontaneously, and attended better to their grooming. From this she concluded that activities designed to stimulate the proprioceptive and vestibular systems might be useful in the treatment of certain types of schizophrenia. Furthermore, King has stated repeatedly that the improvements gained from sensory integrative treatment are permanent because they change the way the central nervous system operates; research has not supported this view, however.

Before we explore the treatment principles and activities that King and others have recommended, it should be noted that sensory integrative treatment has been found effective only in persons with certain diagnoses. King recommends its use with all schizophrenias except the paranoid type. She has used it with depressed adolescents but does not think it suitable for persons with mania (52). It has been attempted with clients who have dementia with no evidence of significant therapeutic benefit (58). Because of its powerful and occasionally unpredictable effects on the central nervous system, a sensory integrative treatment program must be designed and monitored by a occupational therapist. Assistants can help by carrying out the treatment once it is designed. At present, there is no conclusive research evidence to support the use of this model with the psychiatric population, although it seems to show positive effects with pediatric learning-disabled clients (67).

Two major treatment principles should be kept in mind when choosing activities and carrying out a sensory integrative program. The first is that attention should be focused on the outcome of the activity or on the objects used in it rather than on the movements. In other words, the person must move without having to think about it. For example, if a ball is thrown at someone, he moves. He may try to catch it or just dodge it, but in either case he moves quickly and without much conscious deliberation (36). In contrast, to learn tap dancing, a person must consciously observe, think out, and imitate a motor pattern demonstrated by the teacher. Some activities that focus attention on objects or outcomes include stepping or jumping over ropes placed close to the ground, playing with a parachute or balloons, tossing a large ball overhead, walking a balance beam, spinning in a desk chair, noncompetitive ball games, and obstacle courses (36, 57). These and other activities are discussed in more detail in Chapter 22.

The second treatment principle is that the activity must be pleasurable. The person should have fun doing it, as evidenced by smiles, laughter, or playful behavior (36). This can be facilitated by staff members themselves showing pleasure in the activity. People with chronic schizophrenia are likely to have failed at many things in their lives and consequently have fragile self-esteem. Staff should avoid criticizing or trying to improve clients' performance and should focus instead on helping the clients enjoy themselves, praising their efforts, and having a good time themselves.

The goal of any particular sensory integration program depends on the needs of the clients. In general, however, these programs are directed at five main areas: balance, posture, range of motion, spontaneity of motion, and correction of abnormal hip and shoulder positions. The following are examples of activities that are suitable for or that can be adapted to meet these goals:

- *Balance.* Activities that incorporate hopping, skipping, or standing on one foot. Where available, bicycle riding, cross-country skiing, and roller skating can also be effective provided the clients are capable of attempting them safely.
- *Posture.* Activities that require straightening the back and lifting the head, such as holding up a parachute or throwing a ball into the air.
- *Increased range of motion.* Many ball games and housework activities (e.g., sweeping) can be adapted to improve range of motion.
- *Spontaneity of movement.* Activities that are varied and not entirely predictable and that incorporate chance and surprise, such as follow-the-leader. Clients can be instructed to take turns being the leader or to make up their own variations.
- *Correction of abnormal adduction, flexion, and internal rotation.* Activities that use the opposite motions are needed. Abduction, extension, and external rotation of the shoulder occur when the parachute is lifted over the head and increase if the hands are held apart from each other. Shaking out bedclothes and throwing a beach ball also involve these motions.

To summarize, sensory integration aims to improve the reception and processing of sensory information within the central nervous system. Vestibular stimulation and gross motor exercises are the preferred activities. To be effective, activities must be pleasurable and not require conscious attention to body movement. Although appealing and exciting, sensory integration meets only some of the needs of persons with schizophrenia, who also need training in daily living, recreational, and vocational skills (52). The following case example illustrates sensory integrative treatment.

CASE EXAMPLE

## Richard

Richard, 18 years old, is an inpatient in a state psychiatric hospital. His diagnosis is psychotic disorder not otherwise specified (NOS). He has been hospitalized since age 14 because his violent temper tantrums cannot be controlled with medication. Because of this, he could not remain in the community residence for emotionally disturbed children where he had lived since age 8. Richard's mother placed him there because she could not control him; he was physically abusive and frequently threw things. He twice bit her so badly that she needed emergency treatment. She says that he was always a difficult child; even as an infant he was floppy and unresponsive and had trouble sucking.

Richard's behavior in the hospital has been erratic. At times he is fairly calm but unresponsive to people around him; he says he is dead and appears to be hallucinating. At other times he makes wild animal noises and attempts to bite and claw staff and patients. His hygiene is very poor; nursing staff are somewhat afraid of him and reluctant to help him with bathing and grooming. Forward flexion of the neck as well as protraction, internal rotation, and limited flexion of the shoulder all combine to limit his ability to raise his arms to carry out grooming and hygiene of the head, neck, and back.

Paulo, the OT in charge of rehabilitation services for Richard's unit, thought he might benefit from a sensory integration treatment program. A behavior modification program attempted over 8 months had produced no improvement. Richard was not cooperative during the evaluation, which consisted of a test of postrotatory nystagmus, gait analysis, drawing double circles on a chalkboard, and imitation of postures. Evaluation took several sessions. Results showed deficits in bilateral motor coordination, a flat-footed gait, and rigidity and limited range of motion in the neck, trunk, hip, and shoulder joints. Richard refused to complete the test of postrotatory nystagmus or the imitation of postures. At times he appeared tactile defensive, jumping when touched. On the basis of the evaluation, Paulo selected the following treatment goals:

- Increase range of motion in the neck, trunk, hips, and shoulders so that Richard gains enough functional range of motion to bathe, dress, and groom himself independently.
- Increase tolerance of others, as evidenced by staying in a group of three (including therapist) for 15 minutes without violent behaviors, so that Richard can be placed in groups to address his other rehabilitation needs.
- Develop other behaviors needed for discharge and community placement.

Paulo instructed Alan, the OTA, in the specific treatment activities, approaches, and techniques for Richard's program. With this supervision and direction, Alan carried out the program, which included mirror play, rolling in a parachute and blankets, tossing a ball overhead and later into a hoop, kickball, and swimming. Treatment, which was one on one, occurred daily for 30 to 45 minutes. Activities were rotated; some (e.g., swimming) occurred only once a week, whereas others (e.g., rolling in blankets) were done almost daily.

After 3 weeks of treatment, Richard appeared more alert and seemed calm enough to be placed in a low-level task skills group. Although he had one serious violent outburst, he was able to tolerate the group. He began to bathe at least every other day and was able to dress himself, shave, and comb his hair. He continued his individual treatment with Alan for 2 more months, during which time sessions were gradually tapered off and replaced with a sensorimotor activities group. In this group Richard is learning to play various noncompetitive games with the other 20 patients and the staff.

Richard's social worker now believes that community placement is a realistic goal and is trying to find an appropriate facility. Paulo has placed Richard in a prevocational training group with the goal of preparing him for employment in a sheltered workshop.

Although this example shows the dramatic improvement sensory integrative treatment can achieve for some, not all patients react so positively or improve so quickly. Some clients do not respond at all for several months but begin to change slowly if treatment is continued (37). Some patients do not improve at all.

The effectiveness of sensory integration for persons with schizophrenia has little research support. In a review of the literature, Hayes and co-workers (20) conclude that little evidence has been found to show improvement in patients' conditions. Reisman and Blakeney (56), in a study of only five patients, demonstrated significant improvement in measures of ward behavior (social interest and reduction of psychopathology) following sensory integrative treatment of just a few weeks' duration. Additional research is needed.

Occupational therapy for sensory integrative dysfunction requires extensive evaluation, which must be selected by the OT and carried out by an OT or by a OTA under an OT's supervision. In addition, the AOTA has taken the position that therapists desiring to use sensory integrative techniques should receive advanced training, because sensory integration is based on more advanced knowledge than is provided in entry-level professional education programs (24).

The role of the OTA within sensory integrative treatment will vary with location, availability of occupational therapists, and the results of future research within existing treatment programs. Certainly, the assistant is not qualified to initiate a program but may be trained by a skilled and appropriately trained therapist to carry out treatment activities and to perform structured parts of evaluations.

## CONCEPTS SUMMARY

1. Successful motor output depends on accurate reception and interpretation of sensory input.
2. Persons with nonparanoid schizophrenia and other types of chronic psychiatric illness may suffer from a defect in reception or processing of proprioceptive and vestibular input.
3. This sensory integrative defect may cause or contribute to other psychiatric symptoms, such as hallucinations, lack of perceptual constancy, psychomotor retardation, and decomposition of movement.
4. Some persons with chronic schizophrenia have visible postural and movement abnormalities such as poor balance, shuffling gait, an S-curved posture, weakness of grip and atrophy of hand muscles, immobility of the neck and trunk, difficulty raising the arms overhead, and a tendency to hold the hips and shoulders in a flexed, adducted, and internally rotated position.
5. Activities that provide increased vestibular, tactile, and proprioceptive input can help reorganize the way the central nervous system organizes and interprets sensory input.
6. Activities selected for a sensory integrative treatment program should not involve conscious attention to movement but should focus instead on the objects used or on the outcome.
7. Activities selected for a sensory integrative treatment program should be pleasurable and should be presented in a noncompetitive, unpressured, and cheerful manner.
8. Improvements gained from sensory integrative treatment are permanent because they involve a change in the way the central nervous system operates.

### VOCABULARY REVIEW

**sensory integration** The process of receiving and organizing sensory information within the central nervous system.

**proprioception** The sensory mechanism for locating body parts in space without visual clues.

**kinesthesia** The sensory mechanism for receiving information about gravity and the weight of body parts and other objects during movement.

**vestibular awareness** The sensory mechanism for receiving information about balance, velocity, and acceleration of the body.

**body image** An internalized image of oneself, one's physical size and attractiveness, and other qualities, such as coordination.

**perceptual constancy** Learned ability to recognize different objects regardless of their position or context. In other words, the ability to see the world and the objects in it as relatively predictable, based on experience.

**decomposition of movement** A symptom associated with psychotic illness in which complex movements are no longer performed automatically but are broken up into their parts.

**corticalization of movement** A symptom associated with psychotic illnesses in which movement requires conscious effort and deliberate planning rather than being automatic or involuntary.

**psychomotor retardation** A general slowing of movement seen in some psychotic illnesses.

**vestibular stimulation** Sensory input to the balance system. Such input may include rocking, spinning, and other movement.

**postrotatory nystagmus** Rapid eye movements normally occurring immediately after vestibular stimulation that includes rotation.

**bilateral motor coordination** The ability to perform activities that involve the use of both sides of the body, particularly when the two sides perform different motions, as in swimming or tying one's shoes.

**tactile defensiveness** A syndrome in which the person has an aversive response to being touched. Touch is perceived as unpleasant (59).

## COGNITIVE DISABILITIES

The theory of cognitive disabilities, developed by occupational therapist Claudia Kay Allen, focuses on the effect of impaired cognition—a frequent symptom of psychiatric disorders—on task performance (1–3, 5). The central concept is that some people with psychiatric and neurological disorders suffer from a disturbance in the mental functions that guide motor actions. (We have already discussed some of the perceptual disturbances that accompany schizophrenia.) Allen states that "just as physical disabilities restrict the physical ability to do a voluntary motion action, a cognitive disability restricts the cognitive ability to do a voluntary motor action" (2). In other words, a person's mental disorganization can impair performance of tasks such as leather lacing and getting dressed.

Allen believes that the reason some persons with psychiatric diagnoses cannot perform these activities correctly is that they have a cognitive disability. She further states that cognitive disabilities may prevent some people from successfully adapting to life outside a hospital or supervised living situation. In other words, task performance, even on seemingly unrelated tasks such as crafts, reflects ability to function and to take ordinary care in the community. Persons with impaired task performance may be at risk of injury to self or others because they do not understand cause and effect and do not anticipate ordinary dangers, such as fire danger from storing too many flammable objects in the home (5). One might question whether crafts are the best task to test performance; why not use ordinary familiar activities, such as dressing or cooking? Allen uses crafts precisely because they are unfamiliar to many people. Familiar tasks may have been overlearned—that is, practiced so frequently that they have become habits. An unfamiliar task, such as a craft, gives a better measure of how well the person can solve problems and process new information.

To appreciate the subjective experience of a cognitive disability, think of how you feel when you have a fever. Everything seems extraordinarily difficult; it is hard to make sense of what people are saying; studying for a test may be impossible; even following the dialogue on a television show can be a challenge. This is the sort of experience people with cognitive disabilities have all the time. Cognitive disability can occur to various degrees with diagnoses such as schizophrenia, affective disorders, dementia, substance abuse, traumatic brain injury, and cerebral vascular accidents.

Allen (2) originally defined six levels of cognitive ability and disability related to task performance. These range from level 1 (severe impairment) to level 6 (no impairment). These have been further expanded into 26 modes, permitting greater sensitivity in rating task performance. A decimal system organizes the modes within the original six levels (e.g., level 4.4, level 5.0) (4). For simplicity's sake, the following discussion is limited to the original six levels.

Those functioning at levels 1 through 4 have difficulty living unassisted in the community because they cannot perform the necessary routine tasks, such as paying bills, obtaining adequate nourishment, and finding their way to an unfamiliar place. The lower the cognitive level, the more difficulty the person has and the more assistance he or she requires.

Cognitive level is assessed by observing the motor actions the person performs during a task and by inferring the sensory cue that the person was paying attention to at the time. In other words, the therapist watches what the person does (motor action) and tries to identify what sensory information provoked or started that action. The sensory cues progress from internal at the lowest cognitive levels to external and more complex and abstract at the higher levels. Motor actions are automatic at the lowest level and become more refined at higher levels. Table 3-2 outlines the motor actions and associated sensory cues for the six levels.

Identification of a person's cognitive level requires careful evaluation, which must be interpreted by an OT, although the OTA may be asked to perform some parts of the evaluation. Instruments used in this model include the Routine Task Inventory 2 (RTI-2), the Cognitive Performance Test (CPT), the Allen Cognitive Level Screening (ACLS) test, the Large Allen Cognitive Level Screening (LACLS) test, and the Allen Diagnostic Module (ADM). The RTI-2 is an activities of daily living screening instrument that covers 32 specified tasks and 8 unspecified ones in which the person's performance is to be observed or reported. The RTI-2 may be completed by any of three methods: patient's self-report, caregiver's report, or observation of performance. The RTI-2 may not provide an accurate assessment of cognitive level because daily practice and habitual performance make many tasks routine and habitual. The tasks are shown in Table 3-3. For each of the tasks, the behaviors typical of the cognitive levels are described. For example, using a map is typical of level 6 and not knowing one's destination is characteristic of level 3. The RTI-2 may yield a falsely high score because performance of activities of daily living does not involve new learning. The RTI-2, which can be administered by an OTA, is discussed further in Chapter 15.

Individuals scoring at or estimated to be capable of scoring at levels 3 through 5 on the RTI-2 may be evaluated with the Allen Cognitive Level (ACL) test. The person is asked to imitate the therapist's demonstration of leather lacing stitches, graded in complexity from the running stitch (level 3) to the single cordovan stitch (level 5). A person's performance on this test must be interpreted cautiously because visual deficits and drug side effects can need care & supervision for safety

**TABLE 3-2 COGNITIVE LEVELS: MOTOR ACTIONS AND ASSOCIATED SENSORY CUES**

| ACTION | LEVEL 1: AUTOMATIC ACTIONS | LEVEL 2: POSTURAL ACTIONS | LEVEL 3: MANUAL ACTIONS | LEVEL 4: GOAL-DIRECTED ACTIONS | LEVEL 5: EXPLORATORY ACTIONS | LEVEL 6: PLANNED ACTIONS |
|---|---|---|---|---|---|---|
| Spontaneous motor actions | Automatic | Postural | Manual but not goal directed | Goal directed | Exploratory (experimentation, trial and error) | Planned |
| Imitated motor actions | None | Approximate imitations | Manual or manipulative | Copy or reproduction of an example, rote learning | New steps are imitated | Often unnecessary; actions can be initiated without demonstration |
| Examples of motor action | Sniffing, withdrawal from noxious stimuli, swallowing | Walking, gesturing, calisthenics | Picking up or touching objects, stringing beads | Chopping carrots, sanding wood | Spacing of tiles, blending of makeup colors | Budgeting, building a project from a diagram |
| Attention to sensory cues (inferred from observation) | Subliminal (dimconscious awareness) | Proprioceptive (movements and position of body), effects of gravity | Tactile (touchable cues), objects that can be touched and moved | Visible (what is not in plain sight is ignored) | Related (relations between two visible cues) | Symbolic (abstract or intangible) |
| Examples of sensory cues | Hunger, thirst, or discomfort | Posture, gesture, motion | Texture, shape | Color, size, discomfort | Overlapping, color mixing, spatial relations | Evaporation, electrical current,heat, time, gravity |

Adapted with permission from Allen CK. Occupational Therapy for Psychiatric Diseases: Measurement and Management of Cognitive Disabilities. Boston: Little, Brown, 1985:34.

**TABLE 3-3 ACTIVITIES ANALYZED ON RTI-2 AS BEHAVIOR DISABILITIES**

| 10 SELF-AWARENESS DISABILITY | 11 SITUATIONAL AWARENESS DISABILITY | 12 OCCUPATIONAL ROLE DISABILITY | 13 SOCIAL ROLE DISABILITY |
|---|---|---|---|
| .0 Grooming | .0 Housekeeping | .0 Planning, doing major role activities | .0 Communicating meaning |
| .1 Dressing | .1 Obtaining, preparing food | .1 Planning, doing spare time activities | .1 Following instructions |
| .2 Bathing | .2 Spending money | .2 Pacing and timing actions | .2 Contributing to family activities |
| .3 Walking, exercising | .3 Shopping | .3 Exerting effort | .3 Caring for dependents |
| .4 Feeding | .4 Doing laundry | .4 Judging results | .4 Cooperating with others |
| .5 Toileting | .5 Traveling | .5 Speaking | .5 Supervising independent people |
| .6 Taking medications | .6 Telephoning | .6 Following safety precautions | .6 Keeping informed |
| .7 Using adaptive equipment | .7 Adjusting to change | .7 Responding to emergencies | .7 Engaging in good citizenship |
| .8 Other | .8 Other | .8 Other | .8 Other |
| .9 Unspecified | .9 Unspecified | .9 Unspecified | .9 Unspecified |

*RTI-2,* Routine Task Inventory 2.

impair performance (2). An enlarged version, the LACLS, with larger, more widely spaced holes and larger lacing material that is more easily grasped is also available to be used with the elderly and with persons with poor vision. An OTA who has established service competency may administer any of these tests. The CPT evaluates cognitive level by observing the patient's performance in structured tasks, such as dressing for wet weather, shopping, and making toast. Although it is recommended that the CPT be administered by an OT, the OTA may develop service competency after sufficient supervised practice.

The ADM was developed to provide alternative tasks to evaluate and reevaluate cognitive levels and to avoid the practice effect (tendency to perform better as the task is practiced) of repeated use of the ACLS and LACLS. The ADM offers 29 activities that have been analyzed and clinic tested against the 52 modes. An ADM task such as placing mosaic tiles can be used to verify an ACL score obtained by one of the other instruments, and the variety of ADM tasks allows for tracking changes in cognitive level (e.g., when medications take effect).

Allen describes each of the levels in great detail. Only an OT can use this model to evaluate the person and plan interventions. The assistant may conduct parts of the evaluation and may carry out the treatment. The following descriptions, which are brief, summarize and illustrate only the six original levels (2, 5):

- *Level 1.* The person seems mostly unaware of what is going on and may be in bed with the side rails up. The person pays attention for only a few seconds but carries out automatic habitual motor routines, such as self-feeding when food is presented. The patient is very slow to respond to the therapist's request or cue but may respond by rolling over or holding up a hand, for example.
- *Level 2.* The person seems to be aware of movement and position and of the effects of gravity. The person sits and initiates some gross motor actions. Someone at this level is not aware of social context and may wander off. The person may assume bizarre positions or perform strange-looking movements.
- *Level 3.* At this level the person is interested in what is going on. Easily distracted by objects in the environment, the person enjoys touching them and manipulating them. The person engages in a simple repetitive craft or other activity but is likely to be surprised to see that something has been produced. The person has difficulty understanding cause and effect except in his or her own simple actions. The person may be easily disoriented and may get lost. Figure 3-4 illustrates the repetitive actions of a person at level 3, who would not stay focused on the task of setting the table and would instead enjoy repeating the placing of utensils in a line.
- *Level 4.* The person is able to copy demonstrated directions presented one step at a time; can visualize the goal of making something; and is interested in doing simple two-dimensional projects, such as mosaic tile trays with a checkerboard pattern. However, the person does not plan for such details as spacing between the tiles. The person tends to rely on prior learning and finds it easier to imitate a sample than to follow a diagram or picture. The person cannot recognize errors and may not be able to correct them when they are pointed out. The person does not understand that objects can be hidden from view (e.g., may not look under the bed for shoes). Similarly, the person does not notice glue sticking to the bottom of a tile tray.
- *Level 5.* The person shows interest in the relationships between objects. However, the relationships must be concrete and obvious. Some examples are overlapping edges in paper folding or woodwork, space between tiles, and matching colors in makeup or clothing. The person is interested in the effects that can be produced using the hands and may vary the pressure or the speed of hand motions. The person can generally perform a task involving three familiar steps and one new one. New steps must be demonstrated. The person at level 5 may appear careless because of inability to anticipate the possible consequences of actions. For example, the person may damage a garment when removing the price tag or label by pulling too hard or cutting through the fabric. The person who functions at level 5 may benefit from social skills training to improve attention to the nuances of expected social behavior. Allen believes that level 5 is sufficient for a person of lower educational and occupational background to function in the community, although she warns that the level 5 person may not take ordinary and reasonable care regarding the rights of others.
- *Level 6.* The person appreciates the relationships between objects even when they are not obvious. Some examples are anticipating that a dark-colored, hand-dyed garment may bleed when washed and planning ahead to have enough money for infrequent expenses, such as car repairs or doctor bills. At level 6, the person is able to anticipate errors, reason why they may occur, and plan ways to avoid them. Level 6 is associated with higher levels of education, occupational background, and socioeconomic status.

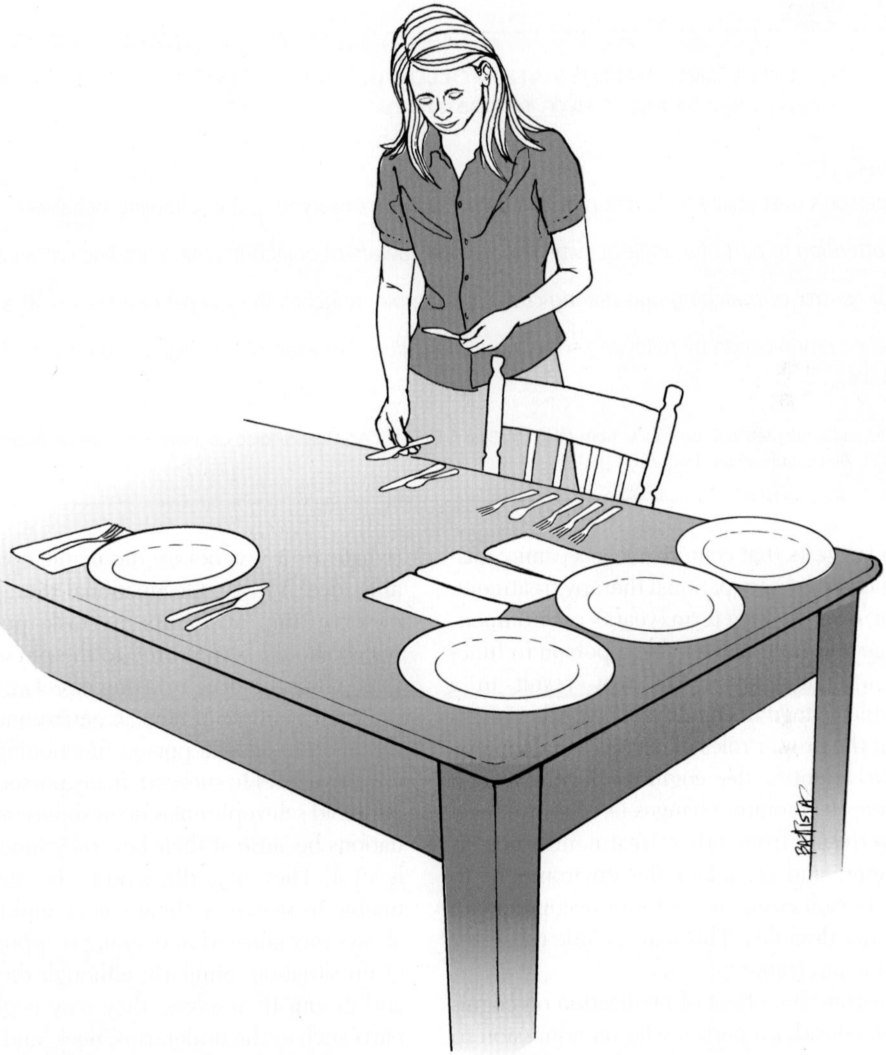

**Figure 3-4. Allen's Level 3.** A repetitive action with disregard for a goal. (Adapted with permission from Allen CK. Occupational Therapy for Psychiatric Diseases: Measurement and Management of Cognitive Disabilities. Boston: Little, Brown, 1985:88.)

Since first publishing in 1985, Allen and colleagues have elaborated the six levels, creating sublevels within them. These sublevels are termed *modes*. Modes are defined in the following format: ". . . pays attention to [_______], motor control of [_______], and verbal communication by [_______]" (4). An example of a mode is given in Box 3-1. The mode shown, 4.2, is the level at which Allen judges a person sufficiently competent for discharge to the street, since the person is able to ask for help.

**BOX 3-1**

## MODE 4.2: ENGAGING ABILITIES AND FOLLOWING SAFETY PRECAUTIONS WHEN THE PERSON CAN DIFFERENTIATE THE PARTS OF THE ACTIVITY

### Abilities

The person's best ability to function at this time has been observed in the following behaviors:

*Pays attention to part of a single activity*, For example, aware of objects in plain sight and within 24 inches.

*Motor control of matching one striking cue*, For example, matches the sample one feature at a time.

*Verbal communication by following social rituals inflexibly*, For example, recognizes the rules of give and take.

Adapted and condensed with permission from Allen CK, Blue T, Earhart CA. Understanding Cognitive Performance Modes. Ormond Beach, FL; Allen Conferences, 1995;77.

Allen suggests that cognitive levels cannot easily be changed by occupational therapy treatment. However, over the long term (years), environmental change and time may enable a person to function at a higher level; this may result in a measurable change in cognitive level. Allen maintains that the proper roles of occupational therapy are to *(a)* identify the cognitive level through evaluation, *(b)* monitor changes in cognitive level that may result from other treatments such as medications, and *(c)* adapt the environment to help the person compensate for or accommodate to his or her disability. This may include caregiver instruction and training.

To illustrate the effect of medication on cognitive level, consider a person who on admission to an inpatient service is overactive, has trouble concentrating even for brief periods, is distracted by objects in the environment, and has little awareness of his or her own effect on others but is able to do repetitive manual tasks like stringing beads. Such behavior, which is characteristic of level 3, is typical of a person with mania. Someone with this diagnosis may be given lithium carbonate; when this drug reaches therapeutic levels, the person's cognitive level returns to the premorbid level (whatever it was before the manic episode, probably level 5 or 6). Occupational therapy staff can observe improvements in task performance, which should be reported to the physician as evidence that the drug is taking effect (2).

As an example of how an environment must be modified to allow a person functioning at a lower cognitive level to succeed, many persons with nonparanoid schizophrenias need supervised living situations because at their best they function only at level 4. They may dress oddly because they are unable to match clothing colors, and they do not always recognize what clothing is appropriate for a given situation. Similarly, although they can wash and groom themselves, they may neglect hidden parts such as the underarms, neck, and back of the head. They may burn themselves on hot cooking equipment and cannot budget money and pay bills. They may not be able to manage their own medication, forgetting to take pills or to get prescriptions refilled. For all of these and many other reasons they need assistance and supervision. Depending on what is available, the person may live in a group home or supervised residence or in an apartment with other clients. In the latter case, daily visits from a supervisor are advisable.

Another example of environmental modification or compensation is setting up supplies and tools for activities in a manner that allows for the person's disability. At levels 3 and 4 patients are easily distracted by anything visible. Consequently, supplies that are not needed until the later stages of an activity should be placed on a separate table. Also, patients should have individual sets of their own tools and supplies. By contrast, at level 5 a person can be expected to share tools and to focus only on the supplies needed for the current step, although supplies for other steps may be present. An extended discussion of how to modify activities, the task environment, and the manner of presentation for patients using the Allen Cognitive Level system appears in Chapter 23.

Allen's theory of cognitive disabilities is summarized in nine propositions (2):

1. *"The observed routine task behavior of disabled patients will differ from the observed behavior of nondisabled populations."* Persons with cognitive disabilities perform less well than others in activities needed for independent community living.
2. *"Limitations in task behavior can be hierarchically described by the cognitive levels."* In other words, the degree of disability is more severe at level 4 than at level 5, at level 3 than at level 4, and so on.
3. *"The choice of task content is influenced by the diagnosis and the disability."* Although people functioning at level 6 typically prefer some balance of work, self-care, and leisure activities, those functioning at lower levels may find work too difficult and prefer crafts instead. Crafts allow lower-functioning persons to produce something tangible as a result of their efforts; these tangible products may compensate in some way for the loss of self-esteem from not being able to work in competitive employment.
4. *"The task environment may have a positive or a negative effect on a patient's ability to regulate his or her own behavior."* In general, tasks that are unstructured and creative tend to make lower-functioning persons feel worse. Because the directions are not clear, those who lack good internal organization have no way to organize their efforts and may become confused and frightened. An example is asking someone like Richard (previous case example) to draw a picture of himself. He is likely to reject the task totally, to perform it in a perfunctory fashion (by drawing a stick figure, for example), or to produce something bizarre that reflects his hallucinations and other symptoms (for example, drawing a huge mouth with jagged teeth). When someone appears uncomfortable with a task because it is beyond his or her capabilities, the therapist should adjust the directions or the steps involved and sometimes should substitute a different task altogether.
5. *"People with cognitive disabilities attend to those elements of the task environment that are within their range of ability."* This is another way of saying that persons ignore whatever they do not understand or cannot make sense of. For example, those functioning at level 4 or 5 cannot be expected to construct a project from a three-dimensional plan, such as a working drawing or mechanical diagram; they have not the slightest idea of how to proceed from such directions, although this would be a reasonable task for someone at level 6. Similarly, persons at level 4 may not recognize that they can get up and look in a closet or ask the therapist for a tool; because they cannot see the tool, they assume it does not exist or is unavailable.
6. *"Therapists can select and modify a task so that it is within the person's range of ability through the application of task analysis."* In other words, the therapist can restructure the directions, materials, or nature of the activity so that the person can perform it. As an example, when

teaching the sanding of wooden kits, the therapist can expect persons at level 6 to sand with the grain once the concept of grain is explained. Persons at level 5 can be told to sand up and down, the long way or other similar wording; after a few experiences of sanding and more verbal instruction, they should be able to understand and apply the concept of grain. Persons at level 4, on the other hand, because they can follow only demonstrated directions presented one at a time, have to be shown the motion to use with the sandpaper. They have to be instructed to turn the project over and sand the other side. Persons functioning at level 3 can sand once the motion is demonstrated but may sand back and forth as well as up and down and have difficulty learning to sand in just one direction. Similarly, unless the therapist or assistant intervenes, they may continue sanding until they have reduced the project to toothpicks, because they do not recognize the purpose of the sanding or that they should stop at a given point.

7. *"An effective outcome of occupational therapy services occurs when successful task performance is accompanied by a pleasant task experience."* In other words, the therapist or assistant should help patients feel good about what they have done, both during the process and afterward. In part, this is achieved by presenting only achievable tasks. A person faced with a task that is too difficult is likely to feel overwhelmed, ashamed, frustrated, or angry. Sometimes it is helpful to select an activity that the person has performed well in the past and feels good about. When a new task is introduced, it should be analyzed and presented at the person's level of comprehension (see proposition 5).
8. *"Steps in task procedures that require abilities above a person's level of ability will be refused or ignored."* This is self-explanatory. Someone who cannot do something will find a way to avoid it. For example, a person at level 4, when shown how to braid the upper edge of a basket, instead substitutes a less involved finishing method, such as making simple loops. He or she cannot follow the over, under multistrand demonstration of braiding.
9. *"The assessment of the cognitive level can contribute to the legal determination of competency."* Because persons functioning at level 4 or below have identifiable problems that prevent them making sound judgments about their own welfare, assessment of a person's cognitive level may be useful in a court of law. Persons at level 1 and 2 typically behave so bizarrely that their disabilities are obvious, but the person functioning at level 3 or 4 may appear reasonably intact, especially if he or she has good verbal skills. At these levels of disability, there is serious question about a person's competence to manage financial affairs or to stand trial for a crime.

In summary, the theory of cognitive disabilities provides a system for classifying a person's ability to carry out routine tasks needed for successful community adjustment. The theory provides instruments for evaluation of cognitive level and prescriptions for how to modify tasks, environment, levels of assistance, and therapeutic approach for those with levels of disability that are incompatible with independent functioning. The following case example illustrates the theory of cognitive disabilities:

**CASE EXAMPLE**

## Marvin[7]

Marvin has been hospitalized twice in the past month. On the last admission, his diagnosis was adjustment disorder, based on his report of a recent separation from his wife. During the current admission, it was learned that Marvin and his wife have been separated for 5 years, that his wife lives out of state, and that Marvin is concerned about his two children. He has threatened to harm his wife. The social worker has

[7] This case is adapted from case example 17 in Allen (2).

been unable to locate Marvin's wife or anyone else who can verify his story.

Marvin is 45 years old, tall, overweight, and sloppily dressed. He needs a shave. He says that he knows eight foreign languages, which he learned in his 20 years as a business consultant. He is able to speak some of them, according to staff fluent in foreign languages. His diagnosis is major depressive episode with suicidal ideation. On the ward, he has shown a good appetite at meals, has slept soundly, and does not appear depressed. Marvin scored at level 3 on the Allen Cognitive Level test. He was placed in a basic skills group. During his first week in this group the following behaviors were observed:

- When asked to cut apart strips of mailing labels, he held the scissors upside down but was able to perform the task.
- When asked to cut rags into 7-inch squares, given a sample, he cut pieces of varying sizes ranging from 10 to 18 inches. None of the pieces was square. When this error was pointed out to him, Marvin apologized and his eyes appeared wet. He then tried to correct his error by trimming the edges but did not attempt to trace the sample size on to the squares or otherwise measure them.
- After satisfactorily completing a découpage project, Marvin attempted to attach the hanger to the front of the plaque but had the attachment prongs facing up and was using the round end of a ball-peen hammer.

In accordance with the misuse of scissors and hammer and the failure to recognize the proper positioning of the hanger, the OT recommended that the patient be evaluated for organic brain syndrome. Misuse of common tools is not usually seen in depression but is often a feature of organic mental disorders. Marvin's teary-eyed apology for cutting the rags incorrectly was seen as evidence to support the diagnosis of depression. The therapist also recommended that Marvin be placed in supervised living because he was indeed functioning at mode 3.4.

As this case example illustrates, assessment of cognitive level is very useful for diagnostic and discharge planning purposes.

In the two decades since Allen first published her theory, research and development have supported and developed some aspects of this practice model (14, 15, 25, 44, 51, 54, 62). In addition, Allen and colleagues have provided detailed and specific treatment guidelines for persons at each level (4, 5, 40–42); the model seems most often used with regressed persons who have dementia. Chapter 23 explores some of the basic guidelines.

The Allen Cognitive Level model has been criticized by some clinicians for inadequately considering the capacity of the severely impaired to improve in function over time. The brain is remarkably plastic (able to reshape itself and to recover functions after injury) even in adult life. It appears that functional abilities and cognitive levels do increase for many persons in the months and years following injury and that these increases are not owing to medication or other somatic intervention. This is true of persons with traumatic brain injury and also for some of those with severe and persistent mental illness. Many people are uncomfortable with the characterization of persons at levels 5 and 6 and consider that social class and culture account for some behaviors, which may be appropriate in the sociocultural context in which they were acquired.

## CONCEPTS SUMMARY

1. The observed routine task behavior of disabled persons differs from the observed behavior of nondisabled populations.
2. Limitations in task behavior can be hierarchically described by the cognitive levels.
3. The choice of task content is influenced by the diagnosis and the disability.

4. The task environment may have a positive or a negative effect on a person's ability to regulate his or her own behavior.
5. Persons with cognitive disabilities attend to the elements of the task environment that are within their range of ability.
6. Therapists can select and modify a task so that it is within the person's range of ability through the application of task analysis.
7. An effective outcome of occupational therapy services occurs when successful task performance is accompanied by a pleasant task experience.
8. Steps in task procedures that are above a person's level of ability will be refused or ignored.
9. The assessment of the cognitive level can contribute to the legal determination of competency.

## VOCABULARY REVIEW

**cognitive disability** Lack or impairment of ability to carry out motor actions, caused by a disturbance in the thinking processes that direct motor acts. Cognitive disability can be observed in the way a person performs routine tasks.

**cognitive level** The degree to which the mind is capable of responding to task demands. Allen identifies six cognitive levels, ranging from level 1 (severe impairment) to level 6 (no impairment).

**routine tasks** Activities of daily living, such as grooming, dressing, bathing, walking, feeding, toileting, housekeeping, preparing food, spending money, taking medication, doing laundry, traveling, shopping, and telephoning.

**task demands** The degree of complexity present in the materials, tools, and skills needed to perform a task. Task demands vary from simple (eating a sandwich) to complex (providing for adequate income at retirement).

**task abilities** What the person can do successfully; the tasks or parts of tasks that the person can complete adequately in the present state.

**task environment** The people, objects, and spaces in which the person performs a task. Psychological and emotional aspects of the environment must be considered along with physical aspects.

**task directions** Oral, written, or demonstrated instruction about how to perform a task.

**environmental compensation** Modification of the environment to permit successful completion of a task. An example is seating a distractible person away from other people.

**Routine Task Inventory 2 (RTI-2)** A checklist of task behaviors in 32 specified and 8 unspecified categories, used as a guide for observing and classifying a person's task abilities and cognitive level.

**Allen Cognitive Level (ACL) test** An evaluation in which the person is asked to imitate the therapist's demonstration of leather lacing stitches graded in complexity from the running stitch to the single cordovan stitch.

**competence** A legal term meaning having sufficient mental ability to manage one's own financial affairs, safeguard one's own interests, and understand right and wrong.

**practice effect** The tendency to perform better as a task is practiced.

## THE MODEL OF HUMAN OCCUPATION

The *model of human occupation,* developed by Gary Kielhofner and his colleagues beginning in 1976 (9, 30, 31), provides a broad view of human occupation in relation to health. Based on concepts introduced by Mary Reilly and others in the 1960s and 1970s, this model analyzes and describes the development of occupational behavior. It considers the roles of culture and of environment in shaping occupation and addresses specifically the health-maintaining and health-restoring aspects of activity. It emphasizes the effects of choice, interest, motivation, and habits on human activity. The model is particularly useful because it can be applied in all areas of occupational therapy practice and can be combined with other models.

The central organizing principle of the human occupation model is that humans have an innate (inborn) drive to explore and master their environments. A related idea is that doing, exploring, and taking action help organize and maintain us in the world. This process of exploring, creating, and controlling the environment is termed *human occupation.* The natural human tendency to engage in activity and the ways in which this tendency can be nourished or thwarted are what the human occupation model seeks to understand and explain.

This model views the individual as an *open system.* An open system can be affected by things around it (the environment) and can also affect things around it. A pond is an open system: It makes the land around it green with vegetation but can be damaged by chemicals in the runoff from the land. In contrast, a *closed system* cannot affect or be affected by its environment. As an open system, a human acts on the environment, takes in information from the environment, and ignores other information.

By continually acting and receiving information, people change their actions and adapt to their environment. For example, to open a new bottle of prescription medication, a woman might try to turn the cap and discover that this does not work. A family member might suggest that she push down while turning; she may find that this does not work either. Then she might read the directions and take in the information printed on the cap. By carrying out the series of actions described in the directions, she can finally open the bottle. This sequence of taking action, reflecting on information received, and then altering the action to be more effective is essential for developing *occupational adaptation,* which is defined by Kielfhofner as "the construction of a positive occupational identity and achieving occupational competence over time in the context of one's environment" (31, p. 121).

Any single occupational performance will differ from countless similar performances by the same person at other times and may include innovative outcomes and new occupational behaviors. Humans bring to each occupational performance the full depth and complexity of their experience, and the performance changes as a result. In the cap-opening example, the woman might get someone else to open the bottle and then, having had the bottle opened, transfer its contents to a more convenient container. Or she might write a letter to the manufacturer or sit down and sketch a better design idea. In each of these responses, new occupational behaviors emerge. These behaviors are entirely new and not an obvious outcome of the interaction of individual, task, and environment. Occupational behavior is thus continually created.

We are used to thinking of ourselves as actors and as the originators and source of our own occupational behavior. The model of human occupation conceptualizes this somewhat differently: *Occupational behavior is the outcome of an interaction among the person, the occupational task, and the environment.* The person brings to the situation his or her own capacities and inclinations for action, but the task itself and the environment provide opportunities, demands, and constraints that also shape behavior. So, in this sense, the behavior is not our behavior but a product that results from the interaction of the self, the task, and the environment. Minor changes in any of the three variables may result in major changes in occupational behavior. An example is the shift from walking fast to running when trying to catch a bus; a minor change in the speed of the bus (or a change in a traffic light from green to red) will motivate the person to start to run.

Engaging in occupation changes the physical and mental structures of the person who engages in it. For example, over time, the fingers of someone who plays the piano become opened and appear more elongated, smoothly muscled, and sensitive; they look totally different from those of the mechanic, whose hands express years of tool use and appear more heavily muscled, compact, square, and knobbed. Similarly, the experience of writing a research paper in grade school—with its subtasks of reading, taking notes, categorizing, organizing, and writing—becomes part of the mental structure of the student. This first experience of studying and reorganizing a body of information becomes the foundation for performing related tasks in the future; and, with repetition, the process becomes highly elaborated and efficient. Here's another example: When relating to other people, the art of listening and responding is acquired and refined by experience and repeated practice, so that over time it becomes part of an organized and flexible repertoire of conversational and social behavior. All of these examples show the following:

- Experiencing a given occupation increases one's capacity for engaging in it in the future.
- Repeated experience imprints itself into occupational behavior so that it becomes organized in particular patterns.

In other words, we become what we do, and what we do becomes part of us. But how is action or occupational behavior organized? Kielhofner conceptualizes three subsystems (Fig. 3-5) that interact to produce occupational acts (31). People do things because on some level they choose to do so. The first subsystem, *volition,* relates to this aspect of choosing and the reasons for choosing one occupation over another. People also do things because they have established patterns of doing them, and so they do them again and again; the *habituation* subsystem addresses this aspect. Finally, in order to act people must have the capacity to do so, the physical and mental skills that enable performance; this aspect is expressed in the *performance capacity* subsystem. The three subsystems interact with each other and with the task and the environment to produce occupational behavior.

## Volition Subsystem

Volition, or motivation, is often (but not always) the starting point of any action. Each person has a different capacity for motivation, or volition, because of differences in innate interests and talents and in experiences of what happened in the past when the person tried to do things. A person who has a good voice is more likely to pursue a career as a singer than someone who cannot carry a tune. This is what is meant by innate interests and talents. Previous experiences also affect volition. People learn how other people react and what happens when they try certain actions. For example, if our budding singer's mother listens and applauds every performance, the singer is encouraged.

Kielhofner conceptualizes the volition subsystem as consisting of three elements: *personal causation, values,* and *interests.* Personal causation refers to a person's knowledge and beliefs about his or her ability to have an effect on the world. Does he or she expect to do things well? Control his or her own destiny? Succeed when trying new things?

Values are internalized images of what is good, right, and important (31). Values are commitments to action; they clarify what is important in life, and they may carry a strong emotional pressure to act in ways that are consistent with "the right way to behave."

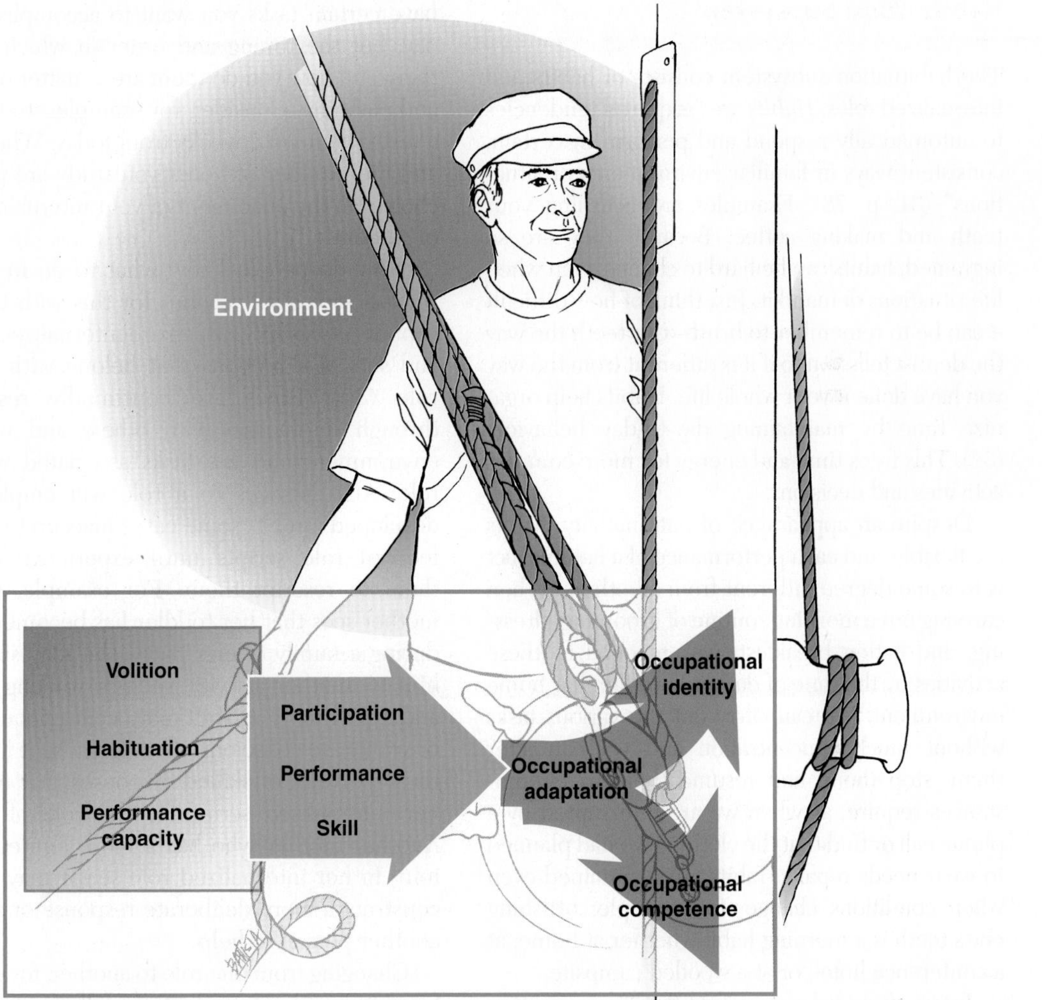


**Figure 3-5. The process of occupational adaptation.** (Adapted with permission from Kielhofner G, ed. A Model of Human Occupation: Theory and Application. 3rd ed. Baltimore: Lippincott Williams & Wilkins, 2002:121.)

Interests are "personal dispositions to find pleasure in certain objects, events, or people" (33). In other words, interests are what people *like.* Interests attract a person to new activities and help broaden and diversify the person's occupational pattern. When people choose an activity that makes them feel good, they feel energized and ready to try other activities. The ability to take pleasure in doing things is just as important to human volition as is the belief in one's own competence (personal causation) and the sense of the importance of one's own efforts (values).

## Habituation Subsystem

The habituation subsystem consists of habits and internalized roles. *Habits* are "acquired tendencies to automatically respond and perform in certain, consistent ways in familiar environments or situations" (31, p. 78). Examples are brushing your teeth and making coffee. Because they are so ingrained, habits can be hard to change even when life situations demand it. Just think of how difficult it can be to remember to brush your teeth the way the dentist tells you to if it is different from the way you have done it your whole life. Habits help organize time by maintaining day-to-day behaviors (32). This frees time and energy for more complex activities and decisions.

Despite an appearance of automaticity, habits are flexible, and each performance of a habitual act is to some degree different from all others. When carrying out a morning routine of grooming, dressing, and eating breakfast, we are cued to these activities by the time of day and our familiar home environment. We can carry out the various tasks without much concentration and yet can alter them, stop them, and resume them as circumstances require, as when we are interrupted by a phone call or find that the clothing we had planned to wear needs repair. Habits are maintained even when conditions change; for example, brushing one's teeth is a morning habit whether at home, at a conference hotel, or at a wooded campsite.

*Internalized roles* represent the "incorporation of a socially and/or personally defined status and a related cluster of attitudes and actions" (31, p. 78). Some examples of occupational roles are worker, student, and homemaker. Each role has certain expected behaviors that go with it; this helps the person construct the behaviors appropriate for the situation. The individual's beliefs and perceptions about these behaviors are the internalized role, which like habits, helps organize daily activities. Internalized roles involve more active choice and decision making than do habits. As a student, you have certain tasks you want to accomplish every day, but the timing and order in which you do them and how you do them are a matter of choice and planning. Consider, for example, studying for a test scheduled 2 weeks from today. When, how, and the number of hours you study are personal choices in the enactment of your internalized role of student.

How do people know what to do in a given role? Sociologists account for this with the concept of *role scripts,* which are internalized images and sets of directions that belong with a given role (30). Roles are continually rescripted through interaction with others and with the environment and the tasks associated with the role. Also, novices to a role will employ less-developed (and in some cases inaccurate or ineffective) role scripts until experience coaches them to rescript them. For example, when a mother sees that her toddler has become restless during a family dinner party, she may shift with him to another activity, such as walking around and exploring. This shift may occur unconsciously or with little conscious effort because it is part of the repertoire of skilled responses that make up her internalized script for the role of parent. Another mother who has a more limited repertoire in her internalized role script may have to construct a more deliberate response or may ask another person to help.

Changing from one role to another, for example from high school student to college student or from homemaker to college student, can be difficult and complex. Role change entails replacing established habits and skills with new ones needed for the new role. Although role change is exciting, it is also stressful and occasionally stressful enough to require psychiatric treatment. One example is the depression and aimlessness that affect some parents (more often women) when their children grow up and leave home. And sometimes a disability forces a role change on someone who might otherwise have continued in an accustomed role.

We have seen that the habituation subsystem consists of habits and internalized roles that organize actions into daily patterns. When behavior is organized in this way, a person's relationship with the social and nonhuman environment is relatively predictable and requires little conscious effort. Not having to think and decide about every aspect of daily activity frees energy for other tasks and involvements.

## Performance Capacity Subsystem

The third subsystem is the performance capacity subsystem, which consists of "the abilities for doing things" (31, p. 81) based on underlying mental and physical capacities and the person's subjective experience of those capacities. In other words, how the person feels about his or her performance affects his or her capacity to perform.

Kielhofner adds to this the concept of the *lived body,* which is the personal experience of understanding and knowing the world through a particular human body. Each person's body is different, with unique talents and capacities and with a history of body experiences. Events, both positive and negative, can affect the body. Examples of such events are athletic training, a traumatic accident, sudden onset of a psychiatric disorder, or a successful experience when attempting something one has never done before (assembling a piece of furniture from a kit). The lived body accumulates experiences and contributes to beliefs about the self.

In summary, the performance capacity subsystem consists of both objective capacity and subjective experience of that capacity.

## Interaction Among the Subsystems

In earlier development of the model of human occupation, the three subsystems were viewed as hierarchical, with the volition subsystem governing the other two (29). In the present model, any of the subsystems can take the lead, depending on circumstances. For example, volition is often the controlling factor; whether or not a person desires to enact a behavior may be the starting point. However, desire may be constrained by limitations in the other subsystems. For example, a person with a C4 spinal cord injury cannot perform grooming and dressing despite the desire to do so and the existence of prior habits. All three subsystems interact and respond to changes in the others, so that an injury to the performance capacity subsystem can impair volition and habits; the person with a spinal cord injury may feel negative and unmotivated because he or she cannot perform customary activities in the habitual way (28).

Similarly, an injury to the volition subsystem can impair the habituation and performance subsystems. A woman who has devoted herself to her husband and has lived her life through his may on his death become very disorganized because her primary motivation is gone.

## The Environment

The environment also influences human occupation. Even subtle changes in the environment can affect the way a person acts—for example, substituting a round table for a long, narrow one increases communication in a group. For optimum occupational performance, the environment should provide the "just-right" level of stimulation. Too little stimulation leads to apathy and mechanical performance; too much causes anxiety and withdrawal. People, objects, noise, color, texture, air quality, and temperature are some examples of environmental features that influence occupational performance. To understand how environment affects performance you need only reflect on the many courses you have taken in school. The teacher, the other students, the furniture, the design and layout of the room, the maps and models and learning aids, and the presence of windows and daylight all influenced your work, although not to an equal extent. Perhaps from your own experience of how environment affected your learning you can gather some ideas about how you might change a person's environment to improve occupational performance.

Improving occupational performance and satisfaction with that performance is the goal of occupational therapy. Although many specific recommendations for evaluation and treatment are discussed in later chapters, none is as important as the underlying principle that unites them. The principle is this: *In an open system, changes in any of the parts change the whole.* In other words, when working with a client who has problems in occupational performance, the therapist and the assistant must be aware that the environment, each of the subsystems, and their components are influencing what is going on (34). If the intervention is to have a positive effect, it has to stimulate a change in the direction of occupational adaptation, behavior that helps the person meet needs and succeed in life situations. How to create this change is a complex question that requires careful analysis; it is best answered by an OT, who has the educational background to evaluate and analyze the subsystems and their relationship to the person's present functioning. The OTA can contribute by carrying out selected portions of the evaluation, participating in the analysis and planning, and performing much of the treatment.

Healthy human occupation occurs in a dynamic relationship with the environment, which ideally should match the interests, skills, and capabilities of the individual. The importance of the environment in shaping behavior cannot be overstated. Kielhofner and colleagues emphatically argue that "the only tool which therapists have at their disposal is to change the relevant environment to support or precipitate a change in the human system" (30, p. 261). We will discuss specific recommendations for changing the environment in later chapters.

CASE EXAMPLE

## Rose

Rose, a 20-year-old mother of two, was admitted to the inpatient psychiatric unit with a diagnosis of depression following a suicide attempt. Over the past 3 weeks, she had begun to neglect the housework and the children. She spent long periods sitting around "thinking." She was able to feed and clothe her two children, a boy aged 4 and a girl aged 2; but she paid little attention to her own grooming. When she was taken to the emergency room by her husband, Larry, her hair was oily and dirty and her clothes were food stained.

Larry and Rose married almost 5 years ago, when she was pregnant with their first child. Because both were still in high school, they lived with Larry's parents until Larry got his diploma; they then moved to a one-bedroom apartment nearby. Since then Larry has been working for his uncle, who installs aluminum siding, and since the birth of the second child he has had a second job pumping gas at night. Rose, who is a year younger than Larry, did not complete high school.

Rose's parents, who are extremely religious, totally disapprove of Rose and Larry and the out-of-wedlock pregnancy. They have not seen Rose since she left their home on her marriage; they have never seen their grandchildren.

During the first day of her hospitalization Rose was quiet and subdued. She isolated herself from other patients but responded when spoken to by them or by staff. After several reminders from nursing, she carried out her morning grooming in a superficial and inattentive manner. She ate little, pushing the food listlessly around on the plate.

The supervising OT, Raquel, assigned James (an OTA) to collect background information. James reviewed Rose's chart, looking through the admitting information, the history, and the nursing notes for any information about Rose's feelings about herself, her interests, past and present roles, habits, and skills.

He then introduced himself to Rose, briefly explained what occupational therapy is and how it might help her, and asked her a series of questions from the *Occupational History Interview* about her childhood, her schooling, and her present life at home. Rose spoke softly, sometimes hesitating, but answered all the questions. She said she was willing to fill out some questionnaires. James left her with the *Role Checklist* to complete on her own. He also gave her a schedule of general activity groups and scheduled a meeting for the following day to collect and review the questionnaires.

Later that same day, after reviewing James's interview notes, Raquel met with Rose and explained that she would be working with James to plan the occupational therapy program. She followed up on some points from James's notes and discussed the *Role Checklist*. She encouraged Rose to talk about her child-care and homemaking responsibilities and asked her about her goals for the hospitalization. The next day, Raquel and James went over the results of all of the evaluations and arrived at the following conclusions:

- *Volition subsystem.* Rose feels that she has no control over her life. She is overwhelmed by the responsibilities of caring for her home and family; she loves her children, but feels she cannot handle them. She checked several group sports activities and computer programming on the interest checklist but says she has no time for these things. On the *Role Checklist* she listed religious participant, friend, and hobbyist as past and future but not present roles.
- *Habituation subsystem.* Rose is having difficulty with her homemaker and child-care roles. She wanted to study computer science in college and to become a computer programmer but now sees this as impossible. She performed well in the student role, completing her junior year in high school despite her advanced pregnancy. She manages her time poorly, not completing household chores before attempting others, does not have a routine schedule for housework, and has trouble managing money (pays bills late, buys unnecessary items).
- *Performance capacity subsystem.* Rose seems to have adequate motor skills but has trouble sequencing and continuing with tasks. She complains that she cannot concentrate. She seems not to plan things before she does them. She is personable and pleasant to others but waits for them to approach her rather than taking the first step (does not initiate or assert). She evaluates her own performance negatively.
- *Environment.* According to both Rose and Larry, her home life is very disorganized. Although Rose rarely leaves home, the small apartment is crowded with furniture, dirty clothes and dishes, unanswered mail, and children's toys. The disorder increased when Rose started to become ill 3 weeks ago. Larry's parents visit about twice a week, and Larry's mother tries to help out but has recently been impatient with Rose, who does not follow through on her advice to keep things organized. Rose and Larry both had friends during high school but have not seen any of them in the past 6 months.

Because Rose's hospitalization insurance allows for only a 1-week stay, Raquel and James arranged for continued care with a community mental health agency that provides occupational therapy services. They contacted a local agency and scheduled an appointment for Rose to visit the center and meet the therapist. James and Rose together outlined a series of goals on which Rose could begin to work while still in the hospital and that she would continue and complete at home:

1. Require that Rose complete self-care routines adequately and on time each day. Increase Rose's sense of self-control by allowing her to choose, with guidance, the occupational therapy groups she will attend during the next few days. Encourage her to try out computer games or simple word processing on the occupational therapy department's computer. Encourage her to discuss her situation with other patients, especially those who are parents, in social groups.
2. Establish a daily routine for self-care, housekeeping, and child care at home, scheduling only necessary tasks and leaving time for leisure.

3. Review Rose's plans for the future. Explore options for her to resume friendships, to return to church activities, and to complete school and help her consider how she might approach these goals.
4. Recommend that the community occupational therapist visit Rose and Larry at home after discharge to evaluate the home environment and discuss ways it could be reorganized. Recommend community follow-up, a parent support group, and a play group for the children. Recommend that Rose be taught streamlined routines for housework and self-care and that she be helped to establish a weekly and seasonal housekeeping and child-care schedule.
5. Support Rose's interest in group sports by helping her explore opportunities for volleyball and softball at the local YWCA and community center.

On the day of discharge, Rose smiled as she said to James, "It seemed so hopeless to me before. Nothing is really different yet, but now I feel like I can make it different. Maybe that's what matters."

This case example illustrates some principles for using the model of human occupation. First, in an open system, all parts affect the others. Requiring Rose to demonstrate adequate self-care routines activates the habituation and performance capacity subsystems. Engaging in these customary occupational routines can support more normal functioning and engagement in other tasks. Second, change in the relevant environment can support or precipitate a change in the human system. Rose's home environment is critical to her ability to become and stay organized; the home visit will provide information so that the therapist can suggest ways to make it more manageable and supportive for Rose. Furthermore, learning simplified housework routines will help her establish efficient habits and will free her time for other pursuits, such as sports or finishing school.

The example also shows the role of the OTA in this model. The assistant carries out the structured parts of the evaluation, gathers data from the medical record, and collaborates with the OT to develop the treatment plan. The OTA works closely with the patient to set treatment goals and schedule activities. Either in the hospital or in the community, the OTA could provide training in household management or leisure planning, could teach child-care and self-care skills, and could help Rose reorganize her home environment.

The model of human occupation gives us a good basic design for understanding the occupational nature of human beings. The description of the model as presented here has been brief and basic and is intended to help the OTA obtain a general sense of the clinical reasoning a therapist might apply to a person's problems. The model itself is much more complex; an entire text has been written to explain it (29–31). In addition, much research has explored the effectiveness of the model and has attempted to develop it further (21, 22, 35, 48) and analyze its value (17). We can expect to witness further changes and growth in the model.

## CONCEPTS SUMMARY

1. Human beings have a natural, inborn tendency to act on the environment, to explore and master it.
2. The human being is an open system. Human beings interact with their environments, affect their environments, and are affected by their environments.
3. Human action in the environment is called human occupation. Human occupation is organized into three subsystems, each of which affects and is affected by the others.
4. One subsystem is volition, or motivation, which initiates action.

5. Another subsystem is habituation, which organizes actions into predictable routines and patterns.
6. The third subsystem is performance capacity, consisting of objective physical and mental capacities for action and the subjective experience of this capacity.
7. Because it is an open system, the system of human occupation is vulnerable to effects from the human and nonhuman environments, which may damage or impair the function of any of the subsystems. These can affect the entire system and can result in problems in occupation. Such problems will benefit from occupational therapy intervention.

## VOCABULARY REVIEW

**open system** Any system that is capable of influencing and being influenced by its environment.

**human occupation** A fundamental aspect of being human, this is the process of exploring, responding to, and mastering the environment through activity. Interactions among the human, the task, and the environment contribute to occupational behavior.

**occupational adaptation** The construction of a positive occupational identity; achieving occupational competence over time in one's environment.

**environment** The human and nonhuman object world in which human occupation is carried out.

**volition** Motivation; the thoughts and feelings that are involved with selecting, enacting, and continuing an occupation or activity.

**personal causation** The individual's sense of his or her own competence and ability to be effective.

**values** Internalized images of what is good, right, and important.

**interests** Personal preferences in activity or people. Interests are pleasurable and motivate actions accordingly.

**habituation** Within the human occupation, the subsystem that contains patterns and routines for organizing actions; these are called habits and internalized roles.

**habits** Automatic or preconscious routines, actions carried out so frequently that they can be done without any conscious effort.

**habit map** An internalized set of rules guiding the carrying out of habits, enabling habitual behavior in different contexts.

**occupational role** A pattern for carrying out productive activity, such as playing child, homemaker, worker, or retiree.

**role script** Internalized images and sets of directions that belong with a given role.

**performance capacity** The subsystem of human occupation that contains the ability to do things.

**lived body** The personal experience of living and doing through a particular human body.

## SUMMARY

This chapter introduces six practice models used by occupational therapy practitioners for interventions with persons who have mental health problems:

- Development of adaptive skills
- Role acquisition and social skills training
- Psychoeducation
- Sensory integration
- Cognitive disabilities
- Model of human occupation

The student or OTA encountering these models in practice may find that occupational therapy practitioners refer to some of these as frames of reference and to others as treatment techniques. These distinctions have meaning to educators and to developers of occupational therapy theory but may be confusing to the entry-level practitioner. What is important, however, is to employ a practice model (or treatment technique or frame of reference) that complements the client's situation. Selection of an appropriate practice model is the responsibility of the OT; the occupational therapy assistant can learn much by observation and discussion with the OT.

## REVIEW QUESTIONS AND ACTIVITIES

1. Name and briefly describe each of the six practice models covered in the chapter.
2. For each practice model, state which of the theories in Chapter 2 would be compatible.
3. With a classmate, create scenarios or situations that illustrate the concepts of each model.
4. Create flash cards for the terms used in each model. Learn the definitions.
5. Use the flash cards for a matching game. Match each term to the practice model with which it belongs.
6. For each case example in the chapter (Judi, Howard, Eloise, Richard, Marvin, Rose), identify one other practice model that might address the client's needs. Explain your choice.
7. Write multiple choice examination questions, each with four possible answers but only one correct one. Write one question for each practice model. Share your questions with your teacher and classmates.

## REFERENCES


1. Allen CK. Independence through activity: The practice of occupational therapy (psychiatry). Am J Occup Ther 1982;36:731–739.
2. Allen CK. Occupational Therapy for Psychiatric Diseases: Measurement and Management of Cognitive Disabilities. Boston: Little, Brown, 1985.
3. Allen CK, Allen RE. Cognitive disabilities: Measuring the consequences of mental disorders. J Clin Psychiatry 1987;48:185–191.
4. Allen CK, Blue T, Earhart CA. Understanding Cognitive Performance Modes. Ormond Beach, FL: Allen Conferences, 1995.
5. Allen CK, Earhart CA, Blue T. Occupational Therapy Treatment Goals for the Physically and Cognitively Disabled. Rockville, MD: American Occupational Therapy Association, 1992.
6. American Occupational Therapy Association. Occupational therapy practice framework: Domain and process. Am J Occup Ther 2002;56:609–639.
7. Ayres AJ. Sensory Integration and Learning Disorders. Los Angeles: Western Psychological Services, 1972.
8. Barris R, Kielhofner G, Watts JH. Bodies of Knowledge in Psychosocial Practice. Thorofare, NJ: Slack, 1988.
9. Barris R, Kielhofner G, Watts JH. Psychosocial Occupational Therapy: Practice in a Pluralistic Arena. Laurel, MD: Ramsco, 1983.
10. Brady JP. Social skills training for psychiatric patients. 1: Concepts, methods and clinical results. Occup Ther Ment Health 1984;4:51–68.
11. Bruce MAG, Borg B. Psychosocial Frames of Reference Core for Occupational Based Practice. 3rd ed. Thorofare, NJ: Slack, 2002.
12. Corbett L. Perceptual changes in schizophrenia. Paper presented at the Neuropsychological Perspective of Sensory Integration in Psychiatry symposium, Chicago, Nov 12, 1981.
13. Crist PH. Community living skills: A psychoeducational community-based program. Occup Ther Ment Health 1986;6(2):51–64.
14. David SK, Riley WT. The relationship of the Allen Cognitive Level Test to cognitive abilities and psychopathology. Am J Occup Ther 1990;44:493–497.
15. Decker MD. Evaluating the client with dementia. Am Occup Ther Assoc Ment Health Special Sect Q Newslett 1996;18(4):1–2.
16. Hagedorn R. Occupational therapy: Foundations for practice—Models, frames of reference and core skills. Edinburgh: Churchill Livingstone, 1992.
17. Hagulund L, Kjelberg A. A critical analysis of the model of human occupation. Can J Occup Ther 1999;66:102–108.
18. Hayes R. Occupational therapy in the treatment of schizophrenia. Occup Ther Ment Health 1989;9(3):51–68.
19. Hayes RL, Halford WK. Generalization of occupational therapy effects in psychiatric rehabilitation. Am J Occup Ther 1993;47:161–167.
20. Hayes R, Halford WK, Varghese FN. Generalization of the effects of activity therapy and social skills training on the social behavior of low functioning schizophrenic patients. Occup Ther Ment Health 1991;11(4):3–20.
21. Helfrich C, Kielhofner G, Mattingly C. Volition as narrative: Understanding motivation in chronic illness. Am J Occup Ther 1994;48:311–317.
22. Henry AD, Coster WJ. Competency beliefs and occupational role behavior among adolescents: Explication of the personal causation construct. Am J Occup Ther 1997; 51:267–276.
23. Hewett FM. A hierarchy of educational tasks for children with learning disorders. Except Child 1964;34:459–467.
24. Hinojosa J. Position Paper: Occupational therapy for sensory integrative dysfunction. Am J Occup Ther 1982;36:831–832.
25. Josman N, Bar-Tal Y. The introduction of a temporal variable to the Allen Cognitive Level (ACL) test in adult psychosocial patients. Occup Ther Ment Health 1997;13(2):25–34.
26. Kaplan K, Kielhofner G. Occupational Case Analysis Interview and Rating Scale. Thorofare, NJ: Slack, 1988.
27. Kelly JA. Social-Skills Training: A Practical Guide for Interventions. New York: Springer, 1982.
28. Kielhofner G. A model of human occupation. 3: Benign and vicious cycles. Am J Occup Ther 1980;34:731–737.
29. Kielhofner G, ed. A Model of Human Occupation: Theory and Application. Baltimore: Williams & Wilkins, 1985.
30. Kielhofner G, ed. A Model of Human Occupation: Theory and Application. 2nd ed. Baltimore: Williams & Wilkins; 1995.
31. Kielhofner G, ed. A Model of Human Occupation: Theory and Application. 3rd ed. Baltimore: Lippincott Williams & Wilkins; 2002.
32. Kielhofner G, Barris R, Watts JH. Habits and habit dysfunction: A clinical perspective for psychosocial occupational therapy. Occup Ther Ment Health 1982; 2(2):1–21.
33. Kielhofner G, Burke JP. A model of human occupation. 1: Conceptual framework and content. Am J Occup Ther 1980;34:572–581.
34. Kielhofner G, Burke JP, Igi CH. A model of human occupation. 4: Assessment and intervention. Am J Occup Ther 1980;34:777–788.
35. Kielhofner G, Forsyth K. The model of human occupation: An overview of current concepts. Br J Occup Ther 1997; 63:103–110.
36. King LJ. A sensory-integrative approach to schizophrenia. Am J Occup Ther 1974;28:529–536.

37. King LJ. Sensory integration as a broad spectrum treatment approach. Paper presented at the Continuing Education Programs of America symposium, Philadelphia, 1978.
38. Lillie MD, Armstrong HE. Contributions to the development of psychoeducational approaches to mental health service. Am J Occup Ther 1982;36:438–443.
39. Litterst TAE. A reappraisal of anthropological fieldwork methods and the concept of culture in occupational therapy research. Am J Occup Ther 1985;39:602–604.
40. Levy LL. Activity, social role retention, and the multiply disabled aged: Strategies for intervention. Occup Ther Ment Health 1990;10(3):2–30.
41. Levy LL. Psychosocial intervention and dementia. II: The cognitive disability perspective. Occup Ther Ment Health 1987;7(4):13–36.
42. Levy LL, Burns T. Cognitive disabilities reconsidered—Rehabilitation of older adults with dementia. In: Katz N, ed. Cognition and Occupation Across the Life Span. Bethesda, MD: American Occupational Therapy Association, 2005.
43. Luboshitzky D, Gaber LB. Collaborative therapeutic homework model in occupational therapy. Occup Ther Ment Health 2000;15(1):43–60.
44. Mayer MA. Analysis of information processing and cognitive disability theory. Am J Occup Ther 1988;42:176–183.
45. Mosey AC. Activities Therapy. New York: Raven, 1973.
46. Mosey AC. Psychosocial Components of Occupational Therapy. New York: Raven, 1987.
47. Mosey AC. Three Frames of Reference for Mental Health. Thorofare, NJ: Slack, 1970.
48. Neville-Jan A. The relationship of volition to adaptive occupational behavior among individuals with varying degrees of depression. Occup Ther Ment Health 1994; 12(4):1–18.
49. Neville-Jan A, Bradley M, Bunn C, Gehri B. The model of human occupation and individuals with co-dependency problems. Occup Ther Ment Health 1991;11(2–3):73–97.
50. Padilla R. Teaching approaches and occupational therapy psychoeducation. Occup Ther Ment Health 2001;17(3–4): 81–95.
51. Penny NH, Mueser KT, North CT. The Allen Cognitive Level test and social competence in adult psychiatric patients. Am J Occup Ther 1995;49:420–427.
52. Posthuma BW. Sensory integration in mental health: Dialogue with Lorna Jean King. Occup Ther Ment Health 1983;3(4):1–10.
53. Pratt CW, Gill KJ, Barrett NM, Roberts MM. Psychiatric Rehabilitation. 2nd ed. Burlington MA: Elsevier Academic, 2007.
54. Raweh DV, Katz N. Treatment effectiveness of Allen's cognitive disabilities model with adult schizophrenic outpatients: A pilot study. Occup Ther Ment Health 1999;14(4):65–77.
55. Reed K. Models of Practice in Occupational Therapy. Baltimore: Williams & Wilkins, 1984.
56. Reisman JE, Blakeney AB. Exploring sensory integrative treatment in chronic schizophrenia. Occup Ther Ment Health 1991;11(1):25–43.
57. Rider BA. Sensorimotor treatment of chronic schizophrenics. Am J Occup Ther 1978;32:451–455.
58. Robichaud L, Hébert R, Desrosiers J. Efficacy of a sensory integration program on behaviors of inpatients with dementia. Am J Occup Ther 1994;48:355–360.
59. Royeen CB. Domain specifications of the construct tactile defensiveness. Am J Occup Ther 1985;39:596–599.
60. Schindler VP. Occupational therapy in forensic psychiatry: Role development and schizophrenia. Occup Ther Ment Health 2005;20(3–4):1–175.
61. Schindler VP, Ferguson S. An education program on acquired immunodeficiency syndrome for patients with mental illness. Am J Occup Ther 1995;49(4): 359–361.
62. Secrest L, Wood AE, Tapp A. A comparison of the Allen Cognitive Level test and the Wisconsin Card Sorting test in adults with schizophrenia. Am J Occup Ther 1999;54: 129–136.
63. Sharrott GW. An analysis of occupational therapy theoretical approaches for mental health: Are the profession's major treatment approaches truly occupational therapy? Occup Ther Ment Health 1985;5(4):304–312.
64. Spackman CS. Methods of instruction. In: Willard HS, Spackman CS, eds. Occupational Therapy. 4th ed. Philadelphia: Lippincott, 1981.
65. Stein F. A current review of the behavioral frame of reference and its application to occupational therapy. Occup Ther Ment Health 1982;2:35–62.
66. Thomson LK. The Kohlman Evaluation of Living Skills. Bethesda, MD: American Occupational Therapy Association, 1992.
67. Vargas S, Camilli G. A meta-analysis of research on sensory integration treatment. Am J Occup Ther 1999; 53:189–198.
68. Whitehead AN. Dialogues with Alfred North Whitehead [Prologue]. In: Bartlett J, ed. Familiar Quotations. 15th ed. Boston: Little, Brown, 1980:697.

## SUGGESTED READINGS

### General

Giroux Bruce MA, Borg B. Psychosocial Frames of Reference Core for Occupational Based Practice. 3rd ed. Thorofare, NJ: Slack, 2002.

### Development of Adaptive Skills

Mosey AC. Psychosocial Components of Occupational Therapy. New York: Raven, 1987.

Mosey AC. Three Frames of Reference for Mental Health. Thorofare, NJ: Slack, 1970.

### Role Acquisition and Social Skills Training

Brady JP. Social skills training for psychiatric patients. 1: Concepts, methods and clinical results. Occup Ther Ment Health 1984;4(4):51–68.

Gutman SA. Brain injury and gender role strain: Rebuilding adult lifestyles after injury. Occup Ther Ment Health 2000;15(3–4) 1–147.

Gutman SA, Leger DL. Enhancement of one-to-one interpersonal skills necessary to initiate and maintain intimate relationships: A frame of reference for adults having sustained traumatic brain injury. Occup Ther Ment Health 1997; 13(2):51–67.

Mosey AC. Activities Therapy. New York: Raven, 1973.

Schindler VP. Occupational therapy in forensic psychiatry: Role development and schizophrenia. Occup Ther Ment Health 2005;20(3–4):1–175.

### Psychoeducation

Luboshitzky D, Gaber LB. Collaborative therapeutic homework model in occupational therapy. Occup Ther Ment Health 2000;15(1):43–60.

### Sensory Integration

Gorman PA. Sensory dysfunction in dual diagnosis: Mental retardation/mental illness and autism. Occup Ther Ment Health 1997;13(1):3–22.

King LJ. A sensory-integrative approach to schizophrenia. Am J Occup Ther 1974;28:529–536.

Simpson LD. Seeing the forest for the trees: Treating adults with mental retardation through structurally based manual therapy. OT Pract 1996;1(11):40–45.

### Cognitive Disabilities

Allen CK. Occupational Therapy for Psychiatric Diseases: Measurement and Management of Cognitive Disabilities. Boston: Little, Brown, 1985.

Allen CK, Earhart CA, Blue T. Occupational therapy treatment goals for the physically and cognitively disabled. Rockville, MD: American Occupational Therapy Association, 1992.

Levy LL, Burns T. Cognitive disabilities reconsidered—Rehabilitation of older adults with dementia. In: Katz N, ed. Cognition and Occupation across the Life Span. Bethesda, MD: American Occupational Therapy Association, 2005.

### The Model of Human Occupation

Helfrich C, Kielhofner G, Mattingly C. Volition as narrative: Understanding motivation in chronic illness. Am J Occup Ther 1994;48:311–317.

Johnson H, Kielhofner G, Borell L. Anticipating retirement: The formation of narratives concerning an occupational transition. Am J Occup Ther 1997;51:49–56.

Kielhofner G, ed. A Model of Human Occupation: Theory and Application. 3rd ed. Baltimore: Lippincott Williams & Wilkins; 2002.

CHAPTER 4

# The Occupational Therapy Practice Framework

***Labour is blossoming or dancing where The body is not bruised to pleasure soul. Nor beauty born out of its own despair, Nor blear-eyed wisdom out of midnight oil.***

William Butler Yeats (8)

## CHAPTER OBJECTIVES

After studying this chapter, the reader will be able to:

1. Contrast the domain and process sections of the *Occupational Therapy Practice Framework* (*OTPF*).
2. Discuss the relationship between the *OTPF* and the *International Classification of Functioning, Disability, and Health* (*ICF*).
3. Appreciate the value of using the *ICF* to supplement the *OTPF*.
4. Define and give examples that illustrate terms and concepts of the *OTPF* and *ICF*.
5. Give examples of psychosocial concepts that are addressed in the *ICF* but not in the *OTPF*.
6. Compare each of the practice models or theories from Chapters 2 and 3 with the concepts and ideas of the *OTPF*.
7. Apply terms and concepts of the *OTPF* and *ICF* to case examples.

This chapter concerns the *Occupational Therapy Practice Framework: Domain and Process* (*OTPF*) (1), currently the core document outlining the scope, focus, and process of the occupational therapy profession. The *OTPF*, published in 2002, replaced an earlier document, the *Uniform Terminology for Occupational Therapy*, 3rd edition (*UT*-III) (2). The *OTPF* is significantly different from the *UT*-III and previous versions of the *Uniform Terminology*. The author assumes the reader has some familiarity with the *OTPF*.

Before continuing with this chapter, read the following three case studies. When reading the cases, think about the occupations of each individual, the health status of each, and any possible interaction between occupation(s) and health.

CASE EXAMPLE

## Betty

Betty[1] lives with her husband in a row house in a big city. She has a history of heart disease and has a pacemaker. She has smoked a pack of cigarettes a day for 55 years, although she has been advised many times to quit. Betty, now 76 years old, retired 11 years ago from her job as a bookkeeper in an ironworks company. She has no hobbies. She spends her days staring out the window and says she cannot do more because of her health conditions. She sleeps poorly and at night wanders around the house checking doors and windows to be sure that they are locked. She has difficulty with the stairs owing to her limited strength and stamina. Betty's chief activities out of the house are getting her hair done once a week and going to church on some Sundays. Her athletic 77-year-old husband, Mark, goes to the gym every day and is busy with volunteer activities and hobbies of his own. He is frustrated with Betty's inactivity but has "given up talking to her about it because she doesn't want to change." Mark does most of the cooking and the housework because Betty says she is too ill; Betty says "I'm sick. I'm depressed. Leave me alone."

CASE EXAMPLE

## Judith

Judith is also 76 years old and lives a few blocks away from Betty. The two women do not know each other. Judith lives in a house that she co-owns with Dennis, who is 77. They are not married and live in separate apartments in the house; they are friends from work. Judith and Dennis are former teachers and each has been retired for more than 15 years. Judith has a history of bipolar disorder, controlled with medication. She spends her days in a variety of activities alone and with other people. She travels by public transportation to another part of the city to make recordings for the blind. She attends theater and dance events weekly. She takes yoga classes, does gardening, and entertains friends. She is a mentor to young teachers, and they often visit her home to discuss their work.

CASE EXAMPLE

## Dennis

Dennis, who lives in the lower floor of the house he co-owns with Judith, has asthma, chronic obstructive pulmonary disease, and cardiovascular disease. He takes a number of medications. Because his stamina is limited, he structures his days so that he can do the activities he most enjoys. He swims three times a week in an indoor swimming pool and then lunches with friends. He volunteers at the botanical garden in the winter, in the reference library. In the warmer months, he volunteers in the community garden two blocks away, talking with children from the schools

[1]Betty and the other case examples in this chapter are fictionalized composite characters drawn from the author's experience.

and camps who visit the site. When the weather is nice, he sits out on the front steps of the house and converses with passersby. He admits that some days are difficult and that he's frustrated by his lack of energy, but he makes an effort to keep going and to create opportunities for the social contact that he craves. For example, he plays Scrabble and pinochle with Judith and chats with her while she is gardening. He also enjoys each small trip to the grocery store and drugstore, where he jokes around with the cashiers.

## STRUCTURE OF THE *OCCUPATIONAL THERAPY PRACTICE FRAMEWORK*

The two main sections of the *OTPF* are the *domain* and the *process*. The process section describes how the services of occupational therapy are designed and provided, through the stages of evaluation, planning, and intervention; the process will be discussed in more detail in Chapter 14 and later chapters.

The domain section, which is the main focus of this chapter, provides a structured explanation of the concepts and ideas and functions that occupational therapy addresses. The *OTPF* was developed to be compatible with the *International Classification of Functioning, Disability, and Health* (*ICF*) (7), a core document of the World Health Organization (WHO). Compatibility with the language and ideas of the WHO and other major health care organizations and providers aids in communication of ideas among professions.

The domain is composed of six categories, arranged in three levels (Fig. 4-1). At the top is *performance in areas of occupation;* the ability to engage in performing occupations represents occupational health. This is the goal of all occupational therapy intervention. At the second level are acquired characteristics of the individual that support engagement in occupation: the *performance skills* and *performance patterns.* At the third level are three kinds of factors that influence the development or enactment of skills and patterns: *contexts, activity demands,* and *client factors.*

Additional detail about the terms used in the OTPF is found in the original document (1), and you are encouraged to consult it frequently. Use Table 4-1 to locate specific information in the OTPF.

## THINKING ABOUT MENTAL HEALTH PRACTICE

Occupational therapy provides services to individuals who have difficulty engaging in occupations. Why would occupational engagement be a problem for a person who has a mental health problem? Before reading further, go back and look at the case of Betty and write down what you think is interfering with her engagement in occupations. Then continue reading this section.

**TABLE 4-1 LOCATION OF *OTPF* ASPECTS, TERMS, AND CATEGORIES**

| ASPECT, TERM, OR CATEGORY | LOCATION[a] |
|---|---|
| Areas of occupation | Table 1, pp. 620–621 |
| Performance skills | Table 2, pp. 621–622 |
| Performance patterns | Table 3, p. 623 |
| Context or contexts | Table 4, p. 623 |
| Activity demands | Table 5, p. 624 |
| Client factors | Table 6, pp. 625–627 |

[a]Table and page numbers refer to American Occupational Therapy Association. Occupational therapy practice framework: Domain and process. Am J Occup Ther 2002;56:609–639.

**Performance in Areas of Occupation**

Activities of Daily Living (ADLs)
Instrumental Activities of Daily Living (IADLs)
Education
Work
Play
Leisure
Social Participation

**Performance Skills**

Motor Skills
Process Skills
Communication/Interaction Skills

**Performance Patterns**

Habits
Routines
Roles

**Contexts**

Cultural
Physical
Social
Personal
Spiritual
Temporal
Virtual

**Activity Demands**

Objects Used and Their Properties
Space Demands
Social Demands
Sequencing and Timing
Required Actions
Required Body Functions
Required Body Structures

**Client Factors**

Body Functions
Body Structures

**Figure 4-1. Domain of occupational therapy: engagement in occupation to support participation in context(s).** Note: ADLs are also referred to as basic activities of daily living (BADLs) and personal activities of daily living (PADLs). (Reprinted with permission from American Occupational Therapy Association. Occupational therapy practice framework: Domain and process. Am J Occup Ther 2002;56:609–639.)

Many factors can impair or limit occupational engagement, including the following:

- Inexperience with performing certain occupations, or lack of role models for occupational performance
- Absence or weakness of necessary performance skills
- Presence of dominating or nonproductive habits and patterns that interfere
- Absence of (or failure to develop or sustain) useful habits and patterns
- Difficulty understanding what is required in a given context
- Pressures from the context that exceed the person's abilities
- Inability to respond to the demands of an activity (task–person mismatch)
- Problems in specific body functions or structures that interfere with occupational engagement

Helping someone engage in occupations requires investigation into the reasons why that person is having trouble engaging appropriately. To illustrate, Betty (from our first case example) engages in few occupations. Our investigation about her lack of occupational engagement might consider the following:

- *Performance in areas of occupation*
  - Does she know, or has she been exposed to, other retired women who might serve as role models?
  - Does she have any activities in which she used to participate that she might want to attempt again?
  - What activities might she be interested in that she has not done before?
- *Performance skills*
  - Does she have the motor skills (strength, endurance, pacing) to begin to participate?

    - Does she have the process skills (knowledge, planning, organization) to begin to participate?
    - How do her communication and interaction skills support or fail to support participation?
- *Performance patterns*
    - What useful habits support performance of occupations?
    - What habits are poorly developed or weak?
    - What nonproductive or dominating habits interfere with performance?
    - How did loss of the worker role affect her ability to perform occupations?
    - How did adoption of the role of sick person affect her ability to perform occupations?
- *Contexts*
    - In what contexts does Betty participate?
    - And what are the demands and supports that come with these contexts?
    - What other contexts are available to her?
- *Activity demands*
    - What are the demands of going to the hairdresser and going to church?
    - What is the match or mismatch between Betty's skills and other occupations she might be interested in attempting?
- *Client factors*
    - Which mental functions are intact? Which, if any, are impaired (e.g., level of arousal, sleep, motivation, attention, range of emotions, self-control)?
    - Which movement-related functions are intact? Which, if any, are impaired?
    - Which cardiovascular, hematological, immunological, and respiratory functions are intact? Which, if any, are impaired?

## Objective and Subjective Aspects of Performance of Occupations

There are many other questions we might consider. Mental health practice, as we have seen in Chapters 2 and 3, concerns the internal psychological and affective (feeling) states of the individual as well as the behavior(s) that person displays. Thus there are subjective (internal, not outwardly visible) aspects to occupational engagement as well as the objective (behavioral, visible) aspects. Motivation, energy level, and mood are some internal or subjective aspects. Skill in performance is an external or objective aspect. For occupational therapy practitioners, the focus of concern is the person's ability to function in, and to perform effectively and with personal satisfaction in, occupations that are necessary or interesting to that person. Our concern embraces both the objectively visible evidence of occupational performance and the person's subjective experience.

Traditionally, for many other health care professions, the exclusive focus of mental health practice has been the internal subjective experience of the person, such as the person's insight, feelings, conflicts, and neurotic thinking. In the object relations approach discussed in Chapter 2, we saw one example of this.

A different focus of mental health professions with a medical orientation has been on the biological functions that appear to be responsible for mental health problems, or at least some aspects of these problems. Some of these aspects are brain functioning, neurotransmitter mechanisms, and organic mental disorders. The neuroscience approach (see Chapter 2), has this focus.

The *OTPF*, because it corresponds to the language of the *ICF*, gives occupational therapy practitioners a way to "speak the language" of other health care providers while still maintaining the focus on occupational engagement, which has traditionally been the centerpiece of our practice. The *OTPF* and the *ICF* include concepts and terms related to medical and biological functions, psychological functions, and the ability to participate in occupations. The *OTPF*, however, has reduced the information about psychological and psychosocial functions compared to the *UT*-III. The *ICF* expands on the psychological functions cited in the *OTPF*, as the examples in Table 4-2

**TABLE 4-2 CATEGORIES AND TERMS FROM THE *ICF* THAT EXPAND ON THE *OTPF* IN RELATION TO MENTAL HEALTH**

| CATEGORY | TERM | DEFINITION | CLASSIFICATION CODE |
|---|---|---|---|
| Temperament and personality functions | | General mental functions of constitutional disposition of individual to react in a particular way to situations, including set of mental characteristics that makes individual distinct from others | b126 |
| | Extraversion | Mental functions that produce a personal disposition that is outgoing, sociable, and demonstrative as contrasted to being shy, restricted, and inhibited | b1260 |
| | Agreeableness | Mental functions that produce a personal disposition that is cooperative, amicable, and accommodating as contrasted to being unfriendly, oppositional, and defiant | b1261 |
| | Conscientiousness | Mental functions that produce personal dispositions such as being hardworking, methodical, and scrupulous as contrasted to mental functions producing dispositions such as being lazy, unreliable, and irresponsible | b1262 |
| | Psychic stability | Mental functions that produce a personal disposition that is even tempered, calm, and composed as contrasted to being irritable, worried, erratic, and moody | b1263 |
| | Openness to experiences | Mental functions that produce a personal disposition that is curious, imaginative, inquisitive, and experience seeking, as contrasted to being stagnant, inattentive, and emotionally inexpressive | b1264 |
| | Confidence | Mental functions that produce a personal disposition that is self-assured, bold, and assertive as contrasted to being timid, insecure, and self-effacing | b1266 |
| | Trustworthiness | Mental functions that produce a personal disposition that is dependable and principled as contrasted to being deceitful and antisocial | b1267 |
| Energy and drive functions | | General mental functions of physiological and psychological mechanisms that cause individual to move toward satisfying specific needs and general goals in a persistent manner | b130 |

*(continued)*

**TABLE 4-2 CATEGORIES AND TERMS FROM THE *ICF* THAT EXPAND ON THE *OTPF* IN RELATION TO MENTAL HEALTH (*Continued*)**

| CATEGORY | TERM | DEFINITION | CLASSIFICATION CODE |
|---|---|---|---|
| | Energy level | Mental functions that produce vigor and stamina | b1300 |
| | Motivation | Mental functions that produce incentive to act; conscious or unconscious driving force for action | b1301 |
| | Appetite | Mental functions that produce a natural longing or desire, especially natural and recurring desire for food and drink | b1302 |
| | Craving | Mental functions that produce urge to consume substances, including substances that can be abused | b1303 |
| | Impulse control | Mental functions that regulate and resist sudden intense urges to do something | b1304 |

Modified from World Health Organization. International Classification of Functioning, Disability, and Health. Available at: www.who.int/classifications/icf/en. Accessed Dec 2006.

illustrate. The reader is encouraged to study and learn these and other terms from the *ICF* to aid in communicating with other health care providers. The *Illustrations Library of the ICF* (6) provides visual images that may help in understanding.

## CONCEPTS RELEVANT TO MENTAL HEALTH PRACTICE

The occupational therapy assistant (OTA) would expect to encounter mental health disorders in traditional mental health practice settings such as psychiatric hospitals, clinics, and community mental health centers. But, as should be evident from the case of Betty, these problems also occur in persons whose original diagnosis is a physical health disorder. How can the OTA use the *OTPF* effectively to analyze the occupational performance of persons with mental disorders? The following discussion gives an overview by briefly introducing each of the sections of the *OTPF*, beginning with the functions and structures of client factors and ending with performance in areas of occupation. Owing to the scope of this text, only selected terms and concepts are discussed. The reader is encouraged to use the *OTPF* for further analysis.

### Client Factors

Client factors consist of body functions and body structures that support the ability to engage in occupations.

#### Body Functions

Impairment of *mental functions* occurs in many mental health disorders. The person may be overaroused or excited or may be lethargic and slow to respond (*consciousness functions, level of arousal*). Someone who has dementia or an organic mental disorder may be unaware of the date, place, or people present; this is called disorientation (*orientation functions*). As in the case of Betty, sleep disorders may occur, resulting in too few or too many hours of sleep or in a disturbance in the pattern (the person may sleep poorly at night and fall asleep during the day).

*Temperament and personality factors* are aspects of how a person interacts with others and with the world (Table 4-2). These factors greatly affect occupational performance; they color the way the person is seen by others. The person who is introverted (introversion is the opposite of *extraversion*) will behave in a shy, withdrawn, and reserved manner; these behaviors may interfere with success in school and at work. An absence of *agreeableness* may be expressed through oppositional behaviors, making the person hard to get along with and impairing success in social participation. The person lacking in *conscientiousness* will be viewed as indifferent and irresponsible. The person who has a deficit or impairment in *psychic stability* experiences difficulties with other people as a result of to unpredictable and moody behaviors. A person who is lacking in *openness to new experiences* may be seen as having little imagination and being not much fun. A person who has an impairment of *confidence* will be viewed as insecure and timid. The person who has not developed *trustworthiness* will not be trusted by others and may be seen as a criminal.

*Energy and drive functions* are disturbed in some mental health disorders. The person's *energy level* may not be sufficient to initiate and complete the activities that make up occupations; the person who is depressed may have trouble just getting out of bed, completing grooming and hygiene, and getting dressed. Or the person may be overexcited and display excessive energy. As discussed in Chapter 3, *motivation* is needed to drive action; impairment of motivation may stop the person from beginning or continuing activities. *Appetite* is necessary to provoke eating and drinking liquids essential for physical survival. Disorders of appetite are common in mental health disorders and may range from the apparent absence of appetite (as in anorexia and other eating disorders) to overeating and obesity. People with depression also typically experience disturbed appetite. *Craving* for substances such as alcohol and drugs leads to substance use and abuse disorders and may complicate recovery from physical disorders. The inability to stop oneself from acting on impulse, or impairment of *impulse control*, occurs with several psychiatric disorders. For example, the impulse may be to spend more money than one has, to engage in unsafe sex, to abuse substances, to gamble, to steal, or to commit other crimes.

Specific mental functions such as *attention, memory,* and *perception* are altered in some disorders. Someone who has a psychotic disorder will typically pay more attention to internal stimuli, such as thoughts and imagined images, than to what is going on in the environment. A person may have problems with the ability to continue attending to a task (sustained attention) and to be unable to perform two or more tasks at the same time (divided attention). Memory (especially short-term memory) is deficient in dementia. In major mental disorders, misinterpretation of sensory stimuli may lead to hallucinations, a disorder of perception.

Deficits in *logical thinking skills* (*thought functions*) accompany some mental disorders. Sometimes the deficit is temporary and is relieved by medication or other treatment; in other cases, the deficit is permanent. Observers look to task performance or spoken language for evidence of a person's thinking. A psychologist may test for the ability to identify objects (*recognition*), the ability to put objects in appropriate groups (*categorization*), or the ability to apply a concept or idea from one situation to another that is similar (*generalization*). These mental functions (or absence thereof) can also be observed in task performance, in the handling of objects, and in the approach to an activity. In severe mental disorders, *awareness of reality* is impaired to the point that such individuals have very different notions about reality (e.g., thinking that earmuffs conduct one's thoughts into space). The speech of persons who have mental disorders may be disturbed, showing an absence of logical and coherent thought or appropriate thought content. What the person says may not make much sense and may seem very disconnected.

*Higher-level cognitive functions,* such as *judgment, concept formation, time management, problem solving,* and *decision making,* are impaired to varying degrees in mental disorders. Most serious, in dementia, the person gradually loses the ability to perform these functions. In schizophrenia and depression, there are sometimes problems with time management and judgment.

Mental functions of *language* reflect the ability to understand and use language to receive information and to express oneself. In some forms of schizophrenia and in autistic disorders, there are deficits in these functions.

Impairments in *calculation functions* (the ability to perform simple arithmetic needed in daily life transactions) may be evident. In some cases this is the result of an absence of learning; in others, it reflects difficulty sustaining attention and concentrating adequately to complete a calculation.

Research shows that the mental functions of *sequencing complex movement* (motor planning) are impaired in some forms of schizophrenia (3). *Psychomotor functions* may be abnormal as in the case of psychomotor agitation (restlessness and constant moving about) or psychomotor retardation (extreme slowing of movement).

Having feelings and not knowing how to control these or express them appropriately is one example of a disturbance in *emotional functions;* the person may explode or act out when unable to express herself. Alternately, in some disorders, an absence of emotion occurs; the person feels very little. Others see this person as cold or just odd.

*Experience of self* refers to one's ideas about the self, including one's body. The person who has an eating disorder generally has an altered *body image,* believing himself to be fat when in fact he is overly thin. Those with depression may have a negative view of themselves and their own qualities, indicating poor *self-esteem.*

Impairment of *sensory functions* may be present. Hallucinations, discussed earlier, are sensory experiences of things that are not there, such as voices and sounds, people, and crawling sensations on the skin. Psychiatric medications sometimes affect sensory functions in an adverse way, causing blurred vision, ringing in the ears, or disturbed taste, for example.

*Neuromuscular and movement-related functions* are affected by psychiatric medications that may cause tremors, rigidity, and other impairments of movement.

## Body Structures

Although not immediately obvious, some mental health disorders may include a physical component involving a defect or impairment of body structure. These defects may be a bodily aspect of the disease itself, as in the case of brain changes associated with dementia and with some schizophrenias. Or the impairments may result from disuse or misuse syndromes in which the person's body assumes limited or misaligned postures after many years; see, for example, the postures shown in Figure 3-3. Postural changes may also accompany depressive and anxiety disorders, as shown in Figure 4-2. In depression, the chest may sink, the shoulders round forward, and the head drop toward the chest. In anxiety, the person may hold the shoulders tensed, jutting the chin out and moving the head forward of the body, and protruding the eyes. These postures, initially an expression of the feelings or mood of the individual, may become rather fixed and difficult to release if they are maintained over time.

Psychotropic medications used to treat mental disorders may affect body structures. Weight gain is associated with several of the major drugs. Movement disorders such as tremors can become permanent. Photosensitivity, or extreme sensitivity to sunlight, is another common adverse effect. These adverse reactions are described further in Chapter 8.

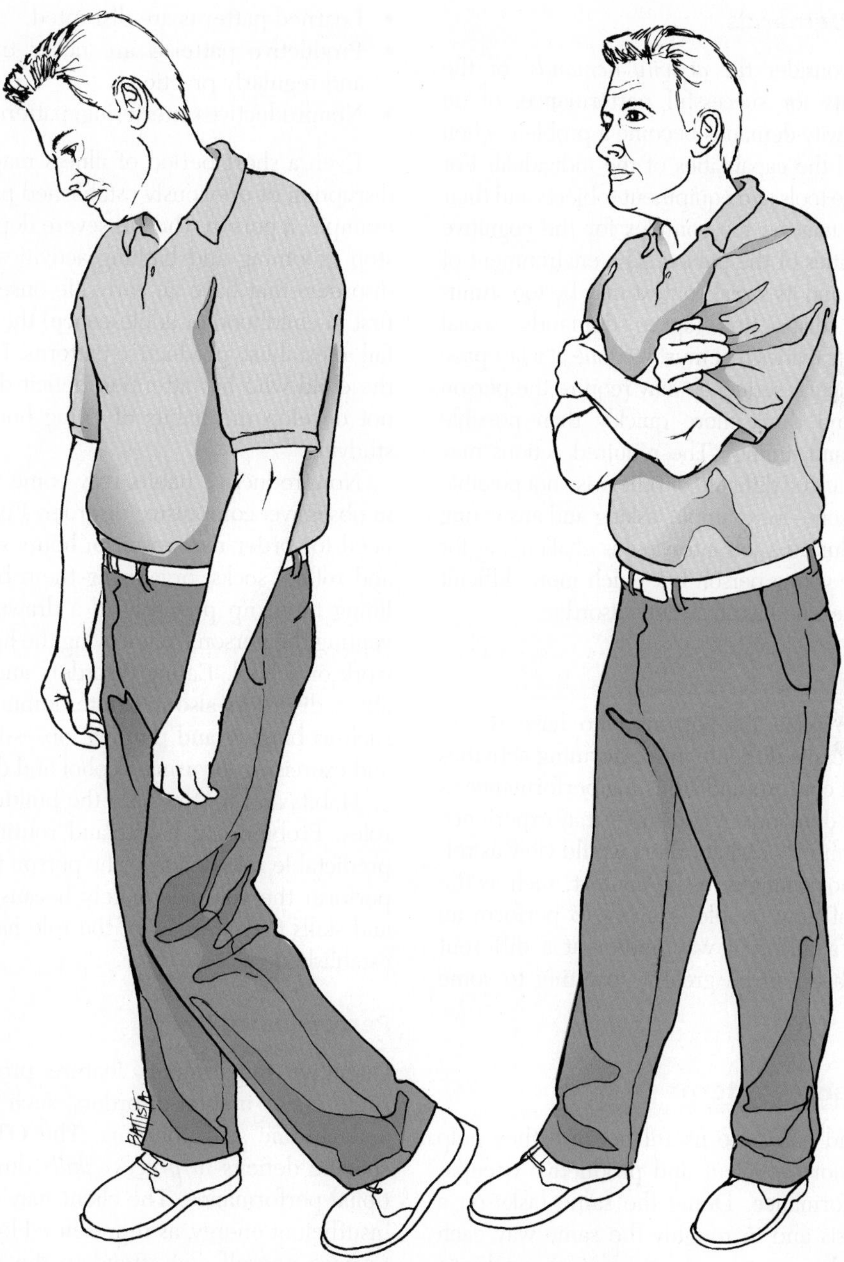

**Figure 4-2. Postural habits associated with depression (left) and anxiety (right).**

## Activity Demands

Next, we consider the *activity demands,* or the requirements for successful performance, of an activity. Activity demands become a problem when they exceed the capabilities of the individual. For example, the tools and equipment (objects and their properties) may be too complex for the cognitive mental abilities of the person. The environment of the activity and its social context may be too stimulating and distracting (space demands, social demands). Activities that must be done at a fast pace or in a particular sequence may require the person to move and think more quickly than possible (sequence and timing). The required actions may be unfamiliar, too difficult, or otherwise not possible for the person—for example, asking and answering questions during a job interview is challenging for the average young person but much more difficult for someone who has an anxiety disorder.

## Contexts

A common issue for persons who have severe mental illness is difficulty in performing activities in different contexts and adjusting performance as the context demands. A consumer may experience great discomfort at what others would view as relatively minor changes in the context, such as the presence of new people. Having to perform an activity in a different way and/or at a different time or place can be greatly upsetting to some consumers.

## Performance Patterns

*Routine* and *habit* are useful because they help generate more efficient and productive occupational performance. Doing the same tasks on a regular basis and in roughly the same way each time provides practice, structure, and regularity, allowing the tasks to become fairly automatic. The mind no longer needs to attend in a concentrated way. Problems of habit and routine that accompany some mental disorders occur when:

- Learned patterns are disrupted.
- Productive patterns are never truly learned and regularly practiced.
- Nonproductive (interfering) patterns dominate.

Even a short period of illness may result in a disruption of previously established patterns—for example, a person who has severe depression may stop grooming and bathing activities. In mental disorders that have an early life onset (occurring first in childhood or adolescence) the person may fail to establish productive patterns. For example, the child who has attention deficit disorder may not develop the habits of doing homework and studying.

Nonproductive habits may come to dominate in obsessive–compulsive disorder. For instance, a need for order may result in hours spent sorting and rolling socks, organizing them by color, and lining them up precisely in a drawer, thus preventing the person from leaving the house to go to work or school. Eating disorders and substance-abuse disorders also generate dominating habits, such as binging and purging, obsessive weighing and exercising, or using alcohol and drugs.

Habits and routines are the building blocks of roles. Problems in habits and routines result in predictable role deficits. The person is not able to perform the role adequately because the habits and skills that are part of the role have not been established.

## Performance Skills

Cognitive impairments feature prominently in some major mental disorders, such as dementia and chronic schizophrenia. The OTA will note specific deficits in *process skills* during occupational performance. The client may demonstrate insufficient energy, as represented by an inability to pace oneself and attend to the task through completion. Problems with eye tracking, the ability to follow objects with the eyes, may contribute to attention deficits. With a deficit in *knowledge,* the client's performance will be characterized by inaccurate use and choice of tools and perhaps a disregard for safety or for the outcome of the task. Poor *temporal organization* will be evident in difficulty starting, continuing, sequencing, or completing the task. Difficulties in *organizing space and objects* can be observed in wasted and duplicate effort in searching for items needed for the task, failure to set up the task before beginning, knocking things over and bumping into furniture, and so on. Deficits of *adaptation* are seen in failure to notice cues associated with the task (such as a burning smell or glue that overruns the borders of the project) and difficulty adjusting to changes in a situation (not observing that one might move over to make space for another person). These few examples illustrate the connection between thinking, or process skills, and effective occupational performance.

In some mental disorders, *communication and interaction skills* are impaired. These impairments affect social behaviors and effectiveness when giving and receiving information from others. Most people learn appropriate *physicality* of communication (the body movements that make for effective social interaction) by observing and imitating others. However, the skills of physicality are not easily learned in some mental disorders such as Asperger's syndrome. Persons with this disorder may find it almost impossible to comprehend and imitate nonverbal elements of communication such as eye contact, standing at a just right distance from others, and making understandable gestures. Giving and receiving information, asking questions, and keeping up one's end of a conversation are all skills of *information exchange,* skills that may be deficient in those who have anxiety disorders. Finally, the communication skills of *relations* involve being flexible in responding to others and being able to go along with a group, work with others, and respect the choices of other people; these skills may be deficient in persons who have impulse control disorders, who may lie or avoid responsibility.

Persons with mental disorders will sometimes have impairments of *motor skills.* Grasp and pinch may be weak, possibly from disuse. The person may have difficulty sequencing motor actions, as in some forms of schizophrenia (3). Problems with coordination are associated with the manic phase of bipolar disorder and with anxiety. Reduced strength may result from adverse effects of medications such as lithium.

## Occupational Performance

Performance of the many activities that make up the seven areas of occupation depends on all of the factors discussed thus far. When working with a client who is having problems engaging in occupations as desired, the occupational therapy practitioner will remember that these problems of performance may originate in body structures and functions, in the context, in the demands of the activity, or in the performance skill (deficits) of the individual. However, predictable deficits in performance of occupations can be observed in persons with major mental disorders.

In carrying out *activities of daily living* (ADLs), there may be failure to perform the activity, or the performance may miss the social standard or show errors. Persons with very severe mental disorders sometimes have poor hygiene and will require reminders. On the other hand, many persons who have less severe disorders will have no problems performing dressing, grooming, hygiene, and other ADLs. The *instrumental activities of daily living* (IADLs) are more complex, but persons with mild disorders generally perform these activities adequately. Those who have severe disorders will have much more difficulty taking care of their living space (*home management and maintenance*), handling money and banking (*financial management*), and responding to *safety and emergency* issues and other IADLs.

Performance in *education* and *work* also ranges from excellent (in higher-functioning individuals who have depression) to unpredictable (in persons who have some personality disorders) to very weak or limited (in persons who have schizophrenia that began in late childhood). Engaging in *play* and *leisure* occupations is a challenge for people with depression because they often don't feel like doing such activities. People with substance-abuse problems typically lack knowledge of leisure activities that don't involve using substances.

*Social participation,* the activities that involve being with and interacting with other people, depends a great deal on both the capacity of the person and the kinds of support available. People with severe depression may not feel like interacting with others. People with social anxiety may be frightened by the idea of interaction. People with dementia may lack sufficient awareness and arousal to interact. However, if family or friends or other supportive people provide sufficient support and stimulation, the quality and satisfaction of social participation may increase.

### Dynamic Interactions Among Person, Task, and Environment

Perhaps the most important idea for the reader to consider from the OTPF is that occupational performance results from an ongoing interaction among the task or activity, the person performing the activity, and the environment (including other people) of the activity. This is shown in Figure 4-3. Relatively minor changes in the environment, such as the presence of one supportive or friendly person or the placement of a screen to block out distractions, may change the performance from very poor to quite satisfactory, with an increase in pleasure and effectiveness. Changes in the demands of the task, such as substituting left-handed scissors or an envelope slitter for standard scissors, can make a frustrating activity suddenly doable. And, if the person takes his or her medication and is able to pay attention longer, this also makes the performance better. The lesson here is that improving effectiveness and satisfaction with occupational performance can be addressed from any of these aspects: the person, the task itself, and the environment. Minor changes can produce big results; careful analysis is needed to determine where and how to make a change.

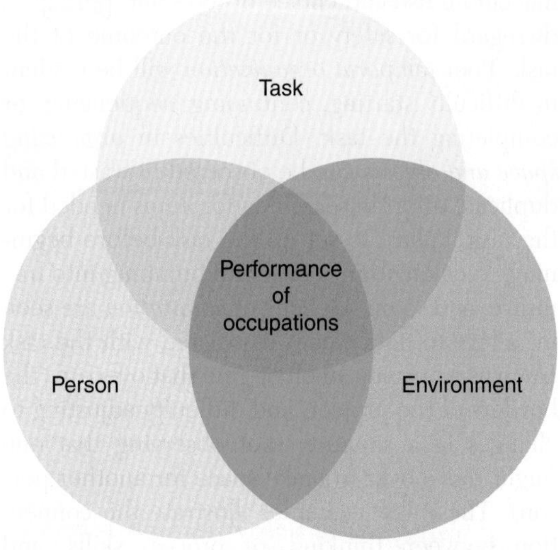


**Figure 4-3. Dynamic interaction of person, task, and environment produces occupational performance.**

## MENTAL HEALTH THEORIES AND OCCUPATIONAL THERAPY PRACTICE MODELS

Now that the *OTPF* has been promoted by the American Occupational Therapy Association (AOTA) as the organizing framework for all occupational therapy practice (10), we need to consider how the *OTPF* works with the theories and practice models prevalent in mental health (4). Because occupational therapy practitioners generally work together with other medical and human services workers, it's useful to think about how the *OTPF* might mesh with theories used by other professions.

### Mental Health Theories

The following brief discussion applies to the 2002 version of the *OTPF;* future versions of the *OTPF* may address some of the issues of incompatibility with the major mental health theories.

- *Object relations theory.* This theory addresses functions of the ego and superego, terms not mentioned in the *OTPF.* It would be difficult for occupational therapy practitioners to apply *OTPF* terms in a setting that uses object relations theories. Only a few terms and concepts are compatible, such as experience of self through body image and self-concept.
- *Developmental theory.* No conflict exists here; the *OTPF* is compatible with developmental theories.
- *Behavioral theory.* The OTPF emphasizes the client at the center of occupational performance. This may be incompatible with strict behavioral models that aim to reinforce desired behavior and limit less desirable behavior. Such behavioral approaches assume that the client will be manipulated by outside forces in order to change. In the *OTPF,* the client selects the desired changes.
- *Cognitive-behavioral theory.* In this approach, the client or consumer is taught to examine his or her ideas and beliefs and to challenge erroneous beliefs. This approach is compatible with the *OTPF,* especially when the outcome of therapy is focused on improved occupational performance.
- *Client-centered therapy.* The techniques used here are also used in the occupational behavior approach from which the *OTPF* was developed. Because the *OTPF* is also client-centered, this kind of therapy is compatible. However, the goals of client-centered therapy are not necessarily aimed at improved engagement in occupation.
- *Neuroscience theory.* Because the structure and function of the brain are client factors (body structure and function), it is at this level that neuroscience best fits with the *OTPF.*
- *Psychiatric rehabilitation.* The *OTPF* is compatible with this approach. As noted in Chapter 2, the authors of psychiatric rehabilitation admit to borrowing from other disciplines and theories. The rigorous activity analysis structure of the *OTPF* is an asset for the occupational therapy practitioner working in psychiatric rehabilitation settings. Analyzing activities and occupations that interest the consumer will yield useful information about the obstacles involved; the occupational therapist (OT) or OTA will be prepared to suggest solutions at the levels of client factors, patterns, skills, contexts, and activity demands.

## Occupational Therapy Practice Models

One of the reasons the *OTPF* was developed was to align practice with current knowledge and thinking about occupation. Occupational therapy practitioners would be encouraged to place occupational engagement at the center of their work with clients. This has not always been the case; in past decades, changes in body functions (strength, range of motion, insight, body image) were sometimes the main goal of occupational therapy intervention. Thus the challenge for OTs and OTAs using any practice model is to maintain a focus on occupational engagement while employing the unique advantages of each practice model.

### Development of Adaptive Skills

The development of adaptive skills practice model concerns mainly the performance skills of the *OTPF* as well as with some of the body functions. Cognitive and sensory integrative skills contribute to both motor and process skills. Dyadic and group interaction also seem to be skill areas related to communication and interaction, but they also overlap with the occupational performance area of social interaction. When working with a consumer who has identifiable deficits in performance skills, this might be an appropriate practice model.

### Role Acquisition and Social Skills Training

Both role acquisition and social skills training fit well with sections of the *OTPF.* These practice models use the approach that skills and habits are acquired through learning within a social environment. Both approaches assume that if the input from the environment is changed, the person's behavior will change. Role acquisition focuses on development of performance skills and performance patterns. Social skills training directs attention to the performance skills of communication and interaction.

### Psychoeducation

The goals of psychoeducation address performance patterns and performance skills. They also engage the person at the level of mental and emotional functions by requiring an investment in setting goals and assuming the role of student, with homework and other assignments. The emphasis on environment, *in vivo* and simulated, in psychoeducation is compatible with the *OTPF.*

### Sensory Integration

Sensory integration approaches can be used with the *OTPF* to improve skills in moving within the environment and perceiving reality; these would be considered body functions and performance skills. The prospect of fun and the playful quality of sensory integrative activities can motivate the person to move and to explore the environment and can directly influence motor and process skills. There may be positive effects on performance of occupations related to play, leisure, and social participation.

### Cognitive Disabilities

The theory of cognitive disabilities intersects with selected aspects of the *OTPF.* First, cognition is both a body function and an essential foundation of the process skills. The theory of cognitive disabilities recognizes that the environment affects task performance and that changing the environment can allow a person to function better. A major emphasis of the cognitive disabilities theory is the fit between task abilities and task demands. In the *OTPF,* the category of *activity demands* is similar to task demands. Task abilities seem to be a blend of *body functions* and *performance skills* in the *OTPF.*

### Model of Human Occupation

The *OTPF* and the model of human occupation (MOHO) approach overlap extensively. The concepts are identical, although the vocabulary used in MOHO occasionally differs from that of the *OTPF.* The easy fit between the two suggests that MOHO may increasingly dominate occupational therapy practice.

## SUMMARY

This chapter has described and discussed in some detail the *Occupational Therapy Practice Framework: Domain and Process* (*OTPF*) (1), a core document of the AOTA. The *OTPF* was developed in order to unify occupational therapy practice around the general outcome of "engagement in occupation to support participation in context" (1). Using the concepts and vocabulary of the *OTPF,* the OT and OTA can analyze the occupational goals and obstacles of clients, with an aim to providing a means to reach goals and reduce the effect of obstacles.

Because mental health treatment traditionally has taken its direction from professions other than occupational therapy, some mental health theories fit poorly with the *OTPF,* and the practitioner working in settings using these theories may find authentic occupational therapy practice challenging to implement. This chapter provides some basic understanding of how theories and practice models may fit (or not) with the *OTPF.*

The reader is encouraged to examine the original *OTPF* document (1) carefully, to keep a copy close at hand, and to take advantage of the resources available to increase understanding. These include the AOTA's website (www.aota.org), the WHO's *ICF* document (7), and other references listed at the end of the chapter (5, 9).

## REVIEW QUESTIONS AND ACTIVITIES

1. Contrast the domain and the process sections of the *OTPF*. Explain the purpose of tailoring the *OTPF* so that it is compatible with the *ICF*.
2. Why should readers examine the *ICF* when providing services that have psychosocial aspects?
3. Explain how the reader can access the *ICF*. Give examples of terms found there, in addition to those included in this chapter.
4. Review the vocabulary from the tables in the chapter. Test yourself on your ability to write definitions for these terms. Test yourself on your ability to give examples that illustrate each term.
5. To what extent, and in what ways, is each of the practice models or theories from Chapters 2 and 3 compatible with the *OTPF*?
6. Return to the three case examples at the beginning of the chapter and outline each case using terms from the *OTPF*. Be sure to include areas of occupation, patterns, skills, and client factors.
7. Using concepts from the *OTPF*, analyze the problems faced by Betty and her husband, Mark. What, if anything, needs to be done? What additional information would be helpful? What questions would you ask?
8. Reread the quote from poet William Butler Yeats at the beginning of the chapter. How does this quote relate to the *OTPF*? What is Yeats saying in these lines?

## REFERENCES


1. American Occupational Therapy Association. Occupational therapy practice framework: Domain and process. Am J Occup Ther 2002;56:609–639.
2. American Occupational Therapy Association. Uniform terminology for occupational therapy, third edition. Am J Occup Ther 1994;48:1047–1054.
3. Delovoye-Turrell Y, Giersch A, Danion J-M. Abnormal sequencing of motor actions in patients with schizophrenia: Evidence from grip force adjustments during object manipulation. Available at ajp.psychiatryonline.org/cgi/content/full/160/1/134. Accessed Dec 2006.
4. Holmquist BB. Incorporating the occupational therapy practice framework into a mental health setting. Am Occup Ther Assoc Ment Health Special Sect Q Newslett 2004; 27(2):1–4.
5. Law M, Baum CM, Baptiste S. Occupation-based practice: Fostering performance and participation, Thorofare, NJ: Slack, 2002.
6. World Health Organization. ICF Illustration Library. Available at: www.icfillustration.com/icfil_eng. Accessed Dec 2006.
7. World Health Organization. International Classification of Functioning, Disability, and Health. Available at: www.who.int/classifications/icf/en. Accessed Dec 2006.
8. Yeats WB. Among school children. In: The Collected Poems of W. B. Yeats. New York: Macmillan, 1933.
9. Youngstrom MJ. Introduction to the occupational therapy practice framework: Domain and process [Continuing Education]. OT Practice 2002;7(16):CE1–8.
10. Youngstrom MJ. The occupational therapy practice framework: The evolution of our professional language. Am J Occup Ther 2002;56:607–608.


## SUGGESTED READINGS


Youngstrom MJ. Introduction to the occupational therapy practice framework: Domain and process [Continuing Education]. OT Practice 2002;7(16):CE1–8

CHAPTER 5

# Human Occupation and Mental Health Throughout the Life Span

***Most people live, whether physically, intellectually or morally, in a very restricted circle of their potential being. They make use of a very small portion of their possible consciousness, and of their soul's resources in general, much like a man who, out of his whole bodily organism, should get into a habit of using and moving only his little finger. Great emergencies and crises show us how much greater our vital resources are than we had supposed.***

WILLIAM JAMES (18)

## CHAPTER OBJECTIVES

After studying this chapter, the reader will be able to:

1. Analyze the motivations for performance of occupation.
2. Outline changes in performance of occupation from childhood through late life.
3. Contrast involvement in work and play occupations at different ages.
4. Identify important achievements in occupational development at various life stages.
5. Recognize psychiatric disorders that typically appear in childhood, adolescence, adulthood, and later life.
6. Describe the effects of mental disorders on performance of occupation at different stages of life.

The desire to act upon the environment and to have an effect is a force that drives and shapes human behavior from birth to death. Occupation, or the expression of this urge through activity, is essential for human growth and development. The focus and specifics of occupation change throughout life as the playing child matures into the working adult, who later retires and is occupied with nonwork activities. The foundation of occupation-related habits and skills formed in childhood profoundly influences all later development. Without occupation, growth is frustrated and impaired.

This chapter considers how performance of occupation develops and changes as the person matures and ages. We will also look at some of the common mental health problems that arise in different life stages, with particular emphasis on the occupational aspects of these disorders and the role of occupational therapy in evaluation and treatment. It is important to remember that mental health problems do not always impair the ability to engage in occupation or to use occupation to further growth and development.

## MOTIVATION TOWARD OCCUPATION

To understand how occupation develops and changes throughout life, we must first consider why humans engage in occupation at all. What are the reasons? And are the reasons always the same? Reilly (31) identified a sequence of three levels of motivation for occupation or action: exploration, competency, and achievement.

- *Exploration motivation* is the desire to act, to explore, for the pure pleasure of it. This is the primary, or first, motivation for action. Infants and small children do things because they are exploring what will happen, but adults do the same thing when they encounter new situations that arouse their interest.
- *Competency motivation* is the desire to influence the environment in a specific way and to get better at it. When motivated by competency, the individual will practice the action over and over again and seek feedback from the environment, including other people, about the effects of the action. Competency is the second level of motivation; it helps sustain actions that were initially motivated only by exploration.
- *Achievement motivation* is the desire to attain, compete with, or surpass a standard of excellence. The standard may be an external one or may be generated by the individual. Achievement is the third and highest level of motivation for occupation. When competent at the action, the person continues to perform it to achieve success according to a standard.

These three levels of motivation—exploration, competency, and achievement—form a continuum that gradually transforms playful exploration into competent performance and ultimately into achievement and excellence. The skills that the child learns through play are later practiced and refined and finally polished and combined with other skills to enable more sophisticated and complex behavior to emerge.

Whenever the individual encounters novelty in the environment, these three levels of motivation are reexperienced in sequence. New situations and unfamiliar environments bring out the urge to explore, then to become competent, and then to achieve. This is as true of the working adult and the retiree as of the preschool child.

Kielhofner (21) argues also that different levels of motivation predominate at different stages in life. He suggests that the child engages in occupation primarily because of a motive to explore, that the adolescent does so to become competent, and the adult, to achieve. He states that older adults are motivated by an urge to explore the past and their own life's accomplishments and to explore their present capabilities through leisure. Let's now take a closer look at this view of how occupation evolves as the individual grows and matures.

## CHANGES IN OCCUPATION OVER THE LIFE SPAN

Human occupation traditionally has been divided into two main categories: work and play. Play consists of activities engaged in for pleasure, relaxation, self-exploration, or self-expression. Work includes all activities through which humans provide for their own welfare and contribute to the welfare of the social groups to which they belong. For the child, play is the dominant form of occupation; for the adult, work is the dominant form. The balance and relationship between work and play change throughout life in certain predictable ways (Fig. 5-1).

The patterns of work and play illustrated in Figure 5-1 are based on an American notion of normal human life and activity. Although anthropological studies show many similarities in patterns of work and play across different cultures, persons who come from other cultural backgrounds may have expectations and experiences that differ from those illustrated. Keeping this possibility in mind, let us now look at the different life stages.

**Levels of Organization of the Occupaional Behavior Career**

The Balance of Work and Play

| | CHILDHOOD | ADOLESCENCE | ADULTHOOD | OLD AGE |
|---|---|---|---|---|
| Waking hours occpied by work and play | | | | |

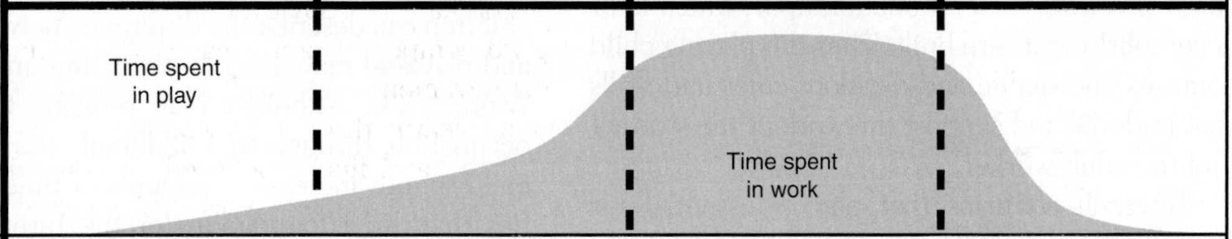


| | CHILDHOOD | ADOLESCENCE | ADULTHOOD | OLD AGE |
|---|---|---|---|---|
| Play yields | Reality is explored via curiosity for rule of competent action. | Competent behavior is learned and experienced in games, personal hobbies, and social events. | Relaxation and recreation support the worker role. Exploration of novel situations allows new roles to be taken on. | Play allows the exploration of past achievements and the unknown future, and maintenance of competence through leisure pursuit of interest. |
| Relationship of play and work | **Exploration** Skills for productivity are acquired and work roles explored through imitation and imagination. | **Competency** Personal and interpersonal competency are developed in a matrix of cooperation, yielding habits of sportsmanship and craftsmanship. | **Achievement** Play supports the worker roles by providing an arena of retreat and rejuvenation. Exploration in novel situations allows the ongoing development of new competency for work. | **Exploration** Retirement leisure signals that the productive obligation to society has been fulfilled. Past work has earned for the person the right to leisure. Leisure replaces work as the major source of life satisfaction. |
| Work yields | Productive behaviors are practiced through chores and in school. | The work role is practiced and the commitment process of occupational choices takes place. | There is entry into worker roles with the requirement of establishing and maintaining a productive and selfsatisfying career. | Retirement brings reduced expectations for productivity and personal capacities for productive action are waning. |

**Figure 5-1. The balance and interrelationship of work and play during the life span.** (Modified with permission from Kielhofner G. A model of human of occupation: 2. Ontogenesis for the perspective of temporal adaptation. Am J Occup Ther 1980;34:661. Copyright © 1980 by the American Occupational Therapy Association, Inc.)

## Childhood

Play is the main occupation of the child. Figure 5-1 shows that in early childhood the child performs no work at all. Gradually, as children are assigned chores and other responsibilities at home and in school, they spend some of their time in activities that must be classified as work. The purpose of play and work in childhood is distinctive. As children play, they explore their environments, learn about reality, and develop rules that are used to guide actions. For example, the child learns that objects fall to the floor when dropped, that a stove is sometimes hot, that a favorite uncle will allow things that Mother will not. These rules about motions, objects, and people (32) are tools that the child uses to guide future action and to develop skills. This childhood learning about how the world works is a foundation upon which later accomplishments are built. Thus the playing child acquires knowledge and develops rules and skills that underlie and support the work of the student and the adult worker.

Research confirms that play is essential for later development (1). Studies of many species show that important neurological connections, such as cerebellar synapses and long fiber tracts, are formed in their greatest numbers during the period when play is most vigorous in the young animal. These connections establish a foundation for skillful, responsive motor actions. Another important function of play for young animals is to practice and rehearse the subtle social behaviors they will need as adults (1). Thus imitation and exploration of future occupational roles are enacted in play. Through fantasy and imitation, the child investigates and experiences various adult roles (mommy, doctor, teacher, and so on). This experience, known as the fantasy period of occupational choice, is the first step in the three-stage process of choosing a career or adult occupation (12).

During play, the child also learns the joy of having an effect on the world and on other people. This helps form an image of the self as personally effective and powerful, thus developing and enhancing a sense of personal causation. The pleasure that the child takes in one activity over another helps form interests that will motivate life choices.

Although the child is not expected to do much work, the productive activities of the child are very important for later development. Studies have shown that industriousness in childhood is associated with job success and personal adjustment in adult life (38). Chores and schoolwork are the major productive activities of childhood. By engaging in these tasks over time, the child acquires habits of industry and responsibility and learns to schedule activities so that time also remains for play. Some tasks, such as handwriting, have clear associations with work. Even very young children can describe the difference between work and play and may describe their time in school as "work" (23). Although play remains the major occupation throughout childhood, the maturing child spends increasing amounts of time in activities that lay a foundation for the future role of adult worker. Habits and routines are developed and established.

## Adolescence

Adolescents, like children, continue to spend more time in play than in work. However, now motivated more by the desire to become competent than by the urge to explore, they choose activities in which practice and the habits of sportsmanship and craftsmanship make the difference between success and failure. Whether the activity is the track team, the chess club, or video games, the adolescent approaches it with determination to master and succeed. The biological changes of puberty interact with the adolescent's use of occupation to motivate a growing interest in social activities that provide opportunities to explore and practice social and sexual behaviors.

Sports, grades, popularity (Finding the balance)

The work of the adolescent, like the work of the child, consists of school and chores. School work becomes more rigorous and more time consuming, in keeping with the adolescent's growing cognitive capacity and discipline. Depending on the parents and the family situation, the chores may also be increasingly challenging. Many adolescents take on part-time jobs, which provide important experiences of what life is like in the adult working world and give feedback about the adolescent's readiness for work.

Adolescents are concerned about what they will do with their lives as adults, and occupational choice is generally viewed as one of the most important developmental tasks of adolescence. The process that began in the fantasy period of childhood enters a new stage, known as the *tentative period.* During this time, the adolescent considers possible adult occupations; this evaluation considers interests and likelihood of success. Finally, the adolescent weighs any choice in terms of personal values and achieved or expected place in the social system. From this overwhelming mass of factors, the adolescent must finally choose a career but may remake this decision several times throughout life.

Once the decision is made, the adolescent begins to work toward it, for example by enrolling in a training program or looking for a job. This begins the *realistic period,* in which the choice of career is examined in light of personal needs for achievement, satisfaction, status, and economic security. For example, if the chosen career is one in which jobs are scarce (e.g., acting) or the pay is low, the person may reconsider this decision and then must come up with alternatives and choose among them.

Thus occupational choice is crystallized and acted upon during adolescence, although for adolescent children of affluent parents the choice may be delayed into early adulthood. By contrast, adolescents from disadvantaged backgrounds may encounter overwhelming obstacles to realizing their occupational choice. In times of high unemployment, the adolescent with few skills may be denied employment or forced into a job that feels demeaning and unsatisfying. Ultimately, the process of occupational choice may be repeated by the adult who decides or is forced to change careers later in life.

## Adulthood

The adult spends many hours in work, leaving little time for play. The work of the adult centers on the occupational role selected through the process of occupational choice. This work, which is not necessarily salaried (consider the homemaker), consumes much time and energy and allows for expression and gratification of the urge to achieve. For many adults, there is the additional work of parenthood.

Adults work to provide for their own needs and those of their families. Beyond this, they work to produce something of value to the rest of society. Having a productive work role is important for the self-esteem of the adult; it bestows a sense of identity, a place in the social hierarchy, and a reason for being. Adults who are unemployed or underemployed (working at jobs that are beneath their capacities) often have negative views of their own abilities and worth. They may see themselves as incompetent and helpless rather than as competent and achieving members of society.

Despite the fact that working adults have little time for play, the time they spend in leisure and recreation serves an important function: It restores and refreshes their energies to work again. The word *recreation* actually means "the creation (again) of the laboring capacity." Different people feel different degrees of need for recreation; some people spend almost all of their time working, leaving only negligible amounts for play, and appear to be quite satisfied and happy. Others limit their work to a specific number of hours precisely because they want to make time for leisure pursuits.

In middle and later adulthood the individual looks toward the future and retirement and begins to explore and plan for this next stage. The major issue is the replacement of work with some other activity that will fill the hours, that will compensate for the loss of the worker role and of the social relationships with co-workers. Jonsson and colleagues (19) analyzed statements of people anticipating retirement and classified them as belonging to three types:

- Regressive (anxious and uncertain, dreading the future)
- Stable (expecting little change—may be either positive or negative)
- Progressive (may be either positive, focusing on new activities, or negative, focusing on getting rid of unpleasant work situation)

Examples of statements reflecting these three styles of response to retirement are shown in Box 5-1. Successful adjustment to retirement may require a reassessment of interests and the development of new hobbies and goals. Without this preparation, the transition from full-time work to retirement can be stressful, even devastating.

## Later Adulthood

During the latter part of life and certainly after retirement, the number of hours spent in work dramatically decreases. Thus vast quantities of time suddenly become available, and decisions must be made about how to fill the hours. Leisure replaces work as the primary occupation, although many retirees continue to serve productive social roles (e.g., as volunteers) that can only be classified as work.

The loss of a work role or of the role of parent and homemaker represents not just the loss of activities that once filled one's day but also of status and social identity. To adjust, the older adult needs goals and occupations that provide satisfaction and opportunities for success and that support a sense of self-worth. Older adults find particular meaning in maintaining leisure activities that have been lifelong interests (17). Each older person

**BOX 5-1**

### SAMPLE STATEMENTS OF PERSONS ANTICIPATING RETIREMENT

*Regressive:* "I can't imagine not going to work. I don't have a plan for how to spend the time."

Stable (positive): "I do so many things now that I will be continuing [golf, volunteer at church], that I think very little will change except maybe I'll have more time."

*Stable (negative):* "Well, you know, I can't say that life will be different. Just more of the same. The same old, dreary routine."

*Progressive (positive):* "I have just been waiting so long for this. I'll have more time for the botanical garden and the arthritis group and travel and just everything that I want to do more of."

*Progressive (negative):* "Definitely retirement will be an improvement for me. My whole body aches after a long day at work, and frankly, I'm a little tired of the whole situation. It will be a relief."

Fictional composites, with acknowledgment to Jonsson H, Kielhofner G, Borell L. Anticipating retirement: The formation of narratives concerning an occupational transition. Am J Occup Ther 1997;51:49–56.

lives in a particular environment, has a particular occupational history, and has specific interests. The ability to continue living with maximum independence in the community is highly individual and requires client-centered support (16).

In the words of the 18th-century poet William Cowper, "Absence of occupation is not rest,/A mind quite vacant is a mind distressed." Thus one of the important tasks of this stage of adult life is to identify and develop interests and challenges that will sustain one's sense of independence and self-worth.

### Occupational Development

Because occupational therapy practitioners are concerned primarily with a person's ability to develop and maintain satisfying occupational patterns, it is helpful to understand the functions, typical patterns, and development of occupation during the major life stages. The child samples and learns about the world through playful exploration, laying a foundation of motor and social skills. The adolescent, acting on the drive to become competent, practices and refines these skills and consolidates them into habits and roles. The adult, wishing to achieve and contribute, makes choices about career and life goals and selectively continues to develop and elaborate the skills and habits cultivated earlier in life. In later life, once career patterns are established and especially after retirement, the older adult may wish to integrate the long-abandoned interests of a younger self. Thus favored activities may be rediscovered and pursued again in later life. New occupations can be discovered and old interests reexplored.

We have said that the ability to engage in occupation is one of the signs of mental health and that mental illness can interfere with a person's ability to carry out daily life activities and to fulfill occupational roles. Let's look now at other significant factors in mental health at various ages and the kinds of mental health disorders that tend to occur at different stages of life.

## MENTAL HEALTH FACTORS THROUGHOUT THE LIFE SPAN

This section is an overview of the mental health needs of clients of various ages and the ways in which occupational therapy intervenes to help them. The section is divided according to six major life stages: infancy and early childhood, middle childhood, adolescence, early adulthood, midlife, and late adulthood and aging. For each stage, normal development and the kinds of mental health problems that sometimes arise are briefly described. The general goals and methods of occupational therapy are identified; and, where relevant, special intervention settings and evaluation and treatment methods are discussed. More detail on specific diagnoses and settings can be found in Chapters 6, 7, and 9.

While reading this section and after finishing the chapter, the reader should examine Table 5-1, which summarizes aspects of human occupation for each age group and lists major mental disorders that typically occur in the respective age groups. A case example later in the chapter illustrates the interactions among developmental tasks (10), the development of human occupation, environmental risk factors, and age-specific vulnerabilities to mental illness.

### Infancy and Early Childhood

Babies start life with enormous needs and wants and absolutely no ability to satisfy them on their own. Parents have to be able to figure out what babies want—whether the infant is hungry or thirsty or needs to be burped or cuddled or changed—and then provide it. To be able to relate to other people later on and to engage in activities that involve others, infants and small children need to learn to trust their parents and then people in general. In addition, they need to learn to communicate their needs and feelings and to control their impulses. Thoughtful interaction and consistent

**TABLE 5-1 SOME ASPECTS OF DEVELOPMENT OF HUMAN OCCUPATION SUBSYSTEMS AND RISKS OF MENTAL DISORDERS BY AGE GROUP**

| AGE GROUP | VOLITION SUBSYSTEM | HABITUATION SUBSYSTEM | MIND–BRAIN–BODY PERFORMANCE SUBSYSTEM | MAJOR MENTAL DISORDERS BY TYPICAL AGE OF ONSET |
|---|---|---|---|---|
| Childhood | Personal causation developing through social interactions and play; values of culture taught; interests enacted through choice of activity | Self-maintenance habits; routines established by parental scheduling; gradual shift to more control by child; student, friend roles learned | Tremendous development of skills trans forming from helpless infant to active agent in worlds of family, play, school; age of exploration and increasing competence | ADHD, PDD, autism, Asperger's syndrome, OCD, ODD |
| Adolescence | Increasing drive for autonomy; considering choice of occupation; weighing parental vs. peer values; shifting interests affected by peer or environ mental pressure | Exploration of roles; role experimentation; expanded; more independent student role; first enactment of worker role; increasing self-regulation; acquisition of habits of time management | Continued development of skills in motor, process, communication, interaction; social relations with peers fostering expanded communication and interaction skills | Schizophrenia, substance-related disorders, mood disorders |
| Adulthood | Maturation of personal causation, interests, values culminating in choice of occupation; values increasingly important in motivating behavior; interests possibly not addressed by work; avocational activities possibly especially fulfilling | Multiple roles (spouse, parent, worker, friend, volunteer, church member); despite role conflict, multiple role involvement satisfying; habits and routines influenced by need to manage time for multiple involvements | Peak abilities; mastery of many work-related skills; declining capacity may come from physical changes leading to reduced energy, need for eyeglasses, hearing aids; continued high level of involvement helping sustain greatest capacity and skill level | Schizophrenia, mood disorders, substance abuse |
| Later adulthood | Sense of efficacy possibly challenged by diminished physical capacity; importance (value) of work possibly declining as family and social values increase; opportunity in retirement to pursue interests more rigorously | Potential loss of major roles and role companions through retirement, physical disease, death (work role, spouse role, friend role); family roles and social roles increase in importance; habits of a lifetime well established; new habits hard to acquire | Age-related changes in musculoskeletal, neurological, cardiopulmonary systems varying in intensity; adjustments, adaptations to continue using skills (e.g., energy conservation, pacing, rest periods); adaptive equipment, environmental aids helping sustain skills | Alzheimer's, vascular, and other dementias; depression; polysubstance abuse (prescription medications, alcohol) |

*ADHD,* attention deficit-hyperactivity disorder; *PDD,* pervasive developmental disorder; *OCD,* obsessive–compulsive disorder; ODD, oppositional defiant disorder.

Data from Kielhofner G. A Model of Human Occupation: Theory and Application. 2nd ed. Baltimore: Williams & Wilkins, 1995.

discipline by the parents help the child acquire these skills. A stable, secure, and predictable environment is one of the most important factors in helping the child at any age to develop trust in self, other people, and the world in general.

While all of this psychosocial development is going on, the child is developing in other ways too. Sensory abilities are becoming more refined, motor skills better coordinated, and perceptual and cognitive abilities more complex. The child constantly uses and refines developing abilities to learn more about the world and how to interact with it.

It is unusual for mental health problems to be diagnosed in infancy and the preschool years. Often problems that are brought to the attention of psychiatric professionals are quite severe. Some of these problems are believed to have biological causes, meaning that the behavioral or emotional disorder is caused at least in part by something physical within the body or the brain.

Attention deficit disorder (ADD), attention deficit-hyperactivity disorder (ADHD), and pervasive developmental disorder (PDD) are in this category. The child with ADD or ADHD has a shorter attention span than is normal for a child of similar age. Jumping from activity to activity, often with a high level of energy (hyperactivity) but with an apparent inability to concentrate long enough to finish many of the tasks attempted, the child leaves a trail of chaos and confusion. It is not hard to imagine how this can interfere with learning.

PDD is a cluster of disorders occurring in very early childhood and impairing the ability to develop in many areas. Infantile autism is one example. This is a disorder in which the very young child fails to respond to other people, often ignoring them completely. Autism is believed to have an underlying biological component, and research supports this view (30). Children with autism differ from other children in the way they process and understand sensation (39). The child is usually slow to develop language skills, the learning of which seems to rely upon interactions with others. In addition, children with autism may exhibit strange mannerisms, such as wiggling their fingers in front of their eyes, and bizarre interests, for example in bright lights or spinning objects.

Occupational therapy for children with these disorders often focuses on sensorimotor or sensory integrative treatment approaches, which are believed to affect the underlying biological problem. Occupational therapy assistants (OTAs) may carry out such treatment only under the direct supervision of occupational therapists (OTs) who have special training in these approaches. Psychoanalytic (object relations) methods are sometimes used instead, but these also require direct supervision and special training. A more behaviorally oriented treatment approach focuses on the development of self-care skills (e.g., shoe tying) through direct instruction and reinforcement.

Building a trusting relationship and modifying the environment to enable success are often the twin foundations of intervention with children. Baron (3) presented a case study of a 4-year-old boy who had oppositional defiant disorder (ODD). A structured play experience with the occupational therapist over many weeks helped this child give up his resentful and argumentative behavior and develop a more spontaneous and genuine approach to play. Key elements of this treatment included a slow and careful building of trust through brief, frequent, one-on-one play with activities selected by the child from a limited choice given by the therapist; modification of the social play environment so that competition was reduced; and teaching and reinforcement of social skills such as taking turns.

Another serious mental health problem of early childhood is reactive attachment disorder, in which the child stops responding to other people because he or she has been neglected or ignored; this sometimes leads to failure to thrive, a condition in which the child may stop eating and withdraw totally. In such cases, the most intensive work is with the parents, teaching them how to provide more affection and better care.

Very small children with mental health problems are seldom treated as inpatients. Because of the important role of parents and family life in a child's development, the philosophy is to keep the child with the family whenever possible. Therefore, children may attend day treatment centers, special preschools, or programs at community mental health centers or may be treated at home, often with the parents participating. Chapter 9 contains more information on this topic.

Occupational therapy for infants and small children with mental health problems is considered a very demanding and complex area of practice (6). In addition to emotional and social deficits, it seems that children with mental health problems are more likely than other children to have developmental motor delays (22). The occupational therapist uses special developmental assessments and data collection instruments, such as the play history (4, 36), to evaluate the child's abilities, interests, and needs. Treatment programs are usually highly individualized, although they may take place in groups. Groups provide an experience of working with others, sharing, waiting, and taking turns—skills that prepare the child to succeed during the school years.

Some of the goals of treatment with this very young population are developing trust and social interactions, increasing gross and fine motor coordination, improving sensory processing and perceptual skills, and facilitating spontaneous play. In addition to sensorimotor and sensory integrative methods, play therapy and expressive art activities are sometimes used to help children develop and express their fantasies. OTAs who wish to work in this area need training beyond their basic education and should receive extensive supervision from a qualified OT.

## Middle Childhood

During the grade school years, the child refines growing abilities in many areas. The roles of student and contributing family member are gradually adopted. The child develops a more sophisticated awareness of social norms and expectations and of the needs of others, learning to delay gratification for increasingly long periods. In addition, the child becomes physically better coordinated and more intellectually sophisticated. Vast amounts of knowledge and increasingly complex skills are acquired through schoolwork and peer relationships.

The child continues to need the love, support, and encouragement of parents and family to feel secure enough to attempt new challenges. Some mental health professionals believe that the family has such an effect on the mental health of the child that it may be the cause of emotional and behavioral problems. Others believe that the family is a factor but that other factors, such as biological predisposition and experiences at school and elsewhere, are also involved. Yet others suggest that the peer group is the most influential factor (14).

Fortunately, mental health problems in middle childhood are infrequent, although more common than in early childhood. Among the problems that are seen in children during these years are conduct disorders, in which the child behaves in an antisocial fashion (e.g., stealing, cutting school), and other disorders that show up in physical behaviors (eating problems, stuttering, bedwetting, and so on). These behaviors may merit a diagnosis of ODD. Drug and alcohol problems may also appear at this age. ADHD often continues into middle childhood or makes its first appearance at this time. Some children have difficulty learning in school and may be diagnosed with learning disabilities.

Symptoms of obsessive–compulsive disorder (OCD) may appear in middle childhood. The child with OCD may be fearful and anxious and may use ritual behaviors (such as ordering, checking, or touching things) to cope with these feelings. The ritual behaviors interfere with success in school and may prevent the child from making friends. This disorder is generally treated with medication.

Asperger's syndrome may be first diagnosed in middle childhood. This is considered a higher-functioning autistic disorder on the spectrum of PDD. The person with Asperger's syndrome is typically highly intelligent but socially awkward. The person has great difficulty learning how to communicate with others, does not understand how other people feel, and cannot understand social cues. Figure 3-1 illustrates this disorder in an adult. The good to excellent academic skills and high level of analytical intelligence associated with Asperger's syndrome are assets for the person. Children with this disorder can achieve success in school and on the job provided they learn to compensate for their difficulties with social cues. Like children with autism, those with Asperger's show clear sensory processing deficits (9).

Children of school age are treated on an outpatient basis and hospitalized only when they are so out of control that they may harm themselves or someone else. They may be seen in school settings, in day treatment settings, or in after-school programs. The *Occupational Therapy Psychosocial Assessment of Learning* (*OT PAL*) may be used to observe and measure the child's ability to function appropriately for his or her age in the classroom (28, 37). Typically, the occupational therapy staff works with other professionals, such as the special education teacher, the speech therapist, the child life specialist, and the school psychologist. The goals of treatment may include increasing trust and social relatedness; developing cooperation; improving self-esteem and self-awareness; enhancing self-control; developing body awareness and sensorimotor skills; and improving coordination, perceptual skills, and cognitive abilities.

Occupational therapy assessment and intervention for school age children logically should first address the occupational roles of the child: family member, friend, player, student, and so on (7). Children and their families can learn how to better use the environment to make it easier for the student to do homework and chores successfully. Segal and Hinojosa (33) point out that families and situations require individual analysis and individualized support.

Occupational therapy treatment models vary with the setting and its philosophy but may involve sensory integrative, behavioral, psychoanalytic, and environmental approaches. Children with ADD or learning disabilities may be taught progressive relaxation and stress management techniques. Computer games have been used to evaluate cognitive and perceptual problems and as rewards or reinforcers for participating in other treatment activities (11). As with the treatment of small children, occupational therapy intervention in middle childhood is considered a complex specialization, and one in which the OTA will benefit from additional training and supervision.

## Adolescence

The most important task of adolescence is to develop an identity separate from one's parents—a social and sexual identity that will support an independent life. Occupational choice (discussed earlier) is a process that contributes to the development of identity in adolescence. Other important experiences center around the peer group of other adolescents. Through a variety of interactions and relationships with others of similar age, the adolescent explores values and interests and develops social skills. It is not unusual for an adolescent to experience insecurity, mood swings, loneliness, depression, and anxiety in response to hormonal and physical changes and the increasingly demanding expectations of others. These are normal responses to a challenging life adjustment. Sometimes, however, the problems are severe.

Major psychiatric disorders such as schizophrenia and mood disorders (mania and depression) often make their first appearance in adolescence. Schizophrenia (see Chapters 3 and 6) is a disorder that is poorly understood but that manifests itself in extreme personal disorganization. Its psychotic symptoms, hallucinations and delusions, can usually be controlled only with prolonged use of powerful medications. But even with medication, many people who have schizophrenia have difficulty setting goals or structuring their time; their sense of self-identity is frequently impaired. The newer, so-called atypical antipsychotic medications are more effective in helping with these problems. However, these more expensive drugs are not always prescribed to persons who receive health care through Medicaid. When schizophrenia occurs as early as adolescence, it interferes with further psychosocial development; in other words, the developmental task of forming a separate identity is extraordinarily difficult, and later development suffers as a consequence.

Mood disorders (mania and depression) may also first appear in adolescence. They have a better prognosis, or predicted outcome, than does schizophrenia. Nonetheless, they are serious disorders, and suicide is a growing risk among adolescents, especially those with mood disorders.

Substance-related disorders are mental health problems that arise from use or excessive use of drugs, alcohol, inhalants, or other mind-altering substances. Adolescents may fall into substance abuse after experimenting with drugs or alcohol to be accepted by their peers. Some adolescents who have other mental health problems use these substances as self-medication to deaden their feelings of anxiety or depression.

Because forging a personal identity is the major task of the adolescent, gender identity may be a source of confusion. Experimentation with various sexual roles can be an expression of personal preference but may also be a way of acting out against one's parents.

Eating disorders affect some adolescents. Anorexia nervosa (abnormal loss of appetite and thinness) and bulimia nervosa (purging after binging) are more common in girls than boys. Real or perceived social pressure to look thin is a contributing factor. These conditions are discussed in Chapter 6.

Although adolescents may be treated in outpatient or community settings, it is not unusual for them to be hospitalized, especially when they are psychotic and in need of medication. Separate wards or adolescent services are provided wherever there are sufficient numbers of adolescent clients to justify the expense. Most adolescent inpatient services use milieu therapy (see Chapter 7). The adolescent who is trying to develop a separate identity will often act out or rebel against authorities (e.g., treatment staff). If the staff is too permissive or inconsistent, the adolescent fails to grasp the boundaries of reasonable behavior; on the other hand, if the staff is too punitive and restrictive, the adolescent may become withdrawn and confused. Staff who work with adolescents are usually trained on the job to support the adolescent's independence while setting firm limits on unacceptable behavior.

Occupational therapy for adolescents is a specialized practice area. The therapist may use specialized evaluation instruments such as the *Adolescent Role Assessment* (5) to learn how the adolescent is adjusting to school, family life, and friendship. The *Adolescent Leisure Interest Profile* (*ALIP*) is a newer evaluation to assess leisure interests (15). Goals of treatment may include development of self-esteem and self-identity skills, development of occupational choice, training in daily living skills, development of sensorimotor skills (especially in relation to body image), and acquisition of prevocational and leisure behaviors.

In selecting activities for adolescents, occupational therapy staff must consider current fashions in activities and technology. Franklin (11), for example, reported that adolescents responded more favorably to a computer-based values clarification program than to a traditional paper-and-pencil version. Baron (2) incorporated computers for word processing and graphics design into the tasks available to adolescent members of a newspaper treatment group. In this group, the variety of job tasks and the structure and limitations provided by the leader helped members acquire and develop a sense of internal control and direction.

In working with adolescents who have mental health problems, the OTA may lead self-care and other activities of daily living (ADLs) groups, provide sessions on sex education and birth control, or run vocational programs such as work groups and assembly lines. Because adolescents are still in school most of the day, occupational therapy and other clinical services are scheduled around consumers' schoolwork. Students with mental health problems may present behavior problems in school; occupational therapy practitioners can help identify the cognitive deficits and other factors responsible and can work with the student to develop less-disruptive and more appropriate ways of coping (8).

In general, the OT or OTA working with the child or adolescent who has mental illness will focus on the young person's "occupations and interests of choice rather than the disorder" (13, p. 2). This is a client-centered practice in which the occupational therapy practitioner asks the young person to identify goals that are personally important. The OT or OTA then creates strategies and interventions to work toward those goals; the young person is continually involved in evaluating whether the plan is working and in determining future goals of interest.

## Early Adulthood

The years from 18 to approximately 40 are filled with challenges and opportunities. Young adults, having completed the process of occupational choice, strive to obtain employment and succeed in their chosen careers. Having attained a sense of identity as a separate person, young adults are able and eager to develop friendships and intimacies with others. The search for a marital or intimate partner is a primary task of this age group. Young adults with children are faced with the new role responsibilities of parenthood. Thus early adulthood is a period characterized by a search for intimacy with others and a desire to achieve and contribute to the future in some way, whether through a career, raising children, or both.

Many of the clients seen in mental health settings fall into this age range. Young adulthood is the period during which many of the major psychiatric disorders of adult life are first noted. Also, for those who are insecure in their jobs or in their personal and sexual or family lives, this can be a period of severe stress and difficult adjustment. Varying levels of employment and uncertain job security can impede occupational success. The fact that there are more women than men in the population means that more women cannot find marriage partners. This is compounded by fears of infection by human immunodeficiency virus (HIV) and other sexually transmitted diseases (STDs). The rise in infertility problems, some a consequence of prior STD infection, in this age group means that many couples cannot have their own biological children. Persons who are HIV positive may fear rejection on the job and in society. All of these factors are potentially stressful and may lead to mental health problems. Individuals with limited coping skills and limited exposure to effective role models may act out their stress and anxiety through domestic abuse and violence, substance abuse, or road rage (aggressive driving).

Among the mental health problems and psychiatric disorders often seen in young adults are adjustment reactions, alcohol and drug abuse, schizophrenia, mood disorders, eating disorders, anxiety disorders, and various personality disorders (see Chapter 6 for more information on diagnoses). Adjustment reactions or disorders are maladaptive or ineffective reactions to life stress; instead of dealing with the stress in a positive way (i.e., by trying to solve problems and rise above the situation), the individual may feel depressed or anxious or function poorly at work or in social situations. It is believed that these people do not have an underlying psychological problem, but rather are reacting to stress. Occupational therapy intervention for people who have adjustment disorders focuses on helping them identify and work toward specific goals. A crisis intervention approach (described in Chapter 7) may be used.

Alcohol and drug abuse is more prevalent among young adults than among adolescents. Alcoholism is a disease that has many definitions; what all of these definitions have in common is excessive or uncontrolled use of alcohol, whether daily or episodically. Alcoholics typically deny that they have a drinking problem; denial prevents them from seeking help or accepting it when it is offered; and this is considered part of the disease. Another problem alcoholics have is with their use of time, they spend their leisure hours drinking and often have no other consistent leisure pursuits. Alcoholics tend to become increasingly dependent on alcohol and are likely to have job problems and end up losing their jobs and relationships.

The goals of occupational therapy for alcohol and drug problems usually include development of self-awareness and self-responsibility, identification of personal goals, vocational assessment and work adjustment, and development of time-management and leisure-planning skills. In particular, recovering alcoholics need to learn new activities and routines for their spare time to replace the empty hours once filled with drinking. Frequently, the occupational therapist and assistant work with a treatment team that may include medical staff, creative arts therapists, psychologists, and alcohol counselors. Programs and occupational therapy approaches to persons with alcoholism and other substance abuse disorders are discussed in more detail in Chapters 6 and 9.

Eating disorders include anorexia and bulimia. Anorexia is a disorder in which the person (usually female) literally starves herself, believing that she is fat even though she is emaciated. Bulimia, also mainly affecting women and girls, is a disorder in which the person goes on eating binges and then makes herself vomit. It is believed that anxiety about self-control versus control by others is one of the factors in both of these conditions. Occupational therapy usually includes assessment and modification of the person's habits and beliefs related to eating and food, education in nutrition and cooking, sensorimotor and expressive activities for development of a more positive body image, and training in daily living skills. Chapter 6 contains more information on these disorders and on occupational therapy approaches to treatment.

Many of the young adults seen in mental health settings have a diagnosis of either schizophrenia or mood disorder. For some this is a continuation of a disease first diagnosed in adolescence, with multiple hospitalizations since then. Others have their first episode during their 20s or 30s. Some individuals are controlled with medication, so that the person leads a fairly normal life free of severe episodes that require hospitalization. However, most cases of schizophrenia and mood disorders become classified as *chronic,* meaning that the disease continues throughout life. These conditions are commonly viewed as serious and persistent mental illness (SPMIs).

Clients with a SPMI are considered very challenging. Some have alcohol and drug disorders and borderline and other personality disorders in addition to schizophrenia or an affective disorder. Although such individuals may have limited skills for independent living, they are usually street smart, able to survive on their own in a marginal way. Large numbers of the homeless are in this group. Many of these people reject the stigma or label of mental illness, refuse to identify themselves as ill, and move in and out of treatment on personal whim. Involvement in criminal activities is not unusual; these clients may as easily be imprisoned as hospitalized (34).

Obviously, not all young adults with SPMIs share these characteristics. Some respond well to a structured environment and accept the role of patient or client. The challenge is to motivate such clients to do their best within the limits of the disability. Others are very difficult to manage and hard to keep in a program. These clients decide what to do based on what they want at the moment. If the therapist will not give in right now, the client is likely to walk out and not come back until no other option remains.

High-functioning young adults with SPMIs are more receptive to help as long as it is provided in a manner that meets self-esteem needs and aspirations. The person is likely to be well educated and to hold very specific career goals. Such individuals do not want to be identified as patients but will actively participate in a treatment program if it is provided somewhere that is not identified as a hospital or part of the mental health system,

A psychoeducational approach is often used with these consumers. When skills are presented in this format, the person can perceive them as education rather than therapy, thus supporting the identity of self as a person rather than a patient (34).

Occupational therapy goals for young adults focus on the development of adult life skills and the fulfillment of personal aspirations. Typical goals include completing one's education, identifying vocational interests and aptitudes, acquiring prevocational and vocational skills, obtaining and maintaining employment, developing daily living skills, improving social skills, developing coping skills, identifying and developing leisure interests, and structuring leisure time. The therapist performs the evaluations and formulates the treatment goals and plan, working closely with the client.

The OTA may provide tutoring or academic assistance while the person works toward a general equivalency diploma (GED) or other educational goal. Other roles for the OTA include running classes or training programs for daily living skills, social skills, leisure skills, and job search skills and day-to-day supervision of work-oriented programs.

## Midlife

Ferol Menks, an occupational therapist, defines midlife as "the point in the life cycle when the individual realizes that time is limited and that he or she cannot accomplish everything hoped and planned for" (26). The goals that were selected and pursued during the early adult years may have been reached or may seem unattainable. Around age 40 the adult begins to reevaluate life's direction, feeling that this may be the last chance to make major changes.

Erikson (10) conceptualizes the major task of the middle adult years somewhat differently, terming it the crisis of *generativity versus stagnation. Generativity* is a "concern in establishing and guiding the next generation." Adults in the middle years who are unable to direct this energy successfully will feel stagnant or purposeless, cut off from the stream of human achievement that extends into the future.

One obvious avenue for achieving generativity is through one's children, but this path is not open to everyone and for many does not by itself satisfy this urge. For those who are working, this need may be transformed into a concern with nurturing the careers of younger workers. Some adults seek out ways to contribute their expertise and energies through church or community organizations.

The adult at midlife assesses whether work has been satisfying and worthwhile. If the work is found lacking either in opportunities for further achievement or in personal satisfaction, the individual may move into a second career. This may necessitate a return to school, a transition that some find stressful.

Additional developmental stresses center around the process of aging. During this period, the adult undergoes a decline in physical capacities, a change in sexual energies, and significant cosmetic deterioration (wrinkles and so on). Women go through menopause, and men's sexual potency declines. All of these changes signify that one is no longer young. Different people react differently to this. Some seek cosmetic surgery, subject themselves to intense exercise programs, look for younger sexual partners, and attempt to stay the forces of time. Others accept these changes gracefully as a condition of life and move on to other concerns.

Typically, the children of adults in this age group are teenagers. Dealing with the rebellion and turmoil of adolescent children can be a challenge and joy or a significant stress, depending upon the adult's coping skills. Eventually these children mature, leave home, and create lives and families of their own; some adults find this prospect alarming because it means the end of their own roles as parents. Midlife adults also are frequently faced with the needs of their own aging parents, who may be dependent in some way on their care and whose deterioration is a reminder of the inescapability of death. Adults caught between the demands of their aging parents and demands of their own children have been named "the sandwich generation."

Thus the stresses on the midlife adult are multiple. Successful negotiation of this stage entails understanding and accepting the aging process and identifying and pursuing goals in work or family or community life that enable one to contribute to the future in a way that feels significant to the individual.

It is helpful to categorize midlife adults who have mental disorders into three groups. The first group consists of those who have had mental health problems for many years—problems that have continued and often worsened as they aged. The second group comprises persons with various adjustment disorders, those who are unable to master or resolve the crises and stresses of adult life and who resort to maladaptive behaviors such as drug and alcohol abuse, overeating, or withdrawal. The third group consists of individuals who are developing dementias such as Alzheimer's disease. Each of these groups has different treatment needs.

Many of the middle-aged adults who have had mental health problems for many years are somewhat burned out. This means that they have little energy and seem passive and almost indifferent to what goes on around them. They will go along with treatment programs but do not seem to have much invested in their own progress; getting through each day seems enough of a challenge. Not every person in this category is burned out, however. Some are career patients who have come to identify themselves in the patient role; they use the mental health system to meet their needs for physical safety, food, shelter, and economic assistance. Occupational therapy interventions for adults with chronic disorders of long standing focus on improving and maintaining daily living skills, providing opportunities for productive work in a sheltered environment, and facilitating as much independent function as the person can manage.

The second group, those with adjustment reactions to the crises and stresses of adult life, need assistance in identifying and resolving the issues that confront them. As was mentioned earlier, crisis intervention is a widely used approach. Menks (25) has described a *conflict resolution model* in which the occupational therapist guides the client through five steps that begin with identifying the problem and end with implementing a plan of action. The problems addressed are varied, ranging from how to use leisure time to how to compensate for a career that feels demeaning and pointless to how to cope with divorce or the death of a spouse.

In the third category are people with primary degenerative dementia, a kind of organic brain syndrome that is progressive. Alzheimer's disease, which is in this category, may show its first signs as early as age 40. Memory impairment or forgetfulness is usually the first symptom; the person first has trouble remembering details (dates, names, facts), and the memory loss becomes more profound as the disease progresses. Gradually so much of the memory is lost that the victims cannot complete simple activities because they do not remember that they started them. There are personality changes as well; though these are not always noticeable in the early stages, the behavior of persons with dementia becomes less social and more inappropriate over time. Ultimately, they lose physical neuromotor control over their bodies, become incontinent and less mobile, and die.

Because the symptoms of Alzheimer's disease progress slowly at first, the person in the early stages of the illness can usually continue customary activities with a few minor adjustments. For example, at work the person may have to be supervised more closely than before or switch to duties that require less attention to detail. Similarly, family members have to compensate for cognitive deficits in the home. The patient who is the cook in the family needs supervision to make sure he or she does not cause a fire. Occupational therapists and assistants work with these early-stage individuals and their families in the home wherever possible. The goals of intervention are to assess what areas and activities are causing difficulty for the person, to evaluate current strengths and deficits, and to help the family adapt the environment and provide the social support the person needs.

It is important that persons with Alzheimer's disease remain at home or in the accustomed environment for as long as possible, because they are better able to function in familiar environments than in new ones (24). In the later stages of their illness, these individuals cannot remain in the community because they need either medical care or round-the-clock supervision. They are most frequently placed in nursing homes, although some are hospitalized in large public institutions. Occupational therapists and assistants provide services that help them remain alert and function to the best of their present capacities. These might include reality orientation (described in Chapter 22), sensory stimulation (e.g., olfactory and tactile stimulation), and physical activities (exercise, ball play, dancing). Memory training is sometimes used with those who are higher functioning—that is, are in the early or middle stage of the disease.

## Late Adulthood and Aging

The most important psychosocial task of older adults is believed by many experts to be the development of an understanding and appreciation for what they have accomplished during their lives. Erikson (10) has called this the crisis of *ego integrity versus despair.* Erikson believed that in order to feel that life has been worthwhile, the older adult needs to see the self as only a small part of the human community, which will endure beyond one's own death.

In addition to this major developmental task, the older adult often must deal with significant life stress. One's aging body, retirement and the loss of a career role, the deaths of spouses and cherished friends, economic worries, and the loss of one's home are just a few of the stresses that may press on the older adult's diminished energies. New hobbies, new friendships, and new roles as volunteer or grandparent may compensate for some of these losses, but many older adults find it difficult to make these adjustments.

Shimp (35) reminds us that many of our cherished "truths" about older people are in fact myths. While many retirees are satisfied and relieved to give up their productive roles, many others happily undertake volunteer and paid jobs into their 90s. Also, the notion that the aged cannot adapt to life stresses needs careful examination in each case. Even a severe stress such as acute-care hospitalization can be endured and managed successfully, given sufficient motivation and hope.

Depression is the most common psychiatric diagnosis in the elderly population. A person in a very deep or severe depression can become so withdrawn and self-involved as to appear demented (cognitively impaired); for this reason, the condition is sometimes misdiagnosed as an organic mental disorder. In some cases, the depression is masked by multiple physical complaints—aches and pains, stomach problems, and so on—that may cause physicians to completely miss the underlying depression. When the depression is finally recognized and properly treated, usually with medication, the person's attention and cognitive functions return to normal. After depression, Alzheimer's disease and other organic mental disorders are the psychiatric conditions most commonly diagnosed in the aged population. Coincidentally and confusingly from a diagnostic point of view, depression is often a symptom of organic mental disorder.

Occupational therapy may be provided to the older adult in the home, in a geriatric day center, or in a hospital or nursing home. The purpose of occupational therapy is to help the older adult maintain or achieve a feeling of competence or self-reliance and to prevent further deterioration in functioning. Environmental adaptations made by the occupational therapy practitioner can allow higher-functioning individuals to continue living in their own homes; this is very important for maintaining their sense of self-identity and a personal daily routine. In addition, the therapist or assistant may provide leisure counseling, assist in the development of hobbies, and facilitate social involvement.

Occupational therapy interventions for the older adult in a nursing home or geropsychiatric unit are similar to those described earlier for the midlife adult with Alzheimer's disease. The OTA may use reality orientation and remotivation or reminiscence techniques and life-review activities (described in Chapters 20 to 22) or instruct nursing staff and volunteers to do so. Other aspects of occupational therapy intervention for this group are described in Chapter 9.

Because not all residents in a nursing home function at such a low level, the occupational therapist must plan programs that allow people with different capacities to participate and that provide challenges to each person at his or her own level. The therapist begins by assessing how well each person functions in terms of social, physical, and cognitive functioning and self-care skills. The *Parachek Geriatric Rating Scale* (27, 29), which is sometimes used for this, may be administered by the OTA. The Parachek scale allows the observer to rate 10 functions in the three categories of physical capabilities, self-care skills, and social interaction. The scoring system and treatment manual that accompany the scale assist the therapist in assigning residents to groups based on functional level as determined by their scores on the rating scale. Parachek recommends that crafts and cognitive activities like games and puzzles be provided for higher-functioning residents, simple group activities and self-care for those with scores in the middle range, and sensory stimulation for those with the lowest scores. She recommends physical activities for all three groups and adapts the activities to compensate for more limited function in the low-scoring group. Allen Cognitive Level tests, described in Chapter 3, may also be used, along with the Allen approach to cognitive disabilities.

The OTA who works with the geriatric population must be very receptive to the needs and concerns of the older individual. It is important to respect and accommodate the habits and beliefs that the person has built up over a lifetime. Because they have lost so many of the things that were once important to them, older people often fear the loss of their identity and self-direction and may feel threatened when a health professional pushes them too far too fast. Also, because of a general slowing of physical capacities, older people may respond less quickly and usually need more time to answer questions and learn new things. Finally, the older individual thinks often and deeply about the past and enjoys telling stories about it; this recounting is an important psychological process for establishing a sense of ego integrity. It is important for the OTA to recognize the value of this reminiscence and encourage it.

## SUMMARY

We can think of life as a puzzle or a project that can be worked out only by traveling down a path that is not always clear. A turn in the road may bring us face to face with obstacles that must be dealt with before we can proceed. As the quotation from William James at the beginning of this chapter suggests, obstacles and crises often stimulate us to reach deeper into ourselves and thus grow and develop. We each have our own tools (our native talents and acquired skills) to help us work out the puzzle and to clear the path. Sometimes, though, the obstacle seems unconquerable, and this is when mental health problems arise.

Problems can occur at any age at any point along the path; some individuals are more vulnerable to these problems than are others. The role of the mental health professional is not to solve the problem or clear the path but to enable people to tackle and master their own obstacles so that they can clear their own way and proceed. To do this well, we must know as much as we can about human development, because this forms the underlying structure of each person's path;

knowledge of major developmental milestones and tasks helps us predict a person's capabilities at each point in the life span and alerts us to possible stresses and vulnerabilities.

We must also know as much as possible about occupation and its development in the human being, and we must value it highly. Occupation is an essentially human tool for tackling the puzzles of life. It gives us a sense of purpose and competence, channels our energies, and sustains our forward movement. Without occupation there is no progress; everything stops. When occupation is disordered and when occupational roles are poorly grasped and weakly lived, life becomes chaotic. Disability or disease may impair the ability to use occupation, depriving the individual of a vital link to living ordinary life. The role of occupational therapy is to restore this ability, to enable and support each person's ability to use this powerful tool to solve life's puzzles, to master stresses and obstacles, and to propel the self on the path to the future. The following case example illustrates the interactions among developmental tasks, the development of human occupation, environmental risk factors, and age-specific vulnerabilities to mental illness and provides an opportunity for the reader to explore these issues further.

## CASE EXAMPLE

### Ericka

Ericka is a 17-year-old black, single student in a large city high school. She was recently arrested for a felony, charged with putting a younger girl in a choke hold while two others tore the gold chains from the victim's neck.

Ericka is the 6th of 14 children of an unmarried drug-addicted mother. Ericka was born addicted to crack cocaine. She received therapy in the neonatal intensive care unit (NICU) and later through several early intervention (EI) programs. At one time, Ericka attended a school for emotionally disturbed (ED) children; but at age 11 and in the 5th grade, she was mainstreamed into a public school, where she received special services outside the normal classroom in which she was placed. At present, she is in 10th grade in a special education classroom. She is a poor student but attends school consistently. Teachers report that she does not sit still easily and that she is quickly distracted. She has limited social skills (has trouble negotiating, enters situations without trying to understand them first, interrupts, and so on), and has no close friends. The female police officer who arrested her said that Ericka indicated that the girls from the gang were her "friends" but that Ericka also said they had been friends for just a couple of weeks, during which time the other girls encouraged Ericka to bully and overpower victims for them.

Ericka is tall for her age (5 feet, 11 inches). She lives with her great-grandmother because both her parents are now deceased. The great-grandmother, aged 62, says she has tried to keep Ericka under control and that she is afraid Ericka has begun, with her new friends, to use marijuana and drink beer.

#### Case Study Questions

- Discuss the developmental task(s) of Ericka's age group.
- Identify the environmental risk factors for Ericka.
- For what mental disorder(s) does Ericka seem to be at risk?
- Based on the information provided, discuss Ericka's mastery of the occupational roles that are normal at her age.
- Following from the model of human occupation, what else would you like to know about Ericka?
- How would you begin to engage Ericka in a discussion of goals she might value or want to work toward?

## REVIEW QUESTIONS AND ACTIVITIES

1. Contrast the motivations for exploration, achievement, and competency.
2. Define *work–play balance* and discuss the amount of time spent in work and play at different stages of life.
3. Briefly describe the occupations of the child, the adolescent, the adult, and the late-life adult.
4. Identify important achievements in occupational development at each of the following life stages: childhood, adolescence, adulthood, and late adulthood.
5. Trace the development of the worker role from childhood through retirement.
6. For each of the major life stages identified in the chapter, list the psychiatric diagnoses that are common to that stage. For each diagnosis on your list, write down the effects of the disorder on the ability to function in performing occupations of play, work, education, leisure, ADLs, instrumental activities of daily living (IADLs), and social participation. Where the information is provided, also note the occupational therapy intervention that is recommended.
7. Ericka, introduced in the case study, is now 17 years old. Write a description of her as you imagine she might be at 27, 47, 67, or 87 years of age. Emphasize her occupational functioning. Write a best-case and a worst-case scenario. (This may be done as a class project, with different groups taking different ages.)

## REFERENCES


1. Angier N. The purpose of playful frolics: Training for adulthood. New York Times, Oct 20, 1992, C1–8.
2. Baron KB. The model of human occupation: A newspaper treatment group for adolescents with a diagnosis of conduct disorder. Occup Ther Ment Health 1987;7(2): 89–104.
3. Baron KB. The use of play in child psychiatry: Reframing the therapeutic environment. Occup Ther Ment Health 1991;11(2–3):37–56.
4. Behnke CJ, Fetkovich MM. Examining the reliability and validity of the play history. Am J Occup Ther 1984;38:94–100.
5. Black MM. Adolescent role assessment. Am J Occup Ther 1976;30:73–79.
6. Burnell DP. Children with severe emotional or behavioral disorders. In: Clark PN, Allen AS, eds. Occupational Therapy for Children. St Louis: Mosby, 1985.
7. Coster W. Occupation-centered assessment of children. Am J Occup Ther 1998;52:337–344.
8. Dirette D, Kolak L. Occupational performance needs of adolescents in alternative education programs. Am J Occup Ther 2004;58:337–341.
9. Dunn W, Myles BS, Orr S. Sensory processing issues associated with Asperger syndrome: A preliminary investigation. Am J Occup Ther 2002;56:97–102.
10. Erikson E. Childhood and Society. New York: Norton, 1963.
11. Franklin DA. comparison of the effectiveness of values clarification presented as a personal computer program versus a traditional therapy group: A pilot study. Occup Ther Ment Health 1986;6(3):39–52.
12. Ginzburg E. Toward a theory of occupational choice. In: Peters HC, Hansen JC. Vocational Guidance and Career Development. New York: Macmillan, 1971.
13. Gray K. Mental illness in children and adolescents: A place for occupational therapy. Am J Occup Ther Ment Health Special Interest Section Q 2005;28(2):1–3.
14. Harris JR. The Nurture Assumption: Why Children Turn Out the Way They Do. New York: Free Press, 1998.
15. Henry AD. Development of a measure of adolescent leisure interests. Am J Occup Ther 1998;52:531–539.
16. Horowitz BP. Occupational therapy home assessments: Supporting community living through client-center practice. Occup Ther Ment Health 2002;18(1):1–17
17. Howie L, Coulter M, Feldman S. Crafting the self: Older person's narratives of occupational identity. Am J Occup Ther 2004;58:446–454.
18. James W. Letter to W. Lutoslawski, May 6, 1906. In: Beck EM, ed. Bartlett's Familiar Quotations. 15th ed. Boston: Little, Brown, 1980.
19. Jonsson H, Kielhofner G, Borell L. Anticipating retirement: The formation of narratives concerning an occupational transition. Am J Occup Ther 1997;51:49–56.
20. Kielhofner G. A Model of Human Occupation: Theory and Application. 2nd ed. Baltimore: Williams & Wilkins; 1995.
21. Kielhofner G. A model of human occupation: 2. Ontogenesis from the perspective of temporal adaptation. Am J Occup Ther 1980;34:657–663.
22. Kramer LA, Deitz JC, Crowe TK. A comparison of motor performance of preschoolers enrolled in mental health programs and non-mental health programs. Am J Occup Ther 1988;42:520–525.
23. Larson EA. Children's work: The less considered childhood occupation. Am J Occup Ther. 2004;58:369–379.
24. Liu L, Gauthier L, Gauthier S. Spatial disorientation in persons with early senile dementia of the Alzheimer type. Am J Occup Ther 1991;45:67–74.
25. Menks F. Challenges of mid life: An occupational therapy conflict resolution model. Occup Ther Ment Health 1980;1(4):23–32.
26. Menks F. Changes and challenges of mid life: 1. A review of the literature. Occup Ther Ment Health 1980; 1(3): 15–28.
27. Miller ER, Parachek JR. Validation and standardization of a goal-oriented, quick screening geriatric scale. J Am Geriatr Soc 1974;22:224–237.
28. Nave J, Helfrich CA, Aviles A. Child witnesses of domestic violence: A case study using the OT PAL. Occup Ther Ment Health 2001;16(3–4):127–135.
29. Parachek JF. Parachek Geriatric Rating Scale. 3rd ed. Phoenix, AZ: Center for Neurodevelopmental Studies, 1986.
30. Peterson TW. Recent studies in autism: A review of the literature. Occup Ther Ment Health 1986;6(4):63–75.
31. Reilly M. Play as Exploratory Learning. Beverly Hills, CA: Sage, 1974.
32. Robinson AL. Play: The area for acquisition of rules for competent behavior. Am J Occup Ther 1977;31: 248–253.
33. Segal R, Hinojosa J. The activity setting of homework: An analysis of three cases and implications for occupational therapy. Am J Occup Ther 2006;60:50–59.
34. Sheets JL, Prevost JA, Reihman J. Young adult chronic patients: Three hypothesized subgroups. In: Hospital and Community Psychiatry Service of the American Psychiatric Association. The young adult chronic patient: Collected articles from H&CP. Washington, DC: APA, 1983.
35. Shimp S. Debunking the myths of aging. Occup Ther Ment Health 1990;10:101–111.
36. Takata N. The play history. Am J Occup Ther 1969;23(3):314–318.

37. Townsend S, Carey P, Hollins N, et al. The Occupational Therapy Psychosocial Assessment of Learning. Chicago: Model of Human Occupation Clearinghouse, University of Illinois at Chicago, 2000.
38. Vaillant GE, Vaillant CO. Natural history of male psychological health: 10. Work as a predictor of positive mental health. Am J Psychiatry 1981;138:1433–1440.
39. Watling RL, Deitz J, White O. Comparison of sensory profile scores of young children with and without autism spectrum disorders. Am J Occup Ther 2001;55: 416–423.

## SUGGESTED READINGS

Fazio LS. Tell me a story: The therapeutic metaphor in the practice of pediatric occupational therapy. Am J Occup Ther 1992;46:112–119.

Glogoski-Williams C. Recognition of depression in the older adult. Occup Ther Ment Health 2000;15(2):17–34.

Gray K. Mental illness in children and adolescents: A place for occupational therapy. Am J Occup Ther Ment Health Special Interest Section Q 2005;28(2):1–3.

Jackson J, Carlson M, Mandel D, et al. Occupation in lifestyle redesign: The well elderly study occupational therapy program. Am J Occup Ther 1998;52: 326–344.

Jamison KR. An Unquiet Mind. New York: Vintage, 1995.

Kaysen S. Girl, Interrupted. New York: Vintage, 1993.

Larson EA. Children's work: The less considered childhood occupation. Am J Occup Ther 2004;58:369–379.

Levinson DJ. The Seasons of a Man's Life. New York: Ballantine Books, 1978.

Maiorana R. Early recognition and management of alcohol problems: Occupational therapy treatment. Am Occup Ther Assoc Ment Health Special Interest Section Newslett 1984;7(2):1–2.

Mallinson T, Kielhofner G, Mattingly C. Metaphor and meaning in a clinical interview. Am J Occup Ther 1996;50: 338–346.

Sheehy G. Passages: Predictable Crises of Adult Life. New York: Bantam, 1978.

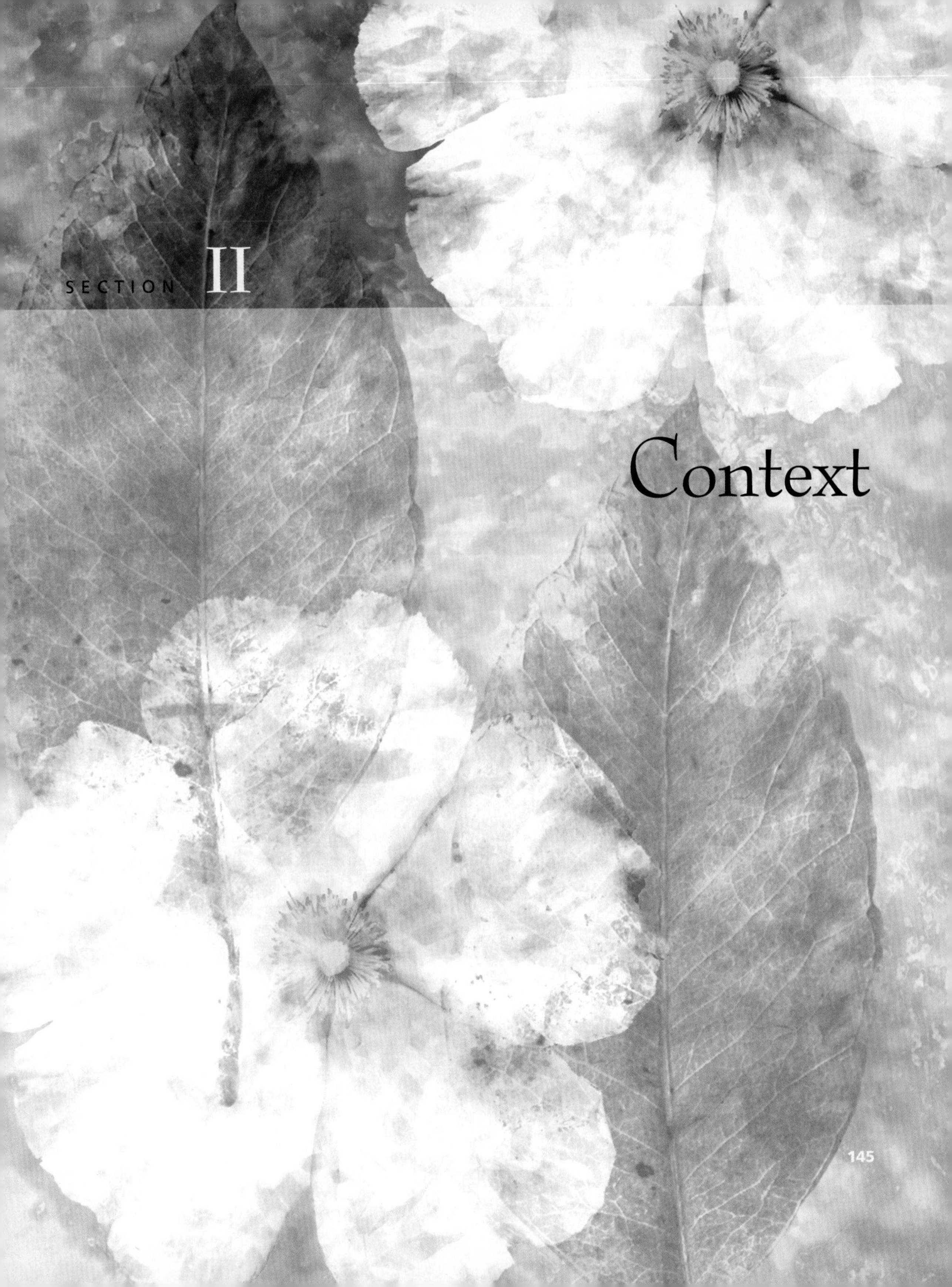

SECTION II

# Context

CHAPTER 6

# Understanding Psychiatric Diagnosis: The *DSM-IV-TR*

***The diagnosis of disease is often easy, often difficult, and often impossible.***

PETER MERE LATHAM (42, P. 463)

## CHAPTER OBJECTIVES

After studying this chapter, the reader will be able to:

1. Identify the purpose of the *Diagnostic and Statistical Manual of Mental Disorders*, fourth edition, text revision (*DSM-IV-TR*).
2. Name and describe the five axes of the *DSM*.
3. Understand the *DSM* system as an evolving system.
4. Explain how the information in the *DSM-IV-TR* can be useful to the occupational therapy practitioner.
5. Name and describe major mental disorders affecting clients seen in occupational therapy.
6. For each major mental disorder, state the treatments used by psychiatrists.
7. For each mental disorder, describe the effects on performance of occupation, the typical problems addressed by occupational therapy, and the interventions used.
8. Explain what is meant by *comorbidity* and discuss how comorbidity affects occupational therapy intervention.
9. Describe the plans for *DSM-V* and the relevance of the proposed changes to occupational therapy.

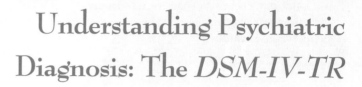

The occupational therapy assistant (OTA) in a mental health setting will most often work with clients who have received a psychiatric diagnosis. Understanding how such diagnoses are reached can help the OTA understand how clients are viewed by other staff, who may be more concerned about clients' symptoms and expressed feelings than about their ability to function in everyday life and major occupational roles. To appreciate how occupational therapy (OT) fits within the treatment team in a mental health setting, one must first appreciate the larger framework of psychiatric diagnosis.

The American Psychiatric Association defines diagnosis as "the process of determining, through examination and analysis, the nature of a patient's illness" (23, p. 62). This definition implies that diagnosis is an ongoing process rather than a final verdict. As was suggested in Chapters 2 and 3, the behaviors and complaints that are grouped together as mental illnesses are not well understood. Evidence supports the hypothesis that abnormalities in the chemistry and structure of the brain are involved in many psychiatric disorders. Increasingly, the major mental illnesses are being seen as brain disorders. Most scholars also believe that the social environment, particularly during development, also plays a role. Stress and life circumstances may also cause or contribute to mental illness.

Clients entering the mental health system are usually assigned, within the first few weeks, a diagnosis from the *Diagnostic and Statistical Manual of Mental Disorders,* fourth edition, text revision (*DSM-IV-TR*). This chapter introduces the reader to the major concepts and overall structure of the *DSM-IV-TR*. The reader will learn some of the underlying assumptions of psychiatric diagnosis. We will explore the structure and organization of the *DSM-IV-TR* and the features of some major diagnostic categories commonly encountered in OT practice in mental health. For each diagnostic category, we will briefly outline some of the problems typically addressed by OT, and the kinds of interventions used.

Throughout this chapter, we will refer to the diagnostician—the individual responsible for the psychiatric diagnosis. Depending on the practice setting, this may be a psychiatrist, a physician with another practice specialty, a psychologist, a psychiatric nurse practitioner, or a psychiatric social worker.

## PSYCHIATRIC DIAGNOSIS: AN EVOLVING SCIENCE

From the 1800s, when all mental disease was categorized as idiocy, to the mid-20th century, when a few diagnostic categories were listed in the *International Classification of Disease* (*ICD*), very little information was available to guide the diagnostician in determining the cause and nature of a person's mental health problems. The *Diagnostic and Statistical Manual, Mental Disorders* (*DSM-I*), published in 1952, was an attempt to offer more structure. Since that time, the *DSM* has undergone many revisions in an effort to improve the accuracy and usefulness of each diagnosis. The *DSM-III* added four new dimensions, or axes, to the main diagnosis (Axis I). The *DSM-IV* was published in 1994; a revision to the text, the *DSM-IV-TR,* was published in 2000 (8, 9). The *DSM-IV-TR,* the current manual at this writing, retains the axial system of the *DSM-III.* The five axes are as follows:

- *Axis I.* Clinical disorders and other conditions that may be a focus of clinical attention
- *Axis II.* Personality disorders, mental retardation
- *Axis III.* General medical disorders
- *Axis IV.* Psychosocial and environmental problems
- *Axis V.* Global assessment of functioning

Axis I is the main psychiatric diagnosis (e.g., schizophrenia, depression). An individual may be assigned more than one diagnosis on axis I. For some clients, no diagnosis is made on axis I; instead, the main diagnosis appears on axis II (e.g., those who have personality disorders or mental retardation in the absence of any other major psychiatric disorder). The other conditions that might be coded on this axis are *(a)* psychological factors affecting medical condition (e.g., maladaptive health behaviors, coping style); *(b)* medication-induced movement disorders (e.g., tardive dyskinesia; discussed in Chapter 8); *(c)* problems in relationships (e.g., between parent and child); *(d)* problems related to abuse or neglect (e.g., physical or sexual abuse); and *(e)* other factors such as difficulties adjusting to a new culture, problems in school or at work, etc. (8).

Axis II describes a different category of mental disorders. These are not the disease entities of axis I but rather the characteristic styles of adaptation that constitute a maladaptive personality. Some examples are paranoid, histrionic, and dependent. Diagnosticians and social scientists continue to debate the distinction between a personality *style* and a personality *disorder.* Large numbers of people have these personality styles and never make contact with the mental health system, so why are they termed disorders? At what point should the person with a suspicious nature be labeled with an axis II diagnosis of paranoid personality disorder? To account for a range in expression of a personality trait, the diagnostician may simply note this as "paranoid personality features" on axis II without assigning the diagnosis of paranoid personality. Mental retardation may be diagnosed separately on axis II.

Axis III lists general medical disorders. The physician must assign a code from the Centers for Disease Control's *International Classification of Disease,* ninth edition, clinical modification (*ICD-9-CM*) which is derived from the World Health Organization's ICD-9 (59). The aim of this axis is "to encourage thoroughness in communication and to enhance communication among health care providers" (8, p. 27). The developers of *DSM-IV-TR* note that physical problems are stressful and may evoke psychological reactions. Some physical diseases, such as multiple sclerosis, characteristically are associated with psychological symptoms. In older persons, psychiatric symptoms may be the first expression of underlying medical problems.

Axis IV describes problems in the environment, in life circumstances, or in relationships with others. Generally these are negative conditions (e.g., death of a loved one, loss of a job, marital discord). Some positive conditions (e.g., promotion to a higher level at work) may appear on this axis if they cause the individual significant stress. The problems are grouped for coding into categories such as housing problems and problems with access to health services.

Axis V provides for the coding of the person's level of functioning at the time of evaluation. Additional ratings may be made (e.g., at admission and at discharge, highest level during the past year). Because OT is concerned with the individual's ability to function in daily life roles and activities, axis V is important to OT practitioners. Information from OT evaluations and observations can assist the physician or other diagnostician in determining the appropriate rating. Axis V is rated on a scale from 0 to 100. A rating of 90 indicates good functioning overall; a rating of 10 is associated with persistent danger to self and others. Axis V is rated with the *Global Assessment of Functioning Scale* (*GAF Scale*), to which the reader is referred for more information.[1]

Figure 6-1 depicts the dynamic interaction among the axes of *DSM-IV-TR.* The five axes act independently but affect each other to create ever-changing conditions—challenges and opportunities to which the individual may respond

[1] The *GAF Scale* and the directions for scoring are available in the *DSM-IV-TR* (9, pp. 33–34).

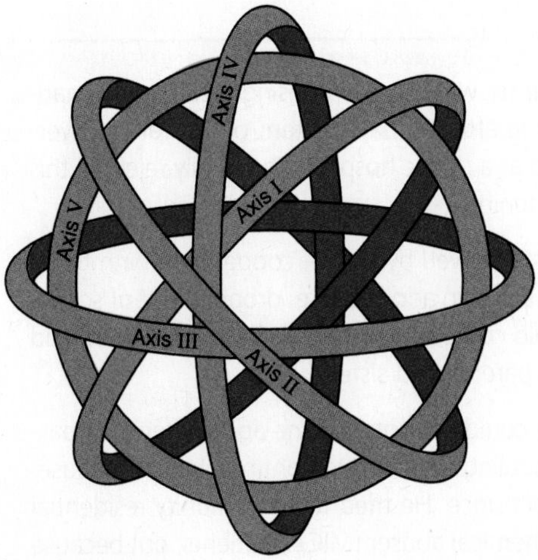


**Figure 6-1. Multiaxial dimensions of psychiatric disorders.**

adaptively or maladaptively. The case example of Matthew, given in Box 6-1, uses the multiaxial (many axes) diagnostic system from *DSM-IV-TR*. This case illustrates how psychiatric disorders may be compounded by chemical abuse, social conditions, and physical disorders. The reader may find it interesting to review the case example of Ericka, given in Chapter 5, from a multiaxial perspective. Multiaxial diagnoses may also be found in the case examples in Appendix A.

As the ongoing revision of successive editions of the *DSM* suggests, the science of psychiatric diagnosis continues to evolve. It is not yet an exact or definitive process. It is not yet as accurate as is the diagnosis of many physical conditions. The

**BOX 6-1**

### MULTIAXIAL *DSM-IV-TR* DIAGNOSIS, "OZONE LAYER"

A 27-year-old white Jewish male named Matthew was admitted through a city hospital emergency room to Garden of Eden State Psychiatric Center in New York City 2 days after the police found him wandering on the street in a neighborhood known for its illegal drug trade. When the police apprehended him, he was naked, shouting, "The ozone layer is gone! God is burning us up for our sins!" and "I am the son of God. I can heal the ozone layer by my touch."

Matthew was restless and required restraint during the initial examination to prevent injury to self and others. He was 40 pounds underweight, poorly nourished, and unkempt, with open sores on his feet and hands and track marks on his arms and feet (suggesting intravenous drug use).

A family history revealed a paternal uncle who had been hospitalized for mental disease in late adolescence and who never subsequently lived outside the hospital. A cousin on his mother's side has had several acute schizophrenic episodes. Matthew's parents and older sister are all professionals. He has had 17 admissions to both public and private psychiatric and drug rehab centers; although the family has been concerned, they have not always followed through with treatment recommendations.

Previous records indicate that Matthew was a difficult child who argued and fought with playmates from an early age. By the time Matthew entered kindergarten, his pediatrician had recommended a psychiatric consultation because of concern about bed wetting, playing with matches, and the near torturing of the family dog. The psychiatrist told the parents that their son had an above-average IQ (133), possessed an ability to take apart and reassemble mechanical devices (clocks, radios)—remarkable in a child of his age—and was developing a severe and chronic behavioral disorder. Various therapies during childhood had poor results; Matthew was first hospitalized at age 13 when he tore the house apart

*(continued)*

**BOX 6-1 (Continued)**

after a teacher asked him to rewrite a composition. Because he was already abusing alcohol and marijuana, his parents agreed to inpatient treatment. On discharge after 90 days (extent of insurance coverage), the hospital recommended that treatment be continued at a public hospital. The family rejected this recommendation because they found the public facility frightening.

This was the first instance in a repeating pattern of treatment followed by lack of cooperation with treatment recommendations. Matthew moved into the hard-drug scene in adolescence, dropped out of school in 10th grade, and ran away from home many times. He would come home and ask for food, a bath, and money. When refused money, he would try to steal from his parents and sister.

When Matthew was 19 years old, the family told him that he could not come home again after their parents-of-addicts support group confronted them with their enabling their son to continue his drug abuse. Matthew has been living on the street for much of the 8 years since. He tried five community residential rehabilitation programs for drug abusers and for mentally ill chemical abuser (MICA) patients; but because he was unwilling or unable to comply with the rules, the programs were unsuccessful each time. He has since been rejected for treatment by five other residential programs. At times, Matthew has been detoxified and appropriately medicated, which reduced his symptoms. He states that his problems are really simple: "People should just be allowed to do whatever they want as long as they don't hurt others. I could do just fine if the police would mind their own business."

Matthew's Social Security benefits have been discontinued because he failed to report for an annual evaluation. His parents refuse to allow him to return to their home

***DSM-IV-TR* Diagnosis**

| | |
|---|---|
| Axis I | 295.30 Schizophrenia, paranoid type |
| | 305.00 Alcohol abuse |
| | 304.30 Cannabis abuse |
| | R/O 305.50 Opioid abuse |
| Axis II | 301.70 Antisocial personality disorder |
| Axis III | Adult protein energy malnutrition (PEM)—not classified in *ICD-9-CM* |
| | R/O human immunodeficiency virus (HIV) infection |
| Axis IV | Estrangement from family, poverty, loss of Social Security benefits, homelessness |
| Axis V | Current *GAF:* 0 (inadequate information) |
| | Highest *GAF* past year: 25 (unable to function in most areas) |

Adapted from a case example contributed by Hermine D. Plotnick and Margaret D. Rerek.

fact that experts debate the specific classification of the variety of mental disturbances that affect humanity in a manner very different from their classification of physical medical conditions should alone suggest how difficult it is to understand mental disorders.

## THE DIAGNOSTIC CATEGORIES OF THE *DSM-IV-TR*

Information in this section follows the organization of the *DSM-IV-TR*.[2] Selected disorders or categories are summarized. Inclusion in this textbook is based on the prevalence of the disorder and the likelihood that it will be encountered by the entry-level OTA working in a clinical or community setting. Details and descriptive illustrations are used as needed to provide a clearer picture. Typical problems addressed by OT are indicated. For a more scholarly and exact discussion, the reader may consult the references.

The summaries are brief. The reader is cautioned that duration and frequency of symptoms are considered by the diagnostician and are part of the operational criteria for each diagnostic entity. *Duration* refers to "how long" the symptoms have been present. *Frequency* refers to "how often" the symptoms are felt. Also, although some of the operational criteria are listed for each diagnosis, space does not permit a full listing. The reader should consult the current *DSM* for detail when needed.

### Disorders First Evident in Infancy, Childhood, or Adolescence

Only a few disorders first appear in childhood, but they have a profound effect. Occurring early in development, conditions such as autism, learning disabilities, and conduct disorders impair the growing child's ability to perceive and respond effectively to the environment. Thus these conditions significantly affect learning and skill development. There are 10 categories of disorders in this group:

- Mental retardation (coded on axis II)
- Learning disorders
- Motor skills disorders
- Communication disorders
- Pervasive developmental disorders (e.g., autism)
- Attention deficit and disruptive behavior disorders
- Feeding and eating disorders of infancy or early childhood
- Tic disorders (e.g., Tourette's disorder)
- Elimination disorders (e.g., bed wetting)
- Other disorders of infancy, childhood, or adolescence

*Mental retardation* (axis II) is characterized by *(a)* intellectual functioning that is significantly below average as measured on an intelligence quotient (IQ) test, *(b)* deficits in adaptive functioning (in daily life activities and roles), and *(c)* onset before age 18. Generally, the lower the IQ, the greater the impairment in ability to function. Those with severe and profound retardation are likely to have significant impairment in motor functions and skills and physical development and may not be able to walk or self-toilet. Typical problems addressed by OT for a person with this condition may include the following:

- Deficits in self-care
- Impaired social functioning
- Impaired or absent vocational functioning
- Perceptual-motor deficits

A *disorder of learning, motor skills,* or *communication* is diagnosed when impairment is significant enough to interfere with academic or daily life functioning. Children with these diagnoses are typically seen by occupational therapy in early intervention programs and in the schools, where the OT goals address functioning in the student role, in social relations with peers and family, and in choice of work or career. In addition, motor function deficits (e.g., apraxia, incoordination) are also treated by OT. The reader is referred to the *DSM-IV-TR* and OT pediatric texts for more information on these disorders.

The diagnosis of *pervasive developmental disorder* (PDD) refers to autism and similar conditions. *Autism* may be diagnosed together with

[2] Unless otherwise noted, all information in this section is summarized from the *DSM-IV-TR* (9).

neurological or mental disorders or mental retardation. It is characterized by *(a)* marked impairment in social relationships, generally including lack of awareness of others; *(b)* significant impairment in communication, such as delayed or absent speech and the inability to recognize nonverbal cues; *(c)* restricted and repetitive interests and activities, such as rituals and motor mannerisms; and *(d)* delayed or abnormal development. Autistic persons typically show stereotyped movements, such as flapping the hands. It is extremely difficult to obtain and maintain eye contact with autistic persons or to interest them in new activities or features of the environment. Autism is widely believed to be a neurological condition with underlying organic brain disease. Problems addressed by OT include the following:

- Impaired sensory processing and sensory integration
- Perceptual-motor deficits
- Deficits in social interaction
- Self-care deficits
- Delayed or absent vocational functioning

Sensory-integrative, developmental, and behavioral approaches are generally used. Applied behavioral analysis (ABA) is also a popular method.

*Asperger's disorder* has some similarities to autistic disorder, with deficits in social interaction and a very restricted range of interests. However, there is no language delay and no cognitive impairment. The social deficit is the primary feature. People with Asperger's disorder (also known as Asperger's syndrome) possess good to excellent verbal abilities but cannot interact successfully with others. Typically, they have specific interests that they pursue to the exclusion of all others. These interests become preoccupations that dominate behavior. The disorder may not be apparent in early childhood but becomes a problem when the child enters school and is unable to relate effectively to peers and teachers. Typically, the older child or adolescent with Asperger's disorder will desire friendships but will be unable to make friends. The child may be victimized or openly shunned, leading to depression and anxiety.

Asperger's disorder is a lifelong condition that may cause significant impairment in performance of work occupations in addition to the impairment of social interaction. Sensory processing deficits are likely responsible. (22, 62). It is possible that Brown and co-worker's *Adult Sensory Profile* (17) and strategies for modulating sensory reactions by modifying the environment (16) could be helpful for persons with this condition. Pfeiffer et al. (62) suggest that sensory-based treatment may help alleviate anxiety and depression. Certainly, social skills training seems appropriate; however, the sensory deficits and lack of awareness of social cues and nonverbal communication are barriers to understanding how social behavior works. When working with a person with Asperger's syndrome on sensory issues or social skills, the OTA should be using a plan developed and monitored by the OT.

*Attention deficit* and *disruptive behavior disorders* include attention deficit-hyperactivity disorder (ADHD), conduct disorder, oppositional defiant disorder (ODD), and disruptive behavior disorder. Children in this group are hard to handle because of their limited attention span and extremely high energy and activity level (ADHD), deviant and antisocial behavior such as stealing or violence (conduct disorder), or argumentative and resentful behavior (ODD). Diagnoses in this category require a pattern of behavior that is sustained for at least 6 months. Typical problems addressed in OT include the following:

- Inadequate attention span
- Poor impulse control
- Deficient age-appropriate skills for academic, social, and occupational roles
- Social skills deficits

Behavioral approaches and the sensory integrative approach are typically used. Cognitive-behavioral methods may be used with older children. Children in the middle school years (ages 11 through 13) may benefit from assertiveness training and social skills training.

Gutman et al. (30) provide occupational therapy guidelines for interventions with children with *regulatory disorders,* a category in which children with autism, Asperger's, and ADHD might be placed. Regulatory disorders share the common quality of difficulty in modulating or controlling one's response or reaction to sensation in order to interact effectively with the environment. The child may overreact to stimulation or fail to notice things that are important. Moods may fluctuate wildly. The guidelines given include the following:

- *Building a trusting and accepting relationship with the child.* The child may be slow to trust because of previous experiences. Accepting the child as a total package and being interested in the child's perspective is a good start.
- *Helping the child recognize which behaviors are a problem.* It is essential for the child to hear that the *behavior* is not working, rather than that he or she is "bad."
- *Giving the child a vocabulary with which to describe what he or she is feeling.* Typically, the child feels uncomfortable in some way and immediately reacts with a behavior that gets him or her in trouble. If the child can learn to say, for example, "I feel jumpy—Woody's standing too close," then it becomes possible to have Woody move, or have the child move to a less crowded space. Similarly, if the child can recognize that her heart is racing, then she can learn to wait for it to slow down, indicating she is more calm.
- *Helping the child identify situations that will cause problems.* For example, the child can learn that he doesn't like the feeling of zippers in pants or of labels in the necks of shirts and sweaters. The parent can be advised to purchase pants with elastic waists and to remove the offending labels.
- *Building impulse control and frustration tolerance.* When the child feels pushed and doesn't see any alternative, he or she will act out. Teaching the child what is required in different situations (school, church) and helping with gradual building of self-control are important.
- *Building the ability to tolerate change.* Change is part of life, but transitioning from one activity to another is very difficult for these children. Similarly, a change in the environment (a new piece of furniture) may be greeted with a tantrum. Telling the child in advance can be helpful. Also, the child can be rewarded for any successful attempt to control behavioral expressions in regard to change.
- *Helping the child acquire social interaction skills.* Taking turns, asking rather than grabbing, and making eye contact are just some of skills that can be taught. Children need to learn to "use your words" instead of acting out.

The reader is encouraged to consult the original article (30).

All of the disorders first seen in childhood and adolescence shape how the individual grows and develops. The aftereffects can be profound and lifelong. For example, learning disorders create stresses in school, may result in poor self-esteem and feelings of inadequacy and depression, and interfere with acquiring life skills. Persons with ADHD as children may be inclined toward substance abuse and other disorders of impulse control in adolescence. This may lead in turn to promiscuous behavior and sexually transmitted diseases (STDs), low educational achievement, low socioeconomic status, and criminal acts. In other words, a psychiatric disorder in childhood places the person at risk throughout life. The case example of Matthew illustrates the relation between childhood psychiatric history (bed wetting, conduct disorder) and functioning in later life.

## Delirium, Dementia, Amnestic, and Other Cognitive Disorders

A significant decline in cognition (specifically memory) is the main characteristic of disorders in this category. All of these disorders involve temporary or permanent disruptions in the functioning of the brain. In older editions of the *DSM* these conditions were termed *organic* to indicate their origin in an organ (the brain). The *DSM-IV-TR* no longer makes this distinction, because all mental disorders are now believed to have an organic (biochemical or biological) component (69).

*Delirium* is characterized by reduced alertness and awareness, disorganized thinking (impaired memory, incoherent speech), probable physiological cause (e.g., fever, head injury, or recent ingestion of toxic substance), and rapid onset of symptoms. Delirium may last for only a few hours or for several weeks; patients are generally not seen in OT until the delirium has passed.

In contrast to delirium, the major feature of *dementia* is a severe impairment of short- and long-term memory as documented by the mental status examination. Additional criteria for a diagnosis of dementia include evidence of impaired thinking or judgment, social or occupational impairment, absence of delirium, and probable organic cause. Individuals with dementia are seen in OT in mental health settings, physical medicine settings, skilled nursing facilities, and adult day care. Six subtypes are recognized: *(a)* dementia of the Alzheimer's type, *(b)* vascular dementia, *(c)* dementia owing to other medical conditions, *(d)* substance-induced dementia, *(e)* dementia of multiple etiologies (causes), and *(f)* dementia not otherwise specified (unknown or unclassified cause).

*Dementia of the Alzheimer's type* (DAT) manifests in progressive and significant deterioration of intellectual, social, and occupational functioning. In other words, the person gets worse and worse and is less and less able to function in daily life as the disease progresses. On autopsy, the brains of patients with this type of dementia have shown clear and characteristic changes both on the gross level (e.g., size of cerebral ventricles) and the microscopic level (e.g., neurofibrillary tangles).

*Vascular dementia* (formerly called multi-infarct dementia) results from damage to the cerebrovascular system (blood vessels of the brain), usually caused by multiple small strokes. Deterioration in function in this type of dementia is more stepwise or patchy than in the more steadily progressive Alzheimer's type. Functioning varies from day to day; and although there may be significant problems in one area (e.g., memory of names), other areas are relatively intact. Evidence of cerebrovascular disease from physical examination or laboratory tests is also needed for this diagnosis. The progress of vascular dementia can sometimes be slowed by treating the underlying cause (e.g., by taking antihypertensive medication).

*Dementia may also result from other medical conditions*, such as infection with the human immunodeficiency virus (HIV), head trauma, Parkinson's disease, and Huntington's disease. *Some dementias result from substance ingestion* (usually alcohol, but also inhalants, sedatives, and others). Some of these dementias result in permanent memory loss and are termed *amnestic* (for amnesia).

OT treatment of persons with dementia and similar cognitive disorders and syndromes addresses the following problems:

- Memory deficits
- Limitations in judgment and other cognitive functions
- Deficits in social skills
- The emotional reaction to one's deteriorating mental state

Because improvement is not generally expected, therapy seeks to maintain maximum functioning as long as possible through the teaching of compensatory strategies and by careful environmental management (26). An example of a compensatory strategy is to perform a simpler version of the desired activity (e.g., using a microwave to reheat prepared foods rather than cooking on a stovetop).

Labeling drawers with their contents is an example of environmental management. When function declines so far that independence is no longer possible, the OT approach shifts to working with the family or other caregivers to assist them in dealing with the person while encouraging as much independent function as possible (54).

Gitlin and Corcoran (26) give practical and detailed explanations of how to work with individuals and families to modify the environment and provide effective care to person with dementia. Four aspects or layers of the environment are considered: objects, tasks, social groups, and culture. In the *object layer,* the emphasis is on clarifying the environment by removing distracting objects and by organizing and drawing attention to the objects the person is expected to use. In the *task layer,* the directions for the task are reduced to two steps or one step, depending on the needs of the person. Tasks are simplified and made into a consistent routine. In the *social layer,* family members are respected, treated as collaborators in intervention planning, and are helped to meet their own needs. In the *culture layer,* the OT observes, asks about, and learns family norms so that these can be incorporated in the plan of care. The reader is highly encouraged to consult Gitlin and Corcoran (26) for further information. Table 6-1 shows the stages of dementia, the behavioral and functional characteristics, and the caregiving issues.

Some evidence exists that aromatherapy and massage may help reduce behavioral problems (70). Research studies of the effectiveness of training to improve cognitive skills is inconclusive. Further details about related treatment approaches can be found in Chapters 10 to 12 and Chapter 23.

## Substance-Related Disorders

The substance-related disorders include all disorders caused by recreational drugs (including alcohol), prescription medications, naturally occurring substances (e.g., peyote), and environmental toxins. There are 11 classes of substances:

- Alcohol
- Amphetamines and similar drugs
- Caffeine
- Cannabis (marijuana)
- Cocaine
- Hallucinogens
- Inhalants
- Nicotine
- Opioids
- Phencyclidine (PCP) and similar drugs
- Sedatives, hypnotics, and anxiolytics

Two other diagnoses in this group are polysubstance abuse (use of several drugs) and disorders related to use of medications or ingestion of or exposure to toxins. The diagnostician attempts to differentiate between dependence and abuse. *Dependence* implies that the person does not have adequate control over the use of the substance and continues to use it despite clear evidence that it is harmful. Some of the symptoms of dependence include taking the substance in larger amounts than originally intended (e.g., having more than the promised "just one drink"), attempting unsuccessfully to control or reduce substance use, tolerance for greater amounts over time, social and physical problems (e.g., health problems and family conflicts), and preference for the company of other substance users. A diagnosis of *abuse* is made when there is insufficient evidence for a diagnosis of dependence but there are clear examples of maladaptive behavior, as in driving while intoxicated or using the substance when it is clearly against one's own interest (causing one to miss school, for example).

Each substance has a particular pattern of use and a particular group of associated behavioral features. Many substance-dependent and abusive persons abuse or are dependent on more than one substance (polysubstance abuse). Substance-related disorders are life-long conditions, and recurrence and relapse are common; brain

## TABLE 6-1 STAGES OF DEMENTIA, ASSOCIATED CHANGES, AND FAMILY CAREGIVER NEEDS

| STAGE | MEMORY AND COGNITIVE CHANGES | BEHAVIORAL CHANGES | FUNCTIONAL CHANGES | CAREGIVING DEMANDS AND CAREGIVER NEEDS |
|---|---|---|---|---|
| Mild cognitive impairment | Subjective and objective memory loss | Possible anxiety<br>Forgetfulness<br>Some confusion | Isolated, if present, and limited to high-level IADL deficits | Caregiving demands:<br>Mild anxiety<br>Caregiving needs:<br>Education |
| Mild dementia | Loss of new or recent memory<br>Word-finding difficulties<br>Decreased concentration<br>Decreased problem-solving skills<br>Lack of initiative | Mood and personality changes<br>Emotional withdrawal<br>Increased anxiety<br>Depression | Difficulties with functional management<br>Difficulty managing mediation routine<br>Tendency to become lost traveling to unfamiliar places<br>Impaired work and social performance | Caregiving demands:<br>Assistance with IADLs<br>Caregiving needs:<br>Education<br>Behavior management struggles<br>Skills for coping with disease process<br>Financial planning<br>Refund to community resources |
| Moderate dementia | Continued decline in memory<br>Increased confusion<br>Difficulty with personal information<br>Dissertation to time and place<br>Difficulty with new learning<br>Incontinence | Paranoia<br>Hallucinations<br>Delusions<br>Compulsive behavior<br>Repititive behavior<br>Agitation<br>Aggression<br>Restlessness<br>Wandering<br>Withdrawal<br>Apathy<br>Anxiety<br>Inappropriate behavior<br>Depression | Difficulty with self-care, including clothing selection, dressing, bathing, and toileting<br>Difficulty with communication<br>Difficulty with mobility<br>Inability to drive safety | Caregiving demands:<br>Moderate assistance with ADL<br>Total assistance with IADL<br>Caregiving needs:<br>Assistance with increased physical burden<br>Assistance with behavior management<br>Assistance evaluating employment situation<br>Stress reduction techniques |
| Severe dementia | Profound loss of function in all areas<br>Increased amount of time spent sleeping<br>Inability to recognize familiar faces<br>Lost capacity for understanding speech<br>Decreased ability to swallow<br>Incontinence of bladder and bowel | Apathy<br>Restlessnees<br>Increased amount of time sleeping | Profound loss of function of all areas<br>Eventual loss of all mobility | Caregiving demands:<br>Total assitance IADL and most of all ADL<br>Caregiving needs:<br>All above |

Reprinted with permission from Gitlin LN, Corcoran MA, eds. Occupational Therapy and Dementia Care: The Home Environmental Skills-Building Program for Individuals and Families. Bethesda MD: American Occupational Therapy Association, 2005.

changes associated with addictive responses are believed responsible (29).

Substance-related disorders merit an extended discussion for several reasons. First, persons with such disorders typically behave in characteristic maladaptive patterns, which are often reinforced or enabled by those with whom the abuser associates (family, employer). Second, in recovery, persons with these disorders may commit to a 12-step program such as Alcoholics Anonymous. Third, substance abusers have a higher than average incidence of other medical and psychiatric problems. The OTA will certainly encounter alcohol and substance abusers frequently as patients, in settings as diverse as burn units, general medical services, trauma units, physical rehabilitation centers, and mental health settings. Finally, OT has a specific focus with this group; thus the OTA can assume a significant role.

In this section, we describe the various abused substances and their effects, the mental and social characteristics of substance abuse, and OT interventions. We also discuss the various 12-step groups and will briefly consider the question of comorbidity.

## Abused Substances and Their Effects

Alcohol consumption is a fact of life in American society and in most other cultures worldwide. Alcohol abuse is epidemic but socially sanctioned. According to the American Psychiatric Association, alcohol and drug abuse is "by far the predominant cause of premature and preventable illness, disability, and death in our society" (11). In small quantities, alcohol has been promoted as beneficial by the medical profession. Research has shown that a glass of wine a day may protect against premature cardiac and vascular disease. There are varying degrees of *unhealthy* involvement with alcohol. Generally, alcoholics begin drinking in their teens or 20s, and the disease becomes progressive, leading to abuse and ultimately to dependence. More males than females are heavy drinkers. There is a familial pattern of alcoholism, which may have a genetic component. However, one cannot discount the effect of observing, as a young child, the drinking behavior of family members.

Three patterns of alcohol abuse are recognized: regular daily drinking, heavy weekend drinking, and periodic or episodic binge drinking. A person who abuses alcohol but who is not yet dependent on it can go for days, weeks, and even months of abstinence without suffering withdrawal symptoms. Once the disease has reached the dependence stage, however, the individual undergoes withdrawal when alcohol is withheld. Symptoms may include delirium tremens (the DTs), characterized by fever, tremors, ataxia, and even hallucinations. Sweating and high blood pressure are other symptoms of withdrawal.

Chronic excessive alcohol use may lead to lasting neurological damage and dementia. Medical disorders caused by alcohol include liver damage; gastric damage; premature aging; impotence and infertility; and increased risk of heart disease, respiratory disease, and neurological disorders. Depression, which is associated with alcohol abuse, may be either a contributing factor or result of alcoholism. Many alcoholics have been prescribed psychotropic medications (antidepressants such as fluoxetine [Prozac] or antianxiety drugs such as alprazolam [Xanax]) by physicians who were not aware of their alcohol abuse. Children born to alcoholic mothers may have fetal alcohol syndrome, characterized by facial abnormalities, mental retardation, and pervasive developmental defects.

Marijuana is the most widely available illegal drug in the United States. It is often used in combination with alcohol or other drugs. Marijuana impairs a variety of cognitive and perceptual-motor functions, including concentration, judgment, short-term memory, perception, and motor skills. Marijuana may adversely affect reproduction and may exacerbate preexisting heart conditions.

Because it is smoked and because it contains many known carcinogens, it may be more damaging to the lungs than tobacco. It has been linked to depression and is suspected as the primary cause of amotivational syndrome in adolescents. This syndrome is characterized by loss of interest and initiative, difficulty concentrating, and diminished functional performance at school and work (11).

Cocaine derives from the leaves of the South American coca plant. As a white powder, it can be inhaled (snorted) through the nose or dissolved and injected. Crack, a smokable form of cocaine, produces a rapid high. Crack is more addicting than other forms of cocaine because the low that follows rapidly from the high increases the desire for the drug. As with alcohol abuse, cocaine abuse may follow either an episodic or a chronic daily pattern. Cocaine abuse may lead to serious medical problems, including frequent and tenacious upper respiratory infections, heart failure, reproductive problems (e.g., miscarriage), stroke. seizures. personality changes. and violent psychosis. Newborns exposed to cocaine in utero may have the same physical problems as the abusing mother and may have serious birth defects and deformities. Furthermore, they may be irritable and have difficulty bonding to the mother or accepting nourishment (11).

Opioid narcotics, which may be either natural or synthetic, include heroin, morphine, and meperidine (Demerol). Illicit use of these drugs leads to addiction in about 50% of cases. Associated medical disorders include heart problems and the risk of acquiring acquired immune deficiency syndrome (AIDS) or other infections from contaminated needles. Children born to opioid-addicted mothers have withdrawal symptoms and may die of them (11).

Other frequently abused drugs include PCP (also called angel dust), lysergic acid diethylamine (LSD), amphetamines, amyl nitrite (poppers) and other inhalants, and various prescription drugs.

## Psychological Characteristics and Social Factors

According to some experts, alcohol and substance abuse problems may evolve from patterns learned in childhood. Children of substance-abusing parents generally do not have a normal nurturing environment. In some cases, the child is rejected and/or physically or sexually abused by the drinking parent and ignored or smothered by the nondrinking parent. In other cases, the child reverses roles with the parent, providing care for the parents and siblings and taking on cooking and other household chores. Another pattern leading to adult alcohol abuse is having been overprotected in childhood, which restricts risk taking, a major source of self-esteem, and limits the development of necessary social skills (56). While these predisposing patterns are not shared by all alcoholics, they are common to many.

Substance abusers as a group tend to employ a characteristic set of defense mechanisms. Moyers (56) summarized the literature on the *preferred defensive structure* (PDS) of alcoholics. The PDS is a group of strategies for achieving one's goals. *Denial* is the first line of defense, because it permits the substance abuser to ignore the disease and to escape accountability for its consequences. Furthermore, even in sobriety this defense is used to avoid painful confrontation with the consequences of one's actions. *Projection,* or the transfer onto others of one's own feelings, is also used to disguise one's unacceptable negative feelings. For example, the alcoholic who is quite angry but can't face the fact believes a neighbor is angry with him or her, and this "makes" the person drink. *Rationalization,* or giving reasons for drinking, helps the alcoholic distance himself or herself from the compulsion to drink by blaming it on, for example, a spouse or employer. Chapters 10 and 11 give more detail on appropriate and helpful responses to these elements of the PDS.

Another characteristic defense is a preference for *dichotomous thinking.* This either–or, black–white reasoning may have been a way of managing unpredictable experiences in childhood. Dichotomous thinking leads to wild variability in behavior. For example, extreme perfectionism and attention to detail may alternate with sloppy indifference. Another example is swinging from overdependence on staff to withdrawal and aloof independence. Moyers (56) recommends that the person be involved in carefully designed experiences that permit him or her to recognize and explore a middle ground between the two extremes. For example, the patient who is alternately overdependent and too independent needs to recognize differences in situations that call for more or less dependence on others.

Social factors that must be understood for effective work with the alcohol or substance abuser include codependency, enabling behaviors of others, and social and leisure deficits. *Codependency* refers to the unhealthy involvement of a nonsubstance abuser in controlling a substance abuser. Codependent behavior is most common in spouses and immediate family members but may occur in others with whom the alcoholic associates. *Enabling* is a codependent behavior characterized by making it easier for the substance abuser to continue to drink and/or take drugs. Examples of enabling include picking up the slack by taking care of the user's responsibilities (calling in sick for him or her) and providing money and other forms of material support.

While the alcoholic may risk losing a job because of alcoholic behavior, in some cases the employer is an enabler. Certain occupations provide numerous job-related drinking occasions, and excessive consumption is condoned—for example, hangovers are accepted as normal or tardiness is overlooked. Richert and Bergland (66) reported an association between evening or night shifts and alcohol consumption.

After years of spending most leisure hours in drinking-related pursuits, the typical alcoholic has a network of drinking companions, a set of familiar drinking locations, and sometimes a repertoire of drinking-related activities (watching sporting events, gambling or playing cards, and so on). These habits related to the use of leisure time are a major problem for the recovering alcoholic, who must relearn how to enjoy leisure in a sober way.

## Alcoholics Anonymous

Alcoholics Anonymous (AA) is a self-help group whose purpose is to help its members achieve and maintain sobriety. Founded in 1935, AA is entirely funded by member contributions. Membership in AA is based on AA's third tradition, that "the only requirement for membership is a desire to stop drinking" (1). AA is commonly accepted as the most successful program for maintaining sobriety, and professionals who work with alcoholics actively encourage involvement with it.

The foundation of the AA program is the 12 steps. The first 3 steps engage the alcoholic in admitting powerlessness over alcohol and promote willingness to seek help from AA and from other sources. The remaining 9 steps provide a structure for understanding the consequences of one's actions, for mending impaired social relations, for maintaining a sober lifestyle, and for carrying the message of hope and strength to other alcoholics. Every day, all over the world, countless AA groups meet in church basements, hospitals, detention centers, detoxification units, schools, and other public places. The atmosphere in a typical AA meeting is warm and accepting, welcoming of all regardless of social status, and nurturing to newcomers and to returning members who have slipped.

In the decades since the founding of AA, other 12-step groups have sprung up on this model. These include Narcotics Anonymous (NA), Cocaine Anonymous (CA), Debtors Anonymous (DA), Overeaters Anonymous (OA), and Al-Anon and Al-A-Teen for families affected by an alcoholic member.

**BOX 6-2**

**BRIEF INTERVENTIONS IN OCCUPATIONAL THERAPY (FOR THE OTA)**

Occupational profile (evaluation) of all clients

- Routinely include alcohol- and drug-use quantity and frequency questions
- Inquire about effects of substance use on occupational performance and satisfaction
- May assist in administering portions of the occupational profile

Evaluation and interventions for at-risk individuals

- Across all practice areas, be alert to behaviors that may indicate substance abuse (e.g., violence either as victim or perpetrator, drunk driving or driving under the influence (DUI) convictions, multiple fractures or fall history, use of high volume of prescription pain medications)
- Alert occupational therapist to client history or behavior that suggests substance-abuse problems

Wellness, prevention, and community health

- Provide information about substance abuse in health and wellness brochures and programming
- Discuss effects on occupational performance and satisfaction; include coping strategies and information on alternative uses of leisure time

Adapted with permission from Stoffel VC, Moyers PA. An evidence-based and occupational perspective of interventions for persons with substance-use disorders. Am J Occup Ther 2004;58:570–586.

## Occupational Therapy

Occupational therapy for the substance-related disorders should be practical and addressed to the problems of occupational functioning that characterize these conditions. Stoffel and Moyers (71) have reviewed the literature and given specific recommendations for occupational therapy interventions for persons with substance-related disorders. These are shown in Box 6-2. The focus on prevention and early intervention aims to reduce impairment in occupational functioning. Clearly, the sooner the problem is recognized and addressed, the greater the likelihood of a positive outcome. The OTA is encouraged to consider that many persons have abuse and dependence problems with substances and that these persons will be seen in all kinds of practice settings, not just psychiatric ones.

In general, occupational therapy intervention aims to improve functioning and provide skill development in specific areas. Evaluation and intervention focus on these factors:

- Use of time, especially leisure time
- Relapse prevention
- Cognitive and perceptual functions and skill development
- Social interaction, social skills and self-expression
- Daily living skills
- Acquisition, development, and maintenance of valued occupational and social roles

### Time Management and Leisure

Viik et al. (73) found clear differences in occupational functioning between newly sober inpatient alcoholics and those with a year or more of sobriety. Newly sober alcoholics preferred activities associated with alcohol, whereas alcoholics with longer recovery preferred activities associated with sobriety. The *Barth Time Construction* (see Chapter 15) has also been used to obtain information about the alcoholic's use of time generally and of leisure time specifically.

Once in recovery, the substance abuser has few resources for spending the large amounts of leisure time now available. Recovering alcoholics are instructed to avoid people, places, and things that lead to drinking. Some newly sober alcoholics use their leisure time attending several AA meetings per day. This may in turn lead to leisure activities such as an AA softball team or tennis league. OT can help by assessment through the Interest Checklist or similar inventory (see Chapter 15) and by providing opportunities to plan and experience sober leisure activities.

### Relapse Prevention

The general rule of relapse prevention is the avoidance of people, places, and things associated with the abused substance. The person must learn healthy substitutes for situations that would trigger relapse. Furthermore, the person must identify his or her triggers.

Corvinelli (18) states that boredom and apathy are linked to relapse. To prevent relapse, the occupational therapy practitioner must help the person engage with interest in activities. Often, the person's concentration is low, and the OT or OTA must find a way to make the task sufficiently challenging to engage attention. In addition, the person must be engaged in a program to increase skills so that more challenging tasks are possible.

### Perceptual and Cognitive Functions

Perceptual and cognitive functions (tactile perception, figure–ground discrimination, and visual–spatial relations) may be impaired by alcohol and substance abuse and are sometimes evaluated and treated by OT (72). The causes of perceptual-motor dysfunction in alcoholics are not clearly established. In many cases, the deficits disappear or diminish after a period of recovery and abstinence. It is not clear whether rehabilitation has an effect; the evidence suggests that younger persons with shorter time in active alcoholism fare better than older alcoholics in recovering a more normal level of perceptual-motor skill. Computer-based games may help.

### Social Interaction, Social Skills, and Communication Skills

In the areas of social skills and self-expression, substance abusers benefit from learning new ways to cope with feelings rather than resorting to use of the drug of choice. Expressive activities (art, clay, poetry, drama) may assist recovering alcoholics to recognize and convey emotions that they have become accustomed to blocking out by drinking and/or by defense mechanisms such as denial and projection.

Assertiveness training may provide the recovering substance abuser with appropriate skills and successful strategies for interacting with others. Stress management and relaxation skills training encourage understanding of what the individual finds stressful and teaches activities that can promote relaxation. In particular, recovering alcoholics and substance abusers may need skills and interventions to rebuild their relationships with their families (57).

### Daily Living Skills

Many patients in recovery benefit from money management activities. Often a large portion of disposable income has been used for the drug of choice; the person in recovery may have limited ideas about how to budget money and control spending (65). Time management, parenting skills, nutrition and meal planning, food preparation, housekeeping, and use of community resources may also need attention.

### Work

Various areas of work can be targeted for intervention, depending on the person's functional level.

Some higher-functioning substance abusers have had great success in their careers; despite alcohol or drug use, they were reliable and in many cases ambitious and conscientious workers. This group may need information and assistance in planning leisure activities, in developing a social network, and in managing work time so that it does not become obsessive. Another group of recovering patients may at some point in the past have had successful work experiences but have been fired because of alcohol-related or drug-related behavior. This group needs help in redeveloping work habits and skills so that they can reenter the workforce. Résumé writing and job search skills are also appropriate for this group. Yet another group of much lower-functioning patients has little or no experience of success in the role of worker. This group may require a full range of vocational and prevocational assessment and training. OT can address the basic task skills and work-related social behaviors through work groups and volunteer positions. In some parts of the United States, alcoholics with several months of sobriety can obtain vocational testing and training from the Employment Program for Recovering Alcoholics (EPRA), which is associated with AA.

### Comorbidity in Substance Abuse

*Comorbidity* is the diagnosis of two or more psychiatric disorders in the same person. A high percentage of persons treated for a substance-related disorder are also diagnosed with another psychiatric disorder. This has been called *dual diagnosis*, but use of this term is discouraged because implies only two diagnoses (and often there are more). The person may also be termed a mentally ill substance abuser (MICA). The comorbid diagnosis is frequently a personality disorder, coded on axis II. Various studies suggest that between 35% and 60% of persons diagnosed with substance abuse or dependence meet the criteria for antisocial personality disorder (69). Some have criminal records.

Some persons with substance-related disorders also receive axis I diagnoses of schizophrenia or affective disorders. In general, substance abusers with comorbid conditions have fewer skills and correspondingly more functional impairments than do patients who have only the diagnosis of substance abuse. These individuals are more prone to relapse and require more structure than those with a single diagnosis. OT interventions for these patients should be training oriented, teaching daily living skills and task skills and reinforcing appropriate behavior.

## Schizophrenia

Although the common use of the word *schizophrenic* is as a catch-all for bizarre behavior, the actual disease of schizophrenia is believed to be a discrete entity. Only a fraction of the people with psychotic symptoms actually receive a diagnosis of schizophrenia. In many cases, an initial diagnosis of schizophrenia is later revised to another with less serious implications for prolonged dysfunction. In the *DSM-V*, schizophrenia and related (less severe) diagnoses may be grouped together in a continuum. Schizophrenia is characterized by several specific psychotic symptoms, deterioration in functioning from a previously higher level, and a duration of illness of at least 6 months. If a mood disorder is present, the diagnosis of schizophrenia is not made; instead the diagnosis may be schizoaffective disorder.

Some of the psychotic symptoms peculiar to schizophrenia include disturbances in the form and content of thought. The person's thoughts, evidenced by what he or she says, are highly disorganized and unusual, sometimes with the idea that others are inserting and removing one's thoughts or that one's thoughts are being broadcast or controlled by some external force. The person may shift from one subject to another, linking them with transitions that are not logical to others. Hallucinations are common, auditory hallucinations being most typical. The person may report that voices are commanding him or her to perform certain actions. Affect, or expressed feeling, is often flat (unresponsive) or inappropriate to the situation. Motivation to participate in daily life is usually impaired, as is the ability to interact with others. As discussed in Chapter 3, psychomotor disturbances such as decomposition of movement may also be seen.

### Progression

The progression of schizophrenia falls into three phases: prodromal, active, and residual. In the *prodromal phase,* the level of functioning deteriorates. Usually this can be seen in a decline in hygiene and grooming, interaction with others, and overall participation in life. In the *active phase,* the psychotic symptoms become apparent. Sometimes a psychosocial stressor appears to precipitate, or bring on, the active phase. Following the active phase, the *residual phase* consists of the remission of the psychotic symptoms that are most disturbing to others (the person may still hear voices but may no longer act so excited about it) and of a continuation and, in many cases, worsening of impaired functioning.

### Positive and Negative Symptoms

Symptoms of schizophrenia been divided into two classes: negative and positive. *Positive symptoms* include hallucinations, delusions, loosening of associations, and grossly disorganized speech and behavior. These symptoms are seen in the active phase of the illness. Though they may be present in the other two phases, they are not severe or prominent. These symptoms respond to the older type of neuroleptic (antipsychotic) drugs, such as chlorpromazine (Thorazine).

*Negative symptoms* include apathy and generally unexpressive mood (affective flattening), lack of goal-directed behavior (avolition), deterioration of hygiene, diminished functioning and participation in daily life, social isolation, and psychomotor slowing. These are seen in both the prodromal and the residual phases, and they appear to be related to physical changes in the brain, such as ventricular enlargement (52) and decreased metabolic activity in the frontal lobes (27). Some of the newer atypical antipsychotic medications such as clozapine (Clozaril) have helped reduce negative symptoms (69).

### Subtypes

There are five subtypes of schizophrenia. The *catatonic type* is differentiated by extreme psychomotor disturbance. This may be either lack of movement, rigidity of movement, resistance to movement, an excited and apparently purposeless style of movement, or catatonic posturing in which bizarre postures are held. Repeated (perseverative) movement or speech may also be seen. This type is not commonly diagnosed today in the United States.

The *disorganized type* shows incoherent thinking, ineffective and bizarre communication, flattened or diminished affect, and grossly inadequate functioning. The person may grimace, demonstrate strange mannerisms, and otherwise behave oddly. This condition is considered chronic, with a prognosis of continued functioning at a very low level. In the past this type was termed *hebephrenic.*

The characteristic difference seen in the *paranoid type* is more systematized delusional thinking organized around themes of persecution. Other aspects of thinking are usually unaffected. Affect and behavior are also more normal. Persons with schizophrenia of the paranoid type usually function better than those with other types, and most are able to live independently. They may participate effectively in many aspects of community life, all the while harboring systematized ideas that others are out to get them. In general, they tend to recover more completely than do persons with other forms of schizophrenia.

The diagnosis of *undifferentiated type* is used when the criteria for the other types are not completely present. The diagnosis of *residual type* is assigned when active psychotic symptoms are not present but residual negative symptoms (impaired functioning) are found. The *simple type* of schizophrenia is listed in an appendix to the *DSM-IV-TR* but does not fall within the *DSM-IV-TR* classification of a mental disorder. Simple deteriorative disorder (simple schizophrenia) is a "less severe" form of a schizophrenia-like condition, characterized by deteriorating functioning in the absence of a mood disturbance or organic condition and marginalization of the person at the fringes of society. Negative symptoms are more prominent than positive ones. This diagnosis was included in *DSM-I* and *DSM-II* to classify persons who functioned poorly and who did not fit the classical pattern.

Two *DSM-IV-TR* disorders similar to schizophrenia are schizophreniform disorder and schizoaffective disorder. *Schizophreniform disorder* is the classification for disorders lasting less than 6 months that nonetheless have the form or characteristics of schizophrenia. *Schizoaffective disorder* is used to designate disorders that have characteristics of both schizophrenia and mood disorders (both disorganized thinking and behavior and a disturbance of mood).

## Diagnosis, Medical Management, and Drug Treatment

Diagnosis and medical management of schizophrenia advanced significantly since 1990. Most experts now view schizophrenia as a disorder of both the structure and function of the brain (35, 69). Research has identified changes in the frontal cortex, the prefrontal cortex, the temporal lobe, and the basal ganglia (27, 34). Abnormal activity of neurotransmitters, particularly dopamine, has also been documented. These changes may account for some of the information-processing difficulties seen in persons with schizophrenia, who find it difficult to stay organized or on task when distraction is present (15).

Research confirming that schizophrenia is a brain disorder has fueled the search for more effective drug treatments aimed specifically at the malfunctioning parts of the brain. The older class of neuroleptic drugs (see Chapter 8) suppressed the positive symptoms of schizophrenia but had little effect on the negative symptoms. Even when patients took their medications as prescribed, they had difficulty performing the normal tasks of daily life and work. These drugs also had undesirable side effects, some of which were permanent, and so patients also had to cope with drowsiness and blurred vision and, in some cases, with abnormal body movements (tardive dyskinesia).

Newer drugs, termed atypical antipsychotics, have fewer side effects and appear more effective in reducing negative symptoms and cognitive deficiencies. These drugs also have side effects of varying severity (see Chapter 8) but have been preferred by both patients and physicians. The newer drugs act more selectively on the brain receptors than did the older neuroleptics. For example, most of the neuroleptics prevent dopamine from acting at the $D_2$ receptors throughout the brain; this relieves positive symptoms by reducing limbic system activity but causes side effects by incidental activity at the extrapyramidal system. Some of the new drugs block $D_2$ receptors only at the limbic system; other drugs affect different dopamine receptors. Some act primarily on the prefrontal cortex and have no effect on other areas of the brain (60).

Current understanding suggests that early aggressive drug treatment may prevent the severe and persistent deterioration of function seen today in older individuals diagnosed when they were younger. Thus experts urge early detection and treatment with appropriate medications. Too often persons with schizophrenia are prescribed inadequate amounts of medication and receive ineffective or insufficient treatment and for these reasons cannot achieve a reasonable level of health and functioning (44).

## Occupational Therapy

OT evaluation and treatment of patients with diagnoses of schizophrenia varies. It can occur in a range of settings from acute inpatient care to home health care and community treatment. Much depends on the person's level of functioning and specific deficit areas. When approaching a person who has schizophrenia, or any other mental disorder, it is essential to focus on the person's strengths as well as the deficits. Every person has strengths that can provide support in recovery. Some persons with schizophrenia already function quite well. In such cases, intervention is directed at the problems that interfere with specific areas of functioning or with dyadic or group interaction skills.

### Social Interaction, Communication and Interaction, Behavioral, and Daily Living Skills

Social competence (skill in interacting with others) and social presence (behaving appropriately in the presence of others) are often deficient in patients with schizophrenia, particularly in those with early onset of disease (20). A person whose first psychotic episode occurs in adolescence probably has not yet developed a good foundation of communication and interaction skills. It is not known which techniques can best teach or improve social skills in this group, or to what extent, though several different approaches are used (32). Social skills training (see Chapter 3) may improve specific behaviors such as making eye contact, initiating a conversation, and responding to questions. Behavioral coaching and cognitive-behavioral strategies can help the person identify and change problem behaviors. Activity-oriented and task-focused groups can provide a milieu for practicing social behavior in a less pressured environment.

Persons with severe and long-term schizophrenia may perform poorly in basic and instrumental activities of daily living. Hygiene, dressing, and grooming can be coached and retaught; behavioral and cognitive-behavioral methods are generally used. To succeed in living independently or in group settings in the community, some people need specific instruction in homemaking, money management, and community mobility skills. Because of the cognitive impairment and deficient attention that often accompany schizophrenia, safety behaviors and emergency management skills are particularly important. See Chapters 11, 12, and 18 for a more detailed discussion.

### Leisure

Many persons with schizophrenia also benefit from structuring and guidance in use of leisure time. Early onset of disease and recurring episodes may have prevented development of specific leisure interests. Low financial status may mean little disposable income for leisure; persons in this situation may be unaware of free events in the community and will benefit from being taught how to look in local newspapers and bulletin boards for this information. Other options include membership in a psychosocial clubhouse and development of specific low-cost leisure interests and hobbies.

### Work and Productive Activity

Many persons with schizophrenia never attain or regain the ability to function in a job, but many others can work for a limited number of hours per week at a job that matches their competencies and does not demand skills that are absent or impaired. Volunteering as a peer counselor or mentor in a clubhouse or advocacy group is one way to begin. Other volunteer positions and supported employment are other options. When possible, the person should be placed as quickly as possible in a real job with long-term follow-up support; this seems to work better than simulated employment in hospital settings (61). The key is to avoid placing the person with schizophrenia in situations that will cause decompensation—for example, a noisy or argumentative office with high levels of expressed emotion will interfere with the person's concentration. A better choice is a clerical position in a quiet cubicle or in an office with a quiet and low-key staff.

### Parenting

For this group, participation in family life may also be challenging. Because social and cognitive skills are impaired, it is difficult for the person with schizophrenia to provide a safe and nurturing environment for children. Thus the individual often needs regular intervention and support from mental health professionals.

### Cognitive Functions

Attention, concentration, and judgment are impaired in schizophrenia. The OT practitioner may use either remedial or compensatory approaches to help improve the patient's overall performance, especially as it affects daily life (6, 50). The *remedial* approach involves direct teaching or improvement of specific skills, as described earlier for activities of daily living and social skills. Computer games, for example, can simulate problem-solving dilemmas and permit the person to practice and gain skill in areas such as attention to detail and speed and accuracy of response (51). The remedial approach may also employ sensory stimulation, sensory integration activities, tabletop games, and simulations. Use of the remedial approach implies that missing or impaired cognitive skills can be learned. Current research suggests that generalization of training to real life situations may be weak.

The *compensatory* approach substitutes other abilities or provides external supports to compensate for impaired skills. This approach can be used in all cases, both for the person who may in future be able to improve cognitive skills and for the person who may not. The person might use a notebook to record information that would otherwise be forgotten or may rely on another person for reminders, cues, or assistance with specific tasks. The Allen Cognitive Disabilities model endorses the compensatory approach (2). A variety of other approaches are proposed that may prove useful (21, 33, 43).

> **POINT-OF-VIEW**
>
> ***Routines were important to me, especially in the early years of my recovery. Sometimes when everything was falling apart inside of me, it was good to be able to rely on routines that would give form and structure to the chaos I was experiencing.***
>
> Patricia Deegan (19, p. 13).
>
> - What routines are important to you?
> - Can you describe a difficult time in your life when routines were particularly helpful to you?

### Patterns and Routines, Development and Maintenance of Habits

The structure provided by the patterns of habits, routines and roles is very helpful in maintaining a sense of continuity and occupational engagement. Schizophrenia disrupts habit and role patterns in several ways: by distraction through hallucinations and delusions and through apathy and other negative symptoms. The less routine, the less personal satisfaction the person is likely to experience (31).

Time itself becomes disorganized if the person does not have places to go and things to do (work, school, or other organizing environments). A time-use diary that encourages the person to keep track of how time is spent is useful, particularly if followed by an interview with the therapist (13). Also, reshaping the environment to provide more cues that stimulate the person's familiar habits and patterns is appropriate. Haertl and Minato write that clients desire an environment that "reinforces expectations for active engagement in daily life yet promotes free time to make personal decisions about time use" (31, p. 26). Challenging and normal occupations should be available and encouraged; these reduce stigma and provide a source of positive self-evaluation. This means that rather than crafts or sheltered "make-work" situations, the client should be offered and expected to engage in activities of daily living (ADLs), work, leisure, and educational occupations. Living in a group apartment or other peer environment can provide social pressure to engage in housework and other instrumental activities of daily living (IADLs).

### Chronicity of Illness

Schizophrenia follows a course of relapsing and remitting over time; periods of illness alternate with periods of better functioning and fewer symptoms. The person with a diagnosis of schizophrenia is likely to be a long-term recipient of mental health services, seen in both inpatient and outpatient settings for the remainder of his or her life. Enabling the person to remain in the community, functioning at the best possible level, should be the goal. Persons with severe and persistent mental illness tend to require many social and environment supports; it is particularly important to identify potential crises and relapses before they occur and to reinforce and support self-management of medication and medical aspects of the disorder. Assertive community treatment (ACT) is reported to be highly effective in preventing relapse and hospitalization.

OT interventions should provide structure and realistic opportunities to participate in valued roles. Close supervision and side-by-side instruction can clarify the desired behaviors and effectively model coping skills and social interactions (36). Detailed suggestions for specific problem areas (e.g., ADLs; work, parenting, and cognitive skills) may be found in chapters on those subjects.

## Mood Disorders

Mood disorders, as suggested by their name, have disturbance of mood as the primary feature. The mood is depressed, manic (high), or alternating between the two. A single incident of disturbed mood is termed a *mood episode.* A recurring pattern of mood episodes is termed a *mood disorder.*

*Mania* refers to a mood that is elevated (high), expansive (including everyone and everything), and/or irritable. Sleep is often disturbed. The person may undertake many activities that are inconsistent with his or her prior behavior (e.g., spending sprees, travel, attention seeking). Cognitive functions are impaired and the person shows poor judgment. Mania typically occurs in episodes, with periods of improved functioning alternating with manic episodes. Mania is a symptom in several disorders; the reader may find additional material on the behaviors associated with mania in Chapter 11.

*Depression* refers to a mood that is low-spirited, with loss of interest in activities that were previously pleasurable. As with mania, sleep is often disturbed. Appetite may be diminished or increased. Associated symptoms include low energy, suicidal thoughts, feelings of worthlessness, and restlessness or torpor (inactivity). A diagnosis of *major depressive disorder* is given when the person has had one or more major depressive episodes lasting 2 weeks or more. Symptoms include depressed mood most of the day, nearly every day, with associated depressive changes such as those listed above. The person with this diagnosis will also have significant impairment of social and occupational functioning. Energy and initiative are low, cognitive functions are slowed, and participation in ADLs and other occupations typically diminishes. Depression as a symptom, with its associated behaviors, is further discussed in Chapter 11.

*Bipolar disorder* is a condition in which mania and depression alternate. If the episodes have been primarily manic but there has been at least one depressive episode, the diagnosis is *bipolar I disorder.* If the episodes have been primarily depressed but there has been at least one episode of hypomania (increased mood that is more euphoric than normal but not quite manic), the diagnosis is *bipolar II disorder.* The up and down moods of bipolar disorders present constant challenges in occupational functioning.

**POINT-OF-VIEW**

***College is a struggle for me. I have to sit in the back of the classroom to avoid being overstimulated. It's hard for me to concentrate and I have episodes of depression that mark me as an outcast in comparison to my chipper colleagues who love to go to . . . football games, drink cheer with friends and travel to sunny beaches during semester breaks.***

Suzette (Susan) Mack (47, p. 47)

- What challenges would Susan have faced as an occupational therapy student?
- How would you, as a classmate, have felt about her situation?

The major affective or mood disorders are characterized as existing on a continuum, and as possessing a strong genetic component. Members of a sibling group are at increased risk if one member has a diagnosis of bipolar disorder. At the less severe end of the continuum are conditions with milder symptoms. These are as follows:

- *Dysthymic disorder.* A low mood, a milder form of depression
- *Hypomanic disorder.* Elevated mood, a milder form of mania
- *Cyclothymic disorder.* Alternating moods between a mild high and a mild low

Thus, in a sibling group of five, two sisters may be diagnosed with bipolar I disorder, another with cyclothymia, and two may have no diagnosed affective disorder (although one of these is characterized as very upbeat and chatty by friends).

During hospitalization, occupational therapy treatment of mood or affective disorders is primarily directed at symptom reduction. In community settings, the OT and OTA emphasize a return to function in desired occupational roles, with compensations and environmental modifications to reduce stress and improve attention and focus.

## Medical Management and Drug Treatment

Physicians treat mood disorders with medication. For bipolar disorders, the commonly prescribed drugs to stabilize moods include lithium and various anticonvulsants. The wide variety of medications used for depression include selective serotonin reuptake inhibitors (SSRIs), tricyclic amines, and monoamine oxidase inhibitors (MAOIs) (see Chapter 8). Typically, several medications must be tried before one is found that is effective for a particular person. Sometimes a combination of medications is needed.

Several interventions other than drugs are used. The oldest of these is electroconvulsive therapy (ECT). Deep brain stimulation through repetitive transcranial magnetic stimulation (rTMS) is another treatment using magnetic pulses . Bright light therapy (BLT) has been effective for some people; the person sits in front of a bright light box that emits light similar to sunlight, for an hour or more each day, usually in the morning.

## Occupational Therapy

Chapter 11 gives more detail on how the OTA might approach and manage the client who has active depressive or manic symptoms. Following a major episode of either mania or depression, once the symptoms have been reduced, the individual may benefit from OT directed at reestablishing life routines in self-care, work, and social and family life. Some individuals, particularly those with a chronic and lengthy history of illness, benefit from training in specific skills needed for life roles (e.g., parenting, work behaviors).

Persons with disorder on the depression continuum can benefit from cognitive-behavioral interventions aimed at helping them reassess their beliefs about themselves. Habits, routines, roles, and occupational patterns may fall apart during depressive episodes but can generally be reassembled when the depressive mood lifts.

For the person with bipolar disorder, it is important to address social and vocational functioning and cognitive skills, particularly judgment and planning. The person may feel shame and loss of self-esteem after a manic episode, recalling impulsive behaviors that would not have occurred during a time of normal mood. The OTA should help the consumer understand these behaviors as part of the disease process and not as personal failings.

## Anxiety Disorders

The major symptom of the anxiety disorders is anxiety. The category includes panic disorder, phobias, obsessive-compulsive disorders, and post-traumatic stress disorder. In *panic disorder*, the patient has repeated and unexpected panic attacks characterized by such symptoms as shortness of breath, racing pulse, dizziness, and nausea. After many such attacks the patient becomes fearful of further attacks and for this reason is generally anxious. In *agoraphobia,* which often accompanies panic disorder, the patient fears being in strange places (where a panic attack might occur). This can become so severe that the person is unable to leave home.

*Phobias* are characterized by panic attacks that occur in response to a specific stimulus. In *social phobia,* the patient fears situations in which he or she might be exposed to ridicule or appraisal by other people (as in, for example, public speaking). Other common phobias are of snakes, airplanes, school, and heights. Phobias, agoraphobia, and panic attacks all impair functioning by interfering with the performance of tasks related to occupational roles. The degree of impairment may be more or less severe, depending on the extent of the phobia. For example, a severe fear of school may prevent a child from attending; but if less severe, it may just cause anxiety in specific situations at school.

*Obsessive–compulsive disorder* (OCD) is characterized by obsessions and/or compulsions, which are time consuming and distressing to the patient and which interfere with functioning. An *obsession* is an unwanted intrusive thought or impulse (e.g., to drive into a wall). The person attempts to get rid of the obsession but often cannot do so. A *compulsion* is a repetitive behavior performed in response to an obsession. Hand washing and checking or touching things are examples.

*Post-traumatic stress disorder* (PTSD) is an anxiety disorder that follows an event so stressful that it would upset almost anyone who experienced it. Such traumatic events include war (especially combat), natural disasters, and personal violence. The anxiety provoked by the original trauma is reexperienced by intrusive memories, dreams, and flashbacks. An avoidance response characterized by withdrawal, isolation, psychological numbing, constricted expression of feelings, and lack of interest in previously enjoyed activities reduces contact with the world and psychologically wards off the distressing feelings. Other associated symptoms may include hypervigilance (tense alertness), disturbed sleep, impaired concentration, and feelings of guilt. Those with PTSD may self-medicate with alcohol and drugs.

*Generalized anxiety disorder* is diagnosed when the patient is anxious about two or more unrelated situations and no other axis I diagnosis can account for the anxiety. Subjective symptoms, which are similar to those of panic disorder, must have been present for at least 6 months.

### Medical Management

Anxiety disorders are treated by a combination of medication and psychotherapy. Medications are *anxiolytic* (anxiety reducing). Behavioral and cognitive-behavioral methods are used to help the person diminish anxiety.

### Occupational Therapy

OT for anxiety disorders usually involves learning to recognize and use activities that are relaxing. An effort is made to teach the patient the relaxation response and how to achieve it. Individual assessment is used to identify activities that are relaxing for that person. For example, exhausting physical exercise may be beneficial for some, while others prefer yoga or a stretch and relax approach. Also, some people may find it helpful to release fears through drawing or other expressive media, while this may frighten others. When the anxiety is stimulus specific and impairs function, as in agoraphobia, systematic desensitization and/or cognitive-behavioral programs may be used to neutralize the anxiety response. This approach requires additional training.

Persons with post-traumatic stress disorder may benefit from wilderness experiences and rituals such as the Native American sweat lodge; talking with others who have shared the experience is a particularly helpful aspect of these activities. Yet another approach that can be helpful for the PTSD patient is involvement in an activity that is socially productive and involves giving help to others (75).

Trauma on a large scale became a reality in the United States on September 11, 2001. While millions watched on television, those who lived or worked near the sites of the attacks witnessed them in person. Occupational therapists responded creatively and supportively to help clients, students, and themselves process and put in perspective what happened that day. Accounts of these interventions can be found in the references (63, 64).

## Eating Disorders

Eating disorders include several patterns of abnormal behavior in the consumption and retention of food. *Anorexia nervosa* is characterized by abnormally low body weight with refusal to gain weight and a disturbed body image. *Bulimia nervosa* is characterized by binge eating followed by self-induced vomiting or other drastic measures to reduce body size (fasting, use of laxatives). These conditions occur mainly in women and girls; diagnosis in men and boys is uncommon. Some clinicians also include *obesity* (excessive body weight) in the category of eating disorders, but this is not a *DSM-IV-TR* diagnosis.

Anorexia has been recognized as a clinical disorder for more than 300 years (74). Many approaches have been attempted, including behavioral (49) and psychoanalytic (67). Current understanding suggests that some eating disorder patients have had childhood trauma, including in many cases sexual abuse. Roth (68) describes these patients as needing to control themselves and others through their food intake. The typical eating disorder patient was controlled in childhood by an overprotective and intrusive parent who did not permit her to acquire the normal experiences that lead to self-assessment and the development of healthy reality-based self-esteem. Instead, the young girl adopts a false ideal of low weight, behind which she hides her chronic feelings of emptiness and low self-esteem.

As with alcohol abuse, to a significant degree our society promotes the development of eating disorders. The popular press and broadcast media represent the ideal female as muscular, underweight, and unrealistically thin. Dieting, powdered and canned food substitutes, and aggressive exercise are all marketed as desirable for reducing weight to keep up with the popular ideals, themselves highly unrealistic.

## Medical Management

The first goal for eating disorders to is restore physical health. Nutritional supplements are given to stabilize the body chemistry; the person is hospitalized for this. The patient is engaged in a program of behavioral or cognitive-behavioral therapy and may be given medications.

## Occupational Therapy

Occupational therapy focuses on the development of behaviors that support role performance as an adult (cooking and menu planning, reasonable exercise routines, and acquiring and caring for a wardrobe). In addition, OT must address underlying problems related to distorted body image, deficient self-esteem, and limited assertiveness. In a review of the literature, Rockwell (67) found that the following types of activities were preferred by occupational therapists working with eating disorder patients: art therapy, cooking and menu planning, crafts, stress management training, and group discussion and activities.

Art therapy facilitates the identification and expression of feelings and beliefs about the self. This can help the patient with low self-esteem explore the reasons for feeling so inadequate. Body image issues can also be expressed and examined. McColl et al. (48) suggest, however, that such an activity should not be forced on the patient. Because the feelings of ineffectiveness run so deep, the activities that work best are those that the patient selects.

Cooking and menu planning are important activities for this group. Bailey (12) notes that the eating disorder patient typically has extensive knowledge of the calorie content of foods but little knowledge of other aspects of food content, such as vitamins and nutritive value. In addition, a cooking group supports the experience of preparing and consuming normal-size portions of food. For patients with bulimia, cooking groups provide an opportunity to experience in a normal way foods that might previously have led to bingeing (25). The patient can bake a cake and share it with the group, having only one portion herself.

Meyers (53) reported on a case study of one 27-year-old mother of two who had a diagnosis of anorexia and bulimia. This patient felt that crafts gave her positive control. She could use her hands for something more productive and useful than putting them down her throat to force vomiting of food. She saw the craft experience as a "microcosm of real life with many different people working side by side." The patient found the body image group a struggle and had difficulty letting go of her ideal of a smaller size. As she gained weight, she found it painful to accept the change in body shape and the need for larger new clothes.

In the therapeutic relationship with an eating disorder patient, Meyers (53) indicates that unconditional caring must be accompanied by the expectation for change. In other words, while accepting the patient for where she is and valuing her for who she is, all staff must convey the attitude that they expect the patient to work toward a normal weight and to cease self-destructive eating behaviors. Follow-up and contact after discharge from treatment are needed to help the patient maintain weight, respond effectively to stressors, and continue to function in occupational roles (40).

Eating disorder patients present a clinical challenge. Good supervision is a must. Because of the risk of death and physical illness from poor nutrition, these patients must be monitored by medical staff.

## Personality Disorders

As stated earlier in this chapter, all personality disorders are coded on axis II. To differentiate between personality taits and personality disorders, the *DSM-IV-TR* makes the following distinction: Personality *traits* are enduring patterns of perceiving, relating to, and thinking about the environment and oneself that are exhibited in a wide range of social and personal contexts. Only when personality traits are inflexible and maladaptive and cause significant functional impairment or subjective distress do they constitute *personality disorders* (8).

The *DSM-IV-TR* further states that to merit the axis II diagnosis of personality disorder the traits must be stable and of long standing rather than associated with another disorder. This is helpful for distinguishing obsessive–compulsive personality disorder from the obsessive–compulsive disorder grouped with the axis I anxiety disorders, for example. The latter is not rated as a personality disorder.

Before exploring further the classification of the various personality disorders, the reader is cautioned that the personality, whether seen as "traits" or a "disorder," has traditionally been viewed as not easily changed. But the widespread use of the newer antidepressants such as fluoxetine suggests otherwise. Kramer (41) discusses the difference between temperament (inborn behavioral predispositions) and character (acquired behavioral patterns), making the point that persons diagnosed with personality disorders often show marked changes in behavior and "personality" when they are medicated with a SSRI such as fluoxetine. This raises many moral, philosophical, ethical, and diagnostic questions and suggests that characteristic styles of behavior might be attributed to underlying biological factors (errors of neurotransmitter mechanisms) rather than to problems in character development.

The *DSM-IV-TR* classifies the personality disorders into three clusters. Cluster A disorders include paranoid, schizoid, and schizotypal types. Persons with these disorders may appear odd, eccentric, different, or bizarre to others. Bonder (14) suggests that these disorders may have a neurological component and that sensory integrative treatment may be appropriate. Cluster B disorders include antisocial, borderline, histrionic, and narcissistic personality types. The common ground in these disorders is erratic, emotional, self-centered behavior. Cluster C includes avoidant, dependent, and obsessive–compulsive disorders. The common feature is a fearful, anxious, or avoidant approach to life. The personality disorders have been criticized as having a sexist orientation. In particular, the histrionic and dependent labels are more often assigned to female patients than to male ones. The behaviors associated with these labels are normal aspects of the social conditioning of women in some cultures.[3]

*Paranoid personality disorder* is characterized by a tendency to interpret the actions of others as deliberately harmful to the self. Suspiciousness of others, including spouses and others who would normally be trusted, is common. Disturbances in routine may be seen as threatening. For example, rerouting of a bus may be taken personally. Persons with this disorder may have problems functioning at work because of their suspicions of the intentions of bosses and co-workers. OT practitioners may assist the person to learn and use new strategies to deal with problems at work. However, no overall change in attitude should be expected, as the paranoid stance is part of the person's adaptation to life.

[3] For an extended discussion of this point, see Nahmias and Froelich (58, p. 36).

A diagnosis of *schizoid personality disorder* is sometimes given to persons who have very limited social involvement with others. They live alone, avoid social contact, and seem uninterested in the social relations on which most people thrive. OT treatment of persons with this diagnosis may be directed at assisting them to find and fit into a niche in life that is compatible with their personality structure. For example, a job with limited or no need for interpersonal relatedness and a high opportunity for independence may permit the schizoid person to be socially productive while attaining a sense of personal competence and avoiding the threatening situation of being with other people.

*Schizotypal personality disorder* is characterized by the indifference to social involvement seen in schizoid personality disorder, coupled with peculiarities of behavior that are similar to those seen in schizophrenia. The OT approach is similar to that for the schizoid personality, with additional attention to improvement in self-care and the minimal social skills needed for community survival.

*Antisocial personality disorder* is diagnosed for those who have evidence of *conduct disorder* since before age 15 and who show a continuing pattern of antisocial acts after age 18. These acts may include various crimes, deliberate cruelty to animals and people, failure to honor debts, lying, neglect of duties as a parent, and a pattern of impulsivity, among others. Persons with this diagnosis are often seen in the criminal justice system or in the forensic units of hospitals. Because of the developmental aspect of this disorder, they never really have the opportunity to acquire the behaviors, skills, and attitudes needed to succeed in life. Little has been written about OT treatment approaches to this population. Bonder (14) suggests that milieu therapy (see Chapter 7) and a behavioral approach are best suited for use with this group and with other cluster B personality disorders.

*Borderline personality disorder* (BPD) is characterized by unstable and erratic relationships and a fluctuating sense of personal identity; the person has persistent fear of abandonment by others. Moodiness and chronic feelings of emptiness are common. The moodiness is often acted out in impulsive behavior such as overspending, substance abuse, sexual relations, and self-mutilation. Interpersonal relationships are highly intense and dramatic, with the partner in the relationship viewed as alternatively all good or all bad. OT treatment is usually directed at reducing the symptoms with the aim of increasing the person's self-esteem and self-identity.

A program of dialectical behavioral therapy (DBT) developed by psychologist Marsha Linehan (45, 46) has a good record of research evidence to support effectiveness with persons with BPD. The program includes individual psychotherapy with someone trained in the DBT method, combined with skills training in groups. The DBT model combines support for the person's experience of intolerable feelings with an expectation that the person not act on these feelings. The skills groups provide training in mindfulness, interpersonal effectiveness, and emotion regulation. Mindfulness is a technique for training the mind to observe and control its own activities. Interpersonal effectiveness techniques help the person communicate with other people so as to meet his or her own needs while maintaining a two-way positive relationship. Emotion regulation training educates the person about the nature of emotions and provides practical ways of recognizing and responding to emotions. Use of the DBT model requires special training, but with such training, the OTA could be effective in leading DBT skills groups.

Another approach suggested for BPD is the use of sensory stimulation following the Wilbarger protocol, which involves deep pressure brushing, joint compression, and activities that provide rich stimulation (vigorous exercise, yoga) (55). The OTA might assist in providing this program under the direct guidance of the OT.

The central pattern of *histrionic personality disorder* is attention seeking and extreme emotionality.

This diagnosis is more commonly given to women than to men. Typically, the individual with this diagnosis self-dramatizes, seeks center stage in all situations, and is uncomfortable when not the center of attention. While the person may express very strong emotions, these seem overexaggerated to others. Also, the histrionic person expresses global approval or disapproval without the usual details, for example, stating that a colleague is "a sadistic predator" but not providing any examples of incidents that led to this evaluation. This disorder may interfere with functioning in work, especially in positions of any responsibility, because impaired judgment is common. This disorder may be confused with borderline and narcissistic personality disorders. However, as stated previously, this diagnostic category is criticized as a sexist label by feminist scholars.

*Narcissistic personality disorder* is characterized by extreme self-centeredness, shown in lack of understanding of the feelings of others, exploitation of others, grandiosity, and preoccupation with success. Fantasies of success may lead the person with this disorder to undertake unrealistic goals. Little has been written about OT treatment, but one focus might be to identify realistic goals by analyzing and modifying the unrealistic goals previously chosen. However, because a sense of special uniqueness is central to this condition, the person will resist relinquishing the fantasy, however far-fetched. Forcing a confrontation with reality before the person is ready is counterproductive. OT staff should use a gentle and consistent manner with firm limits and expectations.

The essential feature of *avoidant personality disorder* is fear and avoidance of social contact with others. This is an exaggerated form of the shyness or discomfort many people feel in unfamiliar social situations. Typically, the person has no close friends, is easily hurt by the mildest criticism, and avoids being evaluated (however briefly or fairly) by others. Understandably, this interferes with functioning in the work world and in social situations. OT treatment for this and other cluster C personality disorders may be directed at social skills training and realistic self-appraisal.

*Dependent personality disorder* is more commonly diagnosed in women than men. It is characterized by a pattern of submission to the wishes of others and apparent inability to make decisions on one's own. Persons with this disorder seek guidance, reassurance, and support that is out of proportion to the situation. For example, an adult might let her spouse decide what she will eat when they are dining out and will permit or even seek recommendations as to what hobbies or social interests should be pursued. These individuals function well on the job, except when independent decision making is needed. Persons with this diagnosis are not usually seen in OT in the absence of another diagnosis on axis I or II. This is another diagnosis criticized as sexist.

*Obsessive–compulsive personality disorder* is characterized by perfectionism and is more often diagnosed in men than in women. Typical patterns of behavior include a preoccupation with details, inflexible insistence that others do things a certain way, overvaluing of productivity and undervaluing of social relations, miserliness, and overconscientiousness. These patterns can interfere with functioning at work because of the overall tendency to miss the main point, being side-tracked by the details. OT approaches to working with persons showing obsessive–compulsive behaviors are described in Chapter 11.

## APPLICATIONS OF *DSM-IV-TR* DIAGNOSES TO OCCUPATIONAL THERAPY

Occupational therapists and assistants practicing in mental health settings must appreciate the reality of psychiatric diagnosis and its relationship to reimbursement. Without a *DSM-IV-TR* diagnosis of sufficient severity, neither public nor private insurers will pay for treatment, which makes the psychiatric diagnosis an inescapable fact of practice today. The diagnosis provides some information that is useful to OT staff. Each diagnosis has functional implications, and this helps practitioners in targeting the areas that might need attention (e.g., work, social skills). Ratings on axis V give a sense of the individual's relative impairment in functioning. But there are limitations to the diagnosis, and other information is needed to guide OT treatment and evaluation.

Many psychiatric diagnoses share similar presenting symptoms, particularly in the acute phase of illness, before medication has taken effect. Since reduction of symptoms is a primary concern of all of the professions in acute care settings, the information in Chapter 11 provides detail on responding to the various symptoms. However, once the symptoms have remitted, the residual disability becomes the focus of treatment. In some psychiatric disorders, occupational functioning is unimpaired, and it is hard to justify giving OT treatment to these patients. For most, however, occupational functioning is disturbed or unsatisfactory in some objective and describable way. To focus on the rehabilitation of these patients, we need clear problem and goal statements that are within our scope of practice.

Working on multidisciplinary teams, too often OT staff are sidetracked by the theoretical orientation and focus of the treatment team leader. The team leader may be a physician, psychologist, or social worker and may emphasize intrapsychic functioning, family relationships, or social adjustment. OTs and OTAs who lack a clear sense of their role may find themselves undertaking tasks that are outside their scope of practice (scheduling clinic visits and accompanying the patient to appointments at social service agencies). Worse, the OT staff may provide a directionless range of activities from which the patient may choose, as in a summer camp or activity center. While diverting and clearly helpful for patients with large amounts of unstructured leisure time, this is not enough. Each patient must have clearly written goals that can be met through OT, and a program of treatment must be designed to meet these goals. The goals and the program must be reevaluated at intervals.

What continues to be needed is a set of *OT diagnoses* or *practice guidelines* associated with the various *DSM* diagnoses. Ideally, each OT diagnosis would catalog the impairments in human occupation that are typically found in persons with the corresponding psychiatric diagnosis. All OT diagnoses would derive from OT's scope of practice. For example, the OT diagnoses for schizophrenia might include impaired volition, absence of major occupational roles, disorganized or inadequate habits related to self-care and use of time, and skills deficiencies in many areas. Some of these diagnoses (e.g., impaired volition) would be listed for other *DSM* diagnoses, such as depression. A separate manual of protocols for addressing each OT diagnosis would provide details on how to use activities and the social and physical environment to approach each diagnosis. In the 1980s, Kielhofner (37) presented a diagnosis-based system; in a recent editions, he moved to a system based on occupational performance dysfunction (38, 39). The American Occupational Therapy Association has published a few guidelines for practice with selected diagnoses (4, 5, 7), but these predate the publication of the *Occupational Therapy Practice Framework* (3) and have not been updated.

In conclusion, while all staff working with psychiatric patients should be acquainted with the *DSM* system, each profession must focus its energy on its own areas of expertise. With our growing understanding of occupation as the core of our profession, we are well positioned to reaffirm and develop further our role in mental health practice.

## COMORBIDITY

Mentioned earlier in the chapter, *comorbidity* refers to the simultaneous existence of two or more axis I and/or axis II disorders in the same individual. The reader will encounter many combinations of conditions in the clients seen in occupational therapy. Some examples that occur commonly are the following:

- Bipolar disorder and substance abuse
- Bipolar disorder and personality disorder
- Schizophrenia and alcohol abuse
- Eating disorder and other personality disorder
- Anxiety disorder and substance abuse
- Borderline personality disorder and other personality disorder

It is not at all uncommon to encounter a patient record that lists three, four, or even more axis I and II diagnoses simultaneously.

Medical diagnoses are often seen in combination with psychiatric diagnoses, particularly depression and substance abuse or dependence. Patients with coronary artery disease and other cardiovascular conditions, diabetes, gastrointestinal disease, and cancer may also have depression (28). It has been argued that depression predisposes the person to develop these conditions, but it can also be argued that depression is an understandable emotional response to such a diagnosis. Clinicians working in general medical and rehabilitation settings must be alert to signs of depression in order to respond supportively.

Comorbidity presents challenges for mental health professionals working with the client. Prioritizing goals and determining the sequence in which to tackle problems can be a puzzle. Clearly, if medical problems pose a threat to physical health, these require immediate intervention. But there should also be a place for recognizing, discussing, and formulating a plan to help the individual with psychosocial distress so as to provide comfort and optimize occupational functioning.

## DSM-V: PLANS AND POTENTIAL

Plans for the publication of *DSM-V* have been under way since 1994. The American Psychiatric Association projects that it will be published in 2011 but indicates that the date may be later than that (10). The fifth edition will attempt to address some of the concerns that have been raised with the earlier editions (24)—for example:

- *Nomenclature and categories.* The names (nomenclature) of the disorders have come from many different sources and do not consistently reflect what is now known about the disorders and their origins. The overlap between disorders is also a concern.
- *Neuroscience and genetics.* The *DSM-V* should incorporate research that has increased our understanding of the biology and genetics of the mental disorders.
- *Developmental issues.* The *DSM-V* will reflect the changing course of mental disorders throughout the life span and will reconsider the classification of disorders first occurring in childhood.
- *Personality and relational disorders.* Long considered a weak point of the *DSM* system, these diagnoses are not always clear-cut; they overlap with each other and in some cases may be early manifestations of axis I disorders. Furthermore, some of these diagnoses have been criticized as sexist and as culturally and politically biased. The difference between a personality trait and a personality disorder has not been obvious. The *DSM-V* will attempt to resolve some of these questions.
- *Mental disorders and disability.* In the *DSM-III* and *DSM-IV,* diagnosis of major mental disorders has required that symptoms be present for

6 months and that the symptoms cause a clinically significant disability. These two stipulations were meant to differentiate between more mild forms of symptoms experienced by many people who are mentally healthy and the more extreme forms that suggest a disabling illness. However, the requirements for significant impairment and 6 months' duration have meant that the psychiatrist could not diagnosis a serious disorder (e.g., schizophrenia) even when he or she was quite certain that the person's symptoms indicated an early stage of that disease. Furthermore, any two individuals with a given diagnosis may show widely different levels of functioning and disability. One person may live independently, holding a job and having social relationships; the other may be homeless, living on the street and unable to obtain work or education and unable to carry on a conversation or behave well enough to live in a supervised apartment. Clearly, the second person is more disabled and more in need of services. Coding a disability dimension into the *DSM-V* would help bolster the argument for provision of additional services to those most in need.

- *Cross-cultural issues.* Because context, including culture, significantly affects the way mental disorders present themselves, more attention will be given to this in the *DSM-V.*

While all six issues potentially affect occupational therapy, disability may be the most important for purposes of providing appropriate intervention. If the *DSM-V* successfully describes the disability dimension of mental disorders and provides a means for the diagnosing professional to indicate the extent of disability and the level of rehabilitation and community support needed, this will greatly facilitate provision of services to the seriously and persistently mentally ill. Furthermore, it may help in targeting specific services, such as supported living and supported employment, to individuals most likely to benefit.

## SUMMARY

This chapter is a brief overview of the structure and contents of the *DSM-IV-TR,* the current version of the American Psychiatric Association's diagnostic manual for psychiatric disorders, as well as a brief history of prior versions of the manual. The focus of OT intervention for selected diagnoses has been given. This chapter provides guidance and direction to the use of psychiatric diagnosis in the development of OT problems and goal statements. This is seen as an undeveloped area to which the OTA might contribute clinical recommendations.

## REVIEW QUESTIONS AND ACTIVITIES

1. What is the purpose of the *DSM-IV-TR*? How is it used?
2. Name and describe the five axes of the *DSM*. Which axis is most important for occupational therapy? Why?
3. Why and how has the *DSM* system changed over the years? Give examples. Should we expect it to change in the future? Why?
4. What information can the OTA learn from the *DSM-IV-TR* diagnosis?
5. Go through the chapter and make of list of the major mental disorders affecting clients seen in occupational therapy.
   - Describe each disorder.
   - For each, state the treatments used by psychiatrists (and/or other members of the multidisciplinary team).
   - For each, describe the effects on performance of occupation.
   - For each, list typical problems addressed by occupational therapy.
   - For each typical problem, state in general terms the type of occupational therapy intervention.
6. Explain what is meant by *comorbidity*. How does comorbidity affect occupational therapy intervention?
7. Describe the plans for *DSM-V*. Are the proposed changes important for occupational therapy? Why or why not?

## REFERENCES


1. Alcoholics Anonymous World Services. Twelve Steps and Twelve Traditions. 3rd ed. New York: Alcoholics Anonymous World Services, 1953.
2. Allen CK, Earhardt CA, Blue T. Treatment Goals for the Physically and Cognitively Disabled. Rockville, MD: American Occupational Therapy Association, 1992.
3. American Occupational Therapy Association. Occupational therapy practice framework: Domain and process. Am J Occup Ther 2002;56:609–639.
4. American Occupational Therapy Association. Practice Guidelines for Attention Deficit Hyperactivity Disorder/Attention Deficit Disorder. Bethesda, MD: AOTA, 1996.
5. American Occupational Therapy Association. Practice Guidelines for Schizophrenia. Bethesda, MD: AOTA, 1996.
6. American Occupational Therapy Association. Statement: Occupational therapy management of persons with cognitive impairments. Am J Occup Ther 1991;45:1067–1068.
7. American Occupational Therapy Association. Practice Guidelines for Substance Abuse. Bethesda, MD: AOTA, 1996.
8. American Psychiatric Association. Diagnostic and Statistical Manual of Mental Disorders. 4th ed. Washington: APA, 1994.
9. American Psychiatric Association. Diagnostic and Statistical Manual of Mental Disorders. 4th ed. Text revision. Washington: APA, 2000.
10. American Psychiatric Association. DSM-V timeline. Available at: www.dsm5.org/timeline.cfm. Accessed Jan 2007.
11. American Psychiatric Association. Let's Talk Facts about Substance Abuse. Washington, DC: APA, 1988.
12. Bailey MK. Occupational therapy for patients with eating disorders. Occup Ther Ment Health 1986;6(1):89–116.
13. Bejerholm U, Eklund M. Time use and occupational performance among persons with schizophrenia. Occup Ther Ment Health 2004;20(1):27–47.
14. Bonder BR. Psychopathology and Function. 3rd ed. Thorofare, NJ: Slack, 2004.
15. Braff DL. Information processing and attention dysfunctions in schizophrenia. Schizophr Bull 1993;19:223–259.
16. Brown C. What is the best environment for me? A sensory processing perspective. Occup Ther Ment Health 2001;17(3–4):115–125.
17. Brown C, Tollefson N, Dunn W, et al. The adult sensory profile: Measuring patterns of sensory processing. Am J Occup Ther 2001;55:75–82.
18. Corvinelli A. Alleviating boredom in adult males recovering from substance use disorder. Occup Ther Ment Health 2005;21(2):1–11.
19. Deegan PE. Recovery as a self-directed process of healing and transformation. Occup Ther Ment Health 2001;17(3–4):5–21.
20. Donohue MV, Lieberman H. Social competence of male and female psychiatric patients: Sociability, social presence, socialization and age of onset of psychosis. Occup Ther Ment Health 1992;12(1):25–46.
21. Duncombe L. The cognitive-behavioral model in mental health. In: Katz N, ed. Cognition and Occupation across the Life Span—Models for Intervention in Occupational Therapy. Bethesda, MD: American Occupational Therapy Association, 2005.
22. Dunn W, Myles BS, Orr S. Sensory processing issues associated with Asperger syndrome: A preliminary investigation. Am J Occup Ther 2002;56:97–102.
23. Edgerton J, Campbell RJ, eds. American Psychiatric Glossary. 7th ed. Washington: American Psychiatric Association, 1994.
24. First MB. Research Agenda for *DSM-V:* Summary of the *DSM-V* Preplanning White Papers. Available at: www.dsm5.org/whitepapers.cfm. Accessed Jan 2007.
25. Gills GM, Allen ME. Occupational therapy in the rehabilitation of the patient with anorexia nervosa. Occup Ther Ment Health 1986;6(1):47–66.
26. Gitlin LN, Corcoran MA, eds. Occupational Therapy and Dementia Care: The Home Environmental Skills-Building Program for Individuals and Families. Bethesda MD: American Occupational Therapy Association, 2005.
27. Gur RE, Pearlson GD. Neuroimaging in schizophrenia. Schizophr Bull 1993;19:337–353.
28. Gutman SA. Unipolar depression: A literature review of the most current epidemiological theories. Occup Ther Ment Health 2002;18(2):45–79.
29. Gutman SA. Why addiction has a chronic, relapsing course. The neurobiology of addiction: Implications for occupational therapy practice. Occup Ther Ment Health 2006;22(2):1–29.
30. Gutman SA, McCreedy, Heisler P. The psychosocial deficits of children with regulatory disorders: Identification and treatment. Occup Ther Ment Health 2004;20(2):1–32.
31. Haertl K, Minato M. Daily occupations of persons with mental illness: Themes from Japan and America. Occup Ther Ment Health 2006;20(1);19–32.
32. Henry AD, Coster WJ. Predictors of functional outcome among adolescents and young adults with psychotic disorders. Am J Occup Ther 1996;51:171–181.
33. Josman N. The dynamic interactional model in schizophrenia. In: Katz N, ed. Cognition and Occupation across the Life Span—Models for Intervention in Occupational Therapy. Bethesda, MD: American Occupational Therapy Association, 2005.
34. Kane JM. Schizophrenia. N Engl J Med 1996;334:34–41.

35. Kautzmann LN, Schizophrenia, part 1. Am Occup Ther Assoc Ment Health Special Sect Q Newslett 1996;19 (1): 1–4.
36. Kautzmann LN. Schizophrenia, part 2. Am Occup Ther Assoc Ment Health Special Sect Q Newslett 1996;19(2): 1–4.
37. Kielhofner G, ed. A Model of Human Occupation: Theory and Application. Baltimore: Williams & Wilkins, 1985.
38. Kielhofner G, ed. A Model of Human Occupation: Theory and Application. 2nd ed. Baltimore: Williams & Wilkins, 1995.
39. Kielhofner G, ed. A Model of Human Occupation: Theory and Application. 3rd ed. Baltimore: Lippincott Williams & Wilkins, 2002.
40. Kloczko E, Ikiugi MN. The role of occupational therapy in the treatment of adolescents with eating disorders as perceived by mental health therapists. Occup Ther Ment Health. 2006;22(1):63–83.
41. Kramer PD. Listening to Prozac. New York: Penguin, 1997.
42. Latham PM. Collected Works. Book 1. In: Bartlett J, ed. Familiar Quotations. 15th ed. Boston: Little, Brown, 1980.
43. Lazzarini I. A nonlinear approach to cognition: A web of ability and disability. In: Katz N, ed. Cognition and Occupation across the Life Span—Models for Intervention in Occupational Therapy. Bethesda, MD: American Occupational Therapy Association, 2005.
44. Lehman AF. Schizophrenia PORT: Call to consumers and families to take charge of system that fails to provide effective treatments and supports. NAMI Advocate 1998;19(6):1–8.
45. Linehan MM. Cognitive-Behavioral Treatment of Borderline Personality Disorders. New York: Guilford, 1993.
46. Linehan MM. Skills Training Manual for Treating Borderline Personality Disorder. New York: Guilford, 1993.
47. Mack S. Where the rainbow speaks and catches the sun: An occupational therapist discovers her true colors. Occup Ther Ment Health 2001;17(3–4):43–58.
48. McColl MA, Friedland J, Kerr A. When doing is not enough: The relationship between activity and effectiveness in anorexia nervosa. Occup Ther Ment Health 1986;6:137–150.
49. McGee KT, McGee JP. Behavioral treatment of eating disorders. Occup Ther Ment Health 1986;6(1):15–25.
50. Medalia A, Revheim N. Dealing with cognitive dysfunction associated with psychiatric disabilities—A handbook for families and friends of individuals with psychiatric disorders. Available at www.omh.state.ny.us/omhweb/cogdys_manual/CogDysHndbk.htm. Accessed Jan 2007.
51. Medalia A, Revheim N. Using computers in cognitive rehabilitation with psychiatric patients. Paper presented at Institute 08, the American Occupational Therapy Association annual conference, Baltimore, Apr 3, 1998.
52. Meltzer HY. Biological studies in schizophrenia. Schizophr Bull 1987;13:77–111.
53. Meyers SK. Occupational therapy treatment of an adult with an eating disorder: One woman's experience. Occup Ther Ment Health 1989;9(1):33–47.
54. Miller PA, Butin D. The role of occupational therapy in dementia—C.O.P.E. (caregiver options for practical experiences). Int J Geriatr Psychiatry 2000;15(1):86–89.
55. Moore KM, Henry AD. Treatment of adult psychiatric patients using the Wilbarger protocol. Occup Ther Ment Health 2002;18(1):43–63.
56. Moyers PA. An organizational framework for occupational therapy in the treatment of alcoholism. Occup Ther Ment Health 1988;8(2):27–46.
57. Moyers PA. Treating the alcoholic's family. Am Occup Ther Assoc Ment Health Special Sect Q Newslett 1990;13(3):2–4.
58. Nahmias R, Froelich J. Women's mental health: Implications for occupational therapy. Am J Occup Ther 1993;47:35–41.
59. National Center for Health Statistics, Centers for Disease Control and Prevention. International Classification of Disease. 9th ed. Clinical modification. Available at: www.cdc.gov/nchs/about/otheract/icd9/abticd9.htm. Accessed Jan 2007.
60. New treatments for schizophrenia, part 1. Harv Ment Health Lett 1998;14(10):1–3.
61. New treatments for schizophrenia, part 2. Harv Ment Health Lett 1998;14(11):1–3.
62. Pfeiffer B, Kinnealey M, Reed C, Herzberg G. Sensory modulation and affective disorders in children and adolescents with Asperger's disorder. Am J Occup Ther 2005;59:335–345.
63. Precin P, ed. Healing 9/11: Creative programming by occupational therapists [Special issue]. Occup Ther Ment Health. 2006;21(3–4).
64. Precin P, ed. Surviving 9/11: Impact and experiences of occupational therapy practitioners [Special issue]. Occup Ther Ment Health 2003;19(3–4).
65. Raymond M. Life skills and substance abuse. Am Occup Ther Assoc Ment Health Special Sect Q Newslett 1990;13(3):1–2.
66. Richert GZ, Bergland C. Treatment choices: Rehabilitation services used by patients with multiple personality disorders. Am J Occup Ther 1992;46:644–638.
67. Rockwell LE. Frames of reference and modalities used by occupational therapists in the treatment of patients with eating disorders. Occup Ther Ment Health 1990;10(2):47–63.
68. Roth D. Treatment of the hospitalized eating disorder patient. Occup Ther Ment Health 1986;6(1):67–87.
69. Sadock BJ, Sadock VA. Kaplan & Sadock's Synopsis of Psychiatry. 9th ed. Philadelphia: Lippincott Williams & Wilkins, 2003.

70. Smallwood J, Brown R, Coulter F, et al. Aromantherapy and behaviour disturbances in dementia: A randomized controlled trial. Int J Geriatr Psychiatry 2001;16(10): 1010–1013.
71. Stoffel VC, Moyers PA. An evidence-based and occupational perspective of interventions for persons with substance-use disorders. Am J Occup Ther 2004;58:570–586.
72. Van Deusen J. Alcohol abuse and perceptual-motor dysfunction: The occupational therapist's role. Am J Occup Ther 1989;43:384–390.
73. Viik MK, Watts JH, Madigan MJ, Bauer D. Preliminary validation of the assessment of occupational functioning with an alcoholic population. Occup Ther Ment Health 1990;10(2):19–33.
74. Waltos DL. Historical perspectives and diagnostic considerations. Occup Ther Ment Health 1986;6(1):1–13.
75. Wilson JP. Trauma, Transformation and Healing: An Integrative Approach to Theory, Research and Post-Traumatic Therapy. New York: Brunner Mazel, 1989.

## SUGGESTED READINGS

Bonder BR. Psychopathology and Function. 3rd ed. Thorofare NJ: Slack, 2004.

Brown C. What is the best environment for me? A sensory processing perspective. Occup Ther Ment Health 2001;17(3–4):115–125.

Gitlin LN, Corcoran MA, eds. Occupational Therapy and Dementia Care: The Home Environmental Skills-Building Program for Individuals and Families. Bethesda MD: American Occupational Therapy Association, 2005.

Gutman SA. Unipolar depression: A literature review of the most current epidemiological theories. Occup Ther Ment Health 2002;18(2):45–79.

Gutman SA. Why addiction has a chronic, relapsing course. The neurobiology of addiction: Implications for occupational therapy practice. Occup Ther Ment Health 2006;22(2):1–29.

Medalia A, Revheim N. Dealing with cognitive dysfunction associated with psychiatric disabilities—A handbook for families and friends of individuals with psychiatric disorders. Albany: New York State Office of Mental Health, 2002.

Miller PA, Butin D. The role of occupational therapy in dementia—C.O.P.E. (caregiver options for practical experiences). Int J Geriatr Psychiatry 2000;15(1): 86–89.

Spitzer RL, Gibbon M, Skodol AE, et al. DSM-IV Case Book. Washington: American Psychiatric Association, 1994.

Stoffel VC, Moyers PA. An evidence-based and occupational perspective of interventions for persons with substance-use disorders. Am J Occup Ther 2004;58: 570–586.

CHAPTER 7

# Contexts of Intervention, Service, and Care

*I was being admitted to a locked unit of a long-term psychiatric clinic. My belongings were searched, then locked away, and I was stripped and dressed in bed clothes—those horrible green hospital-issued "smock things" that tie in the back with two ill-spaced and sometimes nonexistent ties. Thus clad and dehumanized I was sent to "mingle with the other patients."*

IRENE M. TURNER (62)

## CHAPTER OBJECTIVES

After studying this chapter, the reader will be able to:

1. Name and describe settings in which mental health occupational therapy services may be provided.
2. Describe possible roles for the occupational therapist (OT) and occupational therapist assistant (OTA) in each setting.
3. Differentiate between *care, intervention, service,* and *treatment* and the messages these terms impart.
4. Discuss in general terms the effects of different contexts on staff and consumers.
5. Contrast the role of the OT or OTA in a consumer-operated organization versus a psychiatric setting.
6. Discuss the role of the occupational therapy practitioner in settings employing each of the following models: milieu therapy, family therapy, and psychosocial rehabilitation.

Occupational therapy practitioners work with people who have mental problems in numerous settings, each with its own purpose, treatment philosophy, funding pattern, and population. Some settings, such as the locked unit described in the quotation that opens this chapter, are most restrictive, aiming to reduce the risk of harm to the patient, other patients, and staff. Increasingly, however, persons with mental disorders receive services in the least restrictive environment, such as community housing and competitive employment. In addition, many individuals whose first diagnosis is other than psychiatric also experience psychosocial problems for which they receive services in still other settings. Each environment influences the behavior of its occupants, be they consumers of mental health services or the professionals that provide these services. The roles of occupational therapist (OT) and occupational therapy assistant (OTA) and the ranges of services provided vary accordingly.

This chapter gives an overview of the major types of settings in which services are provided to persons with psychiatric problems and of some possible roles and responsibilities of the OTA within each setting. Concepts from *Occupational Therapy Practice Framework (OTPF)* (3) and the model of human occupation about the effect of the environment on engagement occupation are examined to suggest how particular treatment settings may affect behavior of mental health consumers and staff. Because some settings use theories or practice models other than those described in Chapters 2 and 3, several additional models will be described briefly.

## THE SCOPE OF PATIENTS, CLIENTS, AND CONSUMERS

As discussed in Chapter 6, mental health problems range from transient situational disturbances to severe and persistent illnesses. For mild depression and anxiety brought on by life circumstances, most people seek help from their family physicians and may be referred to treatment with a psychiatrist, psychologist, or social worker. Mild problems are rarely treated by occupational therapists, except in case of sustained difficulty in carrying out daily life activities; even then, verbal therapy with another mental health professional may be the only treatment provided. Most mild mental health problems resolve themselves more or less satisfactorily as the person learns to cope or when life circumstances change. Depending on the funding and programs available in a local area, some occupational therapy services may be available to people with mild mental health problems through community mental health centers, home health services, and prevention programs.

People with more serious and persistent mental illness often do not seek treatment; in many states they cannot be forced to accept treatment unless they are a danger to themselves or others. Because public psychiatric beds are in short supply since deinstitutionalization in 1963 and because mentally ill persons may cause a public nuisance, such persons may be taken by the police to the local jail or may be sentenced to long prison terms. Torrey (60) reports that approximately 10% of prison inmates nationwide are persons with severe and persistent mental illness; in fact, with 3000 severely mentally ill persons housed daily, the Los Angeles County Jail is by default "the largest mental institution in the country" (24). Children with mental illness, particularly boys, are especially likely to be housed in the prison system; the *New York Times* (11) reported that 25% of children in juvenile detention in Louisiana and 20% nationally have serious mental illnesses. In general, psychiatric services in forensic settings are minimal; inmates may experience physical and sexual abuse and receive only limited psychiatric care. Only a handful of OTs and OTAs work in such settings, although interesting program ideas continue to be reported (18, 49, 55).

Alternately, the seriously mentally ill may be hospitalized or referred to an outpatient or community mental health center where occupational therapy personnel work with them as part of a team of professionals. Some of the people admitted to these settings, such as battered women, emotionally disturbed children, homeless persons, and the frail elderly, must deal with social and economic problems as well as mental disorders. Drug and alcohol abusers, persons with personality disorders and eating disorders, and the mildly mentally retarded may also be seen.

Most occupational therapists and assistants who work in psychiatric hospital and mental health community settings provide services to persons with severely disabling psychiatric disorders. Serious mental health problems are often first recognized when the person becomes so symptomatic or disorganized as to require hospitalization or, in the case of substance abuse, admission for detoxification. Often, but not always, this initial hospitalization is the first of a series.

Chronic illnesses (see Chapters 5 and 6) are severe and progressive, with an expectation of decreased ability to function in the community and, in some cases, to lifelong association with the mental health system. Many persons with severe and chronic problems can learn to function adequately in the community with varying degrees of supervision, at least in the early years of their illness; advances in medication and improved understanding of effective treatments have made it possible for many to function well enough to attend school and hold jobs.

Many labels (*patient, client, consumer, member, inmate,* and *resident*) are applied to the people served in psychiatric programs. What do these terms mean and which ones are appropriate in which situations? Box 7-1 gives terms in use at this writing. Terms change with time and custom. Stigma attaches to labels of any kind; the effective and compassionate practitioner is alert and attuned to the preferences and sensitivities of the recipient of services, regardless of the setting.

**BOX 7-1**

**THE RECIPIENT OF MENTAL HEALTH SERVICES: WHAT'S IN A NAME?**

**patient** Suggests a dependent relationship to professional staff; most appropriate when applied to a person who is hospitalized or receiving hospital services as an outpatient

**care recipient** Suggests that the person requires substantial supervision or personal assistance with activities of daily living (ADLs)

**client** Suggests that the person is hiring the clinician to perform a service, much as one might hire a lawyer; sometimes used in day treatment programs

**consumer** Preferred by persons with severe and persistent mental illness because it suggests freedom of choice and voluntary use of mental health services

**member** Preferred by persons who belong to a psychosocial club program

**inmate** Connotes that the person has been jailed; correctly used only in forensic environments

**resident** Used when a person with mental illness lives in a nursing home or other supervised living environment

**survivor** A term used by persons with diagnoses of serious mental disorders to connote their commitment to living with the threat of relapse (similar to *cancer survivor*)

## THE SCOPE OF SETTINGS

It is helpful to see the settings in terms of their purposes and the services offered. The title of this chapter suggests some ideas. At one time, all were termed *treatment settings;* but with increased sensitivity to the needs of those served and of what therapy personnel do to help them, the settings are better differentiated.

*Treatment* is generally considered to refer to medical care for disease, injury, or other medically treatable condition. This term is a poor description for services given in community settings and those that are related to housing, employment, or engagement in occupation. It does make sense when the person is ill and is receiving services designed to heal.

*Intervention* is a broad term meaning "an action undertaken in order to change what is happening or might happen in another's affairs, especially in order to prevent something undesirable" (62). This term may include many of the services provided by OTs and OTAs, but it does imply that something bad might happen if the intervention does not occur. It also suggests that the person for whom the intervention is given does not participate in the decisions.

*Service* refers to "work done by somebody for somebody else as a job (or) a duty" (62). This suggests that the person receiving the service has some control over what is being provided. Service is a useful term to apply to settings in which consumers contract with professionals or in which clients choose goals or outcomes.

*Care* is a term that suggests tending to or supervising someone, as in child care and elder care. The implication is that the person needs the ministrations and supervisions of one or more other persons. This term makes sense when applied to settings serving those with advanced dementia and similarly disabling conditions.

The reader is encouraged to keep an open mind about the settings in which occupational therapy personnel work and to think creatively about which of the terms defined here is most accurate for each setting. Settings include high-security inpatient wards, in which violent or suicidal individuals can be adequately supervised, as well as community settings, in which people who do not need hospitalization are seen.

Most inpatient psychiatric settings have some OTs and/or OTAs on staff; these settings may be large public institutions, nonprofit voluntary psychiatric hospitals, general hospitals, or proprietary hospitals. The aged and those with Alzheimer's disease and other organic mental disorders may be treated in long-term care settings such as skilled nursing facilities, assisted living environments, and the person's home. The criminally insane may be treated on forensic units of large state hospitals. Adolescents and children will be seen in schools, camps, and activity programs.

Occupational therapists and assistants may also work with special groups, such as battered women, sex offenders, child abusers, drug and alcohol abusers, persons with dementia, persons with human immunodeficiency virus (HIV) infection or acquired immune deficiency syndrome (AIDS), and persons with selected personality disorders or eating disorders. It is believed that the special needs of these groups are best met when peers with similar problems are treated together. Separate wards exist also for research into the effectiveness of medications and other treatments for persons with a particular diagnosis (e.g., paranoid schizophrenia, eating disorders, borderline personality disorder).

Outpatient settings include aftercare clinics attached to hospitals with inpatient services, walk-in programs in community mental health centers, psychosocial clubhouses, and social and community agencies. Children and adolescents may be seen in schools or in after-school programs at community centers such as libraries, YMCAs, or YWCAs. Those who are very ill may be hospitalized or incarcerated in long-term treatment centers. Home health agencies sometimes provide occupational therapy services in the home to persons suffering from mental disorders.

Occupational therapists and assistants also work in employment-oriented settings, such as supported employment programs, workshops, and vocational evaluation and rehabilitation centers.

## INPATIENT SETTINGS

Inpatient settings, such as hospital and skilled nursing facilities, provide nursing care around the clock. Persons who need supervision because they are violent or so disorganized that they cannot meet their own needs for food, clothing, and shelter can be protected only in this type of setting. Inpatient settings are generally divided into two subcategories: acute and chronic. Acute inpatient settings provide services on a short-term basis, generally for patients who have become ill suddenly or who have a history of psychiatric illness and have a sudden recurrence of psychotic symptoms. Some acute care settings are locked, so that patients are prevented from escaping and harming themselves or others. Acutely ill patients are discharged as soon as they are medically stable, usually 3 to 21 days after admission.

Chronic inpatient settings, such as state hospitals, provide supervision and services for persons who have severe and persistent mental illness and serious disabilities that impair community living (generally schizophrenia or organic mental disorders). These patients may remain in an inpatient environment for decades; chronic care settings for very disorganized patients are usually locked. Long-term inpatient treatment centers, in which patients who were not so seriously ill remained for months or years, were the norm until deinstitutionalization began in 1963; today's practice is based on the notion that people get better faster in their own communities. Unfortunately, most persons with serious mental illness do not receive adequate care in the community and are frequently reinstitutionalized, sometimes in a hospital and sometimes in a jail. Boxes 7-2 and 7-3 outline the focus on treatment in acute and long-term inpatient settings.

### Large State Hospitals and Other Public Institutions

Public intuitions include municipal, state, and county hospitals and Veterans Administration and U.S. Public Health Service facilities. Funding comes from local, state, and federal governments.

**BOX 7-2**

**ACUTE INPATIENT PROGRAMS: TREATMENT FOCUS**

- Rapid individual functional assessment, mutual collaborative goal setting
- Group programming necessitated by short stay and rapid turnover
- Normal daily routine: mix of activities of daily living, productive activities, leisure activities
- Social participation: social skills, interaction with community and family
- Self-expression and self-awareness activities
- Psychosocial skills: stress management, coping skills, problem solving
- Discharge planning: relapse prevention, symptom identification and reduction, medication management
- Therapeutic social milieu that gives a message of ability and empowerment

BOX 7-3

**LONGER-TERM INPATIENT PROGRAMS: TREATMENT FOCUS**

- Protective environment
- Group programming
- Individual functional assessment for clients with strong rehabilitation potential, mutual collaborative goal setting
- Individual programming (mix of group activities and individual activities)
- Behavior management
- Compensatory treatment for cognitive deficits
- Basic activities of daily living: personal presentation; hygiene, grooming, and dressing; basic communication; nutrition; safe sex and other health information; exercise
- Instrumental activities of daily living: communication (using telephone and phone book, basic literacy), using public transportation, clothing care, handling money, shopping on a budget, food preparation, safety, responses to emergencies, trash and recycling, caring for a home or apartment, stress management
- Leisure: identifying interests, finding free or inexpensive events, developing leisure habits, exercise and sports, games, holiday and social events.
- Work: opportunities for exploration, supported employment, transitional placement, meaningful productive employment, volunteer and part-time jobs
- Social participation: social skills, peer interactions
- Other age-related and/or gender-specific support groups, parenting skills, and so on
- Therapeutic social milieu that gives a message of ability and empowerment.

Most such facilities have inpatient and outpatient services, and many have specialized units for forensic (criminal) cases, addiction and alcoholism, the aged, children, and adolescents. Some are in urban centers. Most are very large, consisting of several buildings on a sprawling campus, often in rural areas. Inconvenient locations make it difficult for family members to visit.

The deinstitutionalization of psychiatric patients, compelled by the Community Mental Health Act of 1963 (PL 88-164), resulted in the discharge of many persons who were previously inmates of large state psychiatric hospitals. The original mission of deinstitutionalization (to liberate patients from confinement and enable them to integrate into community housing and employment) has not been realized; many of those discharged or not hospitalized today are found in correctional facilities, in shelters for the homeless, or on the street.

At present, the population of large public psychiatric centers consists of three main categories: those who are too violent or suicidal to be released, those who have intact families or social support systems but who are so severely impaired and disorganized that they cannot live in the community even with this support, and those who lack social support from family or others and who despite apparently adequate skills have shown on repeated discharges that they cannot succeed in the community without support and structure. Political pressure may force premature discharge of these patients, leading to repeated readmission and a revolving-door pattern.

Yet another group of patients, although competent to remain for long periods in the community, may be admitted for occasional brief hospitalization, often precipitated by stressful life events. Young adult chronic patients (described in Chapter 5) are viewed as more difficult to manage and to treat than their older counterparts.

Public hospitals receive admissions on a geographical basis, in which a region is divided into catchment areas; the person is sent to the particular state, county, or municipal hospital whose catchment area includes his or her place of residence. Large public institutions are typically understaffed, not only in occupational therapy and other activity programs but also in basic medical and nursing services. Sometimes their physicians have no psychiatric training or are recent immigrants whose limited command of English prevents their understanding and being understood by patients and other staff. Funding is erratic, and hiring freezes and shortages of supplies are common. Cyclical fluctuations in budget and staff follow election of liberal or conservative politicians.

Despite these drawbacks, such facilities provide many opportunities and challenges for OTs and OTAs. The variety of diagnoses seen and the possibilities for working with individuals of different ages and severity of illness are challenging. Also, because patients tend to remain for long periods or are frequently readmitted, practitioners can develop long-term therapeutic relationships, can observe the progression of the disease, and can watch the effect of their interventions over time. Also, after a few years of employment, OTs or OTAs may rise to administrative or management positions and influence practice on a larger scale.

Occupational therapy services provided in these settings are comprehensive, hence difficult to describe completely. Hemphill and Werner (29) lamented that all too often the OT role is degraded to that of "activity provider." The activities—crafts, indoor sports, and games—may divert the person's attention but do not develop skills needed to leave the hospital and survive in the community. Instead, OTs and OTAs should focus on rehabilitation with the aim of independent living; appropriate practice models for these settings and populations include the model of human occupation (MOHO) and the psychiatric rehabilitation model (4,16).

As stated previously, inpatient wards may be classified as acute or chronic; on acute wards, the emphasis is on medical treatment and control of symptoms through use of medications. Occupational therapists and assistants may offer general activities to simulate normal patterns of daily living and monitor patients' performance and behavior to determine the effect of the medical treatment and the person's readiness for discharge. On chronic wards, depending on the level of disability among the patients, occupational therapy may offer maintenance of or development of daily living skills, work-related skills, and leisure activities.

Chronic wards are generally understaffed, and the OTA may be charged with providing services for as many as 50 to 100 patients. Intensive services may be available only for patients selected for their rehabilitation potential or readiness, based on stable medical status and results of a comprehensive functional evaluation. The program may be on the ward, in special activity rooms within each hospital building, or in a central activities building elsewhere on the hospital campus. Some large state hospitals use the off-unit programming approach; activities occur in a central location away from the living units. These off-unit sites are ideal for activities like work and school that would be done away from home if one were living in the community.

Because of the emphasis on returning persons with serious mental disorders to community living wherever possible, occupational therapy on both acute and chronic wards emphasizes evaluation of and training in daily living skills. If and when patients are discharged, they may be assigned to a satellite clinic near the person's home, at which they can receive whatever aftercare services they need; these clinics are staffed and administered by the state hospital system.

### Intensive Psychiatric Rehabilitation Services Units

Some states, including New York, have adopted the psychiatric rehabilitation model (5) (see Chapter 2). State hospitals and their affiliated outpatient clinics offer intensive psychiatric rehabilitation treatment (IPRT) units to clients who are medically stable and who might be expected to benefit from more intensive environment-specific training. Occupational therapy practitioners may manage rehabilitation programs or may provide direct services under this model. Interventions focus on developing specific skills needed for the person's target environment, identifying and supplying environmental supports, and providing social supports, such as supervised housing and supported employment.

### Behavioral Units

Hays and Baxley (28) describe a special unit for patients who have persistent behavioral deficits. Diagnoses may be schizophrenia, other psychoses, and traumatic brain injury (TBI). Behavioral or cognitive-behavioral treatment aims to reduce problem behaviors and enhance coping strategies. Thus, for example, the person who constantly makes inappropriate sexual advances is helped to curb the behavior, understand the feelings that precipitate the impulse, learn appropriate boundaries for sexual expression, and substitute coping strategies such as distraction or deep breathing.

### Transitional Services

Transitional services prepare patients to move from the hospital to the community. Some state psychiatric hospitals have quarterway houses on or near the hospital grounds. These live-in settings allow residents to explore the experience of more freedom in the community while receiving direct supervision from trained staff. Once they have demonstrated that they can function under these conditions, residents are discharged to independent community living.

Day care centers provide a place for the newly discharged to obtain continuing support and to connect with staff. Transitional services, such as visits by outpatient counselors and telephone counseling, are provided.

## Acute Care Inpatient Wards

Acute care inpatient wards offer a secure environment in which persons who are seriously ill can be evaluated and treated for a short time; typically this means stabilization and reduction of positive symptoms by medication. Patients are then discharged with or without an outpatient treatment plan or transferred to a long-term unit or other facility such as a state hospital. Acute care wards may be housed in a general hospital, a large private hospital (voluntary or proprietary), or a public institution; they are usually locked for the protection of the patients and the general population. Goals in the acute care setting include observing and reporting patients' performance and response to medication, improving patients' performance in preparation for return to the community, assisting in discharge planning, and helping stabilize behavior (2).

Third-party payers have pressed for shorter inpatient stays; a week or less is typical, leading to an increased emphasis on evaluation and discharge planning. Evaluation may focus on cognitive level, self-care skills, and independent living skills. Lengthy evaluation is impractical when quick results are needed for discharge planning.

Note writing and documentation require much staff time because initial and discharge notes must be written for every patient; with 10 to 20 admissions a week this means that 20 to 40 notes are written every week. Meetings to communicate observations and findings about patients and plan for discharge occur daily; up to half of the staff's time may be given to meetings. Therapists are sometimes frustrated when patients fail to attend groups or must leave in the middle of a group to attend an interview or have a test done.

Even a short stay in the hospital is disruptive to the patient. Robinson and Avallone (53) developed an *activities health* approach based on the idea that activity (function) can be healthy even when the person has serious mental illness. This approach aims to maintain activities health during hospitalization by providing a normal routine selected by the person from a typical array of work, rest, and leisure activities. The program encourages patients to engage in specific and individualized tasks similar to those done before hospitalization. Three other objectives in the activities health approach are to monitor the effects of medication on the person's ability to function, to work with the person to assess activities health and routine, and to recommend services needed to improve everyday functioning after discharge.

Another approach is to provide activity groups to meet general needs of hospitalized patients; the goals may be to build self-esteem, increase awareness of self and others, develop group skills, and/or express feelings (52). Typical activities include games, group sports, and art projects. The purpose is to provide positive experiences, restore patients' confidence in themselves, and increase their interest in and ability to relate to other people. For such activities to be meaningful, they should be linked to specific functional outcomes.

Peloquin (46) developed the *interview/therapy set* as yet another approach to providing evaluation and treatment for large numbers of acute care patients who stay less than 2 weeks. Therapy set is the process of orienting patients to the purpose, goals, and procedures used in a particular treatment. This approach uses three forms—an open letter, an activity guide, and a checklist of goals—to help patients understand the value of occupational therapy and to encourage them to participate. The letter, which describes occupational therapy in simple language, is given to all literate patients as soon as they are well enough to understand it. The activity guide is a self-administered data collection instrument. It is divided into sections consisting of several yes-or-no questions about problems the patient may have; each section ends with a brief description of how occupational therapy can help. The checklist of goals, shown in Figure 7-1, is used to develop individual treatment programs based on objectives identified from answers on the activity guide. The therapist checks off the goals the patient is to concentrate on and the activities he or she is to attend; a copy of the form is given to the patient and another is placed in the chart. The interview and therapy set procedure can streamline evaluation and treatment in an acute care setting.

## Proprietary Hospitals

Proprietary hospitals are private hospitals run for profit; because of their profit orientation, these hospitals may exclude those who do not belong to their sponsoring insurance group or who do not have private insurance and adequate funds. Often only the private patients of doctors on staff are admitted; sometimes these doctors are themselves part owners of the hospital. The treatment team approach, as described in "Acute Care Inpatient Wards" in this chapter,- is less often used in proprietary hospitals; instead, the individual physicians write orders for their own patients, which they intend other staff to carry out. Patients may be treated with a combination of psychotropic medication, electroconvulsive therapy, and various verbal therapies. Physicians' attitudes toward occupational therapy vary from indifferent

OCCUPATIONAL THERAPY GOALS TOWARD IMPROVED FUNCTIONAL PERFORMANCE

NAME: ____________ ROOM: ____________ DATE: ____________

OCCUPATIONAL THERAPY WILL BE WORKING TO HELP YOU IN THE FOLLOWING AREAS, HOPING THAT YOU WILL BENEFIT FROM PURPOSEFUL ACTIVITY.

**With Your Thinking Skills:**

_______ improving your concentration by providing crafts, hobbies, and daily exercises that require you to concentrate

_______ reducing your confusion through activities that provide clear directions for you to follow

_______ building your problem-solving skills through activities and puzzles that encourage you to figure out problems

_______ keeping you alert and thinking in order to prepare you to return to your home and community

_______ helping you reduce racing thoughts through organized and calming projects

_______ providing you with opportunities to organize your thinking and behavior through structured tasks

**With Your Feelings About Yourself:**

_______ boosting your self-esteem through daily successes in activity groups

_______ increasing your self-confidence by having you work independently

_______ increasing your feelings of being in control by having you experience the control you have over yourself physically and emotionally

_______ encouraging you to work through hurt or other upsetting feelings through energetic types of activity

_______ maintaining your work and social skills through a full and balanced daily routine

**With Your Use of Leisure Time and Available Coping Resources:**

_______ teaching you ways to use your free time in a healthier, more satisfying way

_______ encouraging you to look around your community to find groups and activities that can help you better satisfy your personal needs

_______ encouraging you to use a part of each day for spontaneous fun and relaxation

**With Dealing With Other People:**

_______ increasing your comfort level and ability to trust others by involving you in pleasant groups

_______ providing you with the support that comes from belonging to a group

_______ providing you with opportunities to communicate with others

_______ providing you with situations in which you must share, interact, and stay in touch with society's demands

_______ encouraging you to use energetic activities to provide healthy outlets for the strong feelings you are experiencing

**Figure 7-1. Occupational therapy goals toward improved functional performance.** (Reprinted with permission from Peloquin SM. The development of an occupational therapy interview/therapy set procedure. Am J Occup Ther 1983;37:457–461. Copyright © 1983 by the American Occupational Therapy Association, Inc.)

**With Your Ability to Handle Stress:**

_______ reducing your anxiety level through energetic crafts, exercise, and games
_______ teaching you to reduce stress and its symptoms through yoga (11:30)
_______ relaxation techniques (4:15)
_______ relaxing hobbies

**With Your Physical Condition:**

_______ improving your general health, strength, and coordination through chair exercise, yoga, recreational games, sports groups requiring physical activity
_______ keeping you in a good physical condition and functioning at your best level
_______ helping you to reduce physical discomforts such as stiffness, shakiness, and pain, through relaxation exercises
_______ helping you to reduce any unpleasant side effects from your medication or treatment

**Other:**

**In Order to Do the Above, You Should Attend:**

_______ MORNING CRAFTS
_______ RELAXATION (4:15) _______ MORNING EXERCISES (11:30)
_______ RECREATION (6:00) _______ RECREATION/WORKSHOPS (1:00)

Suzanne M. Peloquin, OTR/L
Registered Occupational Therapist

Copy given to patient __________

**Figure 7-1.** ***(Continued)***

to enthusiastic. Departments may provide a range of diversional and therapeutic activities, including discussion groups, games, sports, gardening, task groups, and leisure and socialization experiences. Work-oriented and rehabilitative services may be included if the physicians understand and endorse this approach.

## OUTPATIENT SETTINGS

Outpatient facilities provide services at a central facility for people who live at home. Some outpatient settings, such as satellite clinics and aftercare clinics, are affiliated with hospitals; others are privately administered and get their funding from a combination of private and public sources. All share a philosophical orientation that the person can get better faster and stay out of the hospital longer while living as independently as possible in the community.

Community settings match well with occupational therapy's focus on the natural and normal engagement in occupation. Intervention can occur within the normal environment and can be tailored to the needs of the individual. The focus of case management can shift from medical concerns to habilitation within the community (34). Box 7-4 summarizes the treatment focus of community settings. To be effective in community settings, the OT or OTA must be attuned to political and economic events affecting funding and the direction of treatment. Careful attention to systemwide factors (e.g., reimbursement shifts, grant application deadlines, and legislative constraints and mandates) helps identify forthcoming changes and opportunities for program improvements.

**BOX 7-4**

**COMMUNITY PROGRAMS: TREATMENT FOCUS**

- Careful individual functional assessment, mutual collaborative goal setting
- Individual programming: mix of group activities and individual activities
- Basic activities of daily living: personal presentation; hygiene, grooming, and dressing; basic communication; nutrition; safe sex and other health-related information; fitness goals; exercise
- Instrumental activities of daily living: communication (using telephone and phone book, basic literacy), using public transportation, clothing care, handling money, shopping on a budget, food preparation, safety, emergency responses, trash and recycling, caring for a home or apartment, stress management
- Leisure: identifying interests, locating free or inexpensive events, developing leisure habits, exercise and sports, games, holiday and social events
- Work: opportunities for exploration, supported employment, transitional placement, meaningful productive employment, volunteer and part-time jobs
- Social participation: social skills, interaction with community and family, peer interactions, sexual expression and safe sex
- Other age-related and/or gender-specific support groups, parenting skills, and so on
- Therapeutic social milieu that gives a message of ability and empowerment

## Community Mental Health Centers

Community mental health centers (CMHCs) are very large agencies that provide a wide range of services within residential communities; some have inpatient services for brief hospitalization. Occupational therapists and assistants may be employed by the agencies themselves or by specific programs or services within these agencies, such as vocational rehabilitation, transitional living programs, psychosocial rehabilitation programs, and day treatment centers. Wollenberg (66) describes a program focusing on recovery and wellness and using a collaborative model in which the consumer identifies problems and works with the therapy practitioner to find solutions (wellness orograms are discussed later in this chapter).

Community mental health centers traditionally have been and continue to be dependent on public funding. Widespread development of CMHCs was spurred by the Community Mental Health Act of 1963. CMHCs were intended to provide for the treatment and rehabilitation of the seriously mentally ill within the community. Under amendments passed between 1965 and 1979, the centers were expected to provide inpatient and outpatient services, partial hospitalization, round-the-clock emergency services, and consultation as well as services to children, the elderly, and alcohol and drug users. During those years, federal funding was allotted by service categories, ensuring that a variety of services were available and that special groups such as the elderly and children received attention. The CMHCs eventually moved away from their first mission to address the broad mental health needs of the general population and now appear to resist providing services to the seriously and persistently mentally ill (60).

## Community Rehabilitation Programs

Community rehabilitation programs (CRPs) offer supportive skills training and vocational training in daytime programs (8). Patients sent to CRPs from inpatient units may have difficulty making the transition from the dependent role of inpatient to the more independent role of member of the community. Repeated rehospitalization is a frequent result. The OT or OTA can help ease the transition by analyzing and breaking down tasks, training staff, and making the expectations and demands of this new setting explicit to patients. Individualizing the program to meet needs and interests of particular clients is essential; CRPs may use a block programming model that assumes that every entering client requires exactly the same mix of program ingredients. By serving in the role of consultant, liaison, or case manager, the OT or OTA can ensure that patients receive services appropriate to their individual needs and abilities.

## Partial Hospitalization, Day Hospitals, and Day Programs

Partial hospitalization began in 1933 in the Soviet Union in response to an acute shortage of psychiatric hospital beds (51). Partial hospitalization provides a less costly alternative to inpatient treatment and a transition to community life. Rather than living day and night in a hospital, the patient resides in the community and visits the hospital to receive treatment. Day treatment allows clients to receive training in daily living skills and to develop social interaction skills while they remain in the community where they will ultimately need these skills. This approach has been found to be cost-effective as well as less-restrictive than and clinically as therapeutic as inpatient treatment (26).

The term *day hospital* is synonymous with partial hospitalization and more easily understood. Adult day care, described later in this chapter, is also a partial hospitalization program. Depending on local practices, patients may be referred to day treatment directly from inpatient settings or by therapists or outpatient centers as an alternative to hospitalization.

The goals of partial hospitalization include management of short-term problems, rehabilitation for independent living, treatment of mental disabilities, and support services (26). The staff is interdisciplinary but varies tremendously with availability of trained personnel. The roles and scope of practice of occupational therapy within a partial hospitalization program depend on the mix of professional staff. For example, while a nurse may be better trained to provide information on the uses and effects of medication, the OTA may lead a group about medication management and side effects if no nurse is available. Other roles include provision of rehabilitation groups and individual programming for independent living skills, teaching of problem-solving skills and stress management, and vocational development.

The therapeutic program within a day hospital usually consists of a mix of community meetings, small-group learning sessions, and individual case management. Community meetings encourage patients to take an active voice in deciding program policies, field trips, and other special activities and thus promote leadership and self-assertion. Small-group sessions facilitate the development of skills such as money management, basic hygiene, work habits, health and safety, nutrition and basic cooking, home management, communication, and self-expression. Patients are scheduled for groups according to need and whether they possess prerequisite skills. Groups may be run by occupational therapists or assistants, other activity therapists, social workers, or other staff.

Case management is a method of tracking each patient's progress by assigning specific staff members to be responsible for the overall program of a few patients. Thus every staff member from the psychologist to the mental health therapy aide may coordinate the treatment of one to five patients; this includes setting treatment goals and methods in collaboration with the patient, and various administrative duties such as making sure the patient has enough medication, attends medical appointments, and applies for and receives appropriate public assistance. Where permitted by law, OTAs may serve as case managers.

A typical focus for occupational therapy is vocational services. One such program described by Richert and Merryman (51) was organized around Mosey's levels of group interaction skills (see Chapter 3) and Allen's cognitive levels (see Chapter 3). The authors reported that approximately 90% of the recipients of these services were functioning at cognitive levels 4 to 6. In addition to rehabilitation groups at the various levels of group interaction skills and cognitive levels, the program provided for actual work experience within the hospital setting. Level 4 patients were found to function at the prevocational level, needing structured, concrete, well-supervised assignments. Level 5 patients were in general more capable of independent functioning, with 24% engaged in volunteer work. Volunteer work was used extensively in this program for several reasons. It met the self-esteem needs of those who previously worked at more responsible jobs, and it offered a gradual transition to paid employment. Volunteer work also safeguards the patients' benefit programs, which may terminate if too the person works too many hours of paid employment.

Another approach, reported by Coviensky and Buckley (15), was a structured activities program outside of but linked to the partial hospitalization program. The purpose was to provide a structure of work and play for clients who were too severely impaired to function in less-structured settings. The three components of the program were work, play, and milieu. The work component included volunteer work outside the program (e.g., Red Cross, nursing homes) and tasks and chores within the program (meal preparation, gardening, and so on). The recreational component included varied activities typical of normal adults: games, sports, walks, readings, and the arts. The milieu component was provided through community meetings at the start of each day, consistent expectations applied by all staff equally, and careful design of the environment to provide for both privacy and interaction.

A day program provides services in the community and may be loosely structured and collaborative in its work with clients. Some day programs are classified as continuing day treatment programs (CDTPs). Tomlinson (59) describes a day program that empowers clients by encouraging them to take charge of their own medication, determine for themselves whether and when they should attend, negotiate their own goals, and so on. Clients receive individual functional assessments, collaborate on setting goals, and participate in a milieu that provides social interaction and multiple occupational opportunities (e.g., to explore use of a computer or art supplies and to attend groups focused on exercise, social skills, medical issues, leisure, literacy). Clients, depending on diagnosis, may need compensatory or remedial treatment for cognitive deficits and impulsivity; this is particularly important in safety and communication. Many clients in day programs have severe and persistent mental illness and lack the social and verbal skills to benefit immediately from traditional verbal psychotherapy; OTs and OTAs may serve as case managers and may consult with other staff to identify areas in which a more task-based or activity-focused approach might better engage the client.

## CONSUMER-OPERATED PROGRAMS

In recent years, persons with mental illness have founded organizations and programs for their own advocacy and self-help. The *consumer movement* advocates for consumer involvement in decision making and program development. In historical terms, this is a natural outcome of consumer dissatisfaction with the stigma attached to medically based programs and the poor level of community services following deinsititutionalization.

Consumer organizations may provide a range of services, possibly including employment services, case management, crisis counseling, drop-in or self-help centers, peer counseling, financial services, consumer-run business, self-help groups, and housing projects (58). Swarbrick and Duffy (58) describe occupational therapy involvement in a consumer-operated self-help center. The self-help center provides a place for consumers to help themselves and each other through peer counseling, to socialize and enjoy leisure activities, to learn about mental health issues, and to plan and engage in advocacy and networking activities. The occupational therapist serves as a consultant and collaborator.

Rebeiro (50), a Canadian therapist, gives advice for OTs and OTAs considering partnering with consumer-operated programs and organizations, identifying specific qualities that are helpful in establishing effective relationships:

- *Advocacy.* Including advocating for individual clients, advocating for groups of clients, and teaching clients to advocate for themselves
- *Client centeredness.* Placing the needs and goals of the clients first
- *Risk taking.* Being willing to expand into uncharted territory and to give up the unequal power relationship of therapist and client
- *Establishing common ground.* Finding ways to make connections and help clients see their goals as shared ones rather than individual ones
- *Nontraditional.* Accepting the absence of the kinds of structure found in medical settings; understanding that documentation may mean keeping research notes or writing advocacy letters (rather than progress notes)
- *Redefining* professional *(being professional in a nonprofessional way).* Keeping to the values and ethics of the profession while relating on a human-to-human level.

## Psychosocial Rehabilitation: The Psychosocial Club

Psychosocial rehabilitation, which began in 1948 with the founding of Fountain House, is an environmental approach designed to improve the ability of persons with severe and persistent mental illness to maintain themselves in the community by providing support, meaningful work experience, and the opportunity to associate with others. It has been defined as "a therapeutic approach that encourages a mentally ill person to develop his or her fullest capacities through learning and environmental supports" (7). In keeping with the philosophy that people with chronic mental illness can direct their own affairs, the persons who attend psychosocial rehabilitation programs are called "members." Members participate equally with staff in running essential functions such as meals, activities, and clerical support. This multidisciplinary approach may involve professionals as well as paraprofessionals trained on the job, peer mentors (other members) and volunteers. Because of the similarity of terms, *psychosocial rehabilitation* may be confused with *psychiatric rehabilitation.* Although some overlap exists, these are separate movements that are sometimes conflated (blended or mixed together) by practitioners of psychiatric rehabilitation (65). Psychosocial rehabilitation, in its original form, has more in common with consumer-operated organizations than with the medical model or psychiatry. Box 7-5 provides the treatment focus of clubhouse settings.

Psychosocial rehabilitation focuses on the social rather than medical aspects of mental illness. Thus, although psychotropic medications and consultation with the psychiatrist may be available, these are seen as adjunctive rather than essential services. Comprehensive psychosocial rehabilitation centers, such as Fountain House in New York City, typically provide five basic categories of service: socialization programs, daily living skills counseling and training, vocational rehabilitation

BOX 7-5

**PSYCHOSOCIAL CLUBHOUSE: TREATMENT FOCUS**

- Clients called "members"
- Empowering social milieu (members and staff are equals)
- Staff as resources rather than authorities
- Peer counseling and mentoring
- Client-directed goals and plans
- Individual programming: mix of group activities and individual activities
- Basic activities of daily living: personal presentation; hygiene, grooming, and dressing; basic communication; nutrition; exercise
- Instrumental activities of daily living: communication (using telephone and phone book, basic literacy), using public transportation, clothing care, handling money, shopping on a budget, food preparation, safety, emergency responses, trash and recycling, caring for a home or apartment, stress management
- Leisure: identifying interests, locating free or inexpensive events, developing leisure habits, exercise and sports, games, holiday and social events
- Work: opportunities for exploration, supported employment, transitional placement, meaningful productive employment, volunteer and part-time jobs
- Social participation: social skills, interaction with community and family, peer interactions, sexual expression and safe sex
- Other age-related and/or gender-specific support groups, parenting skills, and so on

and transitional employment, transitional living arrangements, and case management.

Socialization programs are at the heart of psychosocial rehabilitation. By participating in organized activities and casual lounge programs, members acquire and maintain social and leisure skills and meet others with similar needs and interests. Informal activities such as playing pool or cards, watching television, reading, and chatting are typical of lounge programs. Organized activities may include cooking, sewing, home repair, crafts, and theater trips. Depending on facilities and funding, other activities such as swimming, skiing, camping, and hiking may be available. Programs that provide only socialization and not the other elements of psychosocial rehabilitation (described later) are sometimes called *psychosocial clubs* or *clubhouse programs,* but these names are also used for the more comprehensive programs as well. Membership is seen as voluntary.

Daily living skills programs may include opportunities for self-assessment, counseling with particular problems, and training in desired skills. After many years of illness, usually including several hospitalizations, the person with chronic mental illness may have no habits or routines for performing the chores and tasks the rest of us take for granted. By providing information, advice, and opportunities to learn and practice new skills, the daily living skills counselor enables members to acquire such skills as using public transportation, caring for an apartment, shopping for and caring for clothing, and shopping for and cooking food. This is a role for which the OTA is particularly well prepared.

Prevocational rehabilitation and transitional and supported employment are services aimed at helping members acquire job-related skills and obtain jobs in the community. Prevocational rehabilitation helps members become acculturated to basic work habits and the social rules typical of community work settings. Members attend work groups where they perform jobs needed by the center or contracted for by the center with businesses in the community. They are expected to behave in a businesslike, productive, work-oriented manner and are counseled about behaviors they need to change. Clerical groups, janitorial and maintenance groups, thrift shops, food service, and simple assembly line work are typical activities. After a period of successful performance in a prevocational program, members are placed in entry-level jobs in the community through the transitional employment program. These jobs give members a chance to be productive in a real-life setting; they are not usually meant to become full-time jobs but are seen rather as stepping-stones to other permanent positions. The OTA's strong background in task analysis is good preparation for preparing members for these transitional employment placements (63, 64).

Transitional living encompasses a range of supervised residential arrangements. The quarterway or halfway house or supervised community residence is usually the first step; here members can receive room and board and round-the-clock supervision from trained staff, often paraprofessional *house parents* or *residential counselors.* Usually members are expected to be out of the house during the day, working, looking for work, or attending a day treatment program. During the evening and on weekends they may be supervised as they help prepare their own meals; do the shopping, laundry, housecleaning, and other chores; and organize and carry out leisure and social activities. Supervised apartment programs are the next step; the apartments are usually leased or, less common, owned by the psychosocial rehabilitation program, which sublets them to members. Several members live together in an apartment, sharing housework and other responsibilities. Staff visit periodically to provide counseling and support and to oversee cleanliness and other basic issues.

Occupational therapists and assistants may be disturbed by the role blurring that occurs among staff in psychosocial rehabilitation settings and may fear that their professional identity will be lost as they take on responsibilities, such as case management, that are typically part of other disciplines and as members of other disciplines become leaders of activity groups. To work successfully in these settings, occupational therapists and assistants have to be comfortable taking on management and program-planning roles (32).

Psychosocial rehabilitation embodies concepts from *moral treatment* (see Chapter 1) that guided the early development of occupational therapy; for this reason, OTs and OTAs may find the model a natural fit for their skills. Although other professionals and nonprofessionals may run activity groups that meet the interests of the members, OTs and OTAs possess unique training and skills in task analysis and environmental management. The OT or OTA can, therefore, serve in a consulting role to assist others in increasing the effectiveness of their groups and interventions.

## Fairweather Lodge Program

The Fairweather Lodge (community lodge) Program was begun by Dr. George Fairweather in 1963 in California with the goals of providing emotional support, housing, and employment for members (12). This is a group model in which four to eight people who have been patients share a house and a small business. Each lodge has access to professionals, although there is no live-in staff. The members are responsible for maintaining the home and running the business.

With 90 lodges in 16 states in the United States, this is a model that OTAs may wish to participate in. The model offers a strong message of wellness and normal engagement in occupation (27).

## OTHER COMMUNITY PROGRAMS

Various community programs administered by private nonprofit agencies have been developed with the aim of helping persons with chronic mental illness survive and succeed in the community after discharge from the hospital. Programs administered by independent agencies may concentrate on just one aspect of continuing care, such as leisure and recreation or vocational rehabilitation. Others provide rehabilitative living arrangements, including supportive housing through halfway houses and supervised apartments; members gradually learn the skills, habits, and attitudes they need to live on their own in the community by practicing them under the supervision and direction of staff.

The specific job functions of occupational therapists and assistants employed by these independent agencies vary. The theoretical orientation or practice model of the facility constrains and molds the roles of staff and clients. At one extreme is the psychoanalysis-oriented program, in which the staff assumes an authoritarian (paternalistic) role, with the attendees being seen as dependent (childlike) patients; although becoming increasingly less common, such programs still exist. At the other extreme is the psychosocial clubhouse model (described more completely elsewhere in this chapter), with member clients directing the program, relying on mental health professionals as resources. Occupational therapy practitioners here may fill highly specialized roles, such as placement manager for transitional employment programs or resource manager (a title less depersonalizing to members than case manager) (63, 64).

### Program for Assertive Community Treatment

The National Alliance on Mental Illness (NAMI) describes the Program for Assertive Community Treatment (PACT) as a hospital without walls (44). PACT began in Wisconsin and has functioned continuously since 1972. Round-the-clock services are provided as needed in the community by a team of psychiatric health care providers. Services include *treatment* (e.g., medication, psychotherapy, crisis intervention), *rehabilitation* (e.g., skill teaching in areas such as daily living skills, supported employment), and *support services* (e.g., education of family members, assistance with housing and legal problems). Thus the client remains in the least restrictive environment, preferably the client's environment of choice. NAMI lists the goals of PACT as follows:

- To lessen or eliminate the debilitating symptoms of mental illness each individual client experiences and to minimize or prevent recurrent acute episodes of the illness
- To meet basic needs and enhance quality of life
- To improve functioning in adult social and employment roles
- To enhance an individual's ability to live independently in his or her own community
- To lessen the family's burden of providing care (44)

In the ideal PACT model, the clients are equal members of the team, and they direct and coordinate their own care. PACT offers an opportunity for OTs and OTAs to make a significant contribution in both rehabilitation and support services. Pitts (47) and Auerbach (6) give more detail on the roles of occupational therapists in PACT.

Some consumers have objected to PACT, arguing that it is too medically driven and that it forces them into a sick role. An alternative, called Personal Assistance in Community Existence (PACE) attempts to replace the illness model with an empowerment model, aiming to energize consumers and validate their sense of being able to recover from mental disorders (1). To work in this model, therapists must be willing to give up the idea of "mental illness" and instead focus on helping consumers who are in recovery from "severe emotional distress".

## Prevention Programs

One of the aims of the Community Mental Health Act of 1963 was the prevention of future mental health problems in disadvantaged populations and other groups at risk; despite this stated objective, these programs have not been a consistent priority for federal funding. Ironically, programs sometimes receive funding for start-up costs but are unable to obtain continued funding once they have demonstrated their effectiveness.

Prevention programs described in the occupational therapy literature include those in employee assistance programs (EAPs) (40) and several for children. One provided developmental therapy to preschool children in an early intervention program (21). Activities such as mirror play, sand and water play, various arts and crafts, puppetry, singing, and nature walks were designed to enrich the experiences of children with developmental delays. Another program, which met once a week in a local library and included participation by parents, provided enriching activities to all of the preschool and kindergarten-age children who attended, not only the developmentally delayed (10). A third provided recreational and educational opportunities for 350 children ranging from preschoolers to high school seniors (30).

Another study by Grossman (25) examined risk factors for psychopathology in preschoolers attending a Head Start program. The author suggested a role for OTs in the teaching of parenting skills to mothers under role strain owing to limited personal resources (education, money, skills, and social support). Knis-Matthews (35) designed and operated a parenting program for substance-dependent women. The program taught basic and traditional games, ways to play with children, ways to match the game or activity to the child, and how to use community resources such as parks effectively.

A major emphasis in work with the seriously mentally ill is relapse prevention. Copeland (13) provides suggestions for helping consumers develop a personal action guide to help identify uncomfortable physical sensations and emotional states that might trigger a relapse. Precin (48) gives exercises and worksheets that could be used in relapse prevention programs to identify stressors and acquire coping skills.

Additional models in prevention are in EAPs and smoking cessation. Use of cigarettes and other tobacco products is epidemic among persons with severe and persistent mental illness; besides endangering the health and welfare of the smoker, this habit pollutes the treatment environment and creates a health hazard for nonsmoking patients, staff, and family members. Affirming a positive health attitude by enabling patients to reduce, limit, or eliminate smoking can be one facet of a wellness program (discussed later in this chapter).

Working in prevention programs requires a tolerance for role blurring and an appreciation of the diffuse structure of community programs. Successful workers must be able to create their own programs, sometimes despite community indifference, and provide services flexibly, adapting to the wishes of the people in the community. This is an exciting area of practice in which the OTA could serve in a leadership role.

## Prevocational and Vocational Rehabilitation

Programs that aim to develop the ability to function in a job or joblike situation address a range of very different needs. For example, those persons who have never worked may start in prevocational programs, which help participants acquire work skills by requiring and reinforcing behavior appropriate for a work setting. Once prevocational skills (work habits and attitudes) are acquired, the client may enroll in a vocational program to prepare for a specific kind of work.

Transitional employment placement (TEP) and supported employment (SE) are designed to move clients into the work world at a pace that can be matched to their own rate of progress. TEP provides temporary part-time paid jobs; counselors and job coaches help clients adjust to jobs and may also help adjust job factors to fit individual clients. The goal is to provide a successful experience of work and to prepare the person to move into community employment as possible. Research evidence shows that SE is highly effective for persons with serious mental illness, and employment is an important factor in recover. Many models of SE exist, but the common elements are individualized placement and support from coaches and other professionals (23).

Those who are so severely disabled that they will never be able to enter competitive employment may be placed in a sheltered workshop. Sheltered workshops employ persons whose rate of production is slow; they are often paid on the basis of how much work (how many pieces) they produce. Tasks one might see in a sheltered workshop include sorting, counting, and bagging plastic tableware; assembling ball-point pens; and counting and packaging envelopes. The use of work activities is further discussed in Chapters 13 and 19.

Prevocational and vocational programs and sheltered workshops may be found in both inpatient and outpatient settings and as independent community programs. Often these programs are staffed by paraprofessionals and by certified rehabilitation counselors (CRCs). Occupational therapists and assistants may administer such programs or serve as consultants or group leaders. The ability to analyze, grade, and adapt activities to enable performance is an essential skill.

## HOME HEALTH CARE

Home health care is a rapidly developing segment of the health care market because government and private insurance programs limit inpatient stays. Once discharged, people with chronic or debilitating illnesses prefer to receive services in their homes rather than travel to health care centers. Although most of those receiving home health services have disabilities that are primarily physical, secondary psychiatric disabilities are quite common, especially when the first diagnosis is neurological. It is sad that occupational therapists with a physical rehabilitation orientation may fail to document psychosocial services provided in the home (36). Without documentation, such services are not recognized or reimbursed.

The success of Supportive Care, an independent home health business founded by Susan Maertz (39), shows that supportive home care for elderly persons suffering from decreased mental abilities is viable and desired. The OT assistant may provide memory aids; training in coping mechanisms and crisis management; and supervision of hygiene, grooming, and nutrition.

Another model program, in Portland, Oregon (31), used two occupational therapists on a team with four nurses to provide mental health services in the home. Most of the clients served by this program were found on evaluation to be functioning at Allen cognitive level 4. Level 4 clients need assistance to transfer skills from one environment (hospital) to another (home) and to solve routine problems and thus can benefit from OT intervention.

Psychiatric home care provides a natural environment for intervention and involves the client and family as coequals with therapy professionals (Box 7-6). The client's ability to fit into the home and community is the ultimate test of functional outcomes (22).

BOX 7-6

**PSYCHIATRIC HOME CARE: TREATMENT FOCUS**

- Client-directed goals and plans
- Naturally occurring activities (e.g., unloading groceries, opening the mail) in the customary environment
- Intervention and education as needed
  - Basic activities of daily living: hygiene, grooming, and dressing; nutrition; relapse prevention; safe sex and health-related information
  - Instrumental activities of daily living: communication (using telephone and phone book, basic literacy), using public transportation, clothing care, handling money, shopping on a budget, food preparation, safety, emergency responses, trash and recycling, caring for a home or apartment, stress management
  - Leisure: identifying interests, locating free or inexpensive events, developing leisure habits, exercise and sports, games, holiday and social events
- Social participation: social skills, interaction with community and family, peer interactions, sexual expression
- Education of family and caregivers about the person's illness, medications, and so on

## COMMUNITY RESIDENCES

Community residences constitute a broad category that includes all of the places other than the family home where a person with mental illness may live in the community. *Group homes* are places where residents live together in the community, with varying levels of supervision from staff. Sometimes each resident has his or her own room and bathroom; in other facilities residents may have their own bedrooms but share all other living areas. Some group homes have live-in managers or house parents, and many provide other services through their affiliation with hospitals or CMHCs. *Board and care homes* or *proprietary homes* are a specific kind of for-profit group home; residents sleep in the facility and eat all meals there, but other services may not be available. A survey of board and care homes found that the smaller homes provided more activities, more community excursions, and more opportunities for social productivity than did larger homes (43).

Persons with severe and persistent mental illness who live in large cities are sometimes housed in *single-room occupancy hotels* (SROs) or in welfare hotels or shelters for the homeless; these settings are typically bleak and often very dangerous. And with the continuing housing shortage and destruction of older housing to make room for new development, many former patients are now homeless. Working with the homeless mentally ill on the streets or in shelters is discussed in Chapter 9.

Some community residences are designed to expose the resident to a natural living experience and to provide opportunities to acquire and practice independent living skills. A halfway house is a transitional residence, not a permanent home. It is designed for people with disabilities who are not yet ready to live in the community but who do not need to be confined to an institution. Halfway houses are often associated with hospitals, and some are on hospital grounds, but many others are freestanding or associated with community mental health agencies. The overall program in a halfway house aims to promote independence in the residents. Two very different approaches to this are nurturing and high expectations (20). The nurturing approach sees the halfway house as an intermediate location for someone who is still quite ill and therefore incapable of much responsibility; in this approach the staff runs the house. In the high-expectations approach residents are expected to manage the house and to deal with pressures and responsibilities.

Friedlob and colleagues (20) described a halfway house, staffed by two occupational therapists in California, for veterans with neuropsychiatric disorders. The program design provided three segments of treatment. The first focused on nutrition and interpersonal and housekeeping skills. The second aimed to promote independence, so the focus shifted to vocational skills and community resources. The third segment provided for ongoing supervision of residents as they semi-independently pursued their individual daily routines, which might include school, work, and community recreation. Graduates of the program were invited back once a month to share experiences and get support from fellow graduates and staff. Halfway houses and supervised apartments are discussed again later in this chapter.

Occupational therapists and assistants working in community residences may provide services ranging from recreational, leisure, and socialization activities to training in independent daily living skills and case management.

### Supportive Housing

Supportive housing (known in Britain as supported housing) is an umbrella name for programs that provide support so that persons with disabilities can reside in the community. The housing units themselves are in SROs, single family homes, group apartments, or other. The aim is to provide housing that is mainstream, located within community residential neighborhoods rather than segregated into marginal areas. Government grants assist in covering the costs of the supports, which may include reduced rents or subsidized housing vouchers, on-site drop-in centers, and professional guidance and training in skills needed to live in the community. Nolan and Swarbrick (45) developed a supportive housing home management program to train persons with mental illness in house cleaning and care, safety, repairs, decorating, and use of community resources. They identify common obstacles to success in supportive housing. Working with clients in these settings can be rewarding but requires creativity, persistence, and patience.

### Assisted Living and Residential Care Homes

Assisted living is a special sort of supportive housing designed for those who need help with activities of daily living, such as dressing and bathing, but who do not require skilled nursing in a 24-hour setting. The primary population for assisted living is older adults with physical and or cognitive impairments. The largest assisted living environments have round-the-clock staffing and on-site nursing. Most assisted living residents reside in large buildings (or groups of buildings on a single campus) with a hotel or apartment atmosphere. A residential care home (RCF) serves five to nine individuals and is a smaller version. Even smaller is the adult family home (AFH), which serves four or fewer persons.

## SETTINGS FOR CHILDREN AND ADOLESCENTS

Children with mental health problems are sometimes hospitalized, but the aim is to keep them with their families and in the community. The three typical settings in which the OTA may meet them are home, school, and camp.

Schools are oriented to providing education to large numbers of children. The child with a psychiatric problem will have an individualized education program (IEP), like other children designated as in need of special services. The child will be seen either in the classroom *(push in model)* or in a separate therapy area *(pull out model)*. Goals may be educational (such as improving handwriting or note-taking skills) or cognitive (such as improving focus, attention, organization). Additional goals could address peer group relationships and improving skills for identifying feelings and managing emotional distress. Beck et al. (9) in a study of 373 school-based therapists found confusion about appropriate OT roles and gave specific suggestions for improving psychosocial services.

In the home setting, the family and the culture affect the services provided by occupational therapy. Being observant and asking questions with a sense of curiosity and respect can help the OT or OTA appreciate the unique, rich, complex home environment. The focus of intervention may be homework, chores, play, or other.

Summer camp provides an exciting context for occupational therapy intervention because it represents a vacation from the routines of the school year and an opportunity for the child to explore and reinvent himself or herself. Florey (19) describes camp as a place for transformations, where new experiences and challenges create the possibility of a new sense of self.

Many excellent pediatric reference texts exist for occupational therapy and the reader is encouraged to consult these if working with children.

## ENVIRONMENTAL CONCEPTS

The relationship between the organism and its environment fascinates scholars in the life sciences and social sciences. Basic questions of evolution and development and health and disease may be answered in part by environmental influences. What is the effect of the environment on the human engaged in occupation?

### Concepts from Occupational Therapy

The model of human occupation and other occupational therapy practice models acknowledge that all human activity arises from the human being's basic urge to explore and master the environment. Contexts of intervention and service are different from the natural and manmade environments in which most people spend their time and hence have different effects on the activity behaviors of the people who inhabit them. Before we explore these effects, it is important to review some of the basic concepts of person–environment interaction from the model of human occupation.

All occupational behavior depends on environmental interaction. The person must be able affect the environment. In general, the more complexity and novelty in the environment, the greater the person's urge to explore it. However, if there are too many new, different, and complicated things in the environment, the person may feel overwhelmed and become unable to act purposefully. Dunning (17) identified three features of the environment that affect social and occupational behavior: space, people, and tasks. *Space* includes the size and kind of space, the objects within it, and how they are arranged. *People* includes not only the number of persons but also the roles they fill and their expectations of each other. *Tasks* are defined by objects in the environment that compel certain task behaviors (e.g., a workbench versus a card table) and by social pressures. Through these three features, environments communicate expectations for occupational behavior.

Inpatient settings are remarkably dull compared with typical home, work, and leisure settings. The space typically has fewer interesting objects in it; because of safety precautions, the setting may seem bare. Curtains, carpets, and stuffed furniture may be absent, which creates an atmosphere more like an airport lounge in an underdeveloped nation than any room in an American home. Patients or residents may be prohibited from placing decorations on the walls. The lighting is likely to come from fluorescent ceiling fixtures rather than incandescent floor and table lamps. Overall, the space may feel barren, sterile, and somewhat depressing—even to staff members.

Although there are usually a lot of people around, many of these are staff. It is clear to everyone that the staff tends to perform almost all of the necessary tasks in the setting, including preparing and serving meals, caring for laundry and housekeeping, and preparing and cleaning up after activities. Patients or residents may be involved to a limited extent in any or all of these tasks, but usually under the supervision of staff.

The environmental characteristics of inpatient settings communicate an expectation that patients need to do very little and that they probably will not be able to do even that very well. Many outpatient settings also fail to communicate an expectation that the consumer perform at anything like a normal level.

To help the person with mental illness develop and maintain the skills and behaviors needed to function independently, the OTA may alter some features of the context. Furniture can be rearranged, folding screens placed to eliminate distractions, and walls painted or wall coverings added to the extent permitted. Clients (or consumers or members) should participate in these decisions and do the work when practical. The OT or OTA can control the effect of people in the environment by modifying the role of group leader and the roles of volunteers and students in groups. The less the staff does, the more consumers will do themselves. Making tasks available to consumers often requires working with administrators to change policies; there is no reason consumers should not be allowed or required to do their own laundry, but administrators may feel that this would be inconvenient or inefficient or interfere with ward routine.

Seeing consumers in their homes presents different opportunities to apply environmental concepts. A person's home or any environment (e.g., office) that he or she creates for the self communicates the person's interests and habits to the careful observer. The objects present, the care given to different rooms or parts of rooms, the age of the furnishings and the amount of use they seem to have received, all indicate their relative importance to the individual. For example, Levine (38) describes a home in which the furniture in all of the rooms but the kitchen was 40 years old and quite worn, but the kitchen was freshly painted and had new appliances. Levine inferred that the kitchen was the center of the family's activities.

Usually a person has more control of the environment at home than in the hospital; this increases the sense of personal causation. The therapist is the guest and relinquishes control naturally to the consumer, supporting the person's motivation to control and master the environment.

Another situation that may call for a different application of environmental concepts occurs when the consumer travels with the OTA out into the community. Observing how the person reacts to the different stimulation presented by shops, bus stops, and public agencies may reveal hitherto unsuspected skills and may help the OTA identify what kinds of environmental changes will facilitate independent behaviors.

In summary, demands and opportunities in the environment have a profound effect on human occupational behavior. Inpatient units and many outpatient programs convey only limited expectations for patients to participate and be competent in daily life tasks and occupational roles; OTs and OTAs may increase performance expectations for persons with mental illness by selectively altering features of the environment. Working with consumers in their homes or in various community environments may provide information about which environmental features best facilitate independent functioning for a particular person.

## Many Environments, Many Roles: The Consumer's Perspective

Considering the many environments through which consumers move, it is not surprising that they acquire strategies and roles particular to each. For example, as "patient" in an inpatient setting, the person is expected to be dependent and compliant, to accept a schedule set by others, to take medications, and to perform hygiene tasks on demand. The patient may use coping strategies such as isolation, triangulation (pitting staff members against each other), and overcompliance to maintain a sense of self-direction within a controlling environment.

Once discharged to home, the same person as "family member" is expected to be the spouse, child, sibling, or parent, with all of the history and attendant feelings, modified somewhat by an expectation that the person is not quite well. Many behaviors that appear dysfunctional, such as getting a spouse to make excuses for the nonperformance of the sick person to reduce demands by others, may instead be survival strategies.

As "inmate" in a correctional facility, the same person might be expected to stand at attention for guards, to respond quickly and accurately to directives from persons in authority, and to accede to the bullying of more powerful inmates; in addition, the person must maintain an attitude of alertness and vigilance to avoid victimization. The mentally ill prisoner may forge alliances with stronger inmates, curry favor with guards, or submit to sexual abuse to avoid painful experiences.

Living homeless on the street or in a shelter exposes the person to the risk of violence (including rape), disease (such as HIV infection), theft, malnutrition, hypothermia, and so on. Survival strategies include wearing multiple layers of clothing (to stay warm, to guard one's belongings, and to prevent rape), carrying weapons, eating from bulk trash containers and trash barrels, and sleeping in storm sewers. Begging, busking (playing a musical instrument or singing), and street preaching are customary daily activities for some people living on the street.

These are only a few of the environments in which patients and consumers live and survive. The roles and strategies they adopt are specialized to these environments. Because cognitive deficits often accompany severe and persistent mental illness, clients may not recognize which behaviors or roles pertain to a particular environment or may have difficulty responding to unfamiliar environmental demands, such as may occur in a progressive treatment environment (e.g., demands to set their own goals, to dress and behave in ways that are closer to the social norm). As rehabilitation specialists, we must be sensitive to the histories of our patients/clients and appreciate their considerable skills and life experience. When we engage them in treatment and ask them to function in community programs and housing, we are at the same time asking them to abandon roles that have served them well. Listening carefully to the person's experiences and dreams should be the starting point for setting small mutual goals toward greater community integration.

## Promoting Change at Many Levels

McColl (42) delineates three levels of environmental intervention: the microenvironment, the mesoenvironment, and the macroenvironment. The *microenvironment* is at the client-centered level, the simple person–environment interactions already described; this is the level at which most occupational therapy intervention occurs. The *mesoenvironment* is at the community level and includes community barriers to employment, housing, transportation, and accessibility; this is the level at which consultants and program developers can improve occupational functioning conditions for clients. The *macroenvironment* occurs

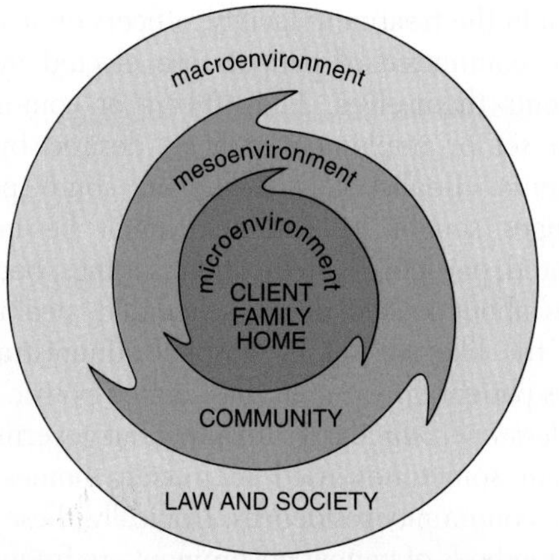


**Figure 7-2. Three levels of environment.** (Data from McColl MA. What do we need to know to practice occupational therapy in the community? Am J Occup Ther 1998;52:11–18.)

at the political and social level, at which consumer advocates and their professional supporters have struggled for social policy changes, such as the Americans with Disabilities Act (ADA).

Figure 7-2 demonstrates the intermeshed nature of these three levels of environmental analysis. Appreciation for and the ability to act at all three levels is essential for OTs and OTAs working in the community. Table 7-1 gives examples of interventions. Note that the creation of opportunities at the macro level (such as legislated requirements for fair housing and equal payment or parity for mental health services) will provide more freedom at the meso level (such as to develop local housing or employment sites) and at the micro level (such as for the individual client to obtain a specific job or housing placement).

Developing community resources at a program level (e.g., for housing or employment) and acting politically to influence policy development are new roles for the OTA. These roles can promote large-scale change and benefit large numbers of persons with severe and persistent mental illness. Many occupational therapy assistant students enter college with extraordinary life experience and job histories that prepare them well to practice at this level. Kluge, a certified occupational therapy assistant (COTA) and a supervisor of several mental health programs in Wisconsin, describes her work over the years as "everything from finding a site for the homes, notifying neighbors, forming advisory committees, rehabilitating and furbishing the homes, hiring, training and

**TABLE 7-1 FOCUS AND EXAMPLES OF OCCUPATIONAL THERAPY AT THREE LEVELS OF ENVIRONMENT**

| LEVEL OF INTERVENTION | FOCUS | EXAMPLES |
|---|---|---|
| Microenvironment | Client and family | Teach compensatory techniques<br>Develop skills<br>Train caregiver |
| Mesoenvironment | Community | Solicit supported, transitional employment<br>Develop housing resources |
| Macroenvironment | Law and society | Assist and support consumers seeking policy changes<br>Lobby legislators for parity and access<br>Teach the public about the needs of persons with severe and persistent mental illness |

Data from McColl MA. What do we need to know to practice occupational therapy in the community? Am J Occup Ther 1998;52:11–18.

supervising staff, students and volunteers, and ensuring compliance with all codes and ordinances" ( (33, p. 33).

## ADDITIONAL THEORIES AND PRACTICE MODELS

Various treatment settings base their therapeutic efforts on various theories. Although the major theories used in the United States today were described in Chapter 2 and the common practice models for psychiatric occupational therapy were presented in Chapters 3 and 4, there are many other theories and practice models that the OTA may encounter on the job; this section briefly describes some of them.

### Milieu Therapy

*Milieu therapy* and a related practice model called the *therapeutic community* are based on the assumption that the treatment unit or day treatment center is a social system. Like other social systems, it has rules, hierarchies, and roles that must be filled if the system is to function. Milieu therapy attempts to give patients as much responsibility as they can possibly handle and to enable them to take charge of their own decisions and day-to-day environment. Because milieu therapy shifts responsibility for decision making to patients, staff who are used to having more authority have to adjust their expectations and behavior (5).

Community meetings and patient government are methods used in milieu therapy. *Community meetings* are scheduled gatherings of all staff and patients that may occur once a week or more frequently. Recent events affecting the patients or staff and plans for the future are typical topics for discussion; disagreements between patients or between patients and staff are often aired and sometimes resolved at these meetings.

*Patient government* is a method for giving patients more control over conditions that affect them in the treatment facility; officers or an executive committee of patients are elected by the patients themselves. The officers or committee then set or implement policies desired by the patients. Realistically, however, some policy changes sought by patients cannot be implemented, particularly in inpatient settings, because rules about locked doors, scheduled mealtimes, and the like are set by hospital administration. Thus patient government has limited power.

*Resident council* is a similar patient government system sometimes used in nursing homes and large community residences. Ironically, these various methods of patient government are frequently included in inpatient units whose overall approach is clearly medical and authoritarian and therefore incompatible with self-determination by patients; this is the very opposite of milieu therapy and is probably confusing for everyone concerned.

The underlying philosophy of milieu therapy holds that each person in the community is capable of contributing in some way to general community life. Therefore, patients are assigned housekeeping and other tasks wherever possible; again, because of bureaucratic and legal restrictions on unpaid labor, it is not possible to enforce a consistent milieu in inpatient settings. The psychosocial rehabilitation approach previously is based on milieu therapy concepts and demonstrates that these concepts are workable in community settings.

### Family Therapy

Family therapy is based on the idea that the patient's illness is intimately connected to family relationships. The patient's behavior is seen as an expression of demands and opportunities presented by the family. According to family therapy theories, any approach that attempts to treat the patient's illness without treating the family is misguided and doomed to failure.

Various theories give various explanations of the relationship between the patient's illness and the family system. At one extreme, some theories hold that the patient's illness is not his or her own but rather the symptom of a sick family; the family uses the patient as a safety valve to express its unconscious conflicts and psychopathology. This extreme view is much in disfavor today. Other theories take the view that regardless of causation, the patient's illness creates such a strain on other family members that they need support and guidance to learn to maintain their own self-esteem and integrity while responding effectively to the patient. All family therapy approaches view the patient and the family as an interactive social system; what happens to one family member reverberates and affects all of the others. The family and the patient are treated together, sometimes by two therapists.

Few occupational therapists practicing in mental health use family therapy as their major practice model, yet most acknowledge and support family therapy concepts. For example, when helping a consumer acquire independent daily living skills, the therapist might (with permission from the consumer) talk with the family about what the person is able to do independently; otherwise the family may continue to do things for the person that the person should be doing. Similarly, families overcome with grief, guilt, and frustration about the disabilities of the patient may benefit from objective advice and information provided by knowledgeable mental health professionals. Family caregivers deserve special attention and support and benefit from interventions designed for their needs (see Chapter 9).

When occupational therapists practice in a setting in which family therapy is the prevailing model, they may find that the administrators view certain methods used in occupational therapy as incompatible with the overall philosophy of the setting. Sensory integration may be considered too "medical," for example. In some family therapy programs with a strongly psychoanalytic orientation, efforts by OTs and OTAs to increase the independence and skills of the identified patient may be viewed as undermining the family system.

## Stress Management

Defined medically, stress is a condition that affects humans and other biological organisms when equilibrium is disrupted by outside forces. These outside forces are called *stressors*. A *psychosocial stressor* is an event or situation that the patient or client experiences as emotionally or psychologically stressful—for instance, learning that one's electricity is about to be turned off for nonpayment of bills. Open systems theories, of which the model of human occupation is one example, assume that biological organisms require a certain amount of stimulation from stressors to develop and function. When the demands from stressors are too great, however, the organism can be overwhelmed and unable to function.

Stress management is an educational approach that teaches people about stressors and the effects of stress and trains them in techniques for controlling psychological and emotional stress. Most stress management programs begin with an assessment of recent psychosocial stressors and reactions to them; positive events (e.g., getting married or getting a promotion) as well as negative ones can be stressors. Participants are asked how they react to each stressor; specific behaviors, such as overeating or sleeping too much, are identified. Depending on the participant's needs as identified through evaluation, the individual is instructed in skills and coping techniques. Some of these include meditation, relaxation exercises, yoga, exercise, assertiveness training, relaxation, and time management. Participants may attend groups in which they learn to explore and share feelings about stressful life events. The specific value of occupational therapy in stress management programs is its unique ability to assess dysfunctional patterns of occupational behavior and restore more natural and adaptive patterns through purposeful activities. Cognitive behavioral approaches that teach how to look at events more positively seem helpful (37).

Some stress management programs are administered by occupational therapists or are co-directed by them with professionals from other disciplines. One model provides for continuity between the hospital and the community to ensure transfer of skills (14). Often OTs and OTAs use stress management techniques in combination with other treatment methods—for example, training in independent daily living skills can be enhanced when participants are taught to be reasonably assertive with shopkeepers and to use relaxation techniques to reduce stress when frustrating things happen. Stein and Cutler (56) describe a stress management program and provide worksheets and protocols. Precin (48) also created worksheets that address stress management.

## Crisis Intervention

Crisis intervention is a practice model that aims to help people cope in the midst of crisis. The client can walk in during clinic hours and receive advice, support, and resources to solve the immediate problem. People in crisis tend to be overwhelmed by feelings and sometimes are confused, passive, and unable to act. They may abandon their usual activities and develop maladaptive behaviors such as denying reality, complaining rather than acting, or giving up entirely.

Rosenfeld (54) developed an approach using nuclear tasks and a cognitive-behavioral model to help people in crisis; his approach includes the steps shown in Box 7-7. This model seeks to restore

**BOX 7-7**

### THE NUCLEAR TASK APPROACH TO CRISIS INTERVENTION

**To identify nuclear tasks through evaluation**

- Use expressive activities when indicated to promote expression of affect.
- Seek evidence of task failures and functional deficits that contribute to the crisis.
- Identify uncompleted tasks that disturb and/or motivate the client. Assess the symbolic and realistic value of these tasks for resolving the crisis.
- Assess the client's functional resources. Identify patterns of attribution and activity that tend to promote or diminish effective coping responses.

**To promote performance of nuclear tasks in treatment**

- Help the client see and accept the challenge inherent in the crisis.
- Promote reasonable attributions to counteract the client's negative, harsh, and hopeless self-estimates.
- Undertake graded remotivating activities designed to yield rapid success in affecting uncompleted task elements of the crisis.
- Teach new functional skills and coping behaviors necessary to surmount the crisis.
- Discuss and implement activities that test or signify progress toward recovery.
- Plan daily activity routines that promote a sense of order, control, and certainty, thereby creating islands of comfort and enjoyment in the client's sea of troubles.

Reprinted with permission from Rosenfeld MS. Crisis intervention: The nuclear task approach. Am J Occup Ther 1984;38:382–385.

normal occupational behavior patterns by engaging the client in nuclear tasks. A *nuclear task* is a purposeful activity that requires the person in crisis to marshal his or her resources and get on with life. Rosenfeld identified three types of nuclear task: remotivating tasks, skills and coping tasks, and symbolic tasks. *Remotivating tasks* help the person get started doing something; doing something lets the person move beyond feeling helpless. An example is a woman cleaning out a closet even though she is preoccupied about having lost her job. *Skills and coping tasks* help the person acquire the skills needed to resolve or work on the crisis—for instance, the woman may need to practice interviewing skills or work on her wardrobe and personal presentation before looking for another job. *Symbolic tasks* are activities, usually chosen by the person, that show resolution of the crisis—for example, a couple whose infant died suddenly might, after some time, decide to have a party and include friends who have young children.

Whereas the nuclear task approach is an occupational therapy practice model, other crisis intervention methods are used by other mental health professionals in psychiatric emergency rooms, in hospitals and CMHCs, in satellite and aftercare clinics, and in some home health programs and community agencies. A crisis hotline is one example that may be familiar.

### Wellness Model

Swarbrick (57) developed a psychoeducational wellness model to promote self-management of illness and a positive attitude toward health among persons with mental illness. Clients learn self-management skills in groups. The presentation of information is designed to compensate for cognitive deficits; environmental distractors are controlled. Clients direct the selection of content, ensuring relevance and increasing participation. Specific topics include smoking cessation, AIDS education, substance-abuse awareness, nutrition, dealing with stress, and dealing with boredom. Other wellness models include aromatherapy, gentle yoga, addictions counseling, reiki, and tai chi (41).

## SUMMARY

Occupational therapists and assistants may be employed in many kinds of settings to provide services to persons with mental health problems. Each setting has its own philosophy, and several alternative practice models that might be used in these settings have been discussed. Each setting presents opportunities and demands that affect both staff and patients/consumers and that shape the roles of everyone involved. Recipients of services may be identified as patients, clients, residents, members, inmates, survivors or consumers, with each name designating a different role and level of responsibility for one's own health care. Correspondingly, the role of the helping professional shifts from total direction of patient care to availability as a resource and skilled adviser.

Recognizing that no setting is ideal and that some are more challenging than others, occupational therapists and assistants can make their service contexts more effective by applying concepts of occupation and occupational engagement. Knowledge about how humans interact with their environments can be used to understand the effects of each type of setting on clients and staff. By manipulating some of the variables known to affect human performance, such as environmental demands and availability of interesting objects, OTs and OTAs can facilitate exploratory behavior and competence in consumers, empowering greater independence and confidence.

## REVIEW QUESTIONS AND ACTIVITIES

1. Make a list of the settings described in this chapter, and write a brief definition or description for each.
2. Why do the roles for the OT and OTA change in the different settings? What features of the settings or what factors in the environment make different roles possible or necessary? (*Hint:* consider roles of other people.)
3. Write a short explanation of the differences between *care, intervention, service,* and *treatment.*
4. What message or behavioral expectation does each type of context send? How is the service recipient expected to behave in each type of context?
5. What are the expectations for staff in each type of context?
6. If your family member had a serious mental disorder, what kind of context would you think best? Why?
7. How would the role of the OT or OTA in a consumer-operated organization differ from the role in a psychiatric or medical setting?
8. What would the OTA be doing (job tasks) in a setting that uses milieu therapy? Family therapy? Psychosocial rehabilitation? Discuss each separately.

## REFERENCES


1. Ahern L, Fisher D. An alternative to PACT: Recovery at your own PACE. Am Occup Ther Assoc Ment Health Special Sect Q Newslett 2001;24(4):3–4.
2. American Occupational Therapy Association. Facts about occupational therapy in acute psychiatric admissions [Fact Sheet]. Rockville, MD: AOTA, 1992.
3. American Occupational Therapy Association. Occupational therapy practice framework: Domain and process. Am J Occup Ther 2002;56:609–639.
4. Anthony W, Cohen M, Farkas M. Psychiatric Rehabilitation. Boston: Center for Psychiatric Rehabilitation, Boston University Sargent College of Health Professions, 1990.
5. Appelbaum AH, Munich RL. Reinventing moral treatment: The effects upon patients and staff members of a program of psychosocial rehabilitation. Occup Ther Ment Health 1989;9(3):69–86.
6. Auerbach E. An occupational therapist in an assertive community treatment program. Am Occup Ther Assoc Ment Health Special Sect Q Newslett 2002;25(1):1–2.
7. Bachrach, LL. Psychosocial rehabilitation and psychiatry: What are the boundaries? Can J Psychiatry 1996;41: 28–35.
8. Baxley S. Options for community practice: The Springfield Hospital model. Am Occup Ther Assoc Ment Health Special Sect Q Newslett 1994;17(1):3–5.
9. Beck AJ, Barnes KJ, Vogel KA, Grice KO. The dilemma of psychosocial occupational therapy in public schools: The therapists' perception. Occup Ther Ment Health 2006; 22(1):1–17.
10. Benzing P, Strickland R. Occupational therapy in a community-based prevention program. Occup Ther Ment Health 1983;3(1):15–30.
11. Butterfield F. Profits at a juvenile prison come with a chilling cost. New York Times, July 7, 1998, A1, A14.
12. The Coalition for Community Living. Fairweather Lodge—Frequently Asked Questions. Available at: theccl.org/Fairweather.htm. Accessed Feb 2007.
13. Copeland ME. Wellness recovery action plan: A system for monitoring, reducing and eliminating uncomfortable dangerous physical symptoms and emotional feelings. Occup Ther Ment Health 2000;17(3–4):127–150.
14. Courtney C, Escobedo B. A stress management program: Impatient to outpatient continuity. Am J Occup Ther 1990;44:306–310.
15. Coviensky M, Buckley VC. Day activities programming: Serving the severely impaired chronic client. Occup Ther Ment Health 1986;6(2):21–30.
16. De las Heras CG, Dion GL, Walsh D. Application of rehabilitation models in a state psychiatric hospital. Occup Ther Ment Health 1993;12(3):1–32.
17. Dunning H. Environmental occupational therapy. Occup Ther 1972;26:292–298.
18. Eggers M, Sciulli J, Gaguzis K, Munoz JP. Enrichment through occupation: The Allegheny County jail project. Am Occup Ther Assoc Ment Health Special Sect Q Newslett 2003;26(2):1–4.
19. Florey LL. Transformations in a summer camp: The role of occupations. Am Occup Ther Assoc Ment Health Special Sect Q Newslett 1999;22(3):2–4.
20. Friedlob SA, Janis GA, Deets-Aron C. A hospital-connected halfway house program for individuals with long-term neuropsychiatric disabilities. Am J Occup Ther 1986;40:271–277.
21. George NM, Braun BA, Walker JM. A prevention and early intervention mental health program for disadvantaged pre-school children. Am J Occup Ther 1982; 36:99–106.
22. Glantz CH, Richman N. OTR-COTA collaboration in home health: Roles and supervisory issues. Am J Occup Ther 1997;51:446–452.
23. Gray K. Evidenced-based employment services for persons with serious mental illness. Am Occup Ther Assoc Ment Health Special Sect Q Newslett 2005;28(3):1–2.
24. Grinfeld MJ. Report focuses on jailed mentally ill. Psychiatric Times, July 1993, 1–3.
25. Grossman J. A prevention model for occupational therapy. Am J Occup Ther 1991;45:33–41.
26. Gusich RL, Silverman AL. Basava day clinic: The model of human occupation as applied to psychiatric day hospitalization. Occup Ther Ment Health 1991;11(2–3): 113–127.
27. Haertl K, Minato M. Daily occupations of persons with mental illness: Themes from Japan and America. Occup Ther Ment Health 2006;22(1):19–32.
28. Hays C, Baxley S. The roles of the state psychiatric hospital and the occupational therapy practitioner. Am Occup Ther Assoc Ment Health Special Sect Q Newslett 1998; 21(1):3–4.
29. Hemphill BJ, Werner PC. Deinstitutionalization: A role for occupational therapy in the state hospital. Occup Ther Ment Health 1990;10(2):85–99.
30. Jaffe E. The role of the occupational therapist as a community consultant: Primary prevention in mental health programming. Occup Ther Ment Health 1980;1(2):47–62.
31. Javernick JA. Delivering psych services in the home: Do OTs have a role [Focus: Home Care]? OT Week, Sept 3, 1992, 6:14–15.
32. Javernick JA. OTs expand their horizons at Way Station [Focus: Mental Health]. OT Week, Sept 15, 1992, 6:14–15.
33. Kluge N. Breaking the glass ceiling: How an OTA degree aided this multi-program supervisor. Adv Occup Ther Practice, June 19, 1998,22–23.

34. Klugheit M. An appreciation for the role of occupational therapy in community mental health treatment. Am Occup Ther Assoc Ment Health Special Sect Q Newslett 1994;17(1):1–3.
35. Knis-Matthews L. A parenting program for women who are substance dependent. Am Occup Ther Assoc Ment Health Special Sect Q Newslett 2003;26(1):1–4.
36. Kunstaetter D. Occupational therapy treatment in home health care. Am J Occup Ther 1988;42:513–519.
37. Lee H, Tan H, Ma H, et al. Effectiveness of a work-related stress management program in patients with chronic schizophrenia. Am J Occup Ther 2006; 60:435–441.
38. Levine R. The cultural aspects of home delivery. Am J Occup Ther 1984;38:734–735.
39. Maertz S. COTA share. Occup Ther Newspaper 1984;38(4):7.
40. Maynard M. Health promotion through employee assistance programs: A role for occupational therapists. Am J Occup Ther 1986;40:771–776.
41. McClintock AM. An OT's venture into wellness practice. Am Occup Ther Assoc Ment Health Special Sect Q Newslett 2001;24(2):1–3.
42. McColl MA. What do we need to know to practice occupational therapy in the community? Am J Occup Ther 1998;52:11–18.
43. Nagy MP, Fisher GA, Tessler RC. Effects of facility characteristics on the social adjustment of mentally ill residents of board-and-care homes. Hosp Comm Psychiatry 1988;39:1281–1285.
44. National Alliance for the Mentally Ill. Assertive Community Treatment (ACT). Available at http://www.nami.org/Template.cfm?Section=ACT-TA_Center Accessed September 30, 2007.
45. Nolan C, Swarbrick P. Supportive housing occupational therapy home management program. Am Occup Ther Assoc Ment Health Special Sect Q Newslett 2002; 25(2):1–3.
46. Peloquin SM. The development of an occupational therapy interview/therapy set procedure. Am J Occup Ther 1983;37:457–461.
47. Pitts DB. Assertive community treatment—A brief introduction. Am Occup Ther Assoc Ment Health Special Sect Q Newslett 2001; 24(4):1–2.
48. Precin P. Living Skills Recovery Workbook. Boston MA: Butterworth Heinemann, 1999.
49. Provident IM, Joyce-Gaguzis K. Creating an occupational therapy level II fieldwork experience in a county jail setting. Am J Occup Ther 2005;59:101–106.
50. Rebiero KL. Partnerships for participation in occupation. Am Occup Ther Assoc Ment Health Special Sect Q Newslett 2002;25(3):1–3.
51. Richert GZ, Merryman MB. The vocational continuum: A model for providing vocational services in a partial hospitalization program. Occup Ther Ment Health 1987; 7(3):1–20.
52. Rider BB, Gramblin JT. An activities approach to occupational therapy in a short-term acute mental health unit. Am Occup Ther Assoc Ment Health Special Sect Q Newslett 1980;3(4):1–3.
53. Robinson AM, Avallone J. Occupational therapy in acute inpatient psychiatry: An activities health approach. Am J Occup Ther 1990;44:809–814.
54. Rosenfeld MS. Crisis intervention: The nuclear task approach. Am J Occup Ther 1984;38:382–385.
55. Schindler VP. Occupational therapy in forensic psychiatry: Role development and schizophrenia. Occup Ther Ment Health 2005;20(3–4):1–171.
56. Stein F, Cutler SK. Psychosocial Occupational Therapy: A Holistic Approach. San Diego, CA: Singular, 1998.
57. Swarbrick P. Wellness model for clients. Am Occup Ther Assoc Ment Health Special Sect Q Newslett 1997;20(1): 1–4.
58. Swarbrick P, Duffy M. Consumer-operated organization and programs: A role for occupational therapy practitioners. Am Occup Ther Assoc Ment Health Special Sect Q Newslett 2000;23(1):1–4.
59. Tomlinson J. The dimensions of occupational therapy in day programs. Am Occup Ther Assoc Ment Health Special Sect Q Newslett 1994;17(1):56.
60. Torrey EF. Out of the Shadows: Confronting America's Mental Illness Crisis. New York: Wiley, 1997.
61. Turner IM. The healing power of respect: A personal journey. Occup Ther Ment Health 1989;9(1):17–32.
62. University of Southern California Human Subjects Protection Program (HSPP: Policies and Procedures, May 2007. Available at: http://www.usc.edu/admin/provost/oprs/private/docs/oprs/pnp/Policies_and_Procedures_Final.pdf Accessed September 30, 2007.
63. Urbaniak M. Thinking and working "out of the box." Adv Occup Ther 1998;14(26):20.
64. Urbaniak M. Yahara house: A community-based program using the Fountain-House model. Am Occup Ther Assoc Ment Health Special Sect Q Newslett 1995;18(1):1–3.
65. U.S. Psychiatric Rehabilitation Association. Who We Are. Available at: www.uspra.org/i4a/pages/index.cfm?pageid=1. Accessed Feb 2007.
66. Wollenberg JL. Recovery and occupational therapy in the community mental health setting. Occup Ther Ment Health 2001;17(3–4):97–114.

## SUGGESTED READINGS

Burson KA. Reestablishing occupational therapy in a state mental health system. Am Occup Ther Assoc Ment Health Special Sect Q Newslett 1998;21(1):1–2.

Eggers M, Sciulli J, Gaguzis K, Munoz JP. Enrichment through occupation: The Allegheny County jail project.

Am Occup Ther Assoc Ment Health Special Sect Q Newslett 2003;26(2):1–4.

Fazio LS. Developing Occupation-Centered Programs for the Community: A Workbook for Students and Professionals. Upper Saddle River, NJ: Prentice Hall, 2001.

Knis-Matthews L. A parenting program for women who are substance dependent. Am Occup Ther Assoc Ment Health Special Sect Q Newslett 2003;26(1):1–4.

Moeller P. The occupational therapist as case manager in community mental health. Am Occup Ther Assoc Ment Health Special Sect Q Newslett 1991;14(2):4–5.

Pitts DB. Assertive community treatment: A brief introduction. Am Occup Ther Assoc Ment Health Special Sect Q Newslett 2001; 24(4):1–2.

Sheehan S. Is There No Place on Earth for Me? Boston: Houghton Mifflin, 1982.

Swarbrick P, Duffy M. Consumer-operated organization and programs: A role for occupational therapy practitioners. Am Occup Ther Assoc Ment Health Special Sect Q Newslett 2000;23(1):1–4.

Torrey EF. Out of the Shadows: Confronting America's Mental Illness Crisis. New York: Wiley, 1997.

Wilberding D. The quarterway house: More than an alternative of care. Occup Ther Ment Health 1991;11(1):65–91.

Wollenberg JL. Recovery and occupational therapy in the community mental health setting. Occup Ther Ment Health 2001; 17(3–4):97–114.

CHAPTER 8

# Psychotropic Medications and Other Biological Treatments

*Some griefs are med'cinable.*

WILLIAM SHAKESPEARE (8)

## CHAPTER OBJECTIVES

After studying this chapter, the reader will be able to:

1. Identify the major categories of medications used to treat mental disorders.
2. Recognize common side effects of psychotropic medications.
3. Describe appropriate actions to assist consumers dealing with adverse effects of psychotropic medications.
4. Name and describe somatic and alternative therapies used in psychiatry.
5. List responsibilities of occupational therapy personnel in regard to consumers and their medications.

Just 60 years ago people with severe mental disorders could not be effectively treated in a medical sense. The introduction in the 1950s of drugs that could control hallucinations and other psychotic symptoms ushered in a new era in psychiatric rehabilitation. Suddenly, patients who had been unapproachable, out of control, and out of touch with reality were calm and could engage in occupational therapy (OT) and other rehabilitative treatments. In the succeeding decades many more types of psychotropic, or mind-changing, drugs have been discovered and introduced, with remarkable advances having been made since the 1990s. These drugs are effective in reducing symptoms and returning people to their premorbid level of functioning. This chapter presents information on the major types or classes of drugs used in psychiatric practice today, their therapeutic uses, and their side effects. It also describes specific OT interventions to help clients understand how medications influence their ability to function in purposeful activities. The use of electroconvulsive therapy (ECT) and other somatic (body-oriented) treatments is discussed. The reader is reminded that the effectiveness of drug therapy and somatic treatments is attributed to neuroscience concepts described in Chapter 2.

## PSYCHOTROPIC MEDICATIONS

*Psychotropic* means "mind changing." Thus psychotropic medications are drugs that alter, or change, the way the mind works. Many drugs have psychotropic qualities. These include medications prescribed for mental disorders, medications that are prescribed for physical disorders but that produce mind-altering side effects, and other mind-changing but illegal drugs (e.g., phencyclidine [PCP] and lysergic acid diethylamide [LSD]).

This chapter considers only the first of these three groups: the psychotropic medications that physicians prescribe to treat the symptoms of mental illness. Occupational therapy assistants (OTAs) must know about these drugs because they are in a position to observe the effects of the medication on the person's symptoms, engagement in occupation, and performance of everyday activities. OT practitioners can see firsthand whether a person is able to function better today than yesterday or whether side effects such as tremors are interfering with the ability to perform routine tasks. The physician relies on OT and nursing staff and patients' self-reports to monitor how well a medication is working, whether it should be changed, and whether the dosage should be increased or reduced. In addition, physicians rely on staff to support their medical decisions, to encourage clients to comply with taking the medication, and to help clients understand that some side effects are temporary. For these reasons it is important for the OTA to know the classes of drugs, the problems for which they are prescribed, and the common side effects.

Research and development of psychotropic medication is ongoing. By the time this book goes to press, new drugs will be on the market. And, studies will have demonstrated more clearly the effects of existing drugs. Some will perhaps have been removed from the market. Therefore, this chapter provides a basic foundation for approaching the subject and is not an exhaustive guide. The reader must take responsibility for keeping informed about changes in medications, so as to provide appropriate support to consumers. Additional references are provided at the end of the chapter.

### How Psychotropic Drugs Work

Psychotropic drugs alter the neurotransmitter balances in the brain. Their effects are a result of changed levels of key brain chemicals (dopamine, norepinephrine, serotonin). Drugs for schizophrenia (the neuroleptics) work primarily on the dopamine system (Table 8-1), and different neuroleptics target specific dopamine receptors (e.g., $D_2$, $D_3$, $D_4$). The newer medications (termed *second generation* and *third generation*

**TABLE 8-1 THERAPEUTIC AND ADVERSE EFFECTS OF ANTIPSYCHOTIC DRUGS**

| CLASS | GENERIC NAME (TRADE NAME) | THERAPEUTIC EFFECT | SIDE EFFECTS (SELECTED) |
|---|---|---|---|
| Conventional neuroleptics (first generation) | Chlorpromazine (Thorazine)<br>Trifluoperazine (Stelazine)<br>Thioridazine (Mellaril)<br>Mesoridazine (Serentil)<br>Perphenazine (Trilafon)<br>Thiothixene (Navane)<br>Haloperidol (Haldol)<br>Molindone (Moban)<br>Loxapine (Loxitane)<br>Ziprasidone (Zeldox) | Decrease in psychotic symptoms (reduction in hallucinations, delusions, psychomotor agitation)<br>Sedation | **TD and NMS** require immediate medical intervention; signs of TD: **involuntary movements of the face, trunk, extremities;** signs of NMS: **rigidity, catatonia**<br>EPS with abnormal movements remedied by antiparkinsonian drugs (Table 8-2)<br>Others: dry mouth, blurred vision, skin rash, photosensitivity |
| Second-generation neuroleptics | Clozapine (Clozaril)<br>Risperidone (Risperdal)<br>Olanzapine (Zyprexa)<br>Quetiapine (Seroquel)<br>Ziprasidone (Geodon) | Decrease in psychotic symptoms (reduction in hallucinations, delusions, psychomotor agitation)<br>Significantly more effective than traditional neuroleptics in reducing negative symptoms of schizophrenia | Dry mouth, blurred vision, constipation, orthostatic hypotension, seizures<br>All may lead to weight gain and possible **metabolic syndrome** and type 2 diabetes<br>**Agranulocytosis,** fatal unless caught early, occurs in 1–2% of patients taking clozapine, which hence necessitates blood monitoring<br>Olanzapine may **elevate liver enzymes,** causes significant weight gain, elevates cholesterol and blood sugar<br>Stopping medication abruptly after prolonged used will cause unpleasant withdrawal syndromes |

**TABLE 8-1 THERAPEUTIC AND ADVERSE EFFECTS OF ANTIPSYCHOTIC DRUGS *(Continued)***

| CLASS | GENERIC NAME (TRADE NAME) | THERAPEUTIC EFFECT | SIDE EFFECTS (SELECTED) |
|---|---|---|---|
| Third-generation neuroleptics | Aripiprazole (Abilify) | Decrease in psychotic symptoms (reduction in hallucinations, delusions, psychomotor agitation)<br>Significantly more effective than traditional neuroleptics in reducing negative symptoms of schizophrenia<br>Improvement in depressive symptoms<br>Low or no motor impairment effect | Drowsiness, insomnia, akathisia |

*TD,* tardive dyskinesia; *NMS,* neuroleptic malignant syndrome; *EPS,* extrapyramidal syndrome.
Both therapeutic and adverse effects vary. Different drugs in these classes behave differently.
Data from Bezchlibnyk KZ, Jeffries JJ, eds. Clinical Handbook of Psychotropic Drugs. 16th rev ed. Ashland, OH: Hogrefe, 2006; Diamond RJ. Instant Psychopharmacology: A Guide for the Nonmedical Mental Health Professional. 2nd ed. New York: Norton, 2002; and Sadock BJ, Sadock VA. Kaplan & Sadock's Synopsis of Psychiatry. 9th ed. Philadelphia: Lippincott Williams & Wilkins, 2003.

but formerly called "atypical antipsychotic") have selective effects in particular parts of the brain (e.g., the frontal lobes and the limbic system) and fewer side effects from unwanted effects in other parts of the brain. Antidepressants work by altering levels of serotonin and other neurotransmitters; each antidepressant has a slightly different action.

All of the psychotropic drugs come in a form for oral administration. Generally these are tablets, capsules, or extended-release capsules. Some are available in liquid form, and some can be given by injection. Some injectable drugs come in a depot formulation, which is long lasting; the patient is administered the medication only every few weeks. This helps with compliance in patients who have trouble remembering to take oral medications.

## The Psychotropic Drugs and Their Side Effects

Tables 8-1 through 8-6 summarize six major categories of drugs: antipsychotic drugs, antiparkinsonian drugs, antidepressant drugs, antimanic drugs, antianxiety drugs, and psychostimulants. For each category, the brand names of individual drugs are listed in the tables. Drugs in Tables 8-1, 8-3, and 8-6 are grouped by class. The last column in each table lists some of the side effects. Side effects shown in **boldface type** are medically dangerous, either life threatening or indicators of possible permanent damage. These side effects *must* be reported to the nurse or doctor immediately, *and* the OTA must also record in the patient's chart the symptom and the person to whom it was reported.

## Antipsychotic Drugs

Antipsychotic drugs, also known as neuroleptics, are prescribed most often for persons with schizophrenia and other psychotic disorders (Table 8-1). These drugs control psychotic symptoms, such as hallucinations and delusions, and generally bring the person into better contact with reality. The neuroleptics are also used to reduce violent or possibly dangerous behaviors in persons having manic episodes and in drug abusers.

The older traditional drugs of this type have no effect on the so-called negative symptoms of schizophrenia (apathy, lack of interest in other people and one's environment, self-absorption, and lack of motivation). Examples of these traditional neuroleptics are chlorpromazine (Thorazine), trifluoperazine (Stelazine), and haloperidol (Haldol). The newer antipsychotics seem much more effective in reducing negative symptoms. Among the second-generation drugs are clozapine (Clozaril), risperidone (Risperdal), and olanzapine (Zyprexa); people taking these drugs function better overall than do those taking the older traditional neuroleptics. Even more promising is the third-generation drug aripiprazole (Abilify). Note that a recent study (5) showed no difference in effectiveness of the different classes of antipsychotics; Abilify was not included in this study.

However, even with the newer medications, the person who has had a major mental disorder for a number of years is at a disadvantage in learning basic skills for getting along in the world. Furthermore, the newer medications are much more expensive than the older ones, and several of them require frequent blood monitoring to detect the onset of potentially fatal side effects. Thus many persons with psychiatric disorders still are prescribed the traditional neuroleptics. Individuals receiving any of these drugs are very much in need of OT and other rehabilitative services to help them function better in daily life.

Among the many side effects of neuroleptics are movement disorders (extrapyramidal syndrome [EPS]), a tendency to sunburn very easily (photosensitivity), dry mouth, and blurred vision. The second- and third-generation drugs have a lower incidence of EPS (3). Postural hypotension may also occur; the person's blood pressure drops on rising—from lying to sitting or from sitting to standing—causing dizziness or fainting. Many people taking these drugs also have a decrease in sexual interest and may secrete milk from the breast (lactation). Side effects are most unpleasant during the first 10 days of treatment. After this time, movement disorders tend to diminish, although the cholinergic effects (dry mouth and blurred vision) may remain. The general public has a low opinion of antipsychotic medication and its side effects; this may cause problems for consumers who listen to friends or family and who then stop taking their medication (1). A study showed that 74% of patients stopped taking their antipsychotic medications within 18 months (5). Thus the OTA and all other staff need to support the consumer to maintain medication adherence.

Tardive dyskinesia (TD) is the most serious side effect of the neuroleptics and is primarily associated with the older, first-generation, drugs. TD is a movement disorder that may become permanent unless the patient stops taking the medication. The initial signs include facial movements, writhing motions of the tongue, and small writhing motions of the fingers. Any suspected signs of TD should be reported to the physician immediately. Some persons develop permanent TD if their medication is not discontinued soon enough. This movement disorder is very disfiguring and embarrassing, causing social rejection, impairments at work, and depression; and it may provoke suicidal acts (10). Despite this, some persons may be quite unconcerned. If you notice someone who is receiving neuroleptics displaying any behaviors that seem similar to those described here, you should contact the doctor or nurse immediately and document your report in the chart.

Neuroleptic malignant syndrome (NMS) is a rare but life-threatening effect of antipsychotic medication (7). Signs of NMS are extreme rigidity and catatonia, which are sometimes mistaken for a worsening of the psychotic disorder. Any patient taking antipsychotics who suddenly becomes rigid or unresponsive requires medical evaluation for NMS.

## Antiparkinsonian Drugs

Because EPS (parkinsonian movement disorder) is a frequent but unwelcome side effect of neuroleptic medication, antiparkinsonian drugs are often prescribed along with neuroleptics (Table 8-2). Examples of these drugs for medication-related movement disorders are benztropine (Cogentin), biperiden (Akineton), and amantadine (Symmetrel). These drugs reduce the EPS, enabling the person to engage more easily in activities in which physical coordination is a factor. Unfortunately, these drugs may exacerbate dry mouth, blurred vision, dizziness, and nausea.

## Antidepressant Drugs

The major therapeutic value of antidepressant drugs is relief from depression and the risk of suicide and social withdrawal associated with it (Table 8-3). There are three major classes of antidepressant drugs, and new drugs that fit in none of these classes continue to be developed. Each class is discussed separately. Often the physician has to prescribe brief trials of different drugs before the one that produces the desired effect for a particular person is identified. Unfortunately, no one has yet found a way to predict which drug will be effective for a given person.

Chemically, antidepressants can be grouped in two categories: the cyclics and the monoamine oxidase inhibitors (MAOIs). Cyclic antidepressants have recently been reclassified according to their specific effects on brain neurotransmitters (serotonin, norepinephrine, dopamine) (1). The older ones are termed *nonselective* because their effects are more general. Some commonly prescribed nonselective cyclics (formerly called "tricyclics") are amitriptyline (Elavil), imipramine (Tofranil), and desipramine (Norpramin). The newer drugs have selective effects on specific neurotransmitters. The selective cyclics are classified by their neurotransmitter effects, shown in Table 8-3.

**TABLE 8-2 THERAPEUTIC AND ADVERSE EFFECTS OF ANTIPARKINSONIAN DRUGS[a]**

| GENERIC NAME (TRADE NAME) | THERAPEUTIC EFFECT | SIDE EFFECTS |
|---|---|---|
| Benztropine (Cogentin)<br>Trihexyphenidyl (Artane)<br>Biperiden (Akineton)<br>Procyclidine (Kemadrin)<br>Ethopropazine (Parsitan)<br>Orphenadrine (Norflex, Disipal)<br>Amantadine (Symmetrel)<br>Diphenhydramine (Benadryl)<br>Propranolol (Inderal) | Control of EPS caused by use of antipsychotic medications (relief from or reduction of akathisia, akinesia, dystonic reactions, and so on) | Dry mouth, blurred vision, dizziness, nausea, fatigue, weakness<br>Propranolol may cause life-threatening **cardiac symptoms** that require prompt medical evaluation |

[a]Both therapeutic and adverse effects vary. Different drugs in this class behave differently.

*EPS,* extrapyramidal symptoms.

Data from Bezchlibnyk KZ, Jeffries JJ, eds. Clinical Handbook of Psychotropic Drugs. 16th rev ed. Ashland, OH: Hogrefe, 2006; Diamond RJ. Instant Psychopharmacology: A Guide for the Nonmedical Mental Health Professional. 2nd ed. New York: Norton, 2002; and Sadock BJ, Sadock VA. Kaplan & Sadock's Synopsis of Psychiatry. 9th ed. Philadelphia: Lippincott Williams & Wilkins, 2003.

## TABLE 8-3 THERAPEUTIC AND ADVERSE EFFECTS OF ANTIDEPRESSANT DRUGS[a]

| CLASS | GENERIC NAME (TRADE NAME) | THERAPEUTIC EFFECT | SIDE EFFECTS |
|---|---|---|---|
| Nonselective cyclic agents | Amitriptyline (Elavil)<br>Imipramine (Tofranil)<br>Doxepin (Sinequan)<br>Trimipramine (Surmontil)<br>Nortriptyline (Pamelor)<br>Desipramine (Norpramin)<br>Maprotiline (Ludiomil)<br>Amoxapine (Asendin)<br>Clomipramine (Anafranil) | Relief from depression<br>Reduction in suicidal ideation and risk of suicide<br>Increased activity<br>Normalization of sleep, appetite | Short-term: drowsiness, nausea, blurred vision<br>Weight gain, agitation, dry mouth, tremors may occur<br>**Arrhythmia, seizures, urinary retention, postural hypotension, constipation**<br>All potentiate effects of alcohol<br>Suicidal patients may try to overdose; large quantities can be fatal |
| Selective serotonin reuptake inhibitors | Citalopram (Celexa)<br>Escitalopram (Lexapro)<br>Fluoxetine (Prozac)<br>Fluvoxamine (Luvox)<br>Sertraline (Zoloft)<br>Paroxetine (Paxil) | Relief from depression<br>Reduction in suicidal ideation and risk of suicide<br>Increased activity<br>Normalization of sleep, appetite | Fewer side effects than other antidepressants, but sexual dysfunction, anxiety, insomnia, nausea, headaches possible<br>May interfere with metabolism of other drugs<br>Signs of **central serotonin syndrome: confusion, agitation, sweating, shivering, tremor, jerky movements (myoclonus), fever, diarrhea;** requires immediate medical attention<br>**Increased risk of suicidal tendencies, especially in children and adolescents** |

**TABLE 8-3 THERAPEUTIC AND ADVERSE EFFECTS OF ANTIDEPRESSANT DRUGS[a] *(Continued)***

| CLASS | GENERIC NAME (TRADE NAME) | THERAPEUTIC EFFECT | SIDE EFFECTS |
|---|---|---|---|
| Norepinephrine dopamine reuptake inhibitors | Bupropion (Wellbutrin) | Relief from depression<br>Reduction in suicidal ideation and risk of suicide<br>Increased activity<br>Normalization of sleep, appetite<br>Less likely to provoke a switch to manic state<br>May have less negative effect on libido | May cause insomnia, seizures, orthostatic hypotension, dry mouth, and so on |
| Selective serotonin norepinephrine reuptake inhibitors | Venlafaxine (Effexor)<br>Duloxetine (Cymbalta) | Relief from depression<br>Reduction in suicidal ideation and risk of suicide<br>Increased activity<br>Normalization of sleep, appetite<br>May work more quickly than some other antidepressants | May cause increased suicidal thinking<br>May cause sleepiness or insomnia, headache, nervousness, dry mouth, increased blood pressure, decreased libido, nausea |
| Serotonin 2 antagonists/ reuptake inhibitors | Nefazodone (Serzone)<br>Trazodone (Desyrel) | Relief from depression<br>Reduction in suicidal ideation and risk of suicide<br>Increased activity<br>Normalization of sleep, appetite | Sleepiness<br>May exacerbate preexisting heart disease<br>**Priapism (painful, long-lasting erection)** is a serious side effect requiring immediate medical care |
| Noradrenergic/ specific serotonergic antidepressants | Mirtazapine (Remeron) | Relief from depression, symptoms of depression as for non-selective cyclics.<br>Helps reduce anxiety.<br>May have faster onset of effects than other antidepressants. | Fatigue, sleepiness, impaired psychomotor functioning, dry mouth, constipation, sexual dysfunction |

*(continued)*

**TABLE 8-3 THERAPEUTIC AND ADVERSE EFFECTS OF ANTIDEPRESSANT DRUGS[a] *(Continued)***

| CLASS | GENERIC NAME (TRADE NAME) | THERAPEUTIC EFFECT | SIDE EFFECTS |
|---|---|---|---|
| Monoamine oxidase inhibitors | Isocarboxazid (Marplan)<br>Phenelzine (Nardil)<br>Tranylcypromine (Parnate)<br>Moclobemide (Manerix)[b] | Relief from depression<br>Reduction in suicidal ideation and risk of suicide<br>Increased activity<br>Normalization of sleep, appetite<br>May be effective in ADHD<br>Classified as reversible (RIMA) or irreversible MAOIs | Signs of possible **tyramine reaction: sweating, palpitations, headache** (from mild to severe), **increase in blood pressure;** requires immediate medical attention<br>**Postural hypotension, vomiting** and **nausea, drowsiness,** and **weakness** necessitate medical evaluation<br>Other possible: dizziness, dry mouth, tremors, constipation |

[a]Both therapeutic and adverse effects vary. Different drugs in this class behave differently.

[b]A reversible inhibitor of monoamine oxidase A. Not marketed in the United States.

*ADHD,* attention deficit-hyperactivity disorder; *RIMA,* reversible inhibitor of monoamine oxidase A; *MAOIs,* monoamine oxidase inhibitors.

Data from Bezchlibnyk KZ, Jeffries JJ, eds. Clinical Handbook of Psychotropic Drugs. 16th rev ed. Ashland, OH: Hogrefe, 2006; Diamond RJ. Instant Psychopharmacology: A Guide for the Nonmedical Mental Health Professional. 2nd ed. New York: Norton, 2002; and Sadock BJ, Sadock VA. Kaplan & Sadock's Synopsis of Psychiatry. 9th ed. Philadelphia: Lippincott Williams & Wilkins, 2003.

Prominent among the selective cyclic antidepressants is the group of selective serotonin reuptake inhibitors (SSRIs). The SSRIs include fluoxetine (Prozac) and sertraline (Zoloft). SSRIs produce fewer side effects; but sexual dysfunction (reduced interest, difficulty reaching orgasm) commonly affects people taking these drugs. Furthermore, sometimes the SSRIs become less effective over time, and the person again becomes depressed, requiring a switch to a different medication.

Compared with the nonselective drugs, the selective cyclics generally have fewer and less-severe side effects (4). All antidepressants take time to begin to work; most do not begin to take effect until at least 7 to 10 days after they are first ingested, and they reach full effectiveness only after 3 weeks. As the drug begins to take effect, the OTA will notice a gradual increase in the depressed person's ability to function. Common side effects of cyclic antidepressants include dry mouth, blurred vision, and constipation (these can be relieved with lemon drops, magnifying glasses, and bran, respectively). Epileptic seizures may also be precipitated in susceptible individuals. When stopped, all antidepressants produce withdrawal symptoms; therefore, the drug should be tapered off gradually under physician supervision.

MAOIs produce an antidepressant effect by interfering with the breakdown of certain brain chemicals. Two commonly prescribed MAOIs are isocarboxazid (Marplan) and phenelzine (Nardil). These drugs may be given to people who have shown a poor response to tricyclics. MAOIs also take up to 3 weeks to reach their full effect, and they can be prescribed only for those who are willing to follow a strict dietary regimen. The amino acid tyramine interacts with MAOIs to cause a hypertensive crisis (sudden increase in blood pressure), which may lead to cerebral hemorrhage and death. Tyramine is found in aged cheese, wine, beer, yogurt, tea, coffee, avocados, bananas, soy sauce, pickled herring, yeast, protein extract, raisins, dates, and other foods; and persons who are taking MAOIs must avoid them. OT practitioners who work with clients in food preparation should avoid foods that contain tyramine when persons taking MAOIs are participating and should obtain a complete list of forbidden foods from a physician, nurse, or clinical dietician.

Central serotonin syndrome can occur when the person is simultaneously receiving an MAOI and an SSRI, but it can also occur in those taking an SSRI alone. Signs of this syndrome are confusion, agitation, shivering, fever, sweating, myoclonus (jerky movements), and incoordination. Such symptoms should be reported to medical staff for evaluation (4).

## Antimanic Drugs

Mood-stabilizing drugs act to reduce intensity of mood swings and control the symptoms of mania (Table 8-4); they are prescribed for affective disorders with manic symptoms. The first group of drugs in Table 8-4 (e.g., Eskalith, Lithonate) contains lithium carbonate, a common metal salt. Lithium is toxic; frequent blood tests are performed to ascertain the level of lithium in the blood. During the first 2 or 3 weeks of receiving lithium, many people have uncomfortable side effects such as diarrhea, dry mouth, frequent urination, drowsiness, and fatigue. These side effects usually diminish with time, and clients should be encouraged to stick it out until this happens. The only lasting side effect seems to be a fine hand tremor, which is sometimes controlled by having the client take another drug, propranolol, simultaneously. Gross bilateral hand tremors and ataxia, jaundice (yellowing of the skin or eyes), diarrhea, and vomiting are signs of possible overdose and should be reported to the physician immediately and documented.

The other major group of medications used for bipolar disorder are the anticonvulsants, also shown in Table 8-4. The mechanism by which anticonvulsants control moods is not clear but may be related to the neurotransmitter γ-aminobutyric acid (GABA) (2). Often, the patient is also prescribed an antipsychotic drug at the same time.

## Antianxiety Drugs

Antianxiety drugs are used to control anxiety in disorders that are not psychotic (e.g., neuroses, personality disorders) (Table 8-5). These drugs are sometimes called the minor tranquilizers to differentiate them from the major tranquilizers, or neuroleptics. The benzodiazepines (Valium, Xanax) can be addicting.

## Psychostimulant Drugs

Medications prescribed for attention deficit disorder (ADD) and attention deficit-hyperactivity disorder (ADHD) are shown in Table 8-6. Psychostimulants are drugs that stimulate and increase mental and physical activity. Paradoxically, they have the opposite effect in children. Their most common clinical application is control of hyperactivity in children with ADD. Side effects, which include impaired growth, tics, and insomnia, must be carefully monitored. Newer medications, such as atomoxetine, seem to control the distractibility of ADHD without having severe adverse effects.

**TABLE 8-4 THERAPEUTIC AND ADVERSE EFFECTS OF MOOD-STABILIZING DRUGS**

| GENERIC NAME (TRADE NAME) | THERAPEUTIC EFFECT | SIDE EFFECTS |
|---|---|---|
| Lithium (Eskalith, Lithane, Lithonate, Lithotabs, Lithizine, Lithocarb, Lithobid, Lithuril, Cibalith-S) | Decrease in manic symptoms: reduces activity level, stabilizes mood, normalizes sleep, decreases speech production, reduces irritability, increases attention span, improves judgment | **Diarrhea, nausea, vomiting, confusion,** and **slurred speech** may indicate **toxic reaction,** requiring immediate medical intervention |
| | May help reduce depressive symptoms | Fine hand tremor, an early side effect, diminishes in time<br>Weight gain, metallic taste, fatigue, thirst |
| **Anticonvulsants**[a] | | |
| Carbamazepine (Tegretol) | Decrease in manic symptoms | Excessive sedation, nausea, motor incoordination<br>May cause birth defects, liver and heart damage<br>**Aplastic anemia,** rare but dangerous |
| Valproic acid (Depakote, Depakene) | | Nausea, vomiting, indigestion, sedation<br>**Liver toxicity** (look for yellow skin or eyes), rare but dangerous |
| Lamotrigine (Lamictal) | | **Severe, potentially fatal skin rash** |
| Gabapentin (Neurontin) | | Excessive sedation |

[a]Most of these medications were originally used to control seizures, but are now used for bipolar disorders to reduce mood swings and reduce episodes of mania and depression

Data from Bezchlibnyk KZ, Jeffries JJ, eds. Clinical Handbook of Psychotropic Drugs. 16th rev ed. Ashland, OH: Hogrefe, 2006; Diamond RJ. Instant Psychopharmacology: A Guide for the Nonmedical Mental Health Professional. 2nd ed. New York: Norton, 2002; and Sadock BJ, Sadock VA. Kaplan & Sadock's Synopsis of Psychiatry. 9th ed. Philadelphia: Lippincott Williams & Wilkins, 2003.

## The Role of the OTA

Clients with mental health problems are often prescribed more than one type of medication. For example, a neuroleptic may be used with lithium to reduce acute psychotic symptoms of mania. Not only are different psychotropic drugs used in combination with each other but clients who have medical problems are generally taking other medications as well. Because drugs interact with each other, the physician is especially careful to prescribe only medications that are compatible with ones the person is already taking. Use of drugs that are not prescribed or not documented in the medical record (e.g., those prescribed by the family physician for a medical problem) should be reported to the psychiatrist in charge of the case.

**TABLE 8-5 THERAPEUTIC AND ADVERSE EFFECTS OF ANTIANXIETY (ANXIOLYTIC) DRUGS**

| CLASS | GENERIC NAME (TRADE NAME) | THERAPEUTIC EFFECT | SIDE EFFECTS |
|---|---|---|---|
| Benzodiazepines | Diazepam (Valium)<br>Lorazepam (Ativan)<br>Clorazepate (Tranxene)<br>Clonazepam (Klonopin)<br>Halazepam (Paxipam)<br>Alprazolam (Xanax)<br>Flurazepam (Dalmane)<br>Temazepam (Restoril)<br>Triazolam (Halcion) | Reduction of anxiety and tension<br>Reduction of symptoms of alcohol withdrawal<br>Relief of muscle spasm, insomnia (drugs vary in effects on insomnia) | Addictive, but less so than alcohol[a]<br>May cause dizziness, drowsiness, memory problems |
| **Others** | | | |
| | Hydroxyzine (Atarax)<br>Buspirone (BuSpar) | Reduction of anxiety and tension<br>Buspirone may be used in higher doses to treat depression | Fewer side effects than benzodiazepines |

[a]Diamond RJ. Instant Psychopharmacology: A Guide for the Nonmedical Mental Health Professional. 2nd ed. New York: Norton, 2002.

Data from Bezchlibnyk KZ, Jeffries JJ, eds. Clinical Handbook of Psychotropic Drugs. 16th rev ed. Ashland, OH: Hogrefe, 2006; Diamond RJ. Instant Psychopharmacology: A Guide for the Nonmedical Mental Health Professional. 2nd ed. New York: Norton, 2002; and Sadock BJ, Sadock VA. Kaplan & Sadock's Synopsis of Psychiatry. 9th ed. Philadelphia: Lippincott Williams & Wilkins, 2003.

**TABLE 8-6 THERAPEUTIC AND ADVERSE EFFECTS OF MEDICATIONS FOR ATTENTION DEFICIT DISORDERS**

| CLASS | GENERIC NAME (TRADE NAME) | THERAPEUTIC EFFECT | SIDE EFFECTS |
|---|---|---|---|
| Psychostimulants | Methylphenidate (Ritalin)<br>Dextroamphetamine (Dexedrine) | Reduces hyperactivity<br>Improves attention span<br>Reduces impulsivity | May increase rather than reduce these symptoms, causing insomnia, loss of appetite, paranoia, anxiety and agitation<br>Pleasurable high may lead to abuse |
| Atomoxetine | Atomoxetine (Strattera) | Treatment of symptoms<br>Less likely to provoke excited mood or euphoria<br>Not a controlled substance | Insomnia, dizziness, nausea and abdominal pain, anxiety, blood pressure irregularities |

Data from Bezchlibnyk KZ, Jeffries JJ, eds. Clinical Handbook of Psychotropic Drugs. 16th rev ed. Ashland, OH: Hogrefe, 2006; Diamond RJ. Instant Psychopharmacology: A Guide for the Nonmedical Mental Health Professional. 2nd ed. New York: Norton, 2002; and Sadock BJ, Sadock VA. Kaplan & Sadock's Synopsis of Psychiatry. 9th ed. Philadelphia: Lippincott Williams & Wilkins, 2003.

Although OTAs cannot prescribe medications or reduce their undesirable side effects, they can help clients learn to identify, tolerate, and adapt to the way their bodies respond to these side effects. Table 8-7 lists selected side effects and provides strategies the OTA can employ to help clients deal with them and function better. OT staff can also assist by monitoring individual compliance with prescribed drug regimens and by observing and reporting to the physician any undocumented drugs, including street drugs or alcohol, that the person may be taking.

Furthermore, OT practitioners can help by encouraging compliance with drug regimens. Like anyone prescribed a drug with unwelcome side effects, the person with mental illness may find the cure worse than the disease. Feeling like a zombie, feeling restless and wound up, or having no sex life is not pleasant. Even though a medication may be controlling the symptoms of

**TABLE 8-7 DRUG SIDE EFFECTS AND RECOMMENDED OCCUPATIONAL THERAPY ADAPTATIONS AND INTERVENTIONS**

| SIDE EFFECT | ADAPTATIONS AND INTERVENTIONS |
|---|---|
| Extrapyramidal syndrome | In general, report all symptoms to physician or nurse when first observed and then report changes as they occur |
| Parkinsonism: muscular rigidity, tremors, drooling, shuffling gait, masklike face | 1. Use gross motor activities that involve rotation of head and trunk<br>2. Avoid activities that require patient to work against resistance |
| Akathisia: restlessness, muscular tension (often worse in the legs than the arms) | 1. Help patient select activities that allow for movement, getting up and down, and so on<br>2. Avoid activities that require prolonged sitting or standing still<br>3. Put patient at a separate table if persistent movement is disruptive to others |
| Dystonia: painful, sudden muscle spasms, often localized to neck, jaw, eyes, or back; patient may arch back, roll eyes, and so on | 1. Help patient engage in activities that do not require fine coordination or attention to detail<br>2. Avoid use of power tools, sharps, and so on |
| Akinesia: muscular weakness and fatigue, reduction of movement | 1. Permit breaks in activity<br>2. Avoid activities in which patient must work against resistance or for a long time |
| Tardive dyskinesia (movement disorder thought to be caused by prolonged use of neuroleptics): movement patterns may be choreiform (jerky, twitching) or athetoid (writhing); often include facial distortions such as tongue thrust, lip smacking, tics, and chewing; early signs include facial tics, slight but definitely abnormal eye or lip movements, rocking, swaying | 1. *If new,* notify physician at once; side effects can be reversed if caught early but, if neglected, may become permanent<br>2. *If chronic* and if patient is aware and concerned, provide support and encouragement; allow patient to verbalize embarrassment and discomfort |

**TABLE 8-7 DRUG SIDE EFFECTS AND RECOMMENDED OCCUPATIONAL THERAPY ADAPTATIONS AND INTERVENTIONS *(Continued)***

| SIDE EFFECT | ADAPTATIONS AND INTERVENTIONS |
|---|---|
| Postural hypotension: patient feels faint or blacks out when rising from lying to sitting or from sitting to standing; caused by effect of gravity | 1. Notify physician<br>2. Teach patient to sit up slowly, stand up slowly; stand close and be prepared to support patient at waist; do not try to support patient by grabbing arm<br>3. Encourage patient to use furniture and other supports to maintain balance<br>4. Avoid activities that involve sudden postural changes<br>5. Avoid gross motor activities to reduce sudden movements |
| Dry mouth: patient feels thirsty | 1. Allow patient to get water whenever thirsty<br>2. Have hard (sucking) candies available; lemon drops are best; some people prefer sugar-free breath mints<br>3. Teach patient about dehydrating effect of caffeinated drinks and alcohol |
| Blurred vision: vision may be blurry or double vision may occur | 1. Help patient select activities that do not involve fine visual attention<br>2. In gross motor activities, use mats and soft equipment to avoid injury<br>3. In crafts, use large pieces that are easily seen (e.g., 1-inch mosaic tiles)<br>4. Provide magnified reading glasses (several levels of magnification) to be used in OT clinic |
| Hand tremors: rhythmic involuntary hand movements (see also *ataxia*). | 1. If patient is on a new trial of a lithium-based mood-stabilizing medication and tremor is gross, notify physician; gross bilateral hand tremor may be a sign of drug toxicity<br>2. Fine hand tremors are common in patients taking lithium for a month or more; help patient learn to compensate by stabilizing elbow or arm to prevent tremor<br>3. If patient is taking a neuroleptic and tremor has a writhing or wormlike appearance, notify physician; these movements may indicate tardive dyskinesia |
| Ataxia: failure of muscle coordination, manifested as clumsiness when a motor action is attempted (e.g., walking or doing a craft) | 1. If patient is on a new trial of lithium-based antimanic medication, notify physician immediately, as this may be a sign of drug toxicity<br>2. Prepare to provide support when patient gets up out of a chair or turns corners while walking<br>3. Help patient select and engage in activities in which incoordination will not interfere with success |

*(continued)*

**TABLE 8-7 DRUG SIDE EFFECTS AND RECOMMENDED OCCUPATIONAL THERAPY ADAPTATIONS AND INTERVENTIONS *(Continued)***

| SIDE EFFECT | ADAPTATIONS AND INTERVENTIONS |
|---|---|
| Nausea | 1. Have soda crackers, graham crackers, and bread available<br>2. Over-the-counter antacids are sometimes recommended by physician; because these preparations may interfere with action of some antipsychotic and other medications, physicians' approval is required |
| Photosensitivity: patient is extremely sensitive to effects of sun and will sunburn after brief exposure; most commonly seen in patients who are taking certain neuroleptics | 1. Teach patient about photosensitizing effect of medications<br>2. Have patient wear sunscreen, long sleeves, hat, and sunglasses; be sure patient applies sunscreen to tops of feet, backs of hands, earlobes, top of head (bald men)<br>3. Keep time in sun as brief as possible<br>4. Observe patient closely for signs of sunburn |

a mental disorder, the person may consider the overall effect not worth it. Furthermore, sometimes family members (e.g., the spouse of the person with diminished sexual interest) are opposed to the person's taking medication. The OTA can help by gentle guidance and by engaging the client in discussion and reflection about the day-to-day benefits of the drug, and the dangers of relapse and what that would be like. The person who complains about side effects deserves a listening ear and a sympathetic response.

## OTHER BIOLOGICAL TREATMENTS

Biological, or somatic, treatments are those that act on the body to produce an effect on the mind. These include ECT and psychosurgery. ECT is sometimes incorrectly called "shock therapy." The person is given a muscle relaxant, after which an electrical current is briefly applied to the temples, causing a convulsion. No one is certain why this treatment is effective, but it does relieve severe depression and reduce the life-threatening risk of suicide in 80% to 90% of depressed individuals who fail to respond to drug therapies. Usually 8 to 12 ECT treatments are given, every other day over several weeks. The only side effects are occasional headache immediately after a treatment and short-term memory loss lasting a few weeks. The person usually does not remember the treatment at all, and the only permanent memory loss may be of events in the few days before the treatment. Clients receiving ECT are often confused and may not remember (for example) who the OTA is or that they were working on a particular project in occupational therapy. Guidelines for responding to this type of confusion and memory loss are described in Chapter 11.

Psychosurgery was a common treatment in previous decades,[1] when it was erroneously believed that surgically cutting the connections between the prefrontal cortex and the hypothalamic area of the brain would relieve mental

[1]For a detailed and sobering discussion of the history of psychosurgery, see Valenstein (9).

symptoms. This procedure, called a prefrontal lobotomy, often left the patient with impaired judgment and a complete lack of motivation. Psychosurgical techniques are occasionally practiced today for relief of seizures and of intractable depression or violence.

Recent additions to somatic therapies for mental disorders include vagus nerve stimulation (VNS), repetitive transcranial magnetic stimulation (rTMS), and magnetic seizure therapy. VNS was originally approved to treat seizures. A stimulator is implanted in the chest to stimulate the vagus nerve, a part of the autonomic nervous system. In rTMS an electrical magnetic impulse is applied in short bursts to the patient's forehead or scalp; this is considered a more mild form of ECT (6). The same apparatus is used for magnetic seizure therapy, but higher frequencies are used to cause seizures. All of these stimulation techniques are in the development phase.

Bright light therapy (BLT) uses timed exposure to ultraviolet filtered light (similar to sunlight) to treat depression. The patient sits in front of a light box in the morning for 30 minutes. Eye irritation and skin irritation may occur if the light is not filtered. Patients cannot use this therapy if they are taking medications that make them photosensitive.

## HERBAL AND ALTERNATIVE THERAPIES

A variety of herbs, vitamins, and other naturally occurring substances have been used to treat mental disorders. Kava kava (a root from the Pacific Islands) may have some effects in reducing anxiety. St. John's Wort (an herb) has been used in Europe for depression. A compound called S-adenosylmethionine (SAMe; a substance that occurs naturally in the brain) also seems to be effective in treating depression. Valerian (an herb) shows positive effects in patients with insomnia. These and other substances should be used cautiously because dosage and quality control vary by manufacturer and batch. Consumers who are interested in using alternative therapies should be advised to inform their physician and to follow medical advice (3).

## SUMMARY

Psychotropic medications affect the way the mind works. Physicians frequently prescribe these drugs and other somatic treatments, such as ECT, for people with mental health problems. Although psychotropic medications have great value in reducing or controlling the symptoms of mental illness, unpleasant side effects may also occur. For many persons with psychiatric illness, the choice is between a side effect and symptoms of a mental disorder, either of which will interfere with their ability to carry out everyday activities. The OTA must be aware of the different kinds of medication and their effects, both therapeutic and adverse. By observing the client closely day after day, the OTA can notice the effects of medication on functional level; this information, when communicated to the physician, aids in the proper adjustment of dosage level. In addition, the OTA can adapt activities to enable clients to succeed despite drugs' side effects, can educate clients to the effects of these drugs, can listen sympathetically to complaints about side effects while encouraging compliance with drug regimens, and can teach strategies to deal with side effects.

Any information on psychotropic medications may rapidly become obsolete. New drugs are under development, and unsuspected side effects of drugs recently released to the market are sometimes reported. Keeping current with psychopharmacology requires regular review of the literature and use of research and Internet sources to obtain current information.

## REVIEW QUESTIONS AND ACTIVITIES

1. Make a list of the major categories of medications used to treat mental disorders.
2. For each major category of psychotropic medication, list the common side effects.
3. For each side effect listed in Table 8-7, identify an appropriate response or action.
4. List the somatic therapies used in psychiatry, and describe them briefly.
5. Name some herbs and other nutritional substances used as alternative therapies; explain what they are used for.
6. Briefly list the responsibilities of occupational therapy personnel in regard to consumers and their medications.
7. *Challenge question:* If a consumer told you that he was going to stop his prescribed medications and instead take kava kava, how would you respond? What additional actions would you take? Explain your thinking process.

## REFERENCES


1. Ajdacic-Gross V, Burns T, Helbling J, et al. Attitudes to antipsychotic drugs and their side effects: A comparison between general practitioners and the general population. Available at: www.medscape.com/viewarticle/551197. Accessed Feb 2007.
2. Anticonvulsants in psychiatry. Harv Ment Health Lett 2004; 20(10):5–7.
3. Bezchlibnyk KZ, Jeffries JJ, eds. Clinical Handbook of Psychotropic Drugs. 16th rev ed. Ashland, OH: Hogrefe, 2006.
4. Diamond RJ. Instant Psychopharmacology: A Guide for the Nonmedical Mental Health Professional. 2nd ed. New York: Norton, 2002.
5. Lieberman JA, Stroup TS, Swartz MS, et al. Effectiveness of antipsychotic drugs in patients with chronic schizophrenia. N Engl J Med 2005;353(12):1209–1223.
6. Magnetic stimulation of the brain: An update. Harv Ment Health Lett 2005;22(2):4–6.
7. Sadock BJ, Sadock VA. Kaplan & Sadock's Synopsis of Psychiatry. 9th ed. Philadelphia: Lippincott Williams & Wilkins, 2003.
8. Shakespeare W. Cymbeline. In: Barlett J, ed. Familiar Quotations. 15th ed. Boston: Little, Brown, 1980.
9. Valenstein ES. Great and Desperate Cures. New York: Basic Books, 1986.
10. Yassa R, Jones BD. Complications of tardive dyskinesia. Psychosomatics 1985;26:305–313.


## SUGGESTED READINGS


Diamond RJ. Instant Psychopharmacology: A Guide for the Nonmedical Mental Health Professional. 2nd ed. New York: Norton, 2002.

PDR Health Drug Information. Available at: www.pdrhealth.com/drug_info/index.html. Accessed Feb 2007.

CHAPTER 9

# Who Is the Consumer?

***No people are uninteresting. Their fate is like the chronicle of planets.***

**YEVGENY YEVTUSHENKO (91, P. 85)**

## CHAPTER OBJECTIVES

After studying this chapter, the reader will be able to:

1. Appreciate the range of persons and groups served by occupational therapy in mental health.
2. Identify differences of approach to children, adolescents, adults, and the aged.
3. Recognize the role of the family and of family support.
4. Discuss the needs and responsibilities of family caregivers.
5. Appreciate the ways in which cultural difference can affect care.
6. Recognize the effects of economic deprivation on mental health.
7. Discuss the psychosocial issues affecting persons whose primary diagnosis is not psychiatric.
8. Recognize the psychosocial consequences of chronic pain.
9. Distinguish the recovery perspective from the medical view of psychiatric illness.

This chapter addresses occupational therapy intervention for diverse groups that were introduced in Chapters 5 to 7. It considers age groups that are often treated separately—children, adolescents, and the elderly. It also addresses the needs of family members (parents, siblings, partners, spouses, and children) of persons with severe and persistent mental illness, especially family caregivers (family members who provide care to the identified patient). Because culture affects so deeply our notions of what is normal and not normal and because cultural transition is considered stressful, this chapter considers cultural differences and the immigration experience. Also included are the poor and the homeless, among whose numbers are found disproportionate numbers of mentally ill persons. And finally, the chapter addresses the psychosocial needs of persons diagnosed with conditions that are primarily physical—physical disabilities, acquired immune deficiency syndrome (AIDS), and chronic pain.

## POPULATIONS BY AGE GROUP

Children, adolescents, and the aged may be treated in separate facilities or programs designed to meet their particular developmental needs. These include outpatient and inpatient programs, community-based programs, and special residential programs. Occupational therapy (OT) interventions for these groups focus on age-appropriate occupational roles and the skills that support them.

### Children

Children are most often seen in the community—that is, at home or at school. Children with psychotic disorders or severe behavior problems may need to be hospitalized, usually in a children's hospital or a children's ward; these facilities have their own staff, which may include one or more OT practitioners as well as teachers, child psychologists, speech and language pathologists, and the usual medical staff. Children who have enough control over their behavior to live in the community may reside with their parents or in special residences and attend a special school for the emotionally handicapped. Children with milder problems are enrolled in regular public or private schools and receive treatment in the school and/or in after-school programs on an outpatient basis. Many children receiving OT services in the schools for other reasons (e.g., learning disability, developmental disability) can benefit from attention to their psychosocial and psychological needs (7, 44, 75, 84).

Working with children requires broad and detailed knowledge of child development and the roles of activities and play in the child's life. Knowledge of sensory integration theories and methods is useful, along with training in applied behavioral analysis (ABA). ABA targets specific behaviors (e.g., sitting down) with a highly structured training regimen. In an ABA program several helpers and the family work with the child intensively, repeating the same instructions and giving the same reinforcements for at least 8 hours a day. Newer methods include functional behavioral analysis (FBA) and positive behavioral support (PBS). FBA looks at the student's behavior, what purposes it may serve, and how best to intervene. PBS considers how the environment may be used to strengthen and support the student. The aim is to recognize a potential problem situation and prevent problem behavior by intervening early. Clearly communicating group rules, appropriately praising, and redirecting the student's focus are some examples of supports (17, 78). The reader is encouraged to consult the references for further details.

Another sensory-based intervention is the Alert Program (75, 90), in which students are taught to identify their level of excitement or arousal and to manipulate it through sensory input. This is especially important for middle school students who are sometimes in trouble in school because they are either inattentive or, on the other hand, so keyed up that they are disruptive to the class.

Mosey's levels of group interaction skill may be applied to children who lack age-appropriate skills for relating to peers in the classroom (1). Children who have no friends and limited social skills benefit from the opportunity to interact with peers in groups, with leadership from a skilled therapy practitioner. Activity-based group treatment closely simulates the normal play groups of childhood and can help these children learn and practice effective social skills (7, 16).

OT programs for children may focus on consultation to parents or teachers to help them provide play and self-care experiences that will interest the child and facilitate development of specific skills (Box 9-1). Practitioners may work in the home, in early intervention (EI) programs or in the schools in programs mandated by the Individuals with Disabilities Education Act (IDEA). In the schools, interventions must be "educationally relevant;" OT is but one of several disciplines working together with a special educator to develop for each disabled child a complete individualized education plan (IEP). In the schools, OT has come to be identified strongly with fine motor interventions; practitioners tend to focus first on fine motor skills, such as handwriting and scissor use. Coping, communication, sensory regulation, and social skills for group and interpersonal interaction should also be part of the IEP for students with problems in these areas. OT groups and individual sessions are usually worked in around the school schedule; another model is for the practitioner to consult with the teacher or carry out the program in the classroom with the assistance of the teacher. Evaluation and intervention should focus on the occupational experience and functioning of the child in the roles of student, player, friend, family member, and so on. Coster (19) provides a model for this sort of occupation-centered assessment.

Children whose mental disorders are so severe as to require hospitalization need a different approach. Sholle-Martin and Alessi (81) described a role for the occupational therapist in inpatient child psychiatry; the role focused on the evaluation of occupational behaviors and of aspects of the model of human occupation (MOHO). Using the Vineland Adaptive Behavior Scale (VABS) and other instruments, the OT can screen for

**BOX 9-1**

**CHILDREN WITH PSYCHOSOCIAL PROBLEMS: TREATMENT FOCUS**

- Occupation-based assessment and intervention, focusing on age-appropriate roles (player, friend, self-maintainer, family member, student)
- Mutual collaborative goal setting, including child, family, and (whene relevant) teacher
- As needed, group programming for development of social skills and play behaviors
- Child-centered positive supports: environmental strategies to promote success, sensory regulation such as Alert, intervention and redirection to prevent disruptions
- As needed, special interventions (applied behavioral analysis, sensory integration)
- Education of and consultation with parents regarding appropriate expectations, behavior management, and so on
- Scheduling compatible with school schedule and needs of family

problems in occupational functioning and work with the team to analyze the interaction of the illness with the ability to function in self-care, work (school, chores), and play. In this model, the occupational therapy assistant (OTA) can carry out evaluations as directed by the OT, contribute to discussion of the child's occupational functioning, and help formulate discharge recommendations.

OT practitioners may work in the community with parents of children who have been discharged from the hospital after a stay for treatment of a psychiatric disorder. Development of age-appropriate skills may lag because of the disorder, and parents may not know what to expect from their child or how to help. Expectations may be set too high or too low. OT practitioners can identify the child's skill level and suggest and model appropriate play (32). Another approach is the multifamily parent–child activity-based therapy group, which gives an opportunity for children with mental disorders and their parents to do activities with other children and parents in the same situation. Activities suggested by the therapist are simple but require some assistance from parents. Parents can get support from others, engage their children in a spontaneous and natural way, and learn techniques for responding positively and effectively to their children (69). Olson (68) states that parents can learn positive and supportive parenting in occupation-based groups with their children, but that this requires vigilance and persistence from the group leaders because families may have long-term negative expectations and behavior patterns.

A common problem among children and adolescents with major psychiatric disorders is sensory sensitivity (misperception of normal tactile stimulation, such as finding tickling unpleasant) (71). Because so much handling and touching occur in the parent–child relationship and because the parent is in a better position to control and limit sensory input than is the child, the OT practitioner can teach the parent about compensatory techniques (e.g., not to tickle, to remove labels from the necks of garments, to reduce environmental stimulation). Leading psychoeducation groups on this and similar topics is a possible role for the OTA.

## Adolescents

Adolescents may be seen by the occupational therapist in the schools or may need inpatient treatment for schizophrenic or depressive disorders (for which adolescence is often the age of onset), for alcohol or drug abuse problems, for eating disorders, for lifelong disturbances originating in childhood psychiatric disorders, or for transient disturbances brought on by life events. Adolescents who have psychiatric problems also must deal with the biological and emotional upheaval of puberty and the identity conflicts of the adolescent period. Staff members may act as surrogates for parents or may be viewed as parent-like authorities. Adolescents may have to work through many challenges as they attempt to exercise more freedom and take increasing responsibility for their own lives. Milieu therapy (see Chapter 7) is often applied in adolescent inpatient and residential settings.

The role of the occupational therapist in an adolescent program usually includes evaluation of current and premorbid occupational functioning (Box 9-2). The therapist may delegate selected evaluation tasks to the OTA. Henry and Coster (43) list the major evaluations used. An evaluation of leisure interests for adolescents has been developed (42). The OTA may be involved in providing a meaningful range of structured therapeutic activities that approximate occupations enjoyed by adolescents in the community at large. Ideally, these should be activities identified by the adolescent as important, but often the person has trouble identifying interests even with the aid of an Interest Checklist. The person may lack confidence and fear failure. With limited social skills

**BOX 9-2**

### ADOLESCENTS WITH PSYCHOSOCIAL PROBLEMS: TREATMENT FOCUS

- Occupation-based assessment and intervention, focusing on age-appropriate roles (player, friend, self-maintainer, family member, student, worker)
- Mutual collaborative goal setting, empowering adolescent to set goals for self, including family and (when relevant) teacher
- Attention to the development of occupational choice for education, training, and career
- As needed, group programming for development of communication and social skills
- Education in special needs of this age group (sexuality, gender identity, prevention of substance abuse)
- Education of and consultation with parents regarding appropriate expectations, behavior management, and so on
- As appropriate, sensory regulation programming such as Alert
- Scheduling compatible with school schedule and needs of family

and little history of success, this should not seem surprising. Lancaster and Mitchell (52) describe a program for adolescents that gradually introduces new activities and facilitates development of communication and social skills. Paper and pencil exercises, structured group exercises, and tasks such as cooking are used. A study by Oxer and Miller (70) showed that providing choices of activities and objects facilitates participation.

Prevocational and vocational activities and training in social skills and daily living skills are often included; sensory regulation (Alert) and cognitive treatments for learning disabilities may be used with some groups. Leisure and physical education activities are essential. To promote free exchange of feelings and ideas about body image and self-esteem, it is recommended that boys and girls be seen, at least some of the time, in separate groups for physical activities such as weight training, aerobics, or yoga (61). Information about human sexuality and universal precautions may fall under the scope of OT in some settings.

Many adolescents benefit tremendously from role modeling and direct training in simple household tasks such as cleaning, cooking, home maintenance, and clothing care. Weissenberg and Giladi (89) reported on a home economics day program in an adolescent day hospital. Once a week for an entire day the adolescent clients planned, organized, and carried out meal preparation for the center. This let them learn and practice skills and habits in a realistic situation but with normal time pressures and performance expectations individually tailored to the capacities of the clients.

Adolescents experiencing the first onset of schizophrenia will generally have difficulty functioning in school and peer situations owing to sensory distractions from hallucinations and other perceptual distortions. When the teenager was previously functioning well, others may believe that he or she is simply not trying hard enough. Educating teachers, classmates, and family to the nature of brain disorders can help adjust unrealistic expectations (23). These adolescents may benefit from accommodations such as a shorter school day with a later start, a distraction-free setting for study hall, a smaller classroom, and one-on-one tutoring.

Stress management training, sensory regulation programs, and strategies from Allen's cognitive disabilities approach may be useful.

Working on an adolescent service requires the ability to tolerate and set limits on provocative and rebellious behavior while supporting reasonable attempts at independence. This is sometimes difficult for younger students and staff, who may identify too closely with issues teenagers are confronting. Adolescents can be quite skillful at manipulating adults and creating conflict though a defense mechanism known as *splitting* or *triangulating.* It's important that staff communicate well with each other so that they can serve the needs of adolescents effectively. The key personal qualities needed to work well with adolescents are firmness, patience, flexibility, persistence, and a sense of humor.

## Elders

Aged persons with mental health problems (dementia and depression are the most common psychiatric diagnoses) may be seen in their own homes, in community senior centers, in nursing homes, or in other inpatient settings. Community geriatric centers may provide activity programs, counseling, and meals; most participants do not have lifetime brain disorders (e.g., schizophrenia) but rather periodic or chronic depression or anxiety because of losses associated with aging. The centers may be housed in their own facilities or more typically within another community agency, such as a YMCA or church.

Some larger settings provide continuity of services from psychiatric inpatient to community aftercare (36). Such a comprehensive array of services, if well coordinated, maximizes independent functioning and permits each person to be served in the least restrictive environment (Box 9-3). This is especially important for this age group, as older people tend to sustain many losses (physical, social, economic) and for this reason are under considerable stress. The patient may be admitted first for acute care and at this level be introduced to ward-level groups that address specific needs such as decreasing anxiety, promoting understanding of and adjustment to the hospital environment, and providing information and skills needed for successful community functioning (e.g., obtaining benefits).

**BOX 9-3**

**ELDERS WITH PSYCHOSOCIAL PROBLEMS: TREATMENT FOCUS**

- Occupation-based assessment and intervention focusing on relevant age-appropriate roles (self-maintainer, leisure participant, friend, family member, homemaker, volunteer)
- Mutual collaborative goal setting, encouraging elder to identify valued goals, including family or other caregiver when relevant
- Collaborative approach to intervention (e.g., elder asked to consider whether a suggested intervention is acceptable)
- Education in special needs of this age group (e.g., safety, fall prevention, nutrition)
- Wellness and lifestyle redesign
- Reconnection with previously enjoyed leisure activities
- Education of and consultation with caregiver regarding appropriate expectations, behavior management, and so on

At the next level, the person is encouraged to attend activities at a senior center on the hospital grounds. The third level is placement as an outpatient in the geriatric day center. Finally, at the fourth level, the consumer living in the community visits the center periodically and receives limited services at home.

Some centers offer evening and night respite care, for example from 7:00 P.M. to 7:00 A.M., giving families a chance to get a good night's sleep while the ill member stays overnight at a fully staffed program that can accommodate the nighttime restlessness so common in persons with dementia. The patient can sleep, of course, but if awake can participate in activities such as horticulture, card games, or listening to music.

Adult day care (3, 22, 37, 67) is a community-based, long-term service model for the elderly. A partial hospitalization program, adult day care provides a group setting for leisure activities, avocational skills development, and social activities. Adaptive equipment and environmental modifications are provided to maximize functioning for clients who have physical and mental impairments. In adult day care, depending on state and local regulations, the OTA with sufficient service competency may take on a managerial role; as director of programs and services, the OTA may direct the activities of other activity therapy personnel and can create an occupation-oriented activity model.

Older persons who have brain disorders with extensive functional losses (e.g., schizophrenia or organic mental disorders) are usually restricted to nursing homes and the geriatric wards of large public institutions, where they can receive skilled nursing and medical services. Occupational therapy is often provided by OTAs, with the therapist serving as part-time consultant; services may include orientation to the facility, reality orientation, memory training and assistance, sensory awareness, environmental modification, and training in daily living skills and use of assistive devices. An activity program, including social and recreational programming, music activities, and exercise and craft programs may be provided by OT practitioners or by recreational therapists or activity leaders.

One of the challenges of nursing home care is creating an atmosphere in which expectations and opportunities for independence are matched to the capabilities of the residents. Too often tasks that the resident is able to do (slowly perhaps, or only with supervision and cuing) are done for the resident because the staff is unaware, unwilling, or unable to take the time to allow the resident to contribute. Working as an activity director, the OTA can promote maximum independent performance in residents and can communicate to other staff the resident's real capabilities.

Older persons will experience age-related declines in memory functions and a general slowing of responsiveness, particularly in short-term memory. The OTA should give the person time to respond, and should anticipate that the person may have some difficulty recalling recent information (55). Reassurance that these are normal effects of aging, and providing training in mnemonics (such as acronyms or other memory tricks) can help these clients function more comfortably. Adaptations to the environment to organize tasks and make objects easier to find also help. However, any changes must be agreeable to the person and not forced on him or her by the therapy provider.

## FAMILY MEMBERS

The medical model focuses on the patient as the recipient of services and the center of intervention efforts. In a systems model, such as the model of human occupation, the perspective enlarges to include the person's environment; hence the family and the social support system. OT practitioners increase their effectiveness when they include the family in their clinical thinking and intervention efforts. While family involvement is common for OT practitioners in the practice areas of physical disabilities and developmental disabilities, it has been rare in mental health practice (47). The social worker is the mental health professional traditionally designated to work with the family. In today's health care environment, team treatment necessitates significant transdisciplinary interdependence; thus all team members must be sensitive to and ready to respond to family needs and issues. Working with families requires commitment and flexibility to schedule meetings when they are convenient for the family, sometimes in evenings and on weekends.

This can seem overwhelming to the entry-level practitioner, who may reason, "It's hard enough to concentrate on the patient's problems; how can I include the family too?" Billing, documentation, and justifying the communication with the family as real work are related concerns (53). It takes time for new practitioners to become skilled at communicating with families and to recognize that family members can yield useful information about the patient, help support and maintain the person at optimum functioning, provide care in the home, and in other ways reinforce the treatment. An OT practitioner's involvement with the family may take many forms, ranging from no involvement (traditional medical model) to family as informant to family as assistant therapist to family as collaborator or team member or even as director of therapy. Each of these forms of family participation requires specific skills and knowledge from the practitioner (10).

Families need help from mental health professionals because they must adjust to the situation of having a mentally ill family member, because they carry the greatest burden of care, and because they can be the most important and positive support in helping the person function. Families need to be partners in the planning and intervention process. Family involvement can be hampered by Health Insurance Portability and Accountability Act (HIPAA) regulations, in that the consent of the identified patient is required, unless the person is a minor. Family members can serve as advocates and case managers and care providers; to perform these roles they need education about the disease process and about any compensations or modifications they can provide that will make things better. With sufficient information and guidance about possible options, family members will devote time and energy to securing reimbursement, housing, supported employment, and other supports for the ill member. But this will happen only if they are involved in a systematic and collaborative manner (50).

Before we consider how OT practitioners can work effectively with the family or even the specifics of how family members can aid in treatment, we must first acknowledge that relatives of a person with a mental disorder face significant challenges and stresses. It is disturbing and difficult to accept that one's loved one has a lifelong mental illness that may result in chronic disability. Among the many issues faced are the following:

- Guilt and fear
- Grief and feelings of loss over the relationship
- Uncertainty about setting limits
- Uncertainty about personal responsibilities and boundaries
- Fear of becoming sick oneself (if a genetic relative)
- Fear of having children who may develop the illness (80)
- Fear that the family member will wander off or become homeless (87)

## Parents

The parents of a mentally ill person, whether the identified patient is a child, an adolescent, or an adult, may feel tremendous guilt and responsibility; mothers especially may feel guilty, wondering if their own health habits during pregnancy contributed to the illness in utero. Some parents may deny that there is any problem. It is important to understand and to reassure parents that the major brain disorders (schizophrenia, affective disorders, attention deficit-hyperactivity disorder) are biological, *not* caused by upbringing.

Parents may feel intense sadness when their child is compared with peers who are not mentally ill; the child's inability to proceed on a normal life course (relationships, career, children) is an ongoing loss. Parents may have difficulty setting realistic limits and expectations because it is hard to differentiate between illness-driven behaviors, for which the person is not responsible, and voluntary actions, which can be controlled.

### Siblings

Siblings react differently, depending on their age at the time of the patient's onset of illness and their own resources. Feelings may include confusion over the ill sibling's behavior, fear of possible violence, anger and resentment over the preferential treatment and parental attention given the ill sibling, sadness over the loss of the relationship, worries that one might become ill oneself, concerns about future liability and custodianship for the ill sibling, and worries about genetic risks to one's own offspring. As already discussed, siblings may take on a lifelong custodial responsibility, which in itself becomes a major occupational role (see "Family Caregivers," later in this chapter). A disproportionate number of siblings of the mentally ill enter helping professions, working specifically with the mentally ill; their childhood may have prepared them to tolerate strange behaviors and to read cues exceptionally well (80). On the other hand, siblings and children of the mentally ill may have difficulty with assertiveness or with setting boundaries on inappropriate behavior, having experienced so much of it.

### Spouses and Partners

Spouses and partners of persons who become mentally ill may wonder whether they have made a bad choice and whether they should leave the relationship. Guilt, fears of personal responsibility in causing the breakdown, grief over the lost relationship, and concerns about any children are common. Spouses may have difficulty setting limits and expectations for the ill spouse, not understanding which behaviors are the result of illness and which are not.

### Children

Children react differently, depending on their age and level of cognitive development. Very young children may not recognize that the ill parent's behavior is abnormal, because it is the only thing they know. Older children recognize more clearly the absence of nurture and the loss of a nurturing relationship. Some may wonder if they caused the parent's illness by their own misbehavior; indeed, some ill parents accuse them of this. Others step into the role of custodian, caring for the ill parent and fulfilling that person's household responsibilities. Children may be afraid of the ill parent who threatens or who is violent or unpredictable.

Children in families with a mentally ill parent or sibling may take on roles of custodian, bystander, or adversary (80). The *custodian* serves as a miniparent, is super-responsible, and fills in for the ill or preoccupied parent. The *bystander* is more detached; less central to meeting the needs of the family, he or she can coolly analyze the situation or may just try to stay out of the way. The *adversary* acts out the unexpressed tensions of the family; those in this role may be seen as trouble-makers. It is not surprising that the adversary may be the one to bring the family to the attention of those who can help; by getting in trouble in school or with the law, adversaries attract intervention.

## FAMILY CAREGIVERS

The caregiver is the person in the home who provides physical and emotional care to the ill person. Typically, the caregiver is female—based on the general social expectation of the nurturing role of women—but men also serve as caregivers, typically for spouses or partners with dementia or with AIDS. Perceived value of caregiving as a role varies by culture; black women are more likely than whites to take on the role because it is highly valued in their culture (80). There may be more than one caregiver, with responsibilities shared by a split schedule or by a division of responsibilities. The role of caregiver cannot be assigned by outsiders; the health professional cannot assume that someone wants to take on this job, which carries significant stresses and requires great personal sacrifice. Caregivers can feel neglected and burdened; with limited skills and energy, the caregiver can feel overwhelmed. Other family members may resent the caregiver's control of the situation or may expect as a matter of course that the caregiver will remain in the role willingly and indefinitely. On the other hand, many caregivers take on their responsibilities gradually, without relinquishing other roles within the family and the community; they may not even consciously label themselves as caregivers (63).

The OT practitioner can offer the caregiver information, support, and advice. Specifically, the occupational therapist can acknowledge the importance of the caregiver role; encourage caregivers to take care of themselves via support groups, outside activities, and respite care; and assist in finding resources to help with some tasks (63). To do this effectively, the OT or OTA must learn from the caregiver what the family considers important and what compensatory strategies the caregiver has already attempted. Too often, recommendations from therapists are rejected by the family because the recommendations do not address what the family considers important (31). Box 9-4 contains questions that may be useful in revealing how the family views the situation.

Clark and associates (18) have identified four primary types of interactions engaged in by OT practitioners with caregivers: caring, partnering, informing, and directing. *Caring* demonstrates friendliness and support for the caregiver and interest in the caregiver's well-being. *Partnering* engages caregivers in decision making; this includes seeking input from the caregiver and acknowledging and praising independent problem solving by the caregiver. *Informing* focuses on giving, obtaining, or clarifying information. *Directing* aims to engage the caregiver in carrying out the treatment; this may include giving instruction or advice. Box 9-5 provides examples of interactions of each type. Caregivers may perceive directing and informing as bossy; this is most likely when the practitioner comes from or falls into a medical model (18). Each type of interaction has its place in therapist–caregiver relations, and each is made more effective when the practitioner aims for a collaborative relationship that acknowledges and embraces the commitment, expertise, and skills of the caregiver.

In 1979 a group of families began meeting to support each other in coping with the mental illnesses of their loved ones; the group became known as the National Alliance for the Mentally Ill (NAMI). NAMI, which has a toll-free number in the United States, encourages membership by mental health professionals. Research is a priority for NAMI, which conducts surveys and funds major studies. NAMI provides education to families and consumers. An example is a multisession course taught by NAMI members to families who desire help in coping with the behavior of their ill member. NAMI has affiliates in most states and convenes local support groups and larger regional meetings. By joining NAMI and its state affiliates, the OT practitioner can gain a much deeper understanding of consumers and their families.

## CULTURAL DIFFERENCE

Increasingly, OT practitioners encounter patients, clients, and consumers from a variety of cultures. Culture can be confused with race, ethnicity, religion, and other things but it is none of these. *Culture* is the learned patterns of interactions and the shared beliefs of a particular group. For example, North Americans as a group have a shared belief in

**BOX 9-4**

**QUESTIONS FOR EFFECTIVE LIAISONS WITH CAREGIVERS**

To **learn** what is meaningful, ask the caregiver the following:

- What is a typical day like for you?
- What most worries or concerns you?
- How is it now versus before?
- How do you manage your day?
- What are your feelings about the future?
- What are some of your successes here?

To **verify** what is meaningful, ask or say to the caregiver the following:

- Is this how you see it?
- So you are saying that when [______] happens, you get frustrated.
- It sounds as though that really upset you.

To **think** reflectively, ask yourself the following:

- What do I see happening in this home?
- Do I understand the perspective of the family members?
- Are my views the same as those of the family caregiver(s)?
- In what way are my values in this care situation the same or different from those of the family caregiver(s)?

To **plan intervention,** ask yourself the following:

- What does the disability or impairment mean to the patient and family member?
- How does the family member experience the caregiving activity?
- On the basis of an understanding of meaning, what is an appropriate treatment strategy to support the efforts of this family?

Adapted with permission from Gitlin LN, Corcoran M, Leinmiller-Eckhardt S. Understanding the family perspective: An ethnographic framework for providing occupational therapy in the home. Am J Occup Ther 1995;49:802–809.

personal freedom as a right. Box 9-6 shows examples of culturally derived patterns of interaction shared in the culture of the United States. All of these patterns are *learned behaviors* that belong to a particular culture. These behaviors may cause discomfort to persons from other cultures, as McGruder (60) points out. In East Africa, for example, anything less than beckoning with the whole hand in a large and generous gesture is considered insulting. Someone who is accustomed to averting eyes and maintaining a neutral expression feels quite uncomfortable with being smiled at constantly and looked directly in the eye. And a person whose cultural experience of business greetings is a hug or a kiss on each cheek may find a handshake very distant and cold.

Relating effectively to people who have a different set of expectations for social behavior is a skill that can be learned. When a health care practitioner meets with a client of a different culture, the main objectives should be to make the person comfortable, to communicate effectively, and to engage the person in working on a program of care. Yet because of cultural differences, practitioners

BOX 9-5

**FOUR TYPES OF INTERACTIONS WITH CAREGIVERS**

**Caring:** building rapport and alliance with the caregiver

- You are putting a lot of effort into making this work.
- I like the way you've arranged the living room.
- It's a lot of work to care for someone like [______].

**Partnering:** involving caregivers in decision making

- What would you like [______] to be able to do for herself?
- I notice that today you have really solved a lot of problems so that [______] can be safe here while you are at work. That's really good.

**Informing:** gathering information, explaining rationales or treatment procedures, clarifying information

- In what ways does [______] contribute to chores around the house?
- Have you considered taking the knobs off the stove burners when you are not using the stove? This will help keep [______] from trying to use the stove.
- He might accidentally start a fire or burn himself.

**Directing:** instructing and advising the caregiver

- I think he can dress himself if you lay out the clothes and remind him to put each item on. Just saying the name of the garment, like undershorts, can remind him. Would you like to try that?
- If you ask him to do his chores sometimes but let him not do them at others, it will be hard to get him to do them when you are pressed for time and really need him to. Do you see why?

Adapted with permission from Clark CA, Corcoran M, Gitlin LN. An exploratory study of how occupational therapists develop therapeutic relationships with family caregivers. Am J Occup Ther 1995;49:587–593.

may inadvertently behave in ways that confuse, embarrass, or offend the client. Thus it is essential for the OTA student (like other health care practitioners) to observe carefully, to ask questions tactfully and humbly, and to learn the cultures and customs of their clients and colleagues. Even before this, the student may take some time to consider the dominant European-American culture and the assumptions it carries.

Bonder and Gurley (9) point out that older adults are more likely to retain cultural traditions. Thus, to improve health outcomes, it is important to find out what traditions and values are important to the consumer. Because of differences in

BOX 9-6

**EXAMPLES OF CULTURAL NORMS FOR BEHAVIOR IN THE UNITED STATES**

- **Business greeting:** Make eye contact; shake hands firmly and briefly while standing 1 to 2 feet away.
- **Communicating "come with me:"** Make eye contact; arch eyebrows; beckon with flexed index finger with palm up (supinated).
- **General social behavior to strangers:** Smile; be pleasant; say "Have a nice day" or "Have a good one."

the way health and health care are conceptualized in the culture of origin, older adults in particular may not receive optimum care. Furthermore, cultural misunderstandings may interfere with the person following instructions or returning for visits. For example, in Puerto Rican and other Hispanic cultures, the extended family is valued and involved in all aspects of life. Insisting on interviewing an older person of Puerto Rican background in the absence of family members is almost certainly a recipe for disaster. This is only one example. Bonder and Gurley note that an attitude of "cultural curiosity" is essential and that developing specific expertise regarding cultures in one's community of care is useful.

## The Immigration Experience

The population of the United States has increased dramatically through immigration. In 1997, for example, the *New York Times* noted that the proportion of foreign-born persons living in New York City was 36.1%, the largest population of ethnically varied immigrants in its history (83). Since 2000, new immigrants are settling in the suburbs, with a 21% increase in persons of Asian descent living in the suburbs around New York (28). At one extreme some new immigrants resist assimilation into American culture, clinging to their native languages, customs, and cuisines; at the other extreme are those who are eager to become American in every way. Most immigrants seem to tread a middle path. The technology of the information age and the availability of air transportation have made it possible for them to maintain an ongoing relationship with their countries of origin via phone, fax, videophone, e-mail, international money wiring, and frequent visits (83). Furthermore, the immigration of successive generations to the United States may span several decades, with periods of residence alternating between the two countries. It is common for parents to send their children "home" (e.g., to India, Trinidad, Mexico) to learn "proper" behavior or for rigorous schooling. Important life events, such as weddings, births, deaths, and burials, may take place in the country of origin. In other words, an ongoing identification with one's native country may co-exist with an American lifestyle.

The children of first-generation immigrants may undergo stress from the conflicting demands of their parents (and the traditions of the original culture) and the expectations of American peers. This stress is compounded in adolescence, a time for questioning and confirming one's identity. Immigrant parents, in reaction to their offspring's interest in and attempts to adopt American culture and behaviors, may also suffer distress. At one extreme of the generations, the oldest members may stubbornly adhere to native traditions; at the other, the youngest are likely to be listening to popular music and wearing the latest fashions.

Blending and adopting dual or multiple cultures is one way some immigrants cope with this. For example, young people from traditional Indian families may tolerate or even seek arranged marriages for themselves, sometimes marrying a person who is still living in India. A young Indian-American woman may wear a designer suit to work in an investment firm yet wear a *salwar kameez* (long loose tunic over pants) at home. Furthermore, she may live across the hall from her mother-in-law, for whom she prepares traditional Indian foods and to whom she defers in decisions relating to home and family (83).

The OT practitioner working with immigrants should appreciate that there is much to be learned—and that little can be assumed—about the values, customs, and life situations of these clients. In many countries and cultures, the concept of mental illness as we know it does not exist; therefore, to speak about it with the patient and the family as such is counterproductive. Skilled clinicians instead learn to phrase their expectations for the patient and families in ways that can be understood and appreciated by them. For example, a psychiatrist, himself Chinese, speaking with the parents of a bright Chinese high school student who was hallucinating and punching walls, never mentions the possibility of schizophrenia or antipsychotic medication. He instead directs them to have their son take "these little pills every day for a week to help his motivation" (56).

## Cultural Differences in Diagnosis

Mental disorders (indeed physical disorders also) are not thought of in all cultures in the same way as in the United States. Fadiman (27) in a fascinating and award-winning account, tells the story of a Hmong refugee family, living in central California, with a young child who had epilepsy. Because epilepsy is regarded in the Hmong culture as a mystical and sacred trance state, the family was inconsistent in applying the remedies provided by the doctors, nurses, and health care team. Problems of language translation, cultural mistrust, and other factors (on both sides) resulted in a frustrating experience for the medical team. Although the child eventually sustained severe brain damage from high fevers and prolonged seizures, the family did not seem unhappy with the outcome and continued to dress and bathe and clothe and feed the girl in the highest standard of their culture. She held a place of honor in the household.

The *Diagnostic and Statistical Manual of Mental Disorders,* fourth edition, text revision *(DSM-IV-TR)* contains an appendix describing other aspects of culture and a glossary of terms for mental conditions that occur only in certain cultures (5). For example, the term *nervios* is a general term for "emotional vulnerability" used by Latinos. *Susto,* another Latino term, defined as "soul loss," may cause symptoms similar to major depressive disorder.

## Populations in Economic Distress

Too often ignored is the effect of low socioeconomic status and limited financial means. People who do not have much money or education also have a different experience and view of the world from those of the more privileged. This difference in experience and perspective affects their participation in therapy.

### Economic Marginalization and Poverty

Health care practitioners, most of whom come from middle class backgrounds, may have difficulty appreciating the role of economics in the health care of poor people. This is true even for practitioners who share a minority race or ethnic identification with their patients; differences in social class and economic power inevitably lead to disparities in services (8). Not having enough money may mean any or all of the following:

- Missing appointments when there's not enough money for carfare
- Not having a phone at home so not making telephone calls as requested
- Living in a place where it's not safe to be out after dark
- Using a single sink for both kitchen work and bathing
- Doing laundry infrequently and by hand
- Eating for economy rather than for nutrition

OT practitioners working with people who are living in or near poverty should carefully consider the effects of limited financial means on the consumer's and family's response to the treatment; often what looks like uncooperative behavior is instead a combination of the inability to comply for financial reasons and embarrassment or unwillingness to admit it.

Low-income families may look very different from the generic nuclear family, with members of the extended family assuming major roles in nurturing and leadership. Sometimes the key family member is an aunt, grandparent, or cousin because parents may be absent or unable to fulfill their roles; this can be confusing to health care practitioners from more traditional backgrounds, who may wonder where the family is and who may have trouble identifying key people with whom to collaborate (53).

Yet another effect of poverty, especially long-term poverty over more than one generation of the family, is a pervasive sense of helplessness and the expectation that things will never change. Fatalism of this sort causes clients to view as silly or meaningless any attempt to set goals or move beyond their experience. In this situation, the practitioner must carefully observe the consumer's circumstances and encourage the person to take the lead in setting goals; even so, the person may continue to feel like an outsider to the situation and may fail to connect to the idea of making an improvement (51).

## Homeless Persons

Homelessness, an extreme form of economic marginalization, is a way of life for many of the chronically mentally ill who would have been confined to public psychiatric institutions 50 years ago. As discussed in Chapters 1 and 7, deinstitutionalization released psychiatric patients from the restrictive environment of the state mental hospital without providing appropriate community supports. Immediately after deinstitutionalization, released mental patients moved into the least desirable community housing. Owing to the real estate boom and speculation since the 1970s, older low-cost housing is continuously destroyed to be replaced by more profitable, more expensive homes. Lacking both financial resources and cognitive skills, displaced patients have difficulty finding affordable housing. Thus, though "free," many persons with mental illness are materially worse off in the community, where they lack shelter and structure, than they were in public institutions.

Working with the homeless mentally ill person presents many challenges. The fact that the person has no stable, nurturing environment cannot be ignored or wished away. Many of the homeless mentally ill are dual-diagnosis patients, having both psychiatric and substance-abuse disorders. In New York City, it is not unusual to encounter the homeless mentally ill Vietnam War veteran who has multiple comorbid conditions (diagnoses of personality disorder, post-traumatic stress disorder, human immunodeficiency virus [HIV] infection, and multiple substance-abuse problems). Compounding their multiple diagnoses and homelessness, many in this population have serious physical problems, have been convicted of crimes, or have spent time in jail when no other placement was available. Depending on state and local laws, the homeless person who resists assistance and refuses shelter may be allowed to remain on the streets even in freezing and inclement weather.

Homelessness as a lifestyle requires ingenuity: Finding shelter in woods or culverts or overhangs of buildings, scavenging return-deposit bottles, begging, and busking (playing music for tips) all are occupations of the homeless. Those who have had some success at these occupations find it difficult to accept treatment, preferring life on the streets to unpredictable interventions by mental health providers. The homeless person understands and has adjusted to street life. Getting involved with the mental health system risks disruption of established patterns without providing anything better in the long term.

Pritchett (74)[1] described her work as associate director of Project Reachout, a program for the mentally ill homeless in New York City's Upper West Side. Case managers in vans roam through Central Park, looking for likely candidates for the program. Because these individuals are notoriously difficult to engage, staff members approach in a manner that allows the person to keep a distance. Through repeated contacts and offers of sandwiches and other tangibles, the targeted individual can be induced to speak with staff. Once engaged, the person is invited to the offices of Project Reachout. To get into a van with strangers, regardless of what they promise,

[1]Pritchett may be reached at Project Reachout, 593 Columbus Avenue, New York, NY 10024.

requires a considerable leap of faith on the part of the homeless person, who may have experience of forced hospitalization. The staff member who makes the original contact becomes the case manager and provides the person with food, coffee, clothing, showers, and aid in obtaining entitlements. Working on a personal contract, once trust has been established, the worker then introduces the need to take medication. The client must agree to this and follow through before the worker will make a referral to permanent shelter. Once a person has been placed in a shelter, a letter certifying ongoing participation in the project is given each day as a condition of continuing to stay in the shelter.

As soon as clients are brought to Project Reachout, the staff begin interventions to help them move from homelessness to community living. Pritchett remarked that the change from homelessness to a home is "as disorienting as suffering a CVA [cerebral vascular accident], in terms of its effects on lifestyle." Clients are given clean clothing and are encouraged to save their dirty clothes and launder them weekly. A mock single-room occupancy (SRO) hotel room at the center is used to demonstrate how a room in a shelter might be set up and used. A cooking group using communal facilities such as those found in SROs orients the client to kitchen skills and teaches survival skills (that food left around will be stolen). Clients are taken on short shopping trips for food, clothing, and small appliances. Activity groups and training sessions about grooming (haircuts, nail care, and so on) and safety (sex education, sexually transmitted diseases [STDs], use of condoms) are provided.

Various structured leisure and expressive activities are included in the day program. In the early stages, more psychotic clients may remain outside the groups, using the offices of the project as a safe harbor and coffee shop. Pritchett believes that the success of outreach projects depends on tapping into the values of the clients, many of whom would like to work, have a home, and be a "regular" person with a social life and a family. Viewed from the model of human occupation, many of the mentally ill homeless have developed a work identity as entrepreneurs, with a focus of panhandling, collecting and redeeming bottles, and other marginal but materially productive activities. To attract such clients, the outreach program must offer something that meets the same esteem needs. A work program in a church basement and a variety of real-world jobs with stipends have been developed by Project Reachout. Even so, some clients find their prior homeless occupations more attractive than the substitute occupations offered by the project.

Barth (6) points out that honesty is the key to successful treatment of the homeless substance abuser. In the shelter program of the Bowery Residents Committee in New York, clients are required to become clean and dry (to stop using drugs and drinking), or they are not allowed to stay. They are told that their success depends on having a brain and nervous system that can function. Once free of intoxicating substances, clients can begin rehabilitation.

The practitioner must be focused on the homeless person's concerns and perceptions to learn how the client sees the world and to understand what the client feels is important. Issues of particular importance are how the person feels about medication; which ones are working and which are not; whether the person has abused substances, and if so, what it does for him or her; and what the person is afraid of and hopes for. Obtaining answers to such questions requires listening. Often the truth is revealed only after the practitioner establishes a solid relationship with the person (7).

As OT practitioners, our goal is to help people achieve and maintain the highest level of occupational functioning possible for them. Thus we must be creative, compassionate, and flexible in our understanding of the customs and culture of the homeless, and we must adapt our interventions so that mentally ill homeless persons learn something that will actually be useful to them. A major role for OT with the homeless mentally ill is in helping them recognize and resolve problems of everyday living, such as obtaining and taking prescription medications, finding and caring for clothing, and managing money. In every case, the skills taught must be targeted to the specific person's situation (33).

For example, learning safety and problem-solving skills in obtaining food is valued by homeless clients, whereas going to classes on doing laundry using a domestic washer and dryer may seem quite fantastic and irrelevant. Barth (6) described her work with a group of homeless substance abusers in a men's shelter in New York City. One activity especially valued by the group was the preparation in the shelter kitchen of simple food for an Alcoholics Anonymous (AA) meeting. The AA group, in which these men previously felt inadequate, welcomed their contribution, and the result for the homeless men was an instant increase in status and recognition. Another opportunity for status is provided through computer skills access and guided learning, encouraging participants to engage with a technology that may seem alien and intimidating (62).

Homeless families experience extreme disruption of routines and patterns (79). Relations between parents and children are strained when the parent is powerless to provide basic shelter, food, and clothing. Children may attend school sporadically or move from school to school as the shelter residence changes. Women heads of household may lack skills and resources for obtaining work and childcare, for parenting their children, and simply for understanding how to think about goals for themselves (46).

The context of a homeless shelter is challenging for the therapy provider. It is common for residents to have multiple medical and sensory problems that have not been addressed; dental, optical, and audiology care may be needed. In addition, the staff of the shelter need to maintain order and safety; and for this reason, many rules exist that interfere with spontaneity and family authority. Children may be required to be much quieter than they would be in a home environment. Timing of meals and of lights out is institutionalized and not under the family's control (29).

Some occupational therapy interventions offered to homeless families include parenting skills training, parenting skills discussion groups, organizational skills, journaling and self-expression activities, sensory soothing techniques for children who are upset or disruptive, volunteer and paid jobs with part-time and flexible hours, and youth development programs (33, 46, 79).

## SOCIAL PROBLEMS—ENDING THE CYCLE OF VIOLENCE

It is sad that violence has become a daily feature of modern life in the United States, as the television news informs us all too frequently. To imagine a more peaceful world, free of shootings, bombings, beatings, and war is a beginning. But we can also work for peace in many ways in our practice of occupational therapy.

### Domestic Violence

Domestic violence is a complex social problem involving women, men, and families. The Injury Center of the Centers for Disease Control and Prevention (14) has classified the following types: child maltreatment, intimate partner violence, sexual violence, suicide, and youth violence. Addressing domestic violence demands persistent and skillful attention to the dynamics that perpetuate violence.

Women are most often the victims of abuse, but men may also be victimized by women. Violence may occur between same sex partners and between different generations. The victim, the abuser, and the witnesses (often children) are all affected (65). Contrary to popular belief, domestic violence is not restricted to persons of lower socioeconomic status or lower educational levels. Six types of abuse are recognized: physical, emotional, sexual, economic, destruction of property or pets, and stalking (40). When the abuser is the caregiver of a dependent, other forms of abuse are possible: rough handling, neglect, abandonment, violation of rights, infantalization, inappropriate touching, and isolation (40).

The cycle of violence, described by Walker (88) consists of three phases that are repeated: *(a)* buildup of tension, *(b)* violent actions, and *(c)* contrition and appeasement of the victim. The cycle then starts again. Escalation of violence is likely, unless the victim receives appropriate intervention, which almost always involves separation from the abuser, at least for a period of time.

The victim of violence is vulnerable to depression and post-traumatic stress disorder (PTSD). She (most victims are women) is likely to feel terrorized and hypervigilant, always alert to the possibility of another attack. It is quite common for the victim to identify with the abuser or to blame herself. Self-help groups are effective for opening discussion and understanding and for building a sense of community (20).

Occupational therapy interventions should begin with assessment by the occupational therapist. Assessments may focus on roles and habits, safety and support in the environment, the person's sense of volition, and specific skills (39, 48). Interventions may address assertiveness, anger management, emotion identification, daily routines and organization, goal setting and task management, and many other aspects of occupational functioning (40). Victims of intimate partner violence need to acquire skills that will allow them to be employed and self-sufficient and thus able move themselves and their children into a safe and productive lifestyle. Interventions include specific skills training and assistance with supported and competitive employment (41).

Gutman et al. (34) described programming for women victims of domestic violence who possibly had brain injury. The program addressed the areas of safety planning, community safety, safe sex practices, assertiveness and advocacy training, anger management, stress management, boundary establishment and limit setting, vocational/educational skills, money management, housing application, leisure exploration, hygiene, medication routine, and nutrition. Practical daily living skills such as banking, driving a car, using public transportation, using a budget, or finding leisure opportunities are also important (48). Any of these interventions may be provided by the OTA.

Frequently, victims of abuse will not come forward unless asked specifically about such abuse. If the OTA suspects a client is a victim of violence, based on physical injury or other evidence, the client should be asked. Proper and complete documentation of the situation is essential, as is referral to a supervisor or other mental health professional (20). Victims should be provided with information about local and national hotlines and about shelters. State laws require occupational therapy personnel to act on reported abuse (40). For more detailed information on violence prevention programs generally and on occupational therapy interventions, the reader is highly encouraged to consult the references (14, 39–41, 65).

## Youth and School Violence

Homicide is leading cause of death for African Americans aged 10 to 24, the second leading cause of death for Hispanic youth, and the third for American Indians (15). The leading cause of death for white males in this age group is automobile accidents (a different form of violence). Males are more frequently involved in violence than are females. Youth and school violence may be connected to domestic violence. Children who act violently may have witnessed violence in the home. Other factors have been implicated, including authoritarian childrearing, peer associations, and community factors. Programs for prevention of school violence use techniques of peer mediation and conflict resolution, attempting to reduce risk by increasing respect and facilitating communication. Occupational therapy could be a very effective addition to youth violence prevention, by providing alternative healthy occupations for leisure time and by assessing for individual factors (such as cognitive problems or impaired volition) that may predispose youth to violence. Another emphasis might involve teaching emotion identification, assertiveness, anger management, and other specific coping skills.

## MEDICAL PROBLEMS AND PHYSICAL DISABILITIES

There are several reasons we are including physical disabilities in a text on mental health. First, psychosocial factors may be contributing factors in physical disabilities. Second, some physical conditions (traumatic brain injury [TBI], for example) have significant behavioral symptoms. Third, *any* physical disability or disease changes a person's life and requires coping. Because occupational therapists are concerned with the occupational life of the person, we take a holistic view, accounting for psychosocial and cognitive responses even when the major presenting problems seem primarily to be physical.

### Psychosocial Factors

As stated earlier, psychosocial factors may contribute to disability. This is obvious in cases of substance abuse that lead to physical trauma and prolonged disability (e.g., falls, automobile accidents). Consumers benefit from attention to their substance abuse problems and from frank discussion of the risks associated with continued use. Because the abused substance may be central to the person's coping behaviors, resistance to this message is expected. Underlying psychosocial problems (including major mental illnesses for which the person was self-medicating) may also be present. See Chapter 6 for more discussion of substance abuse.

Inadequate psychosocial skills, limited awareness or insight, or poor judgment may contribute to disability. For example, Aja (2) described a case of overuse syndrome in which the worker continued to injure herself because she lacked the coping skills to negotiate a better situation for herself. The patient was a lonely woman who perceived her only social support to be at her part-time job in a print shop. From her perspective, she *had* to continue her self-injurious work because otherwise she would lose her friends. This is a case in which the major intervention for a physical disability was instructing the patient in coping skills, a psychosocial component.

### Psychosocial Consequences

The second reason we are including physical disabilities is that some have associated psychosocial consequences. The most prominent such diagnosis is TBI, in which behavioral disorders frequently result. Depending on the area or areas of the brain affected, the TBI patient may be aggressive or demanding; seductive; inappropriate in communications; impulsive; and inattentive to grooming, hygiene, and basic good manners. The Allen cognitive disabilities model can be employed to assess functional level. The occupational therapist must try to determine which of the patient's behaviors are likely to be changed and which ones are relatively fixed and require compensation. Compensatory strategies are used to limit confusing or irrelevant environmental stimuli and to focus the patient on the desired task or goal. The neurobehavioral approach can be used to change behavior; positive behavior is reinforced and negative behavior is ignored so long as it is not a danger to the patient or to others (82).

Memory impairment can be significant, interfering with the person's ability to benefit from a behavioral approach if the person cannot recognize that a specific behavior led to specific consequences. Alternative techniques such as *antecedent management,* in which a consistent sequence of environmental events or cues is used to initiate and shape behavior, are described by Yuen (92).

## Transformative Life Challenges

The third reason for considering psychosocial aspects of physical disability is that the knowledge of illness and physical disability changes a person's life. The first reaction may be denial, with more complex and intense feelings following. The emotional response to disability and the process of adjustment are described elsewhere (12, 25, 76). In addition to the psychological adjustment, the person experiences grief at loss of functions and faces an adjustment in occupational roles. Sanford (76) writes eloquently of the internal transformations that lead to acceptance and movement toward a new sense of self.

Reading Sanford's words, and learning his history, one is struck by the power of the lived body and the mind to create a future that to many may seem impractical or fantastic. As therapists we must remember that we can serve best as partners and collaborators on our patients' journeys to wholeness and that we must encourage and help them to lead the way.

## Psychiatric Occupational Therapy

Medical/surgical occupational therapy was a recognized specialty within the field until the mid-1970s. Psychiatric occupational therapy practitioners have much to offer medical/surgical patients. Provided psychiatric diagnoses are used and a separate referral is given, patients can be seen on the same day by occupational therapy staff from physical medicine and psychiatry (54). Appropriate interventions may include use of expressive activities such as collage (particularly useful for patients who cannot speak and for those experiencing emotional reactions to their conditions) and production of small craft items as gifts. Activities chosen should be appropriate for bedside and not create a housekeeping problem for nursing staff. When possible, therapy staff should help patients renew connections to valued life occupations and roles (or explore new ones). Leslie (54) reports on an opera singer hospitalized for a liver transplant, who found his way back to health and to his career. The therapist brought a CD of the patient's favorite opera to his room. This led to spontaneous singing (at first very weak and with lots of coughing) but ultimately to requests from nursing staff for songs. Other therapy for the patient included cognitive activities, memory training, and crafts.

A research study showed that hospitalized persons with physical disabilities reported significantly fewer occupational roles in their future than did persons living in the community or hospitalized persons with psychosocial

**POINT-OF-VIEW**

***Then there are the quiet deaths. How about the day you realized that you weren't going to be an astronaut or the queen of Sheba? Feel the silent distance between yourself and how you felt as a child, between yourself and those feelings of wonder and splendor and trust. Feel your mature fondness for who you once were, and your current need to protect innocence wherever you might find it. The silence that surrounds the loss of innocence is a most serious death, and yet it is necessary for the onset of maturity.***

—Matthew Sanford (76), yoga teacher, paraplegic since age 13

- How does Matthew's story embody the recovery perspective?
- Does hearing his story change your view of what is possible for people with disabilities?
- If his disability were psychiatric, would you have a different opinion of his job as a yoga teacher?

disabilities (22). Is this because they were physically incapable of returning to work or of resuming past hobbies? Or is it an expression of hopelessness and depression? Or is it because OT practitioners in physical disabilities settings emphasize the restoration of motor, perceptual, and other physical functions and do not help their patients reconnect to valued former roles or envision new roles for the future?

Physical disability may mean a change in social roles and difficulties with social and community integration. A disfiguring condition involving the face may lead to social isolation. More than anything, the person with a physical disability desires to be accepted and to be a member of the community, treated as normally as possible. But the stigma and associated compensations by others may be tiresome. As one adolescent with a spinal cord injury said, "It sounds so simple, but just have a place for them in the class. It makes it easier to just have a place to go and sit like a normal person, and even aisles, where you can go up and bring your paper up to the desk. It sounds little, but it's not" (64, p. 311).

Community integration is even more difficult for persons with behavioral and cognitive deficits. For example, persons with TBI are often poorly accepted by the community because of their disinhibited sexual behavior, odd manners, difficulty controlling and expressing emotions appropriately, and so on. Poor social skills may prevent the development of new relationships, and the person can become increasingly isolated and more prone to depression. This trend tends to become more pronounced over time (11). Clearly, these patients would benefit from increased rehabilitation efforts in cognitive and social skills.

Recognizing that role change is a generally undesired consequence of physical disability, therapists can help their clients identify and develop meaningful goals by using instruments such as the *Client-Oriented Role Evaluation (CORE)* (86). This evaluation, designed for use by rehabilitation therapists, helps the client and therapist understand the role change that follows the disability.

## Coping Strategies

How does a person respond to and cope with a disability? And how can coping be improved? Gage (30) described the *appraisal method of coping,* or how the person appraises and evaluates the experience. Appraisal consists of evaluating first the event or experience in terms of whether it is positive or negative (primary appraisal) and second the resources available for coping with the event (secondary appraisal). Resources may be personal, social, financial, and so on.

The appraisal is then enacted in one or more of three categories of coping response: emotion focused, problem focused, and perception focused. Emotion-focused responses are used to control the emotional reaction. Problem-focused responses emphasize changing the environment or the interaction with the environment to reduce stress. Perception-focused responses work on changing the person's perception of the event. This cognitive-behavioral analysis (see Chapter 2) is useful for understanding how patients respond to therapy and for predicting how well they will carry over or generalize skills to the community. For example, avoidant emotion-focused responses, such as denial, wishful thinking, and self-blaming, are associated with high levels of stress and poor adjustment (30). This suggests a role for OT in teaching coping strategies that facilitate generalization of skills and community adjustment.

A related concern is the patient's motivation for treatment; with rehabilitation dollars rationed, therapists must quickly evaluate the physically disabled person's rehabilitation potential and estimate achievable functional outcomes. Despite therapists' concern over patients' motivation for treatment, only a small percentage of OT practitioners in physical disabilities settings ask their patients to describe their own goals and set their own priorities for treatment (13, 66). Simply interviewing the patient about goals or conducting a client-centered assessment such as the *Canadian Occupational Performance Measure (COPM)* can yield this information; the OTA may be asked to assist.

## Specific Medical Conditions

In the early history of the occupational therapy profession, specific therapies were often prescribed for specific conditions. This was characterized as a cookbook approach. Bearing in mind that the following recommendations are not recipes to be followed exactly, let's consider two medical conditions in which psychosocial occupational therapy can be helpful.

### HIV and AIDS

AIDS is a complex medical condition involving the progressive destruction of the body's immune system and consequent vulnerability to other diseases, such as pneumonia and Kaposi's sarcoma, a form of cancer. The virus (HIV) that causes AIDS is transmitted through infected blood and bodily fluids, primarily through unprotected sexual contact and intravenously by infected needles. The material in this chapter addresses the psychosocial aspects of AIDS. The physical aspects of AIDS are addressed in most OT textbooks on physical disabilities and in several of the references listed at the end of this chapter. Information on universal precautions and infection control can be found in Chapter 12.

Persons with HIV infection or AIDS constitute a special population for several reasons. First, the risks of disease transmission to the immune-compromised and vulnerable patient and of HIV infection to others require scrupulous attention to infection control measures. Second, persons with AIDS or HIV infection must adjust to the reality of the disease. For some this includes a coming to terms with how their own actions (unsafe sex, intravenous drug use) or the actions of others (spouses and partners, blood banks) exposed them to infection. For many, ongoing grief over the deaths of many friends, acquaintances, and family members compounds this. For all, it means adjusting to the prospect of diminishing function, the role of patient, perhaps the loss of valued roles, physical deterioration, and for those who do not elect or cannot afford to follow the drug treatment regimen, early death. Finally, many persons with AIDS have dementia. AIDS-related dementia is similar to other dementias, often starting with mild signs such as forgetfulness and social withdrawal and leading in time to physical withdrawal, motor paralysis, and total indifference and inability to communicate with others. Approaches to cognitive problems, including dementia, are covered in Chapters 11 and 22.

Although the psychiatric symptoms of AIDS (depression and dementia) respond to the standard treatments (drugs, psychotherapy, environmental and activity modification), these patients require additional attention to the stress and disruption associated with the illness. Viewed from the model of human occupation, AIDS disrupts at all levels. Belief in self often diminishes, valued roles are lost over time, performance skills deteriorate, the sphere of interests shrinks, and the patient's world becomes much smaller. The social reaction of others who fear infection or who are repelled by the patient's behavior accelerates this process. Persons with AIDS may lose their jobs or be denied health benefits. Although legal remedies are available, the patient who faces the prospect of premature death has little reason to believe that the problem can be resolved in his or her lifetime.

Denton (21) proposed roles for OT intervention at three phases in the illness. At *phase I*, or *pre-AIDS*, intervention focuses on psychosocial support and information about disease transmission. The person who is recently diagnosed as HIV-positive benefits from a supportive relationship that permits the expression of grief and anxiety and the development of coping strategies. Stress management and training in problem solving are most effective at this point. Information about safe sex and values clarification about responsibility to keep others safe from infection are crucial. The focus should be on helping the individual to maintain as normal a life as possible and to develop coping skills.

At *phase 2*, or *early to midstage disease*, the patient, now physically ill, requires environmental modifications, adaptive equipment, and other rehabilitation measures. At this time, the patient may value activities that promote a feeling of self-worth and of contributing to the social network, according to Denton. Schindler (77) discusses the importance of helping the AIDS patient continue to participate in valued roles and continue to present himself or herself as a useful and involved member of society. For example, a young woman who is physically wasted and depressed may need assistance to purchase new clothing and to care for her appearance.

Another role for OT with patients at phases 1 and 2 is provision of health-promotion activities. Gutterman (35) describes strong interest among patients in topics such as skin care, nutrition, yoga, therapeutic touch, massage, and alternative holistic health modalities.

At *phase 3*, or *end-stage treatment*, the patient, who is approaching death, benefits from continuing to participate at any level in activities of interest. Expressive media may be helpful in engaging the person to release and explore feelings. Piemme and Bolle (72) recommend that staff working with patients at this stage of illness prevent professional burnout by strategies such as weekly support groups, multidisciplinary meetings, and other activities that allow health care providers to discharge feelings with each other.

The American Occupational Therapy Association (AOTA) provides guidelines for OT interventions with this population (4). Practitioners who work with this population are at risk for burnout and are likely to benefit from learning and regularly using stress management techniques (45).

## Chronic Pain

The OT literature contains relatively little about the patient who has chronic pain. Long-term pain, which may last for decades and vary in intensity, is associated with a range of diagnoses, including birth defects, back injury, spinal cord injury, arthritis, fibromyalgia, and cancer. Commonly and unfortunately, pain is often undermedicated; patients could be much more comfortable if appropriate doses of pain medication were given at closer intervals (49). On the other extreme, recovering substance abusers and others who avoid drugs and alcohol (e.g., for religious reasons) may reject prescribed pain medication (57). From a psychosocial perspective, chronic pain may lead to depression, fatigue, inactivity, isolation, loss of valued occupations, failure to participate in daily life, a sense of helplessness, and so on.

The experience of pain is not well understood; spiritual beliefs and emotional temperament seem to affect pain perception (57). Research and personal reports suggest that involvement in valued purposeful activity related to chosen life roles or hobbies may make pain easier to endure (38, 58, 59, 76). However, long-term pain may cause the person to believe that action and involvement will be painful and impractical. Having patients monitor their pain levels at specific intervals and write down what they are doing at that time may help create an awareness that activity is possible and may be beneficial. A beeper can be used to signal the intervals at which to record these perceptions (49). Perhaps the simplest method is a visual analog scale (Fig. 9-1); patients are asked to mark the line at the point corresponding to their perception of the pain at that moment.

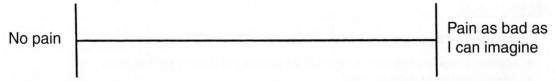


**Figure 9-1. Visual analog scale.** (Reprinted with permission from Engel J. Treatment for psychosocial components: Pain management. In: Neistadt ME, Crepeau EB, eds. Willard and Spackman's Occupational Therapy. 9th ed. Philadelphia: Lippincott-Raven, 1998.)

Engel (26) suggests that OT practitioners may help the pain patient by using the following methods, among others:

- Teaching and reinforcing socially appropriate pain expression (e.g., to involved health practitioners rather than to anyone who will listen)
- Praising and reinforcing social interaction about issues other than pain
- Encouraging appropriate physical activity
- Introducing the patient to support groups
- Teaching distraction as a method of pain management

Using distraction, the pain patient may focus within the self (e.g., meditation, memory) or on a diverting activity (reading, doing a puzzle). Cognitive restructuring, a cognitive-behavioral method for challenging negative automatic thoughts (see Chapter 2), is also recommended. Other approaches to management of pain include progressive muscle relaxation, biofeedback, massage, use of heat packs or cold packs or electrical stimulation, and various stress management techniques.

People who experience chronic pain distinguish between usual or expected pain and unexpected pain (24). It is possible to plan activities around expected pain, because it is predictable. Unexpected pain, on the other hand, comes without warning and disrupts planned activities. People who have ongoing pain problems develop strategies to deal with the two types of pain, according to Dudgeon et al (24). For usual pain, the common strategies are prevention, planning ahead, and making practical decisions. For unexpected pain, the strategies are mind–body dissociation (focusing one's mind elsewhere), relief safety nets (medication and social supports), and reviewing priorities and being persistent. Work simplification, energy conservation, and environmental adaptations may also help.

## UNDERSTANDING AND SUPPORTING RECOVERY

A shift of perspective about psychiatric illness has occurred since 1990, with consumers increasingly embracing a view of themselves as in recovery (not sick, but in recovery from a serious illness). Recovery is a way of life that acknowledges the reality of illness and disability while maintaining hope and working toward meaningful realistic goals and a satisfying life (73). This person-centered, person-directed perspective demands that therapists take a back seat and allow the individual to direct and manage his or her own recovery. Pitts (73) suggests that OTs and OTAs employ specific strategies to support clients in recovery (Box 9-7).

Clients may benefit from concrete help in setting goals, taking control of their health matters, accessing community services, and recognizing their own strengths (85).

## SUMMARY

This chapter presents a brief overview of some special populations that may be encountered by the OTA. It considers children, adolescents, elders, family members, family caregivers, immigrants and

**BOX 9-7**

**GUIDELINES AND STRATEGIES FOR SUPPORTING RECOVERY**

- Maintain a hopeful perspective, believing in the possibility of recovery for every client
- Tolerate uncertainty about the future
- Tolerate slow movement toward goals
- Remember and take note of successes
- Understand that courage and risk taking are required for growth
- See the client as a survivor or hero, not as a patient or victim

persons from other cultures, the poor, the homeless, and persons with diagnoses that are primarily physical. Effective intervention with each of these populations requires additional knowledge that can be found in the references listed at the end of the chapter. OTAs who wish to work intensively with these special populations are encouraged to seek supervision and continuing education.

## REVIEW QUESTIONS AND ACTIVITIES

1. Make an outline from this chapter, listing the persons and groups served by occupational therapy in mental health.
2. Identify differences of approach to children, adolescents, adults, and the aged.
3. Describe some effects on the family of a psychiatric illness in a member of the family.
4. Why does the family need support from health care providers? What kinds of things are helpful?
5. Discuss the needs and responsibilities of family caregivers. How can the OTA help and support the family caregiver?
6. Name specific things the OTA can do to learn about cultural difference and improve the quality of care.
7. How does poverty affect mental health? How does it affect the person's participation in health care?
8. State three reasons why the OTA should consider psychosocial issues affecting persons whose primary diagnosis is not psychiatric.
9. What kinds of problems and goals might occupational therapy address in a medical or surgical hospital?
10. What is the effect of physical disability on engagement in occupational roles?
11. How does chronic pain affect a person psychosocially and in terms of occupational engagement?
12. What strategies can the pain patient use to deal with pain and engage in occupation?
13. How does the recovery perspective differ from the medical view of psychiatric illness.
14. What can the OTA do to support recovery?

## REFERENCES


1. Agrin AR. Occupational therapy with emotionally disturbed children in a public elementary school. Occup Ther Ment Health 1987;7(2):105–114.
2. Aja D. Occupational therapy intervention for overuse syndrome [Case Report]. Am J Occup Ther 1991;45:746–750.
3. American Occupational Therapy Association. Position Paper: Occupational therapy and long-term services and supports. Am J Occup Ther 1994;48:1035–1036).
4. American Occupational Therapy Association. Position Paper: Providing services for persons with HIV/AIDS and their caregivers. Am J Occup Ther 1996;50:853–854.
5. American Psychiatric Association. Outline for cultural formulation and glossary of culture-bound syndromes [Appendix]. In: Diagnostic and Statistical Manual of Mental Disorders. 4th ed. Text revision. Washington, DC: APA, 2000.
6. Barth T. Occupational therapy interventions at a shelter for homeless, addicted adults with mental illness. Am Occup Ther Assoc Ment Health Special Sect Q Newslett 1994;17(1):7–8.
7. Bazyk S. Creating occupation-based social skills groups in after-school care. OT Practice 2006;11(17):13–18.
8. Blanche EI. Alma: Coping with culture, poverty, and disability. Am J Occup Ther 1996;50:265–276.
9. Bonder B, Gurley D. Culture and aging—Working with older adults from diverse backgrounds. OT Practice 2005;4(7):CE1–8.
10. Brown SM, Humphry R, Taylor E. A model of the nature of family-therapist relationships: Implications for education. Am J Occup Ther 1997;51:597–603.
11. Burleigh SA, Farber RS, Gillard M. Community integration and life satisfaction after traumatic brain injury: Long-term findings. Am J Occup Ther 1998;52:45–52.
12. Burnett SB. Personal and social contexts of disability: Implications for occupational therapists. In: Pendleton HM, Schultz-Krohn W, eds. Pedretti's Occupational Therapy Practice Skills for Physical Dysfunction. 6th ed. St. Louis: Mosby, 2006.
13. Carlson JL. Evaluating patient motivation in physical disabilities settings. Am J Occup Ther 1997;51:347–351.
14. Centers for Disease Control and Prevention, Injury Center. Violence Prevention. Available at: www.cdc.gov/ncipc/dvp/dvp.htm. Accessed Feb 2007.
15. Centers for Disease Control and Prevention, Injury Center. Youth Violence: Fact Sheet. Available at: www.cdc.gov/ncipc/factsheets/yvfacts.htm. Accessed Feb 2007.
16. Cermak SA, Aberson JR. Social skills in children with disabilities. Occup Ther Ment Health 1997;13(4):1–24.
17. Chandler BE. Hidden in plain sight—Working with students with emotional disturbance in the schools. OT Practice 2007;12(1):CE1–8.
18. Clark CA, Corcoran M, Gitlin LN. An exploratory study of how occupational therapists develop therapeutic relationships with family caregivers. Am J Occup Ther 1995;49:587–593.
19. Coster W. Occupation-centered assessment of children. Am J Occup Ther 1998;52:337–344.
20. Countering domestic violence. Harv Ment Health Lett 2004;20(10):1–4.
21. Denton R. AIDS: Guidelines for occupational therapy intervention. Am J Occup Ther 1987;41:427–432.
22. Dickerson AE, Oakley F. Comparing the roles of community-living persons and patient populations. Am J Occup Ther 1995;49:221–228.
23. Downing DT. The impact of early psychosis on learning. OT Practice 2006;11(12):7–10.
24. Dudgeon BJ, Tyler EJ, Rhodes LA, Jensen MP. Managing usual and unexpected pain with physical disability: A qualitative analysis. Am J Occup Ther 2006;60:92–103.
25. Early MB. Psychosocial aspects of physical disability. In: Early MB, ed. Physical Dysfunction Practice Skills for the Occupational Therapy Assistant. St. Louis: Mosby, 2006.
26. Engel J. Treatment for psychosocial components: Pain management. In: Neistadt ME, Crepeau EB, eds. Willard and Spackman's Occupational Therapy. 9th ed. Philadelphia: Lippincott-Raven, 1998.
27. Fadiman A. The Spirit Catches You and You Fall Down. New York: Farrar Straus & Giroux, 1998.
28. Fessenden F. The changing face of the suburbs. New York Times, Dec 31, 2006.
29. Finlayson M, Baker M, Rodman L, Herzberg G. The process and outcomes of a multimethod needs assessment at a homeless shelter. Am J Occup Ther 2002;56:313–321.
30. Gage M. The appraisal model of coping: An assessment and intervention model for occupational therapy. Am J Occup Ther 1992;42:353–362.
31. Gitlin LN, Corcoran M, Leinmiller-Eckhardt S. Understanding the family perspective: An ethnographic framework for providing occupational therapy in the home. Am J Occup Ther 1995;49:802–809.
32. Greene S. Child psychiatry and middle childhood: A guide to play for parents. Am Occup Ther Assoc Ment Health Special Sect Q Newslett 1992;15(3):1–2.
33. Griner KR. Helping the homeless: An occupational therapy perspective. Occup Ther Ment Health 2006;22(1):49–61.
34. Gutman SA, Diamond H, Holnes-Parchment SA, et al. Enhancing independence in women experiencing domestic violence and possible brain injury: An assessment of an occupational therapy intervention. Occup Ther Ment Health 2004;20(1):49–79.
35. Gutterman L. A day treatment program for persons with AIDS. Am J Occup Ther 1990;44:234–237.

36. Harwood KJ, Wenzl D. Admissions to discharge: A psychogeriatric transitional program. Occup Ther Ment Health 1990;10(3):79–100.
37. Hasselkus BR. The meaning of activity: Day care for persons with Alzheimer's disease. Am J Occup Ther 1992; 46:199–206.
38. Heck SA. The effect of purposeful activity on pain tolerance. Am J Occup Ther 1988;42:577–581.
39. Helfrich CA, Aviles A. Occupational therapy's role with victims of domestic violence: Assessment and intervention. Occup Ther Ment Health 2001;16(3–4):53–70.
40. Helfrich CA, Lafata MJ, MacDonald SL, et al. Domestic abuse across the lifespan: Definitions, identification and risk factors for occupational therapists. Occup Ther Ment Health 2001;16(3–4):5–34.
41. Helfrich CA, Rivera Y. Employment skills and domestic violence survivors: A shelter-based intervention. Occup Ther Ment Health 2006;22(1):33–48.
42. Henry AD. Development of a measure of adolescent leisure interests. Am J Occup Ther 1998;52:531–539.
43. Henry AD, Coster WJ. Predictors of functional outcome among adolescents and young adults with psychotic disorders. Am J Occup Ther 1996;50:171–181.
44. Hildenbrand WC. Meeting the challenge of psychosocial shifts in service. Am Occup Ther Assoc Ment Health Special Sect Q Newslett 1997;20(3):1–4.
45. Hooley L. Circumventing burnout in AIDS care. Am J Occup Ther 1997;51:759–766.
46. Hotchkiss A, Fisher GS. Community practice for the homeless—OT education at the Mercy Center for Women. OT Practice 2004;14(7):17–21.
47. Humphry R, Gonzalez S, Taylor E. Family involvement in practice: Issues and attitudes. Am J Occup Ther 1993;47: 587–593.
48. Javaherian H. Helping survivors of domestic violence. OT Practice 2006;11(10):12–16.
49. Joe BE. Managing chronic pain and fatigue. OT Week, July 16m 1998, 12–13.
50. Keller J. Helping families to help their loved ones with serious mental illness: A white paper of the National Alliance on Mental Illness of New York State. Available at www.naminys.org/famserwp.pdf. Accessed Feb 2007.
51. Kielhofner G, Barrett L. Meaning and misunderstanding in occupational forms: A study of therapeutic goal setting. Am J Occup Ther 1998;52:345–353.
52. Lancaster J, Mitchell M. Occupational therapy treatment goals, objectives, and activities for improving low self-esteem in adolescents with behavioral disorders. Occup Ther Ment Health 1991;11(2–3):3–22.
53. Lawlor MC, Mattingly CF. The complexities embedded in family-centered care. Am J Occup Ther 1998;52:259–267.
54. Leslie CA. Psychiatric occupational therapy—Finding a place in the medical/surgical arena. OT Practice 2001;6(7):10–14.
55. Levy LL. Memory processing and the older adult: What practitioners need to know. OT Practice 2001;6(7):CE1–8.
56. Lipsyte R. Coping: The two ways of Dr. Hu. New York Times, Aug 30, 1998.
57. Low JF. Religious orientation and pain management. Am J Occup Ther 1997;50:215–219.
58. Lyons M, Orozovic N, Davis, J, Newman J. Doing-being-becoming: Occupational experiences of persons with life-threatening illnesses. Am J Occup Ther 2002;56:285–295.
59. McCormack G. Pain management by occupational therapists. HVD. Am J Occup Ther 1988;42:577–581.
60. McGruder J. Culture and other forms of human diversity in occupational therapy. In: Neistadt ME, Crepeau EB, eds. Willard and Spackman's Occupational Therapy. 9th ed. Philadelphia: Lippincott-Raven, 1998.
61. Melia MA, Weikert K. Evaluation and treatment of adolescents on a short-term unit. Occup Ther Ment Health 1987; 7(2):51–66.
62. Miller KS, Bunch-Harrison S, Brumbaugh B, et al. The meaning of computers to a group of men who are homeless. Am J Occup Ther 2005;59:191–197.
63. Morris AL, Gainer F. Helping the caregiver: Occupational therapy opportunities. OT Practice 1997;2(1):36–40.
64. Mulcahey MJ. Returning to school after a spinal cord injury: Perspectives from four adolescents. Am J Occup Ther 1992; 46:305–312.
65. Nave J, Helfrich CA, Aviles A. Child witnesses of domestic violence: A case study using the OT PAL. Occup Ther Ment Health 2001;16(3–4):127–135.
66. Neistadt M. Methods of assessing client's priorities: A survey of adult physical dysfunction settings. Am J Occup Ther 1995;49:428–436.
67. Norman AN, Crosby PM. Meeting the challenge: Role of occupational therapy in a geriatric day hospital. Occup Ther Ment Health 1990;10(3):65–78.
68. Olson L. Activity groups in family-centered treatment: Psychiatric occupational therapy approaches for parents and children. Occup Ther Ment Health 2006;22(3–4):1–156.
69. Olson L. Parent-child activity-based therapy. Am Occup Ther Assoc Ment Health Special Sect Q Newslett 1992; 15(3):3–4.
70. Oxer SS, Miller BK. Effects of choice in an art occupation with adolescents living in residential treatment facilities. Occup Ther Ment Health 2001;17(1):39–49.
71. Papadopoulos RJB, Staley D. Occupational therapy assessment of neurodevelopmentally disordered children and adolescents. Occup Ther Ment Health 1997;13(1):23–36.
72. Piemme JA, Bolle JL. Coping with grief in response to caring for persons with AIDS. Am J Occup Ther 1990;44: 266–269.
73. Pitts DB. Understanding the experience of recovery for persons labeled with psychiatric disabilities. OT Practice 2004;9:CE1-CE8.

74. Pritchett, J. Address given to the Mental Health Special Interest Group of the Metropolitan New York Occupational Therapy Association, Dec 9, 1992.
75. Salls J, Bucey JC. Self-regulation strategies for middle school students. OT Practice 2003;(8)5:11–16.
76. Sanford M. Waking: A Memoir of Trauma and Transcendence. Rodale, 2006.
77. Schindler VJ. Psychosocial occupational therapy intervention with AIDS patients. Am J Occup Ther 1988;42:507–512.
78. Schultz S. Psychosocial occupational therapy in schools—Identify challenges and clarify the role of occupational therapy in promoting adaptive functioning. OT Practice 2003;8(17):CE1–8.
79. Schultz-Krohn W. The meaning of family routines in a homeless shelter. Am J Occup Ther 2004;58:531–542.
80. Secunda V. When Madness Comes Home. New York: Hyperion, 1997.
81. Sholle-Martin S, Alessi NE. Formulating a role for occupational therapy in child psychiatry: A clinical application. Am J Occup Ther 1990;44:871–882.
82. Sladyk K. Traumatic brain injury, behavioral disorder, and group treatment [Case Report]. Am J Occup Ther 1992; 46:267–269.
83. Sontag D, Dugger CW. The new immigrant tide: A shuttle between two worlds. New York Times, July 19, 1998, A1, A28–30.
84. Stoffel VC. Reducing risks for children and families: How can occupational therapy practitioners be involved? Am Occup Ther Assoc Ment Health Special Sect Q Newslett 1994;17(1):7–8.
85. Taylor RR. Extending client-centered practice: The use of participatory methods to empower clients. Occup Ther Ment Health 2003;19(2):57–75.
86. Toal-Sullivan D, Henderson PR. Client-Oriented Role Evaluation (CORE): The development of a clinical rehabilitation instrument to assess role change associated with disability. Am J Occup Ther 2004;58:211–220.
87. Tryssenaar J, Tremblay M, Handy I, Kochanoff A. Aging with a serious mental illness: Family members' experience. Occup Ther Ment Health 2002;18(1):19–42.
88. Walker L. The Battered Woman. New York: Harper & Row, 1979.
89. Weissenberg R, Giladi N. Home economics day: A program for disturbed adolescents to promote acquisition of habits and skills. Occup Ther Ment Health 1989;9(2):89–103.
90. Williams MS, Shellenberger S. How does your engine run? A leader's guide to the Alert Program for self-regulation. Albuquerque, NM: Therapy Works, 1996.
91. Yevtushenko Y. People: Selected Poems. Baltimore: Penguin, 1962.
92. Yuen HK. Neurofunctional approach to improve self-care skills in adults with brain damage. Occup Ther Mental Health 1994;12(2):31–45.

## SUGGESTED READINGS

### Children

Bazyk S. Creating occupation-based social skills groups in after-school care. OT Practice 2006;11(17):13–18.

Chandler BE. Hidden in plain sight—Working with students with emotional disturbance in the schools. OT Practice 2007; 12(1):CE1–8.

Salls J, Bucey JC. Self-regulation strategies for middle school students. OT Practice 2003;(8)5:11–16.

Schmelzer L. An occupation-based camp for healthier children. OT Practice 2006;11(16):18–23

Schultz S. Psychosocial occupational therapy in schools—Identify challenges and clarify the role of occupational therapy in promoting adaptive functioning. OT Practice 2003;8(17):CE1–8.

### Adolescents

Downing DT. The impact of early psychosis on learning. OT Practice 2006;11(12):7–10.

Olson L. Engaging psychiatrically hospitalized teens with their parents through a parent-adolescent activity group. Occup Ther Ment Health 2006;22(3–4):121–133.

### Elders

Corcoran MA. Occupational therapy intervention for persons with dementia and their families. OT Practice 2002;7(21):CE1–8.

Bonder B, Gurley D. Culture and aging—Working with older adults from diverse backgrounds. OT Practice 2005;4(7): CE1–8.

Levy LL. Memory processing and the older adult: What practitioners need to know. OT Practice 2001;6(7):CE1–8.

### Families

Corcoran MA. Gender differences in dementia management plans of spousal caregivers: Implications for occupational therapy. Am J Occup Ther 1992;46:1006–1012.

Fahl MA. Mental illness and family involvement. Am Occup Ther Assoc Ment Health Special Sect Q Newslett 1996;19(3): 1–2.

Jacobs B. Dual diagnosis: A parent's perspective. Am Occup Ther Assoc Ment Health Special Sect Q Newslett 1997; 20(2):1–4.

Keller J. Helping families to help their loved ones with serious mental illness: A white paper of the National Alliance on Mental Illness of New York State. Available at www.naminys.org/famserwp.pdf. Accessed Feb 2007.

Neugeborgen J. Imagining Robert: My Brother, Madness, and Survival. New York: Holt, 1997.

Olson L. Activity groups in family-centered treatment: Psychiatric occupational therapy approaches for parents and children. Occup Ther Ment Health 2006;22(3–4):1–156.

Schultz-Krohn W. The meaning of family routines in a homeless shelter. Am J Occup Ther. 2004;58:531–542.

Tryssenaar J, Tremblay M, Handy I, Kochanoff A. Aging with a serious mental illness: Family members' experience. Occup Ther Ment Health 2002;18(1):19–42.

## Culture

American Psychiatric Association. Outline for cultural formulation and glossary of culture-bound syndromes [Appendix]. In: Diagnostic and Statistical Manual of Mental Disorders. 4th ed. Text revision. Washington, DC: APA, 2000.

Bonder B, Gurley D. Culture and aging—Working with older adults from diverse backgrounds. OT Practice 2005;4(7): CE1–8.

Fadiman A. The Spirit Catches You and You Fall Down. New York: Farrar Straus and Giroux, 1998.

McGruder J. Culture and other forms of human diversity in occupational therapy. In: Neistadt ME, Crepeau EB, eds. Willard and Spackman's Occupational Therapy, 9th ed. Philadelphia: Lippincott-Raven, 1998.

## Homeless Persons

Cohen NL, ed. Psychiatry Takes to the Streets. New York: Guilford, 1990.

Davis J, Kutter CJ. Independent living skills and posttraumatic stress disorder in women who are homeless: Implications for future practice. Am J Occup Ther 1998;52:39–44.

Lamb HR, Bachrach LL, Kass FI, eds. Treating the Homeless Mentally Ill. Washington, DC: American Psychiatric Association, 1992.

Schultz-Krohn W. The meaning of family routines in a homeless shelter. Am J Occup Ther 2004;58:531–542.

Torrey EF. Out of the Shadows: Confronting America's Mental Illness Crisis. New York: Wiley, 1997.

## Violence Issues

Centers for Disease Control and Prevention, Injury Center. Violence Prevention. Available at: www.cdc.gov/ncipc/dvp/dvp.htm. Accessed Feb 2007.

Countering domestic violence. Harv Ment Health Lett 2004;20(10):1–4.

National Domestic Violence Hotline. 800-799-SAFE (800-799-7233). Website: www.ndvh.org. Accessed Feb 2007.

## Medical Conditions and Physical Disabilities

Fine SB. Resilience and human adaptability: Who rises above adversity? [1990 Eleanor Clarke Slagle Lecture]. Am J Occup Ther 1991;45:493–503.

Gutman SA. Enhancing gender role satisfaction in adult males with traumatic brain injury: A set of guidelines for practice. Occup Ther Ment Health 1997;13(4):25–43.

Leslie CA. Psychiatric occupational therapy—Finding a place in the medical/surgical arena. OT Practice 2001;6(7):10–14.

Price R. A Whole New Life. New York: Atheneum, 1982.

Sanford M. Waking: A Memoir of Trauma and Transcendence. Rodale, 2006.

## Acquired Immune Deficiency Syndrome

American Occupational Therapy Association. Position Paper: Providing services for persons with HIV/AIDS and their caregivers. Am J Occup Ther 1996;50:853–854.

Atchison BJ, Beard BJ, Lester LB, Occupational therapy personnel and AIDS: Attitudes, knowledge, and fears. Am J Occup Ther 1990;44:212–217.

Hansen RA. The ethics of caring for patients with HIV or AIDS. Am J Occup Ther 1990;44:239–242.

Johnson JA, Pizzi M, eds. Productive Living Strategies for People with AIDS. Binghamton, NY: Haworth, 1990.

Marcil WM, Tigges KN. The Person with AIDS: A Personal and Professional Perspective. Thorofare, NJ: Slack, 1992.

O'Rourke GC. The HIV-positive intravenous drug abuser [Case Report]. Am J Occup Ther 1990;44:280–283.

Peloquin SM. AIDS: Toward a compassionate response. Am J Occup Ther 1990;44:271–278.

Sladyk K. Teaching safe sex practices to psychiatric patients. Am J Occup Ther 1990;44:284–286.

## Chronic Pain

Neville-Jan A. Encounters in a world of pain: An autoethnography. Am J Occup Ther 2003;57:88–98.

SECTION III

# Interacting with Patients and Consumers

CHAPTER 10

# Therapeutic Use of Self

***Without the caring elements that ground the therapist-patient relationship and the dialogue that grounds collaborative treatment planning, occupational therapy would be reduced to a sterile science of occupation.***

SUZANNE M. PELOQUIN (10)

## CHAPTER OBJECTIVES

After studying this chapter, the reader will be able to:

1. Define *therapeutic use of self.*
2. Recognize and give examples of therapeutic qualities.
3. Give examples of techniques useful for relating to patients or consumers.
4. Define and give examples of *transference* and *countertransference.*
5. Differentiate among types of dependence.
6. State methods to deal with stigma and with uncomfortable feelings toward patients and consumers.
7. Relate the Occupational Therapy Code of Ethics to the OTAs relationship with persons with mental health problems.
8. Discuss helpful ways to end a therapeutic relationship.

Wanting to help other people is one reason students choose to enter a field like occupational therapy. Although occupational therapists and assistants help people primarily by using activities, they also help them by the way they relate to them, by encouraging them to become more aware of their own abilities and more confident about using them. Relating to people is a skill used by all health professionals and by lawyers, clergymen, and others whose work involves dealing with people. In all of these fields, the abilities to listen and to communicate are essential. Relating to people who have psychiatric disorders requires even greater skill than does relating to other people. People with psychiatric disorders may have had bad experiences relating to other people; this is no less true when they identify themselves as consumers rather than patients. They may be fearful and have trouble expressing themselves. The way we relate to them, what we say and what we do not say in words or in actions, affects them deeply, whether or not we are aware of it.

Being aware of oneself and of the patient and being able to control what one communicates is called *therapeutic use of self.* It is different from other ways of relating to people because the purpose of the relationship is different. The relationship between the patient and the health care worker is not an equal one. Patients expect that the health care worker, in this case the occupational therapy assistant (OTA), will be able to help them with their problems, to make them feel better; the assistant, on the other hand, expects to be able to help patients. The purpose of their relationship is to help patients identify their problems, set reasonable goals, and work toward accomplishing those goals.

## THE THERAPEUTIC RELATIONSHIP

To understand the special nature of the therapeutic relationship it is helpful to consider two important differences between that relationship and a relationship one might have with a friend. The first is that in a friendship each person expects something from the other. By contrast, in the therapeutic relationship, the patient expects to receive help and the therapist or assistant expects to give it, but neither expects the help to be returned. The second is that in a friendship both people are responsible for making sure the relationship is rewarding and mutually satisfying. In a therapeutic relationship, the therapist is responsible for developing and maintaining a good relationship with the patient.

The consumer movement has changed the way therapists and patients think of themselves in the therapeutic relationship. The relationship has evolved to one of collaboration and working together (4, 19). Box 10-1 shows a revised definition that incorporates the consumer perspective. The definition is based on a survey conducted Cole and McLean (4). The survey also found that therapists tied the therapeutic relationship to

**BOX 10-1**

### A 21ST-CENTURY DEFINITION OF THERAPEUTIC RELATIONSHIP

A trusting connection and rapport established between therapist and client through collaboration, communication, therapist empathy and mutual respect.

Cole M, McLean V. Therapeutic relationships re-defined. Occup Ther Ment Health 2003;19(2):49.

functional outcomes, implying that time spent in developing (and being in) the relationship with the consumer positively influences the outcome of therapy.

Relating to patients and consumers effectively, like other skills, comes more easily to some than to others. Fortunately, it *is* a skill, which like any other skill can be developed through effort and practice. Reading about it is only the beginning; like learning to ride a bicycle, it can be mastered only through experience. Still, before attempting to relate to consumers, it is helpful to know something about what is expected. This chapter examines the role that occupational therapy staff typically take toward patients, explores some of the qualities that patients find helpful in therapists, and discusses some techniques the OTA can use to relate to the patient or consumer effectively. It also looks at some of the ways both the patient and the assistant may react to each other. Finally, this chapter considers some of the legal and moral aspects of the therapeutic relationship and discusses how to end a therapeutic relationship. Note that the words *patient, consumer,* and *client* are all used in the chapter; the reader is encouraged to review Box 7-1 to recall when these different terms may apply.

## STAGES IN THE THERAPEUTIC RELATIONSHIP

Tickle-Degnen (14) in a review of the literature, notes that the therapeutic relationship consists of three overlapping stages: *(a)* the development of rapport, *(b)* the development of a working relationship, and *(c)* the maintenance of a working relationship through goal achievement. Different kinds of communication are appropriate to each stage.

In the *rapport-building stage,* it is important to gather information, which also means that the patient will learn about the therapist. It is next important to engage with the patient, to collaborate and to understand how the patient sees this collaboration. Another aspect of this period is learning how to share information with the patient and how the patient is likely to react.

In the second stage, a *working relationship* is built by choosing the therapy goals and tasks carefully and collaboratively. It is important to create a method for responding to success and failure in a way that allows the patient to take control of the information by, for example, keeping a log or record. In this stage, there is also a customizing or individualizing of the working relationship between therapist and patient, so that the patient is comfortable and knows what to expect.

The third period, the *ongoing working relationship,* consists of hard work and is the longest period in the relationship. The relationship will have ups and downs, frustrating moments and triumphant ones. Emotions may be extreme and difficult. It is important for therapist and patient to continue to share information, to use humor and other strategies to deal with feelings, and to adapt goals and strategies to the new realities that begin to emerge. Consumers can manage and tailor their progress by monitoring which methods work and which do not, and by sharing this with the therapist.

## ROLES IN THE THERAPEUTIC RELATIONSHIP

Unlike mental health professionals who help patients primarily by talking with them, occupational therapy (OT) practitioners help patients most often by doing things with them and helping them do things by themselves. The OTA must take on a variety of special roles, at the same time engaging patients in occupation. These roles include instructor, coach, supervisor, role model, problem solver, environmental manager, and group member (3, 7, 18).

When teaching an activity, the assistant is in the role of instructor. He or she analyzes what the clients have to learn, what they already know, their ability to learn, and how they learn best (e.g., demonstration, oral direction). The OTA creates activities and materials that will help clients experience what they need to learn. He or she presents the instructions so that clients can understand them, encourages them to practice, and corrects errors as they make them. The assistant is especially careful to present the "just-right" challenge. By creating conditions in which clients can experience personal accomplishment, the practitioner increases the person's belief in the self as competent and capable (5).

As coach, he or she coaxes clients, supports their efforts, and urges them to do even better. As supervisor, the OTA oversees their efforts, checks the quality of their work, monitors their progress, and supplies them with new tasks and new challenges.

We have already seen that people learn by imitating others. Watching another person is a natural way to learn something new or difficult. Because clients do not always have the skill to serve as role models for each other, the OTA frequently takes on this responsibility. When serving as a role model, the assistant must not only identify what is to be learned but also be able to explain why. He or she must be able to make the person believe that this new skill is important. Finally, the assistant must demonstrate the appropriate skill or behavior and help the person imitate it.

Occasionally, the OTA is asked to model behaviors he or she does not already know and feel comfortable with. For example, an assistant who has little experience with or interest in group sports may be asked to run a volleyball game. If this happens, it might be better to arrange with the supervisor for someone more experienced to lead the game and to learn by assisting the leader. In so doing, the assistant can also serve as a role model who is not afraid to try something new.

The assistant steps into the role of problem solver when he or she helps someone identify problems and set goals for treatment. In this role, the assistant helps the person understand the results of the evaluation. The assistant helps the client choose something to work on first. The assistant also explains why he or she is recommending a particular occupational task or method of doing it; this sets an example for problem solving that the client can later imitate. The assistant tries to involve the client in the process of solving his or her own problems. This may require asking questions rather than making statements; the assistant may already have identified a solution to the problem but does not share it. Instead, the OTA consciously encourages the person to solve the problem by allowing time to do so. The same approach can be used whenever problems arise during the course of an activity.

The assistant also manages the environment and may change the nature of the task, the tools and materials involved, or the social or physical context in which the activity occurs. He or she recognizes that the client's ability to participate in and succeed at the activity is a function of the environment. The OTA observes the environment carefully to see what changes will help the person perform better. In the role of environmental manager, the assistant also tries to show how the environment affects the client and how the client may change it. For example, the assistant may observe that the rock music playing in the background seems to distract the person; the assistant might select instead instrumental music with a slower tempo and softer sounds (e.g., classical guitar or electronic music), then urge the client to consider how he or she feels and performs the activity with the two types of music. The OTA might share with the patient the information that people generally feel more capable when they are more relaxed physiologically, when their heart rate is lower, for example (5).

Finally, the assistant who is running a group often must take on a variety of roles within the group; this is because clients do not always have the skills necessary to perform these roles themselves. For example, the assistant may have to settle disputes between two group members if neither they nor the other members are able to do so. The assistant in doing this is also modeling the appropriate behavior for this role and should follow the guidelines for serving as a role model. Group roles and the role of the assistant as leader of a group are discussed in detail in Chapter 13.

In summary, the occupational therapy assistant is required to assume many different roles when helping clients with activities, individually or in a group. The OTA's success will depend very much on the ability to recognize and step into whatever role is required for each situation. Regardless of the particular role, the OTA should try to embody the therapeutic qualities that have been identified over the years as helpful. As you read about these qualities, try to recall a wonderful relationship from your past and identify specific events that illustrate them. A relative, family friend, counselor, or teacher who listened to you carefully and made you feel special probably demonstrated most of these qualities.

## THERAPEUTIC QUALITIES

In this section, you will learn to recognize some essential qualities of the therapeutic relationship: empathy, sensitivity, respect, warmth, genuineness, self-disclosure, specificity, and immediacy.

### Empathy

Empathy is the ability to understand how the other person feels. The OTA not only should try to see the world from the patient's point of view but should also get this across to the patient. Listening to what the patient says and encouraging him or her to say more about it helps the assistant understand how the patient feels. A patient who believes that the therapist truly understands his or her point of view is likely to communicate more and work harder in therapy. For empathy to be effective, it must be genuine—that is, the practitioner must fully enter into the world of the patient. Empathy requires a kind of experiential bonding, or "being with" the patient (8).

### Sensitivity

In the therapeutic relationship, sensitivity is alertness to the patient's needs and awareness of your effect on him or her. The effective therapist is acutely attuned to the patient's behavior, especially facial expressions and nonverbal behavior. The movements of people's face and body often give a more accurate picture of their true feelings than do the words they use. For example, the OTA might suspect that the patient who claims to be looking forward to being discharged has other feelings as well if the patient bites his or her lip and looks at the floor. These behaviors convey mixed feelings, perhaps fear, sadness, or anxiety. By recognizing this, the assistant can give the person the opportunity to discuss his or her true feelings. If the assistant had taken the patient's words at face value, this might not have happened.

Weinstein (17) describes "the Zen of therapy," or the experience of powerful moments that are mysterious and magical and not easily analyzed. The practitioner who is so involved in the moment as to be truly unconcerned with the self may affect the patient simply by genuineness of concern. In this "being in the moment," spontaneous interchanges with great healing power may occur.

### Respect

The patient requires respect and recognition as a unique individual with personal interests and values that may be quite different from those of the OTA. A man may not, for example, think it particularly important to learn to cook. Perhaps in his culture cooking is seen as woman's work, or maybe his wife or mother cooks for him and he has no interest in it or desire to do it for himself. The assistant should help this patient select a more meaningful activity, unless he really needs to learn to cook because, for example, he must live on his own.

Similarly, patients often choose and enjoy with great pleasure activities that staff may find dysfunctional or unhealthful. For example, the OTA may identify overspending as a problem for a patient who has trouble staying within a budget, although the patient is quite happy with the situation (6). Being "in relationship" with a patient requires that the therapy practitioner willingly look at things from the patient's point of view.

Different cultures have different expectations for what should happen between a patient and a mental health worker. To engage patients from different cultures, the assistant must understand and appreciate the values and traditions to which the person is accustomed. Someone coming from a culture that views health professionals as authorities may be puzzled when asked to participate in goal planning, for example. This means that every time the OTA encounters a patient from a new culture, the OTA has to learn what that culture expects. See Chapter 9 for further discussion of cultural differences.

## Warmth

Warmth is the sense of friendliness, interest, and enthusiasm the therapist conveys. Warmth spreads outward from a person as loving and positive regard. It is shown by smiling, eye contact, leaning forward, touching, and other nonverbal behaviors. Although these behaviors should be genuine, all should be used selectively, depending upon the situation and the patient's ability to tolerate the therapist's warmth. Some people are very uncomfortable about being touched, and the therapist must be alert to this. The way the therapist displays warmth must vary with the situation; smiling is often appropriate when praising someone's efforts but perhaps not when listening to a tearful recitation of problems or when confronting a client who has broken the rules of the group. In the latter two situations, the therapist's warmth is conveyed through eye contact, body position, and tone of voice.

## Genuineness

Genuineness is the ability to be oneself openly. To do this, therapists must first be aware of themselves and be comfortable with who they are. Therapists who have mastered this can say and do what they really mean; their verbal and nonverbal messages say the same thing. They are not afraid of making mistakes or not knowing the answer to every question and are willing to admit it. They do not need to distance themselves from consumers with an artificially professional role; they find it easy to be in the role of therapist without being phony or defensive.

## Self-Disclosure

Self-disclosure is the practice of revealing things about oneself. In a therapeutic relationship the patient is asked to unveil many private facts and feelings. Indeed, patients may be required to reveal so much that at times they feel like specimens under a microscope. By letting the patient know some facts about themselves, OTAs can even the score a little and make the relationship seem more equal. It is important, however, to reveal only as much as is needed to make the person more comfortable. Timing is very important; self-disclosure is most helpful when the patient has asked for it (verbally or nonverbally) and very detrimental when it interrupts the patient in the midst of expressing himself or herself. Also, patients from some cultures may see a therapist's self-disclosure as unprofessional and offensive.

In addition, it is important to know what *not* to disclose. This includes details about one's personal life, such as one's address and phone number. Unfortunately, some patients want to seek out staff after they are discharged, and this can be difficult and sometimes dangerous for the staff member and his or her family. Finally, whatever is disclosed should be for the patient's benefit; the assistant should never burden the patient with his or her own problems.

### Specificity

Specificity is the art of stating things simply, directly, and concretely, focusing only on what is relevant. The effective therapist points out what is happening without labeling it or turning it into an abstract principle or a value judgment. For example, the therapist says, "When you walk away while I am talking to you, I get the feeling you don't want to hear what I have to say," rather than "You're being hostile." When giving directions, the therapist states them in language simple enough to be understood—for instance, telling the patient, "Find the center of the block of wood by drawing lines across from corner to corner" rather than "Find where the hypotenuses of the right angles meet."

Similarly, when helping a patient understand what is happening during an activity, the therapist should identify relevant details and help the person see them. For example, when the patient makes a mistake, becomes upset, and wants to quit the activity, the therapist should help him or her see exactly what has to be done to correct the error.

### Immediacy

Immediacy is the practice of giving feedback right after the event to which it relates. Patients benefit from learning about their successes and their mistakes while they are happening, rather than later, when they or the therapist may have forgotten important details. Immediacy also includes the idea of focusing the patient's attention on the here and now. Patients sometimes become preoccupied with things over which they have no control, like what they will do if they win the lottery or what Dr. Jones said to one of the nurses. The more someone ruminates on things that are not happening and that probably will not happen, the more distanced they become from the here and now, from making real-life decisions and carrying them out. These patients need to become involved in something that is really happening.

To sum up, the occupational therapy assistant should try to cultivate the therapeutic qualities discussed. This is a lifelong project; these qualities cannot be developed overnight. Nor can they be developed by a piecemeal study and practice of their separate parts (e.g., listening, leaning forward, trying to maintain eye contact) (9). Rather, these qualities are acquired only by the struggle to genuinely understand. Once developed, they need constant nurturing, evaluation, and refinement. Research studies have documented that regardless of the health professional's training or theoretical orientation, patients get better sooner and with more lasting results when they are treated by health professionals who possess these traits.

## DEVELOPING THERAPEUTIC QUALITIES

Students and new practitioners may be perplexed by the expectation that they acquire or refine these therapeutic qualities in themselves. From the student's perspective, there may not seem to be a problem. However, we are not always accurate in our assessments of how we seem to others. A gesture or comment that we mean to be warm and understanding may be perceived as pushy and insensitive. How can one resolve this confusion and move toward developing a therapeutic self that is reliable and effective? One key is to improve one's awareness of self. Another is constant examination of one's motives and expectations in relationships with patients.

Many roads lead to increased awareness of self. Some therapy practitioners seek therapy or counseling for themselves, to learn about how they are perceived by others and to understand more about their own ways of being in the world. Another way to learn about the self is to ask trusted and honest colleagues to give feedback; these may be fellow students or teachers or supervisors. An acronym for processing feedback is ALOR (ask, listen, observe, reflect), illustrated in Box 10-2. After the fourth step (reflect), one may circle back and begin with the first step (ask) again. Peer supervision is an especially valuable source of feedback; it is easier for many people to hear the message when it comes from a peer (someone of equal status) than from a supervisor.

Examining one's motives and expectations is part of self-awareness. People who choose a helping profession do so for many reasons (motives). Some motives are a desire to heal others and possibly a desire to heal the self; sometimes a desire to be seen as an expert is part of the motivation (6, 17). Additional motives are added in the training process and in the clinic; these may be a desire to maintain detachment and distance to protect oneself from uncomfortable feelings, a desire to satisfy the requirements of third-party reimbursers, a wish to impress one's colleagues, a desire to prove that a particular approach or technique is effective, and so on. Which of these motives belongs in a therapeutic relationship? Which motives are genuine caring responses to another human being?

In regard to expectations, the self-aware therapist is equally vigilant. Whenever we see a patient or provide a therapy service, we have one or more expectations. Do we know what we expect? And are we fully conscious of what we expect? We may

**BOX 10-2**

**IMPROVING UNDERSTANDING OF SELF AND OTHERS THROUGH ALOR**

| | |
|---|---|
| Ask | *Student to supervisor:* "I am so upset about my interview with Noelani. I was asking her questions and everything was fine and then she just got up and gave me an angry look and walked off. What did I do wrong?" |
| Listen | *Supervisor:* "Well, I wasn't there, so I'm not sure. I have noticed, though, that you sometimes cut people off and finish their sentences for them. You even do this with me. You might try waiting until they finish and then take a breath before you talk again." |
| Observe | *Student* watches self during interactions with friends, patients, colleagues and observes behavior that supervisor described. |
| Reflect | *Student reflects,* "Gosh, I didn't know I did that. I thought I knew what the person was going to say, but now I see that I didn't." |

expect patients to benefit from whatever we do for them or that a particular patient who fits a particular stereotype cannot be reached because the patient is "unmotivated." We may feel disappointed or angry or otherwise negative when our expectations are not met. If we are not conscious of this, we may act it out in ways that are harmful to patients. Thus therapists keep careful watch over their expectations. In summary, therapeutic qualities are developed by seeking and accepting feedback, by learning about oneself, and by maintaining awareness of one's motives and expectations.

## TECHNIQUES FOR RELATING TO PATIENTS

Although self-knowledge and a genuine willingness to enter the patient's world are the foundations of successful therapeutic relationships, it also may help the new practitioner to know some of the specific techniques used by experienced therapists. These are detailed next and rephrased in Box 10-3. Note that these techniques are successful only when applied in the context of a genuinely caring response (9).

**BOX 10-3**

**COMMUNICATION TECHNIQUES**

- Make initial contacts brief.
- Choose words carefully.
- Be comfortable with silence.
- Encourage by minimal response.
- Listen and observe.
- Summarize and focus.
- Ask for clarification.
- Follow through on promises.

1. *When trying to develop a relationship with a new patient, try to make the first contacts brief.* Introduce yourself, explain your purpose for getting to know the patient, briefly describe what the patient may gain from occupational therapy, and set a time for your next meeting. If you place yourself for a moment in the patient's position, you will understand why he or she may feel overwhelmed by meeting so many new people at one time, all of them eager to ask questions. Instead, promote trust by orienting the patient to occupational therapy and providing a schedule for the first few days.
2. *Use language that conveys what you mean and that will accomplish your purpose.* When attempting to get patients to explore their feelings or to give general information about themselves, open questions should be used. Remember that an open question asks for an answer longer than a few words. For example, "What have you been doing today?" is likely to produce a lengthier reply than "Did you go to the exercise group?" On the other hand, a closed question, of which the latter is an example, is more useful when you want to know something specific, like whether the patient has finally gone to the exercise group that he or she has been avoiding. Similarly, avoid suggesting that a choice exists when there really is none. If occupational therapy is a required activity for all patients, asking "Would you like to come to occupational therapy now?" risks angering patients once they learn they have to come. Instead, say "It's time for occupational therapy. We will be meeting in the day room." This gives patients time to collect their thoughts and get ready for the group and makes clear that they are expected to attend.
3. *Be comfortable with occasional silences, your own and the patient's.* Everyone needs time to collect his or her thoughts, and patients may

need more time because their thinking is slowed by the disease process or the drugs they are taking. While you are waiting for the patient to answer, observe his or her nonverbal behavior to determine whether the patient is confused by the question, has not heard it, or is merely trying to compose an answer. In any case, avoid showing that you are impatient or in a hurry by tapping your feet or looking at your watch or the door.

4. *Use minimal responses such as "go on" or "uh-huh" to show that you have been listening and to encourage the patient to keep talking.* At times, patients find it hard to express themselves or to believe that you are interested, and your encouragement will help them. Remember that minimal responses can also be nonverbal, as with leaning forward or making eye contact.
5. *Actively listen to what the patient is communicating.* Words are not everything. Much is conveyed by gesture, by eye movement, by a tilt of the head or a tightening or softening or trembling around the mouth. Watch the patient carefully (without staring) and feel with the person. Pay attention to nonverbal clues as well as to the words used. What is the message in the nonverbal body language? What else is going on? Be ready to tolerate the patient's struggle with uncomfortable feelings. Verbalize what you see. If the patient is fidgeting, say, "I notice you're tapping your nails and twirling your hair." This allows the patient to say, "I always do that when I'm nervous," and thus helps the patient interpret and understand the behavior. Saying to the patient, "You seem nervous" makes the therapist seem the authority and the patient a laboratory specimen.
6. *Try to get the patient to focus on one thing at a time.* Patients may have trouble concentrating and may skip from topic to topic or gloss over something painful to avoid dealing with it. By saying, "I'd like to go back to what you said about banks making you angry because I think it might have something to do with the problem you said you have sticking to a budget," the therapist opens an important topic for a more thorough discussion. Some patients resist this at first or are too anxious to stay on the topic; if so, the therapist should drop the subject and bring it up at another time.
7. *Ask for clarification when you do not understand something the patient has said or done.* Because your purpose is to get the patient to explain further, your request should be phrased so as not to put the patient on the defensive. For example, "Would you repeat that? I didn't hear it" is much easier for the patient to take (and more polite) than "You really have to talk louder if you expect me to answer you." Likewise, when commenting on something a patient has done in an activity, it is better to say, "You've glued the pictures so that they face in different directions. I'm not sure I see why. Can you tell me about it?" than, "Why did you do that?" It is helpful to give specifics and to state your observations in neutral language.
8. *Promise only what you can deliver.* Patients will take at his or her word any staff member who makes a promise and will be hurt if the promise is not kept. Occupational therapy assistants, like other staff, are often so busy that they forget or run out of time to do things they meant to do. The artful therapist will leave a way out by saying, for example, "I'll try to bring you some purple yarn this afternoon if I get out of the meeting in time." The therapist who cannot keep a promise should go to the patient and briefly explain why, indicating whether and when he or she will be able to do it—for example, "I can't find the purple yarn, but I'll ask my supervisor about it tomorrow morning and let you know."

## ISSUES THAT ARISE IN THERAPEUTIC RELATIONSHIPS

In certain respects, relationships between patients and staff are no different from other human relationships. Human beings bring to their associations with each other an array of experiences, emotions, and predispositions. To pretend otherwise is silly. Becoming familiar with the most common emotional issues prepares the occupational therapy assistant to deal with them when they arise.

### Transference and Countertransference

*Transference* occurs when one person, usually the patient, unconsciously relates to the other, usually the therapist, as if that person were someone else, usually an important person in the patient's life. For example, a woman patient may begin to act as if the therapist were her older brother who always took care of her and mediated her conflicts with her friends.

*Countertransference* occurs when the other person, usually the therapist, unconsciously falls into that role. In the example discussed, if the therapist began to do special favors for the patient and step into her quarrels with her peers, this would be countertransference. It would be easy for this therapist to fall into the role unconsciously if he had a younger relative or friend for whom he had played this role in the past.

It is crucial to recognize that transference and countertransference occur on an unconscious level; this makes them very difficult to deal with. If patient and therapist continue to act out the roles prescribed by the transference, the patient in our example will not learn that there are other ways of relating to people who remind her of her brother. The relationship with this therapist will not benefit the patient. If, on the other hand, the therapist can recognize what is going on, he can observe the patient's transference to find out more about how the patient expects other people to act. Once he learns, for example, that one of the things she expects from men is to defend her in conflicts with others, he can bring this up for discussion. He can also, by refraining from entering into conflicts between the patient and her peers, help her explore other ways of relating to people and help her learn to solve problems and conflicts by herself.

There are two ways to identify a transference. The first is to observe your own behavior and study how you relate to patients, especially noting it if you relate differently to (or feel differently about) different patients. The second is to learn from your supervisor and other staff, who have more objectivity because they are not involved in the immediate situation. Students, beginning therapists, assistants, and even experienced staff are sometimes amazed to learn that they have gotten involved in the countertransferential relationship with a patient. Certainly there is no reason to be surprised and even less reason to be ashamed to find out that you have become enmeshed in a patient's transference. The patterns and feelings we have developed over many years of dealing with our families and others close to us are so much a part of us that it is natural for them to be set in motion by patients who remind us of important people from our pasts.

### Dependence

It is quite common for patients to depend on staff members, whom they perceive as having more knowledge, skill, and power than they do themselves. The degree to which patients are allowed or encouraged to depend on staff must be carefully monitored if the patient is ever to learn to be self-reliant. Purtilo and Haddad (11) differentiate three types of dependence, only two of which belong in the therapeutic relationship: detrimental, constructive, and self.

*Detrimental dependence* is excessive dependence by the patient on the health professional. In other words, the patient is capable of doing more, but the patient and the therapist have become entangled in a relationship in which the therapist does things for the patient that the patient could and should do independently. Detrimental dependence undermines the therapeutic relationship, the purpose of which is to help the patient identify and work on his or her problems.

*Constructive dependence* is more productive. The constructively dependent patient relies on the health professional to provide something that the patient cannot manage. For example, a patient with poor daily living skills may need the therapist to say whether or not the patient's clothing is appropriate for a given occasion, such as a party or a job interview.

*Self-dependence* is the ability to depend on oneself, to identify and solve one's own problems. It is synonymous with *independence.* Some patients have trouble seeing their own abilities and strengths and believe they need more assistance from the therapist than perhaps they really do. Others have an exaggerated view of their own capacities or are afraid of depending on another person and for this reason may not ask for help or may decline assistance when it is offered. The OTA should help patients become aware of the extent of their abilities and encourage them to rely on their own resources whenever they can and to ask for help when they cannot.

## Stigma

Stigma is social disapproval. Historically, stigma has been the common response to mental disorders, because of the unusual behaviors associated with these disorders. Animal behaviorists and anthropologists point out that genetic preference may be behind the stigma reaction. In other words, the person who looks and behaves differently from the norm is a poor risk for a mate and not a good prospect for a parent for ones future children. Consequently, the person is shunned and excluded from normal social interactions.

There is an aspect to stigma that is almost involuntary, to gasp when one sees someone with a disfigurement for example. One learns through upbringing not to stare, not to make fun of, and to be nice to people who are different. Professional education aims to help the OTA student learn to respect and work together with people who may be stigmatized by the general population. It is never acceptable for an OTA to shun or otherwise stigmatize a patient. Still, the student will surely have feelings when encountering people who look, behave, and in other respects are different from the normative group. How can one begin to work with these feelings?

Begin first with an absolute conviction that every person is a person, first and foremost. Everyone had a mother and father, who cared for them as best they could and (in most cases) who loved or still loves them deeply. Can you see the consumer with the same love and hope that a parent might see a child? Can you imagine what the consumer's parent would want for him? Can you see in the consumer the same hopes and dreams and human feelings that you have in yourself? Can you imagine that the consumer is your brother or sister?

Next, be honest about your feelings. What are they exactly? Not that you would share them with the consumer, but you might share them with your supervisor. Are you frightened or repulsed? Are you confused? Are you frustrated and angry? Learn to tolerate the discomfort of these feelings and to explore them and recognize them for what they are.

Finally, learn to transcend the discomfort of working with someone who is *other* (a social sciences term for "different" and therefore devalued). See that we are joined together in a common humanity, that *we* is much bigger than *me.* Consider building alliances with consumers, learning from them. Consider what they have to contribute, that they are experts on their own situations, and that they will surely have insights that you would find valuable or important (12).

## Helplessness, Anger, and Depression

Students entering fields such as occupational therapy may fantasize that they will "save the world" by making a big difference in the lives of their patients. However, when they finally begin to work with patients, OTAs are likely to learn that some persons served by occupational therapy are so severely disabled that no amount of intervention can improve their ability to function. Instead, such patients need large amounts of time and attention from staff merely to maintain the few skills they already possess. In addition, patients may have unrealistic hopes and expectations that occupational therapy will help them accomplish things that are simply beyond their capacity at the moment (and possibly ever).

Both patients and therapists occasionally feel helpless, frustrated, and angry about this. The patient may feel that the OTA is not doing enough. The assistant may feel that he or she is doing everything possible but that it is not good enough. If these feelings are allowed to fester, they become open sores that drain the very life out of the treatment relationship. Rather than getting angry at the patient or feeling bad, the assistant should take some positive steps to understand and change the situation. One way is to share feelings with other staff; more experienced staff are likely to have a perspective that the student or new therapist does not; also, a fellow student or junior staff member may be in the midst of a similar crisis and have a lot to share. Another way is to join a support group in the local occupational therapy association.

A third way is to enter therapy or counseling. This is the traditional way for new therapists to learn more about themselves, to release and deal with the troublesome feelings patients can arouse, and to learn firsthand about the therapeutic relationship from the patient's point of view.

Remember always that consumers benefit from open and collaborative relationships with staff, that hope is an essential ingredient in recovery, but that progress can be slow and setbacks many. The OTA can maintain a sense of perspective by focusing on strengths and small achievements, setting realistic goals in a manageable time frame, and keeping an open mind about how one defines success.

## Sexual Feelings

It is quite common for patients to develop sexual feelings toward staff. They may confuse the closeness and warmth of a therapeutic relationship with the intimacy of a sexual one. Dealing with the patient's subtle or not so subtle expressions of sexual needs can be very difficult for students and beginning therapists. The therapist may have to explain firmly but warmly that it is not appropriate to become sexually involved with a patient. The therapist can explain that it is impossible to help a patient work on problems if they are sexually or emotionally involved. If the patient resists this reasoning, the therapist can always simply say, "It's hospital policy."

Dating patients is never a good idea, even after they are discharged. Consider a situation in which a student from a distant state became sexually involved with a patient with a spinal cord injury during a physical disabilities internship. When the student ended her fieldwork and returned home, the patient fell into a deep depression, refused to attend occupational or physical therapy, and developed a lingering respiratory infection.

There are several lessons to be learned from this example. One is that therapists must be aware of their own needs when they are working with patients. It can be tempting to get involved with a patient who seems attractive, especially when one's social life is not particularly satisfying or perhaps is nonexistent. Being away from home, friends, and family may make the student particularly vulnerable to becoming involved.

The second lesson is that sexual relationships with patients can have unpleasant consequences for the student or therapist. The student who became involved with the spinal cord–injured patient was abruptly terminated from her fieldwork. A working therapist would probably have been fired or severely disciplined. When reported to the American Occupational Therapy Association's Commission on Standards and Ethics, the therapist's behavior might have led to public censure, even revocation of association membership (1). Therapy practitioners can also be censured by the National Board for Certification in Occupational Therapy and by licensure boards in individual states and jurisdictions, which may result in revocation of license. There are other sound reasons for being cautious with psychiatric patients; every year there are accounts (although rare) of mental health workers being murdered or harmed by patients with whom they are too closely involved.

The third and most important lesson is that no matter how much fun the relationship was at the time, in the end the patient suffered. Causing unnecessary pain to a patient violates his or her rights, betrays the occupational therapy code of ethics (2), and places the student and the facility at risk for a malpractice lawsuit.

### Fear and Revulsion

Contact with some psychiatric patients can bring up extremely difficult feelings of fear and revulsion or contempt. One fear arises from the risk of contagion from patients who have a communicable disease such as HIV infection or tuberculosis. Any fear of catching a disease from a patient should be discussed with one's supervisor. Application of universal precautions against infection (see Chapter 12) is necessary to protect both patients and staff. However, the fear may still remain. The best way to become more comfortable is to learn all there is to know about the routes of transmission of the disease in question.

Another kind of fear is the fear of the unknown, the unfamiliar, and the different. Again, education and information about differences, be they in cultural practices or sexual preference, can bring the therapist or assistant closer to understanding the patient's view of the world.

One may naturally feel repulsed by a patient who has committed an act of violence against another person. Sometimes one may feel distanced even from the patient who has seen or been the subject of a violent act. When patients confront us with scary experiences, it is natural to want to avoid the feelings they evoke. An honest talk with a supervisor or with another professional who works closely with the patient can help the beginning therapist understand these feelings and develop strategies to keep them from contaminating the therapeutic relationship.

## ETHICS

A code of ethics is a set of principles that guide the practice of a profession. It consists of rules and guidelines about what is considered proper conduct for the professional in his or her relationship with the general public and with the person receiving his or her services. In occupational therapy, the patient is the person to whom the professional has the greatest obligation, one based on the trust implied by the patient's willingness to be placed under the occupational

**BOX 10-4**

**THE SEVEN GUIDING PRINCIPLES OF THE OCCUPATIONAL THERAPY CODE OF ETHICS**

| | |
|---|---|
| Principle 1 | Occupational therapy personnel shall demonstrate a concern for the safety and well-being of the recipients of their services (beneficence). |
| Principle 2 | Occupational therapy personnel shall take measures to ensure a recipient's safety and avoid imposing or inflicting harm (nonmaleficence). |
| Principle 3 | Occupational therapy personnel shall respect recipients to assure their rights. (autonomy, confidentiality) |
| Principle 4 | Occupational therapy personnel shall achieve and continually maintain high standards of competence (duty). |
| Principle 5 | Occupational therapy personnel shall comply with laws and association policies guiding the profession of occupational therapy (procedural justice). |
| Principle 6 | Occupational therapy personnel shall provide accurate information about occupational therapy services (veracity). |
| Principle 7 | Occupational therapy personnel shall treat colleagues and other professionals with fairness, discretion, and integrity (fidelity). |

Adapted with permission from American Occupational Therapy Association Commission on Standards and Ethics. Occupational therapy code of ethics. Am J Occup Ther 2005;59:639–642.

therapy practitioner's care. The guiding principles of the Occupational Therapy Code of Ethics (2) are listed in Box 10-4. A less formal and more specific discussion of the obligations of occupational therapy staff toward the patients in their care follows.

## Patient-Centered Focus

*Place the patient's interests above your own.* The patient always comes first. In a fire or other emergency, patients should be helped to leave the building before staff see to their own welfare. Likewise, in less dramatic situations, OTAs should attend to consumer's needs even if this means they must defer their own. For example, helping a patient to the bathroom is more important than talking to another staff member or to a friend on the phone.

## Goal-Oriented Treatment

*Direct your energies toward accomplishing the treatment goals.* Every encounter with a patient should be related to that patient's problems and goals. An evaluation should be performed and a treatment plan developed and documented as soon as possible, so that the patient can be made aware of the purpose and direction of treatment.

## Patient's Rights

*Respect the patient's rights, including the right to refuse treatment.* The right to refuse treatment is based on the individual's right to determine what is best for his or her own welfare as written in the U.S. Constitution. A patient can be forced to accept treatment only if he or she has been involuntarily admitted to the hospital or declared legally incompetent. Treatment in each of these situations requires a special court order that must be renewed periodically. Patients also have a right to receive treatment regardless of their race, creed, or national origin and regardless of the personal likes or dislikes of the occupational therapy practitioner.

## Confidentiality

*Respect the confidentiality of the therapeutic relationship.* The patient has the right, both morally and legally, to expect that information about his or her condition, personal life, and treatment will be shared only with those directly concerned with his or her care. It is *never* appropriate to discuss this information with anyone outside the treatment facility.

One should refrain from talking about patients, even to another professional, in public places like the elevator, the bus, or the cafeteria. Students and beginning therapists often wonder whether they should share with other staff secrets a patient has told them. Usually they should. Some exceptions are obvious—for example, if the patient is planning a party or a treat for a staff member. In general, however, there should be no secrets from the treatment team. The therapy practitioner must actively support the staff in providing the patient with the best possible care. Reporting a patient's confidence is absolutely necessary when the patient threatens to harm himself, herself, or someone else; such threats should never be taken lightly.

The patient's right to privacy of personal medical information is protected by the Health Insurance Portability and Accountability Act of 1996 (HIPAA) (15). In practical terms, this means that copies of hospital records may not be shared with teachers or classmates, even if all of the apparent identifying information is removed, unless the patient has given express written consent for the one-time use. When writing about a patient for a class assignment or when discussing the patient in a class or seminar, the student must disguise all identifying information so that it is impossible for another person to guess the patient's identity. This means changing details such as name, date of birth, place of birth, and perhaps also the national origin, date of immigration, number of children, and so on. When the person is well known (an entertainer or sports figure), the occupation must also be changed.

When working with an adolescent who is 18 years of age or older, HIPAA rules apply because the person is considered an adult. Before the 18th birthday, information about the child or adolescent may be shared with the parent or guardian; however, to maintain a trusting and genuine relationship with the young person, the therapy provider must advise the patient that the information can (must) legally be shared.

In regard to persons with mental retardation and other cognitive disabilities, HIPAA law permits them to control access to their health information to whatever extent state or local law permits them to act on their own behalf. When in doubt, the OTA should consult a supervisor or more senior health care practitioner in the agency about this and other questions related to HIPAA. The HIPAA website provides extensive information as well as answers to frequently asked questions (16). The reader is highly encouraged to view the site and read the questions and answers.

## Patient Welfare

*Safeguard the welfare of patients under your care.* Although this principle applies equally to all recipients of occupational therapy services, special precautions are necessary when working with psychiatric patients because they may harm themselves or others because of confusion, incoordination, impaired thinking, or inability to control their impulses. In inpatient settings, OTAs must be consistently alert as to where their patients are and what they are doing. They must take care to account for tools, sharp objects, and other materials that could be used in a suicide attempt or an assault. They must make sure that confused patients do not get lost or hurt themselves accidentally. Safety procedures are covered in detail in Chapter 12.

### Continuing Education

*Maintain your own competence to provide occupational therapy treatment.* The patient has every right to expect that the occupational therapy practitioner will provide skillful treatment based on current knowledge in occupational therapy. Consequently, the OTA has an obligation to keep up to date on advances in his or her area of practice. For continuing certification and renewal of certification by the National Board for Certification in Occupational Therapy (NBCOT), all occupational therapy providers must complete units toward certification of competency. In some states, occupational therapy personnel must show evidence of continuing education courses to renew their state licenses or certificates. *Competence* is not synonymous with "years of experience" but is acquired by study and application. Excellent resources for developing and maintaining competency are available at the American Occupational Therapy Association (AOTA) and NBCOT websites and elsewhere (13, 20).

### Standard of Care

*Protect the patient from negligence, abuse, and substandard care.* Most malpractice suits involve situations in which patients were harmed because a health professional failed to attend to their needs or caused them injury directly or indirectly. For example, the OTA could be sued if he or she was responsible for leading or co-leading an activity from which an inpatient escaped and later committed suicide. Similarly, if a patient who was confused as a side effect of receiving electroconvulsive therapy was injured while using a power tool in the workshop, the staff member in charge would be held accountable.

A patient has the right to a reasonable standard of care. This does not necessarily mean the absolute latest in experimental medical technology but rather the kind of care that is usual and considered adequate and customary by most professionals in the field. The patient also has a right to receive treatment only from those who are qualified to give it. OTAs should know and follow their own job descriptions and should refuse to perform tasks for which they are not qualified or trained. Even when following orders, OTAs are still legally responsible for their own actions.

## ENDING THE THERAPEUTIC RELATIONSHIP

Saying good-bye is hard, especially when we have been close to someone. This is no less true of the therapeutic relationship; new therapists are often surprised not only by the strength of their patients' feelings but by their own feelings as well. Many circumstances can bring an end to the relationship between patient and therapist: the patient's discharge, the client's successful accomplishment of goals, a change of job or living situation for consumer or therapist, or a recognition that the client cannot benefit from further interventions. Ending a relationship can be uncomfortable and difficult, but ending it well can resolve unfinished issues and strengthen the person's confidence to deal with the real demands and opportunities that life brings.

OTAs can help consumers learn and grow even at the end of the relationship. One way is to ask clients to take some time to think about what they have gained from the treatment and to have them talk about it. Another is to ask them how they feel about leaving or about the therapist's leaving. If someone is leaving a group or the group is breaking up, the members should each be given time and encouragement to talk about their feelings, to express what they have gotten out of the group, and to say good-bye to each other.

Sometimes new practitioners are concerned that saying good-bye takes too much valuable time away from other therapy activities or from the main business of a group. They should recogn-ize instead that the end of a treatment relationship is at least as important as the beginning. Termination is a potent opportunity to reinforce whatever gains have been made. In addition, it can help prepare the individual to deal with natural losses and terminations in the future.

## SUMMARY

The relationship with the occupational therapy practitioner strongly influences the way patients see themselves and their abilities. At its best, the therapeutic relationship increases patients' confidence and strengthens their will to try new things and become more fully themselves. Such a relationship requires that the occupational therapy practitioner genuinely and unconditionally experience the world through the patient's perspective. While specific therapeutic qualities can be listed and individual communication techniques can be taught, these by themselves are insufficient. To make a connection with another person that is authentic and powerful requires that practitioners be conscious of their feelings and actions and that they take the risk to learn and accept and change themselves. By self-study through counseling and/or supervision and by thoughtful application of ethical principles, the OTA can begin to understand and learn to master this complex and powerful treatment tool.

## REVIEW QUESTIONS AND ACTIVITIES

1. Write your own definition of *therapeutic use of self.*
2. List the roles the OTA may perform in the therapeutic relationship and the situations in which each role is appropriate.
3. List, define, and give an example of each of the therapeutic qualities discussed in this chapter.
4. How do you plan to develop your own therapeutic qualities? Be specific.
5. Which of the techniques for relating to patients discussed in the chapter do you find easy? Which difficult? Discuss.
6. With a classmate, create a scenario that illustrates transference and countertransference.
7. Name the three types of dependence and contrast them with each other.
8. Define stigma. How will you combat stigma in yourself?
9. In regard to helplessness, anger, and depression, what are some constructive aspects of these negative feelings? How can you deal with these feelings in yourself and in consumers?
10. Explain why sexual and other intimate relationships between therapist and patient are forbidden by codes of ethics.
11. What can one do if one is afraid of a patient? Explain the kinds of fear and the ways to cope.
12. Relate the Occupational Therapy Code of Ethics to the OTAs relationship with persons with mental health problems.
13. List and describe helpful ways to end a therapeutic relationship.
14. *Challenge question:* (This is based on an actual situation reported to the author by a student after the September 11, 2001, terrorist attack in New York City). Imagine that you are an OTA working in a community mental health setting. A federal agent approaches you, shows you his identification, and then shows you a picture and asks you if you know the patient. The agent says that the patient, a woman from an Arab country, is wanted for questioning about two of her sons who are suspected of terrorism. The patient is well known to you. The agent presses you to say whether you know her and where he might find her. How do you respond? Explain.

## REFERENCES


1. American Occupational Therapy Association Commission on Standards and Ethics. Enforcement procedure for occupational therapy code of ethics. Am J Occup Ther 2005;59:643–652.
2. American Occupational Therapy Association Commission on Standards and Ethics. Occupational therapy code of ethics. Am J Occup Ther 2005;59:639–642.
3. Barris R, Kielhofner G, Watts JH. Psychosocial occupational therapy: Practice in a pluralistic arena. Laurel, MD: Ramsco, 1983.
4. Cole M, McLean V. Therapeutic relationships re-defined. Occup Ther Ment Health 2003;19(2):24–31.
5. Gage M, Polatajko H. Enhancing occupational performance through an understanding of perceived self-efficacy. Am J Occup Ther 1994;48:452–461.
6. Lyons M. Understanding professional behavior: Experiences of occupational therapy students in mental health settings. Am J Occup Ther 1997;51:686–692.
7. Mosey AC. Activities Therapy. New York: Raven, 1973.
8. Peloquin SM. The fullness of empathy: Reflections and illustrations. Am J Occup Ther 1995;49:24–31.
9. Peloquin SM. Communication skills: Why not turn to a skills training model [The Issue Is]. Am J Occup Ther 1995;49:721–723.
10. Peloquin SM. Sustaining the art of practice in occupational therapy. Am J Occup Ther 1989;43:219–226.
11. Purtilo R, Haddad A. Health Professional/Patient Interaction. 5th ed. Philadelphia: Saunders, 1996.
12. Swarbrick P, Burkhardt A. Spiritual health: Implications for the occupational therapy process. Am Occup Ther Assoc Ment Health Special Sect Q Newslett 2000;23(2): 1–3.
13. Thomson L, Lieberman D, Murphy R, et al. Developing, maintaining, and updating competency in occupational therapy: A guide to self-appraisal. Bethesda, MD: American Occupational Therapy Association, 1995.
14. Tickle-Degnen L. Client-centered practice, therapeutic relationship, and the use of research evidence. Am J Occup Ther 2002;56:470–474.
15. U.S. Congress. Public Law 104-91—Health Insurance Portability and Accountability Act of 1996. Available at: aspe.hhs.gov/admnsimp/pl104191.htm. Accessed Feb 2007.
16. U.S. Department of Health and Human Services, Office for Civil Rights. Medical privacy—National standards to protect the privacy of personal health information. Available at: www.hhs.gov/ocr/hipaa. Accessed Feb 2007.
17. Weinstein E. Elements of the art of practice in mental health. Am J Occup Ther 1998;52:579–585.
18. Willson M. Occupational therapy in long-term psychiatry. Edinburgh, UK: Churchill Livingstone, 1983.
19. Wright CV, Rebeiro KL. Exploration of a single case in a consumer-governed mental health organization. Occup Ther Ment Health 2003;19(2):19–32.
20. Youngstrom MJ. Evolving competence in the practitioner role. Am J Occup Ther 1998;52:716–720.


## SUGGESTED READINGS


Kyler-Hutchison P. Ethical reasoning and informed consent in occupational therapy. Am J Occup Ther 1988;42:283–287.

Peloquin SM. The depersonalization of patients: A profile gleaned from narratives. Am J Occup Ther 1993;47: 830–837.

Peloquin SM. The fullness of empathy: Reflections and illustrations. Am J Occup Ther 1995;49:24–31.

Peloquin SM. The patient-therapist relationship in occupational therapy: understanding visions and images. Am J Occup Ther 1990;44:13–21.

Tickle-Degnen L. Client-centered practice, therapeutic relationship, and the use of research evidence. Am J Occup Therr 2002;56:470–474.

U.S. Department of Health and Human Services, Office for Civil Rights. Medical privacy—National standards to protect the privacy of personal health information. Available at: www.hhs.gov/ocr/hipaa. Accessed Feb 2007.

Weinstein E. Elements of the art of practice in mental health. Am J Occup Ther 1998;52:579–585.

CHAPTER 11

# Responding to Symptoms and Behaviors

*The staff members were very patient with me. I resented their intrusions and their restrictions, but, at the same time, I dimly recognized their actions as evidence of caring and support. Someone sat with me when I could concentrate on a project, such as an embroidery sampler, which I enjoyed although I was not allowed to keep the needle or scissors. I began to feel less like a prisoner because I was given some freedom and because the staff seemed to respect me and care about my getting well.*

IRENE M. TURNER (47)

## CHAPTER OBJECTIVES

After studying this chapter, the reader will be able to:

1. Define *symptom,* and explain why symptoms are useful guides to understanding patient behavior and feelings.
2. Identify the three tools used by occupational therapy practitioners to help consumers experiencing psychiatric symptoms function as best they can and engage in occupation.
3. Describe the following symptoms: anxiety, depression, mania, hallucinations, delusions, paranoia, hostility and aggression, seductive behavior and sexual acting out, cognitive deficits, and attention deficits.
4. For each symptom, identify the diagnoses associated with it.
5. For each symptom, discuss how the occupational therapy assistant (OTA) can use self, environment, and activity to facilitate better functioning for the patient.
6. Identify characteristics of appropriate activities for a person experiencing each symptom and contrast unsuitable activities and explain what makes them unsuitable.
7. Discuss the role of the OTA in promoting wellness and consumer self-management of symptoms.

Imagine that you are entering a locked psychiatric ward to start your first occupational therapy fieldwork in psychosocial dysfunction.[1] An agitated young person approaches you and asks you one question after another: "Who are you? What's your name? Are you the new patient? Are you a volunteer? Did you see the football game last night? Do you like football? I've got season tickets. Wanna go with me tonight?" At the same time you can see two or three other people standing and sitting around the halls, heads hanging, eyes downcast. Another is pacing the hall, touching and trying every doorknob. Meanwhile, your supervisor is right behind you; and while you are grateful for the support, you are also worried that you will say or do the wrong thing to the patients.

Do you think you could handle yourself in this situation? If you are like most people when they begin working with persons with mental illness, you would probably feel anxious and uncomfortable. At times, it seems not only that you don't know what to do but also that you haven't the vaguest idea how to prepare yourself for this experience. You don't even know what questions to ask your supervisor. The purpose of this chapter is to give you a way of thinking about how people with mental health problems act and about how best to respond to them. We first examine why patients (clients, members, consumers) act the way they do, because this helps us understand how to approach them. Then we will discuss some responses you can make to them.

## A FRAMEWORK OF CONCEPTS ABOUT SYMPTOMS

When people who have mental disorders say and do bizarre things, our first reaction may be to label them as "crazy." In doing so, all we have accomplished is to protect ourselves by saying that those people are somehow different from us, that the way they act is not the way normal people act, that their actions make no sense, and that there is no way to understand them. However, if we step back from this reaction and examine the reasons behind it, we may see that we already know a great deal about why patients act as they do.

In most important ways, people with mental health problems are exactly like other people. All people have emotional needs, such as the need to belong and to be accepted by other people, the need to be loved and approved of by those around them, and the need to explore and master their environments. With most people we encounter, it is usually pretty easy to understand what they want from us and how to make them comfortable with us and with themselves. People with serious psychiatric problems may not be so easy to understand. They still have basic needs to be loved and accepted, but the way they express these needs may cause other people to reject them. Other people cannot understand what they want, and they themselves do not always know. Consider the following dialogue between a occupational therapy assistant (OTA) and a client in a community day program:

OTA [observing that client is applying the modeling clay to the front rather than the back of the copper tooling]: Wait. It goes on the other side, like this. [Demonstrates on sample.]

Client [shouting]: You don't know what you're doing. Bogus, bogus, BOGUS! You aren't a therapist! You're so out of it yourself that it's pathetic. Where's a supervisor? I'll get you fired. Out of my way! [Storms off to a corner of the room and lights a cigarette.]

What went wrong here? Why is the client reacting this way? What is he feeling? What should the OTA do about it? One possible interpretation of this client's behavior is that he felt ashamed at not recognizing that he was doing the project incorrectly. After all, it looked simple to him. He interpreted the OTA's comment as a criticism not just

[1] Much of the material in this chapter derives from Early (13).

of his error but of his entire being. He wanted to feel competent; that is why he chose such a simple project. He felt as if he were falling apart, that there were nothing he could do right, not even a very simple thing like copper tooling. Indeed, it seemed to him that he was completely worthless, that he would never be able to leave the hospital and return to his family and his job. So he displaced all of his frustration with himself onto the OTA. He blamed her for his failure because it was too painful for him to face. And all of this happened unconsciously; the client's unconscious protected him from learning the intolerable truth: that he had made the mistake himself.

Do you see that in some ways his reaction seems perfectly natural? Yes, it might be immature or hostile, but it is a reaction we can understand, a reaction that we have perhaps had ourselves in similar situations. We all use defense mechanisms to keep from facing facts that we find threatening. Perhaps you interpreted this client's behavior differently. Many interpretations are possible. The point is that if we take the time and make the effort to grapple with what clients are really feeling and why, we can often see that their reactions make sense, that their behavior does not just come from nowhere, and that in many ways they are no different from us. This may be a scary idea. It raises questions about how sane we are and how safe we are from going "crazy."

Whereas some clients become verbally abusive, as this man did, others withdraw and still others become suspicious. Some may burst into tears and apologize for ruining the project. Such reactions, while understandable, are nonetheless extreme or peculiar. Behaviors like these are termed *symptoms* because they show that some disease or abnormal state is causing the person to act this way. Symptoms may be visible behaviors, such as these, that show underlying problems, or they may be subjective feelings reported by the person, such as a feeling of extreme sadness or a feeling of seeing things as if they were very small and far away.

## Expressing Unmet Needs or Conflicts

To understand the role of symptoms in psychiatric disorders, it may be helpful to recall the concepts of object relations theory (Chapter 2). According to object relations theory, the ego mediates the conflicts among the id (needs and primitive drives), the superego (moral principles), and external reality (real life demands and obstacles). When the ego is not able to solve these conflicts, anxiety results. Anxiety is the most common symptom in psychiatric disorders, and it occurs in a wide range of diagnoses. Anxiety is a state of tension and uneasiness caused by conflicts that the ego is unable to resolve.

Other common symptoms, such as depression, withdrawal, and hostility, are sometimes just the way the person deals with anxiety. It may be helpful to think of these symptoms as maladaptive ego defenses (see Table 2-1). In other words, the person (consciously perhaps, but most often unconsciously) uses the symptom to reduce his or her anxiety. For example, a man who is angry at his boss and frustrated with his job may develop low back pain; this lets him get out of unpleasant situations without having to express his anger directly.

Although symptoms are sometimes effective for avoiding anxiety, they create other problems and may actually increase anxiety. A teenage girl who feels depressed and insecure about her social skills and appearance may withdraw from her peers, eliminating a potential source of anxiety. As she continues to withdraw, however, her peers may consider her less and less socially acceptable, making it harder for her to approach them, hence increasing her anxiety.

Whatever symptom the individual displays, it can help us identify what the person needs and what he or she is compensating for by acting this way. For example, a woman consumer who identifies with a staff member, copying her clothing and hair style or mannerisms, may be compensating for a feeling that she herself is inadequate or inferior. Clients who make excuses for (rationalize) their own behavior may be having trouble accepting themselves and their own responsibilities. And clients who deny feelings or facts that are unpleasant may be protecting themselves from these painful thoughts.

## Symptoms are Not the Disease

Remember, the symptoms are not the disease. They are only the behavioral evidence of the disease. Most of the symptoms discussed in this chapter occur in many psychiatric disorders. The psychiatric disorder, or diagnosis, is associated with a group of symptoms that commonly occur together. This is similar to the way a physical diagnosis is made. For example, the patient who has a fever, a cough, and red spots on his or her chest is diagnosed as having measles because of the symptoms occurring together. Any one of these symptoms by itself or in a different combination of symptoms may lead to a different diagnosis.

A psychiatrist, when evaluating a person and assigning a diagnosis, considers the person's history and presenting symptoms. Although this is similar to the way a doctor might diagnose measles, there is an important difference. Our understanding of psychiatric disorders is not as advanced as that of physical disorders. A psychiatrist can describe how a patient is behaving and can recognize important clues in his history but does not always reach a diagnosis that another psychiatrist would agree with. Indeed, on the next admission the psychiatrist may reevaluate his or her own diagnosis and assign a different one. It is not uncommon for someone to have had different diagnoses on different admissions, especially to different hospitals. You may be wondering whether psychiatric diagnoses are of any use at all. Psychiatrists use diagnoses to select what drugs or other treatment they will use to help the patient.

For your purposes, as an occupational therapy assistant, you may find that a person's diagnosis is not particularly helpful. Instead, you might find that the individual's behavior and/or reported symptoms give you more of a handle on the situation because they give you clues to what the person needs. Also, because symptoms impair functioning in predictable ways, they give you clues to where the person is having difficulty. After all, the purpose of occupational therapy is to help individuals meet their needs, carry on their life activities, and engage in meaningful occupation. By identifying the symptom and deciphering the underlying need, we take the first step toward helping the person satisfy it.

## Responses to Events

It can be useful to look at the behavior as a response to what is going on, or as an expression of needs. Behavior management approaches of this type have been developed for children with autism and emotional disabilities (36, 42), persons with Alzheimer's disease or other dementia, and those with traumatic brain injury. Comprehensive behavior support (CBS) analyses a child's tantrums to determine what needs are being expressed and to meet those needs *before* the behavior manifests again. For example, a child may scream and bite when she is tired and needs to take a break. When the therapist recognizes the early signs of distress and provides an alternate relaxing activity, the screaming and biting can be averted (36). Because it sometimes happens that the child uses the behavior to avoid a necessary learning activity, it may be more effective to switch to another productive activity that is less demanding but that still fits the therapy goals (42). A similar approach for persons with dementia examines behaviors to determine their *antecedent cause* (event that provokes the behavior). By eliminating the cause, the behavior can be avoided (22). The therapy staff must especially identify items in the environment that stimulate challenging behaviors so that these items can be removed (40).

### Personality and Personal Experiences

Often the particular symptoms displayed are more characteristic of the individual's personality than of his or her psychiatric diagnosis. To illustrate, someone with a diagnosis of schizophrenia may show obsessive-compulsive behavior, such as bizarre rituals (touching doorknobs) and obsessive tidiness. Another person, also diagnosed with schizophrenia, may show a different symptom—for example, repeated assaults on others. Although everyone observing the person can identify the symptom or behavior that is maladaptive, psychiatrists often have difficulty agreeing on why someone has that particular symptom and what the underlying process is. For example, research on obsessive-compulsive behaviors points to evidence of brain abnormalities as a causative factor (39).

### Individual Strengths

It is important to remember also that any individual is much more than the bundle of presenting symptoms. Although much behavior may appear to be unreasonable or bizarre, the person usually has some behaviors or qualities that are fairly healthy, which we can call strengths or assets. The person may be able to do crossword puzzles or play basketball well or may spontaneously help others when they have difficulty. An individual's strengths are just as important as his or her symptoms. In fact, they are probably more important because they can help the person control and master the symptoms. For example, when a depressed, withdrawn woman helps another person do a needlework stitch, she feels that she has done something useful. She may be able to stop thinking about her problems for a little while. If she is able to continue doing something at which she feels competent, she will feel more in control, more able to cope with her problems.

As you continue in your reading of this chapter, it is important to remember the concepts we have covered so far:

- Identifying the symptoms and deciphering the underlying need, antecedent event, or environmental stimulus can help in planning interventions.
- Symptoms may be seen as an expression of unmet needs (e.g., for love and belongingness) or of unresolved conflicts.
- Symptoms are not diagnoses. The same symptom may occur in a variety of diagnoses.
- Symptoms are the behavioral or self-reported evidence of underlying psychological or physiological problems.
- Symptoms may be a response to an event or something in the environment.
- Symptoms are sometimes more related to a person's upbringing and underlying personality than to a particular diagnosis.
- Activities selected in response to symptoms should reflect the individual's assets, interests, occupational role, and present level of functioning.

## RESPONSE VARIABLES

The OTA, faced with someone who is behaving oddly and who seems very uncomfortable, has three tools available. We will call these tools *response variables* because we can change them to meet the individual's needs. The three response variables are self, environment, and activity.

### Self

*Self* is the assistant's own personality, the way he or she talks to and acts toward the persons in his or her care. It is synonymous with *therapeutic use of self.* The way OTAs adapt their personalities to meet the client's needs significantly affects clients' self-perception and the occupational therapy process. As specific symptoms are discussed, guidelines will be given for how to approach (modify your personality for) clients with those symptoms. These guidelines are merely suggestions;

they should not be thought of as rules or demands for you to change your personality. In general, your relationships with all clients will depend on a warm, interested, and open-minded approach to them and to their needs. You must be comfortable with yourself and with your own behavior if you wish to reach out effectively to others. Any modifications that you make in your own behavior must feel right to you. To feel comfortable in a therapeutic role it is important not to make unrealistic demands on yourself. No one is perfect or perfectly in control of his or her responses at all times. You will put yourself in the best frame of mind for helping your clients by trying to do the best you can and accepting the fact that you, like everyone else, will make mistakes.

### Environment

*Environment* is the context in which your interaction with the client takes place. It includes the presence or absence of other people, the general noise level, the amount of visual stimulation, the quality of the lighting, the arrangement of the furniture, the ventilation and temperature, and the presence of objects,. Whereas some features of the environment are beyond your control (e.g., central air-conditioning, absence of windows), others may be changed to meet the needs of the client. Sometimes the person needs more stimulation, sometimes less. Sometimes the level of stimulation is good but the type of stimulation should be changed.

### Activity

*Activity* is the thing that you and the client are doing together. It can range from copper tooling to writing a résumé to organizing materials to prepare a meal to looking at newspaper advertisements for apartments. The list is endless. In selecting activities it is important that they be based in occupations valuable to the person. Consider the person's goals, interests, occupational roles, previous skills, and present level of functioning. At times familiar activities offer security by giving someone an opportunity to demonstrate that he or she can do something well. At other times, such as when a client is confused and disorganized, familiar activities can make him or her feel worse because the client either cannot do them at all or cannot do them as well as in the past. The most effective activities are those that the person has chosen, that mean something to him or her, and that support his or her occupational roles. The assistant should encourage clients to choose their own activities, even if the choice is only among two or three options.

## RESPONSE STRATEGIES

The rest of this chapter presents information to help you respond effectively to clients showing particular symptoms. For each symptom you will find discussion of the following:

- *Definition* of the symptom and a discussion of what it may mean for different individuals (i.e., what unmet needs it may be disguising)
- *Diagnosis* or diagnoses in which the symptom commonly occurs
- *Therapeutic use of self* to help the person feel more comfortable and function better
- *Environmental modifications* to meet the person's needs
- *Characteristics of suitable activities* and recommended modifications in activities
- *Examples of specific activities*

These ideas are culled from many oral and written sources in occupational therapy; they do not work with everyone, and they should not be used mechanically. Do not think of these strategies as a cookbook. We cannot approach every person with depression in the same way, no matter what the guidelines say. Every person is unique. Just as when preparing a meal, it is wise to look in the refrigerator before looking in the cookbook, when working with clients it is important to see what they bring to the situation.

Remember also that the most powerful intervention is to educate the consumer about symptom management, so that he or she can monitor symptoms and reduce or eliminate discomforting feelings (11). This will be discussed further at the end of the chapter.

## Anxiety

*Anxiety is a state of tension and uneasiness caused by conflicts that the ego is unable to resolve.* It is one of the most common symptoms seen in psychiatric illness. It is normal for every person to feel some anxiety, particularly when faced with frightening, challenging, or unpredictable situations. The healthy person controls anxiety through the unconscious operation of the various defense mechanisms (see Table 2-1), the purpose of which is to avoid any unpleasant conflicts and the anxiety associated with them. To a certain degree we can think of anxiety as a positive force. It motivates us to attempt new things—for example, your anxiety on first encountering a new client may prod you to approach and try to talk to him or her.

Although everyone feels some anxiety, it becomes pathological (causing illness) only when it is so extreme and so long lasting that it interferes with effective functioning in daily life. Anxiety may occur alone, as the primary symptom, or with other symptoms. Sometimes it causes other symptoms, just as a fever causes malaise, chills, and aches. For example, remember the client dialogue presented earlier in this chapter: We may conclude that the client became angry and hostile because he was anxious about his perceived failure in copper tooling.

We can recognize when someone is anxious by observing body language and listening to what the person says. Some people worry aloud; they talk incessantly about things that may never happen. Others fidget; they tap their feet, jiggle their legs, bite their nails, pull their hair, tug at their faces, drum the tabletop, and pace the halls. Others express fears about certain places or objects. They may be afraid to go outside or to use the toilet. Regardless of the behaviors through which a person expresses anxiety, the therapeutic objective is generally the same: to control or reduce the experience of anxiety so that the person can function.

### Diagnoses in Which Anxiety Is a Common Symptom

As a symptom, anxiety may be found in almost every diagnostic category. The only recognized exception is in cases of social deviancy (antisocial personality). It was once believed that criminals, psychopaths, and other deviant individuals experience no anxiety at all. Current understanding, based on reports from such clients that they feel tense, is that they do feel uncomfortable because they know they are different from other people (5).

### Strategy for Therapeutic Use of Self

Encourage clients to talk about what is bothering them and to express how they feel. Answer their questions if you can but avoid being drawn into extended discussions of physical symptoms and their possible causes. It helps to focus first on what clients are concerned about, listen to their fears, and then gradually redirect their attention to a neutral topic or something more constructive. Different responses are needed for individuals who express their anxiety through rituals, phobias, or constantly demanding attention (Table 11-1).

### Strategy for Modifying the Environment

In general, the environment should be calm, comfortable, and familiar. People who are disposed to be anxious often become more so when overstimulated by too much noise or too many people. A context that is different from what the person is used to may be frightening. Giving such clients a brief tour of the occupational therapy area and a schedule for activities helps them feel more secure and in control.

**TABLE 11-1 FLEXIBLE RESPONSES TO ANXIOUS BEHAVIORS**

| BEHAVIOR | RECOMMENDED RESPONSE |
|---|---|
| **Ritualistic, compulsive** | |
| The patient carries out unnecessary and apparently meaningless actions, such as checking for dust on door sills before crossing them | Never criticize the patient's behavior. Instead, recognize that no matter how ridiculous the ritual may appear, it is one the patient uses to cope with anxiety. You can make such patients more comfortable if you can convince them that you accept them no matter what they do. |
| **Phobic, fearful** | |
| The patient is afraid of things that other people do not find frightening (e.g., going shopping, riding in cars) | Encourage such patients to talk about their fears; help them focus on exactly what makes them afraid. This is especially important when the fear prevents them from accomplishing tasks needed in their occupational role (e.g., a homemaker has to shop for food). |
| **Intrusive, demanding** | |
| The patient constantly demands attention or interrupts when you are working with others | Reassure such patients that you will be available to help them. Give them a definite time and stick to it. Ignore subsequent interruptions but do not become angry with such patients. |

### Strategy for Selecting Activities

Guide clients to choose their own activity; ask clients what things they find relaxing or that take their mind off their worries. Help the client select activities that produce a successful result without excessive attention to detail. A project that the person can work on for a while, get up and move about, and come back to later is ideal. Some anxious persons respond well to activities involving a single motor sequence that is repeated (e.g., quick point); they seem to use the regular pace of the activity to control and calm their own pace. Gross motor activities, such as aerobic exercise or stretching and relaxation, can reduce the uncomfortable physical symptoms that go with anxiety (e.g., tense muscles, neck and back aches, racing pulse). Yoga, tai chi, qi gong and other Eastern practices are beneficial. Meditation, relaxation tapes, or biofeedback can also be used. Stress management techniques such as progressive relaxation, time management, and leisure skills may help the person identify stressors and prevent or reduce anxiety. Social support such as a conversation with a friend or a social gathering can also help. Cognitive behavioral approaches to reduce cognitive distortions (see Chapter 2) helps put worries in perspective. Journal writing, nature walks, and multisensory rooms and other sensory approaches are additional possibilities (9) (Box 11-1).

## Depression

*Depression is a feeling of intense sadness, despair, and hopelessness.* Like anxiety, depression occasionally affects most people. Sadness is an appropriate response to painful losses, such as the death of a loved one, being fired from a job, or being rebuffed by a friend. Most people recover from these sad

**BOX 11-1**

## ANXIETY: EXAMPLES OF APPROPRIATE ACTIVITIES

- *Small woodworking kits.* Those with a small number of pieces (three) are best until you are certain the person can handle more. An exception is the heart basket[a] (shown here), in which many pieces are identical and assembly is obvious if a finished model is provided.

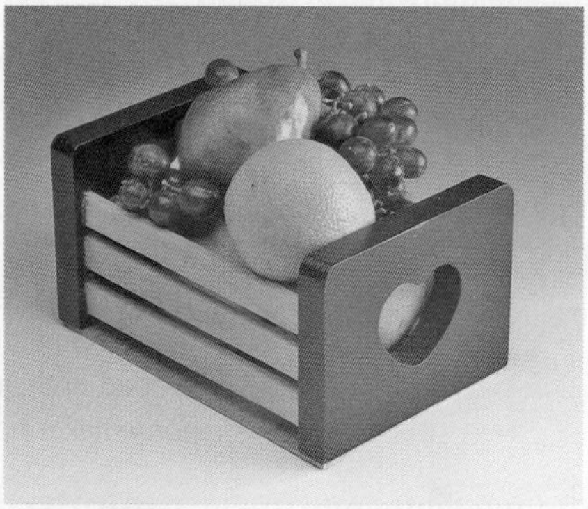

**Heart basket.** The assembly is simple and straightforward; the kit may be sanded and finished over several sessions. The kit requires the help of another person to position and glue the second side of the basket. (Photo courtesy of S&S Arts and Crafts, Colchester, CT.)

- *Simple cooking tasks.* For example making chocolate-chip cookies. There are lots of opportunities for the client to move around while cleaning up or waiting for a batch to be done.
- *Stress management, cognitive behavioral training, and coping skills training.* These can give the person resources to better manage situations that provoke anxiety.
- *Yoga.* This will need physician approval and should be taught by someone who knows the correct body dynamics and techniques. Alternatively, the person can be helped to relax by doing tai chi or qi gong, taking a walk, raking leaves, or doing housework.

[a]Available from S&S Arts and Crafts, Colchester, CT, and other vendors.

feelings and are able to carry on with their lives. Depression becomes pathological when it lasts longer than most people would consider reasonable and when it interferes with ordinary activities.

The depressed person typically shows a cluster of symptoms related to the depression. The most striking is the depressed mood, often accompanied by crying or irritability. Depressed people also tend to have bleak views of themselves and of the world in general and to see the future as hopeless. They feel helpless, hopeless, and possibly worthless and guilty. They usually lose interest in people and activities that previously brought pleasure. Such clients' statements in occupational therapy often betray their low opinion of themselves: "I'm stupid," "Don't bother with me; the other guys need you more," "I can't even do this right." They are easily frustrated and tend to blame themselves for whatever goes wrong.

Other associated symptoms, termed *vegetative signs,* include changes in activity level and biological functioning. Sleeping too much or not being able to sleep, losing one's appetite or overeating, neglect of personal hygiene and grooming, and diminished energy are common. Depressed people's movements and speech may be slowed down (psychomotor retardation) or speeded up (psychomotor agitation). Their mental functions may be dull; they may have trouble concentrating or making decisions and may be slow to respond to questions. They may be easily distracted and unable to pay attention long enough to complete simple hygiene and grooming tasks.

Many theories address the causes of depression. Evidence suggests that a biochemical element may be responsible—for example, low levels of serotonin, a neurotransmitter (brain chemical), have been found in suicidal individuals. It is also possible that the loss of a parent or similar serious loss in early childhood may predispose certain individuals to depression in adulthood. Another theory is that the depressed person has a less stable and secure sense of self than other people and so reacts strongly to even mild criticism and setbacks.

The cognitive therapists Ellis (14) and Beck (6) argue that people become depressed because they think illogical thoughts. For example, a woman who forgets to pick up her husband's shirts from the laundry may think this is just another example of her inadequacy as a wife and may believe that her husband will divorce her or at least criticize her. Cognitive-behavior therapy (see Chapter 2) attempts to help clients identify irrational negative beliefs and to substitute more logical and positive ideas.

Yet another theory argues that depression operates like the defense mechanisms to protect depressed people from feelings that they fear are even more painful. For example, the "anger turned inward" argument is that instead of becoming angry at the cause of the loss (the person who left, died, or rejected the patient), depressed individuals turn the anger against themselves. Because they unconsciously feel it is bad to be angry, they punish themselves by being depressed. Nonetheless, they may still feel guilty about being angry, and this contributes to self-hatred and a sense of worthlessness.

In still another theory, Seligman (43) suggests that depressed individuals may have learned to feel helpless as a result of repeated failures in which nothing they did seemed to change what happened. Depressed people have "learned" that they cannot control their own lives and have decided to give up trying. They attempt to withdraw from other people, seeking physical isolation by sitting alone, wandering off, or staying in bed all day. In this way, they can retreat from a reality that they perceive as threatening, hostile, and unmanageable. The passive and negative behavior of the unemployed, the homeless, and the economically disadvantaged becomes quite understandable when viewed from this perspective.

Seligman concludes that activities that produce an experience of success and self-control will relieve depression. Neville (38) notes that the volition subsystem is impaired in the depressed client, as evidenced by a belief that one's life is not in one's control and that the future is hopeless. Neville, like Seligman, recommends that individuals with depression be exposed to experiences that reinforce their sense of responsibility and self-control.

## Diagnoses in Which Depression Is a Common Symptom

Depression occurs in a wide range of disorders. It is the primary symptom in the affective (mood) disorders. Depression is common in organic mental disorders. It is frequently seen in schizophrenia, in almost all of the personality disorders, and in substance abusers. As previously discussed, it is a normal response to personal loss and so is a common symptom of the various adjustment reactions.

## Strategy for Therapeutic Use of Self

Allow depressed clients to talk about what is bothering them; discussion should focus on exactly how they feel and why. The more they understand the causes of their depression, the more likely they are to be able to do something about it. Engel (16) suggests that the therapist avoid being overprotective and helpful; a matter-of-fact, even-tempered acceptance seems best. The assistant should listen and reflect back what he or she hears such clients saying but should never agree that the situation seems hopeless. Instead, the assistant should provide direction and help with selection of realistic short-term goals and activities that the client can accomplish. The assistant should reinforce good hygiene and grooming and encourage clients to keep up their personal appearance.

Clients who are silent and withdrawn present a special challenge. Often they try to discourage staff contact by becoming more withdrawn or hostile and then fleeing. Assistants should not be tricked by these maneuvers into neglecting withdrawn clients. By approaching them many times, each time for only a brief period, OTAs show that they accept these clients' feelings. As clients become more comfortable, they eventually respond. For example, the OTA may visit the client in the client's customary spot and sit quietly, perhaps commenting occasionally about current events or things that have happened in the neighborhood or the clinic. After several visits, the client may be willing to attempt a simple activity on a one-on-one basis. Later, group activities can be attempted while the one-on-one activity is continued.

In general, therapists should match their tempo to that of the client, whether the client is slow moving or agitated. Therapists should be quite clear when giving any directions to clients and avoid giving them more choices than they can handle. It is better to present only two activity choices at first. Therapists should avoid praising what clients accomplish, rather acknowledging their efforts with a simple comment: "It looks like you've finished that. Is there anything more you'd like to do with it?" Depressed clients are usually well aware of the difference between their present level of functioning and their past abilities, and excessive praise may make them think they must be in very bad shape. Assistants should accept whatever their clients can do at the moment and not pressure them into doing more. It is not unusual for depressed people not to want to keep projects they have made. The project is likely to be poorly executed, showing the person's low energy level and limited attention to detail. The OTA should accept the client's decision to reject the project and should refrain from commenting on it further.

When the depressed individual talks about bad feelings, the assistant should under no circumstances change the subject or try to cheer up the client. These approaches deny the importance of the person's feelings and indicate that the assistant does not accept the client or want to deal with his or her real concerns.

Depressed clients who are receiving medication may be expected to show a decrease in depressive symptoms (symptom remission) within the first 3 weeks of treatment. At this time, clients may have more energy but still feel depressed, and there is a real risk of suicide; the risk is greater for those who have previously attempted suicide. On the other hand, two thirds of suicide attempts are successful the first time (41). Some of the signs that a person may be thinking of suicide include obvious ones like talking about it or wondering aloud what it would be like to be dead. Others that are less obvious are the appearance of feeling much better for no clear reason and giving away personal possessions. For example, the client may present the assistant with an item of personal property. Without rebuffing the client, the OTA should encourage the client to talk about why he or she is doing this.

The OTA who suspects that a client is contemplating suicide *must notify medical staff* (nurse, doctor, or primary therapist). Otherwise, the OTA may hear in the Monday-morning staff meeting that the client jumped off a roof during the weekend. If the client is being seen on an outpatient basis, the assistant should contact his or her own supervisor and the client's primary therapist so that a more skilled person can evaluate whether the client needs to be hospitalized.

### Strategy for Modifying the Environment

The environment should be safe and subdued. In general, the more severe the depression, the less stimulation should be present. It may be necessary to reduce the lighting and the noise level and work one on one to get the client to focus on an activity. Too much stimulation may cause the client to retreat further. This is particularly true for withdrawn clients, who may not be able to tolerate the others in a group. As the client becomes more comfortable, the amount of stimulation should be increased gradually; having more materials, supplies, and sample projects visible will increase opportunities for decision making.

The structure on an inpatient ward limits opportunities for patients to make choices about even simple things. For example, meals consist of whatever is served when the staff says it is mealtime. Patients who are suicidal may not be permitted to wear their own clothing so that staff will know not to let them out of the ward. Showering and shaving may be scheduled at the staff's convenience. This atmosphere can further weaken a depressed person's fragile sense of self-control. Therefore, choices should be presented whenever possible. Merely deciding to rearrange the furniture or hang up a picture can increase the patient's sense of responsibility and competence.

### Strategy for Selecting Activities

Start with simple, structured, short-term, familiar activities. Unstructured activities should be avoided because depression leaves people with little energy to make the necessary decisions. The activities must be short-term ones because the depressed individual typically lacks the attention span for a longer activity and can work only slowly and intermittently. For the same reason, activities that require rapid responses at particular moments (e.g., slip casting) should be avoided unless a staff member or volunteer is available to assist the person. Repetitive activities allow the individual to succeed with minimal new learning because the motions are learned only once and then repeated. Although familiar activities are generally more comfortable, there is a risk that the client will compare present performance with past performance, further damaging his or her self-esteem. Therefore, simple, unfamiliar activities are sometimes preferred, at least initially.

The first activities used should be ones at which the person is guaranteed to succeed. Even a simple task like making a phone call or brushing one's hair can be a first step. Activities are then graded to include more complexity and require more effort as the person becomes more confident and energetic.

In the beginning, the activities should be ones that can be done alone, without the need to interact or share tools or materials with others. Thereafter, opportunities for minimal socialization should be presented as soon as the person seems comfortable. Those who are agitated benefit from activities in which they use their hands; this substitutes productive actions for nonproductive ones like hand wringing and fidgeting.

People who are depressed may avoid crafts, games, and exercise because they seem too pleasurable or too exhausting. Clients with depression may be more able to accept an activity that is useful to other people than to themselves. Staff should try to accept offers of help from depressed clients to reinforce the client's active choice. Some clients respond well to activities that are tedious, menial, and repetitive (peeling potatoes, mopping the floor); the client may be using these activities to work off feelings of guilt. Although clients should be permitted to do these activities when they choose, other activities should be introduced gradually.

Gross motor activities can help to release tension, promote the intake of oxygen, and increase blood flow to the brain. There is ample evidence that activity can relieve depression (49), but the real problem is motivating the depressed individual to attempt it. The person's low energy level is a serious obstacle, but it can sometimes be overcome by simply telling the client that it's time for the activity (e.g., "We are going to the gym now.").

Precautions against suicide and self-abuse should be observed at all times. Although depressed clients may feel more in control if they can use sharp tools without harming themselves, the assistant must stay alert to this possibility. Even seemingly innocuous objects can be used in a suicide attempt—for example, a depressed patient might use a leather belt or macramé project in an attempt at hanging. Particularly in inpatient settings, tools and supplies should be accounted for at the beginning and end of every session and before any patient leaves the room, even to go to the bathroom. Similarly, when working with clients outdoors or in open or unfamiliar settings, the assistant must stay aware of all clients; depressed individuals may leave the group and harm themselves.

Activities that teach chronically depressed persons to manage stress and advocate for themselves are important. This includes leisure skills, assertiveness training, and role-oriented treatment focusing on the roles important to them. These experiences help clients to unlearn helplessness.

Selection of activities depends on treatment goals (Box 11-2). For persons with depression, these may include improving role balance, increasing coping skills, and improving social skills. Engel (16) suggests specific additional activities. Gutman (25) recommends teaching the consumer to monitor herself and her moods and to regulate moods through activity that is arousing or calming (depending on need). Clients can feel discouraged when depression recurs, and psychoeducation about the up and down patterns of mood disorders gives them needed information. Keeping to routines to comply with medication is also important.

## Mania

*Mania is a disturbance of mood characterized by excessive happiness (euphoria), generosity (expansiveness), irritability, distractibility, and increased activity level.* The manic individual appears to be operating at highway speed in a 25-mile-per-hour zone. Everything is speeded up. Manic clients may be hyperactive or agitated. They may speak very rapidly (pressured speech) and skip from topic to topic (flight of ideas). They find it hard to concentrate on any one thing, instead flitting from one to another; they are often involved in many different activities simultaneously. They may express an unrealistic view of their own abilities, believing they can accomplish almost anything (grandiosity). They may get involved in very risky enterprises and endanger themselves or their families by spending money frivolously, taking expensive trips, extorting money from others, and so on. They seem unaware of or indifferent to the consequences of such actions.

People in manic states typically have very poor judgment, which reveals itself in almost everything they attempt. Their style of dress may be eccentric or downright bizarre. They may wear several hats or belts simultaneously or cover their clothing with emblems, buttons, or other decorations. Females (and some males) may wear excessive and poorly blended makeup.

One of the most disturbing qualities of persons in manic states is their attitude toward and effect on other people. They have a lot of energy and commonly flatter others and give them gifts. Because of this an unsuspecting staff member can be drawn into a relationship in which the staff member enjoys the client's mania because it fuels the staff member's own self-esteem.

People with mania are very sensitive to others' vulnerabilities—for example, they may say that

**BOX 11-2**

## DEPRESSION: EXAMPLES OF APPROPRIATE ACTIVITIES

- *Some simple, structured, short-term, familiar activities* include housework, organizing papers or books, folding laundry, simple cooking, sanding, clerical tasks, and sewing. The person's previous interests and occupational roles will guide the OTA in selecting the particular activity.
- *Craft activities* that may be less familiar but are still highly structured include mosaics, copper tooling, leather work, and woodworking. These must be graded down to a fairly simple, short-term level at first. Kits are useful, but the OTA should try the kit first, as many have one or two steps that are not obvious or that require dexterity or timing.
- *Gross motor activities* include aerobic exercise, dance therapy, yoga (shown here), running, swimming, ball games, and walking (especially outdoors).

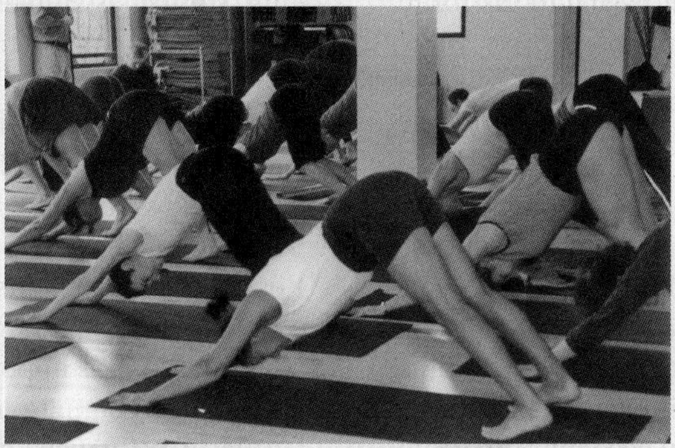

**Exercise and fitness.** Physical health and fitness facilitate wellness and help with regulation of moods. Downward-facing dog *(adho mukha svanasana)* and other yoga poses *(asanas)* help pacify emotions and increase self-awareness and self-control. (Photo courtesy of the Iyengar Yoga Association of Greater New York.)

- *Values clarification, stress management, coping skills training,* and *assertiveness training* may provide resources for addressing specific problems.

they cannot be helped by a certain new therapist because that person just got out of school and does not have enough experience. If the therapist really feels insecure about this, the person may be able to drive the therapist away and manipulate the self-esteem of other staff who feel superior because they have more experience. Using this maneuver (known as splitting) can create staff conflict, which takes the pressure off the client.

Another tactic used by individuals in the manic state is upping the ante. The client starts by making what seems like a reasonable request (e.g., to go out to the hall to smoke a cigarette). Once the request is granted, the person asks for something else, and then something else, until he or she finally makes a request that is completely unreasonable (e.g., to have everyone stop working and take a break). When the therapist refuses to grant the final request, the person becomes angry and abusive, arguing that the therapist is uptight and rigid.

What purpose do these tactics serve? Why is the manic person so ready to manipulate others? Some (28) argue that such individuals are very ambivalent about their need to be taken care of. They need other people but are frightened of depending on them. So they arrange to control and manipulate their caregivers. When such a client finally exhausts the patience of the caregivers and the caregivers take control over the client's behavior, the client has the satisfaction of being taken care of without having to ask for it.

## Diagnoses in Which Mania Is a Common Symptom

Mania is the primary symptom of a manic episode in an affective disorder, but it can occur in other disorders as well. These include organic conditions caused by substance abuse, paranoid schizophrenia, and some personality disorders. Jamison (27), a psychiatrist, has written an interesting and highly readable first-person account of mania.

## Strategy for Therapeutic Use of Self

The manic person's ambivalence about relying on other people raises specific issues for the therapeutic relationship. It is easy to be manipulated by someone who makes you feel special, and the OTA should beware of flattery. Similarly, criticisms of other staff by the client are often the opening gambit in a game of "You're the only one who can help me."

These clients may demand almost constant attention, praise, and approval from staff members. At the same time, their behavior, for which they are seeking approval, is often so bizarre and self-centered that others avoid them. The OTA should be cautious in giving any praise or approval to the person who is manic and should instead firmly and gently focus on how to make the behavior more appropriate. However, it is also essential to avoid criticizing manic clients because they are very vulnerable and easily feel rejected. Some psychologists argue that mania is the flip side of depression. In other words, the low self-esteem and feelings of despair and hopelessness that characterize depression are often just under the surface of the manic person's behavior.

It is important to be calm, matter-of-fact, firm, and consistent with the manic individual. Setting and enforcing limits on what the person can do shows the client that *someone* is in control, even if he or she is not. Such clients may also interpret limit setting as a message that the staff cares enough about them to stop them from hurting themselves.

As these clients' medication begins to take effect and their symptoms diminish, they may become frightened when they remember the bizarre and impulsive things they did when they were ill. Reassuring such clients that these behaviors were caused by the illness can make them feel more comfortable. It is important to recognize, though, that people coming out of a manic episode may face legal or financial problems as a result of their actions during the manic phase.

Getting manic individuals to focus on just one activity is a challenge. They typically make grandiose or unrealistic statements (e.g., "I'm very creative. I know weaving and beading and fashion design. I'm going to weave my own fabric and make a beaded evening gown."). The OTA should not go along with these schemes and should suggest other more realistic activities. The assistant must set firm limits on the use of supplies and materials and not permit the manic person to overrun the clinic. This requires constant alertness and patience; the OTA will have to remind and redirect the client many times over. As the person's mood becomes more stable, expectations for attention span and decision making should be increased (15).

The person is likely to resist rules and expectations for performance, saying in effect, "My way is much more creative. Don't be a drag." It is important not to get emotionally involved in discussing why a project should be done a certain way; instead, firmly and briefly explain what has to be done and show the patient a sample. If the person insists on doing it differently, there is no point in arguing about it as long as no one is endangered. A sense of humor and perspective is very helpful in getting along with manic individuals. Because they are so distractible and have such poor judgment, manic clients should be carefully watched around electrical equipment and other objects that might accidentally cause injury.

### Strategy for Modifying the Environment

Controlling the environment to help the manic patient function is based on a single principle: Manic patients respond to every bit of stimulation present. Therefore, the OTA should eliminate or reduce distractions in the environment to the greatest possible extent. For example, an occupational therapy shop decorated with many finished projects and interesting materials is likely to provoke intense interest in doing everything at once. To avoid this, the assistant should strip the environment of everything but what is essential to the activity. Tools and supplies needed for later steps in a project should be kept out of sight until such time as they are needed.

Remember that *anything* can distract the manic individual. Music, other people, the telephone, the view from the window can all invite the most intense curiosity and involvement. Distractions should be minimized. If possible, have the person work alone, facing a blank wall.

### Strategy for Selecting Activities

Because of the high energy level, activities that permit the manic person to get up and move around are ideal. Short-term activities provide immediate gratification to the person with poor frustration tolerance and inability to wait for results. Allen (2) recommends that craft activities be portable because the client is likely to carry projects around.

Activities should be structured and have three or fewer steps. Activities that are unfocused or creative or that require decisions (e.g., oil painting) should be avoided. Similarly, activities should not require fine coordination or attention to detail. Materials should be controllable, not floppy or unpredictable (e.g., leather or wood rather than clay).

Because the manic person needs to develop a longer attention span, provide activities that involve carryover of skills from one day to the next. For example, whipstitch can be done first on leather and later as an embroidery stitch (fabric is floppier and therefore less controllable than leather).

Clients in a manic state may benefit from gross motor exercise because it allows them to move around and use up excess energy. However, it is difficult for the OTA (or anyone) to deal with more than three or four members in an exercise group if one is acutely manic; more staff are needed for larger groups. In later stages, as medication becomes effective, the person coming out of a manic episode can benefit from exploring ways to create and maintain a balanced daily schedule, including ample time for rest and sleep (15) (Box 11-3).

## Hallucinations

*A hallucination is a sensory experience that does not correspond to external reality.* A hallucinating person sees, hears, feels, smells, or tastes things that are not there. Some common hallucinations are hearing voices, seeing animals or people or lights, and feeling burning or crawling sensations on the skin.

Hallucinations arise from a temporary or permanent defect in the way the brain functions. It is as though a connection were loose or a circuit were overloaded. There is a malfunction in the

**BOX 11-3**

### MANIA: EXAMPLES OF APPROPRIATE ACTIVITIES

As with any other client, it is best to let the manic patient choose the activity. The assistant should present only two or, at most, three choices. Ideas about what activities might be appropriate can be obtained from the person's history or the evaluation.

- *Crafts* that might be used are copper tooling, stringing beads, and sanding and finishing prefabricated wooden projects. Some clients respond well to small leather projects (e.g., wristbands, coin purses with hardware already attached), such as the one shown. The assistant may need to perform one or more of the steps, especially if they involve fine coordination (e.g., ending the lacing, applying a snap). Projects in which the person's name can be part of the decoration appeal to some manic persons.

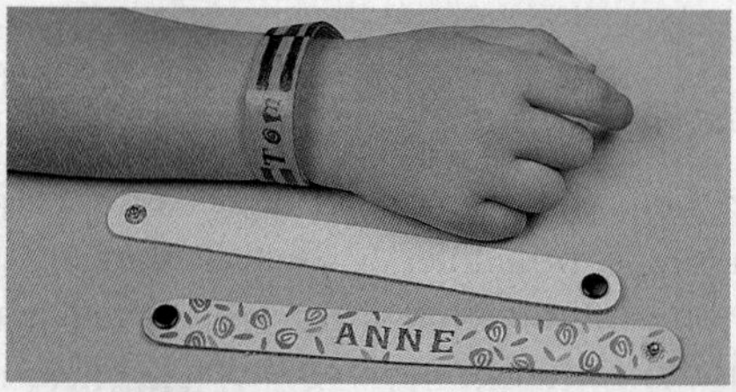


**Small leather wristband.** This is a suitable project for someone in a manic episode or with a short attention span. (Photo courtesy of S&S Arts and Crafts, Colchester, CT.)

- *Semistructured activities* can be used with caution. For example, magazine picture collage will invite chaos unless it is structured; by providing only a few magazines and a pair of scissors at first, then supplying the backing paper after the pictures have been selected and cut out, and the glue only after the pictures have been arranged, the assistant will help the client stay in control of what he or she is doing and obtain a better result.
- *Gross motor activities* such as dance, exercise, and volleyball can help the clients work off energy and use their hyperactivity productively. Sometimes it is easier to work one on one in an exercise activity with the manic person than in a group.
- *Time management, stress management,* and *money management* activities may be of use to persons who have recently experienced a manic episode or who have a history of such episodes.

part of the brain that interprets external sensation and that differentiates between what is happening and what is imagined. Changes in several brain structures and imbalances in several brain chemicals have been suggested as the causes of hallucinations (33).

Auditory (sound) hallucinations occur most often. Hallucinating people may hear voices telling them to do things (command hallucinations) or criticizing them or may hear music or strange sounds or someone calling their name. They may perceive a sound as much louder or softer than it really is. Visual hallucinations are also common and may involve seeing walls move, having one's face look strange in the mirror, or thinking that people look transparent or flat. Gustatory (taste) and olfactory (smell) hallucinations, which are less common, affect patients with temporal lobe epilepsy; usually the hallucinated taste or smell is very unpleasant. Tactile (touch) hallucinations may be of itching or burning or a feeling that insects are crawling on or biting one's skin.

Clients usually find hallucinations troubling, frightening, and uncomfortable. It is not hard to understand this reaction to voices saying awful, threatening things or spiders crawling over one's clothes. However, the client may enjoy hallucinations of voices that praise the client or say he or she has special powers. Similarly, hallucinations that enhance reality are usually perceived as very pleasant. For example, the person may become transfixed by the glittering crystal patterns in an ordinary city sidewalk or by the varied textures and colors on a brick wall. It has been suggested that some individuals rely on their "voices" as a substitute for human relationships; this seems most likely when the voices say reassuring or flattering things.

## Diagnoses in Which Hallucinations Are a Common Symptom

Hallucinations can occur in a wide range of psychiatric disorders and may also accompany a high fever. Some of the psychiatric disorders include schizophrenia (see discussion of perceptual distortions in Chapter 3), manic and depressive psychoses, organic mental disorders, and substance-abuse disorders.

In each of these conditions the type of hallucination may differ. For example, auditory hallucinations are common in schizophrenia; voices may comment on the client's behavior, usually in an insulting way. In schizophrenia, the hallucinations seem unrelated to the person's mood. In manic and depressive disorders auditory hallucinations may also be present, but they are *mood congruent*. This means that the voices say things that are consistent with the person's mood (e.g., telling the depressed person that he or she is bad or to commit suicide).

## Strategy for Therapeutic Use of Self

Therapy staff should try to reassure hallucinating clients and help them understand what is happening to them, saying for example, "I believe that you see rats in the corners, but they are not really there. It's your disease that makes you see them."

Talking in a calm, firm, natural, rhythmic, soothing manner may comfort the person. Assistants should point out any real sensory stimulus that the person seems to misinterpret ("That sound was the central air-conditioning coming on."). They should avoid sarcastic comments, no matter how tempting. For example, when a client says he or she has visitors from another planet, the assistant should not say, "Oh, really? Which one?" Frese (18, 19), a psychologist and a consumer himself, suggests that a helpful reply might be, "How very interesting. Tell me more about it."

At the same time, however, OTAs should refrain from arguing about whether or not the hallucinations are real. Instead, they might redirect a client's attention to some neutral topic or activity and try to draw the person back to reality. They can acknowledge how the hallucination makes the client feel without agreeing that it is real. Because it is impossible to know a person's emotional reaction to a hallucination, the OTA should not assume that the person feels any particular way about it. However, clients who are hallucinating often react aversively to being touched by other people; therefore, the person should be given lots of room.

One report indicates that having the hallucinating client repeat a word or phrase that is comforting and positive may help reduce the length, frequency, and intrusiveness of hallucinations (33). For example, the person might say, "I am safe here," or "I have done the best I can and it is good enough." Other strategies include either increasing or decreasing external stimulation, depending on what works; clients are very interested in exploring these strategies once they trust the practitioner and believe that the strategies may work. The key is for the client to identify simple and successful strategies, practice them, and remember to implement them (19, 32).

Reports (7, 32) suggest that cognitive therapy and other educational approaches may help some hallucinating individuals understand how the hallucinations arise. Persons with paranoid schizophrenia, for example, may be taught to identify "voices" as signals from their own brains; furthermore, they can learn to diminish or block them by wearing a radio headset, for example (7). The OTA who is interested in applying these strategies should read the literature and seek additional supervision and direction.

### Strategy for Modifying the Environment

Many of those who hallucinate do so when they are under stress, especially in environments that are too stimulating for them. Sometimes just moving the person to a quieter, less overwhelming area will make the hallucinations diminish or go away altogether. Therefore, in general, the environment should be calm, quiet, and nondistracting.

On the other hand, clients should not be permitted to isolate themselves from other people entirely because hallucinations may increase in the absence of any other stimulation. In fact, associating with other people, especially conversing with them, tends to block auditory hallucinations and increase focus on reality. MacRae (33) reported that a client successfully limited his hallucinations by going on a planned walk as soon as the voices began.

### Strategy for Selecting Activities

Simple, highly structured activities that encourage involvement and interaction with a few other trusted people are recommended. The structure prevents such clients from drifting away into a private world, and the presence of other people tends to focus them on reality. If possible, the activity should require some minimal interaction with others, if only to ask for a tool. These people should not be permitted to work alone, apart from the group. Activities should not demand attention to detail or fine coordination because the person may still be distracted occasionally by the hallucinations.

Some therapists advocate activities that strongly stimulate the senses. They argue that flooding the person's auditory channels with music or a sing-along may block auditory hallucinations. Allen (1) has observed that hallucinating individuals prefer to work with bright colors, and she believes these somehow interfere with the hallucinations. However, it is also apparent that hallucinations in some persons seem to get worse when other stimulation is increased, as if the hallucination were trying to compete for the person's attention. The most useful information about how a given activity affects a particular individual is obtained from that person. By watching how someone reacts and listening to what he or she says, the OTA can usually learn enough about the effects of the activity to determine whether it is working or how it needs to be changed (Box 11-4).

## Delusions

*A delusion is a belief that is contrary to reality as experienced by others in one's cultural group.* A true delusion is a belief not based on reality. Delusional people may believe, for example, that television shows and newspaper stories have special messages for them or that automobile license plates contain a secret code that they must decipher to save the world. These beliefs are called *ideas of reference.* Or a woman may believe that the FBI is taking thoughts out of her brain (*thought withdrawal*) or putting strange ones in (*thought insertion*). She may feel as if she were

**BOX 11-4**

**HALLUCINATIONS: EXAMPLES OF APPROPRIATE ACTIVITIES**

- *Simple, structured, short-term activities* might include coloring "stained-glass" (nonreligious) pictures, discussing specific current events, preparing lunch, and assembling wood kits. Familiar, necessary life tasks, such as doing laundry or housework, can also be used when relevant to the individual's interests and occupational roles.
- *Activities with strong sensory stimulation* include those involving music or dance, watching films or television, and cooking and eating. Falk-Kessler and Froschauer (17) described a group activity in which clients watched and discussed soap operas with the staff. Because many people with psychiatric disorders tend to watch many hours of television daily anyway, this seemed a way to control hallucinations and create a bridge from their imaginary worlds to reality.

being followed (*delusions of persecution*) or that she had special powers (*megalomania* or *delusions of grandeur*). Other common delusions include *erotomania* (the delusion that someone is in love with you) and *somatic delusions* (belief that something horrible is wrong with one's body).

A delusion is a false belief that is peculiar to the individual. It thus differs from a cultural belief, which although odd may be embraced by an entire nation or ethnic group. For example, people in some Caribbean countries believe that pulling on babies' limbs when they are bathed will make them taller, stronger, and better coordinated when they grow up. As another example, Australian aborigines believe that the "real" world that we experience while awake is less powerful and in a sense less real than the dream world of sleep and drugged states.

Students sometimes find it hard to remember the difference between a delusion and a hallucination. A delusion is an inaccurate thought or idea. (*Hint: de*lusion is a wrong *ide*a.) By contrast, a hallucination is a false perception, sensory experience, or feeling. A person does not have to hear or see something that is not there to have a delusional idea; a delusion may be based on real-life events; it is the interpretation of these events that is odd. For example, the person may think that the newscaster on television who seems to look him or her right in the eye while summarizing a story knows all about the person and is sending a special message. What the person actually sees and hears is no different from what any viewer would see; it is the interpretation that is different.

The content and quality of delusions can give clues about the person's needs. For example, delusions in which one is special are thought to be a defense against feelings of inferiority and inadequacy. Being a target of persecution also conveys a sense of being special that may mask poor self-esteem, but because other people are viewed as dangerous, it also allows such people to distance themselves from others, thereby not risking rejection.

### Diagnoses in Which Delusions Are a Common Symptom

Delusions may be present in any of the psychotic disorders: schizophrenia, bipolar disorder (both manic and depressive phases), and organic mental disorders. They may occur in certain personality disorders (schizotypal personality, paranoid personality), in eating disorders (anorexia nervosa, bulimia), and in persons who have no other known psychopathology.

**BOX 11-5**

**DELUSIONS: EXAMPLES OF APPROPRIATE ACTIVITIES**

Some intellectually challenging verbal activities include board games, current events discussion, crossword puzzles, and word games. Chess and computer games might also be used. Aspects of the person's usual occupation should be incorporated wherever possible—for example, a real estate agent can organize files and develop presentation materials or an office assistant can use a word-processing program. Expressive activities such as dancing or writing poetry are recommended by Frese (19).

Brain disorders, especially injury to the right cerebral cortex, may result in *delusions of misidentification*. In this sort of delusion, the person may feel that someone (spouse, for example) has been replaced by a duplicate or that one's original self has been replaced (12).

### Strategy for Therapeutic Use of Self

As a rule, it is best to avoid discussing the person's delusions because discussion tends to reinforce them. Sometimes it cannot be avoided, however. Whenever possible, try to redirect the person's attention to an activity or something else that is reality based. It is pointless to try to convince delusional people that their delusions are not true; doing so will only alienate and anger them. So listen with interest but keep the focus on what you are doing.

Developing and organizing delusions that, although odd, make a certain bizarre sense requires a fair degree of intelligence and cognitive skill. Relate to the delusional individual as an intelligent adult. Avoid the appearance of being patronizing or frustrated.

### Strategy for Modifying the Environment

The environment should be relatively stimulating and provide opportunities for the person to get involved in real-life activities.

### Strategy for Selecting Activities

All activities should be suited to the person's intellectual level. Because people who develop delusions may have better than average verbal and cognitive skills, activities that use these skills are recommended. Of course, the activities should be appropriate to the person's occupational roles and reflect his or her interests, and the person should be helped to select his or her own activity.

Activities that are in any way related to the person's delusions should be avoided. For example, making wire jewelry might not be the best choice for a woman who believes that part of her brain was replaced by a complicated electrical device during a recent hysterectomy (Box 11-5).

## Paranoia

*Paranoia is a type of thinking in which persecutory and grandiose ideas predominate.* General suspiciousness is usually called *paranoid ideation,* whereas very extreme and unbelievable ideas (such as that the attorney general and the police are out to get one) are termed *paranoid delusions.*

Paranoid individuals feel suspicious of those around them; they are constantly alert and concerned about whether others are harassing them, persecuting them, taking advantage of them, or treating them unfairly. They keep themselves aloof and distant from others, often subjecting family and would-be friends to repeated "tests" of loyalty.

One way to think about paranoia is as a defense against rejection. By believing that others are out to get them, these people protect themselves from rejection. This keeps them from developing relationships in which they fear they may get hurt.

Similarly, they avoid experiencing their low self-esteem by instead thinking that they are special in some way. Paranoid individuals seem to need to believe that they are better, more moral, more self-sufficient than other ordinary people. They are afraid to lose their independence and to have to rely on another person.

## Diagnoses in Which Paranoia Is a Common Symptom

Paranoia is the predominant symptom in paranoid schizophrenia. It is also seen sometimes in psychotic depressions and in paranoid personality disorder. The suspiciousness shown by persons with borderline and narcissistic personality disorders can be considered a kind of paranoia.

## Strategy for Therapeutic Use of Self

Occupational therapy assistants will understand how to approach paranoid persons once they try to look at the world from their point of view. In their way of looking at things, everything is dangerous; anyone or anything can threaten their uncertain sense of self. The OTA should avoid approaching them suddenly, from behind, or in a manner that might be perceived as threatening. It is important not to whisper in these patients' presence because they will believe you are talking about them.

Similarly, any directions or statements made by the OTA should be clear, consistent, directive, and unambiguous. Paranoid individuals are often very intelligent, perhaps more intelligent than many of the staff and, therefore, should be approached as intellectual equals. Arguing with them is pointless; they always win. They often possess extraordinary memories; therefore, it is wise to be truthful and not make promises unless you are certain you can keep them.

Frequently, a paranoid person in an activity group will separate from others and try to strike up a special relationship with a staff member. Some therapists believe that allowing and encouraging this special relationship helps the person adjust faster to the group. The person can be given a special role (passing out supplies, taking attendance) that makes him or her feel important. The paranoid individual is threatened by competition, so competitive games and situations in which one person is compared with another should be avoided. These people should be given the message that they are important and that they should focus on themselves and not worry about what other people are doing.

The question of who is in control of a situation is a real concern for the paranoid individual. OTAs must be careful to stay in charge of the situation and not let such patients run away with the show. For example, these patients may want the other patients to sit in assigned seats (usually away from them); by refusing this request outright, the OTA may alienate paranoid clients; but by giving in to them, the OTA suggests that these patients have a great deal of power. In such a case, artful practitioners work out a compromise that gratifies the paranoid person's need to be alone while still affirming the therapist's own control of the situation—for example, the practitioner may seat the patient at a separate table but let others sit wherever they wish.

## Strategy for Modifying the Environment

The paranoid client is easily threatened by changes in the environment; therefore, the environment should be kept as stable and reliable as possible. When changes are anticipated (e.g., a new paint job, a rearrangement of furniture for a special event), the client should be prepared in advance.

Many paranoid patients deliberately isolate themselves from other people. This is a self-protective measure that the OTA should tolerate and support until the person feels more comfortable. Social contact should never be forced on paranoid individuals. After an initial period of isolation, they should be encouraged to join others in a group; usually they will first take on the role of a watchful observer or "special assistant" described earlier. Gradually, after repeated exposure to the same people, the paranoid client may begin to relate more spontaneously.

Because the paranoid person is easily threatened and frightened, there is some potential for violence. Staff should follow the safety guidelines recommended for the hostile and aggressive client.

### Strategy for Selecting Activities

Activities must be ones the person can control. Structured activities involving controllable materials (e.g., leather work) are recommended. Before presenting any activity, the OTA should make sure that it is appropriate for the person's intellectual level and complex enough to engage and maintain his or her interest. In the beginning, activities should be individual and done independently without need for help or instructions. Most paranoid patients can follow diagrams and written directions. Unless there is reason to suspect that the person is suicidal or assaultive, it is best to hand over the tools at the beginning of the session rather than requiring him or her to come and ask for each one individually (Box 11-6).

## Anger, Hostility, and Aggression

*Anger is a strong feeling of displeasure. Hostility is an unfriendly and threatening attitude directed toward other people. Aggression is an attack on a person or object; aggression can be verbal, physical, or both.* Before discussing some of the reasons clients are angry, hostile, or aggressive, it is important to distinguish aggression from assertiveness, with which it is sometimes confused. Assertiveness is the direct expression of feelings and desires; it has come to be synonymous with "sticking up for oneself." There are situations in which a person must be both assertive and aggressive. For example, in New York City parking spaces are at such a premium that it is quite common for two drivers to want the same space. What should the driver who arrived first do? To secure the space, it may be necessary to get out of the car and argue about it. Most New York City car owners consider this assertiveness appropriate.

Another important consideration is that some cultural groups condone aggressiveness by men, especially when avenging real or fancied insults to women. Although the degree of aggressiveness displayed may seem extreme or silly to someone from a different social class or cultural background, it is accepted and even expected in some cultures.

When the OTA is working with individuals who are verbally or physically aggressive, it is important to distinguish between ordinary (culturally endorsed) self-assertiveness and inappropriate aggression. Although almost everyone feels angry at times, sometimes with good reason, most people can control their feelings and avoid acting them out. Those who are unable to express their feelings in words may resort to violence; this is true especially if the person has a history of being abused as a child or being violent as an adult.

Clients who become verbally abusive or physically violent may be expressing any of a variety of unmet needs. They may feel threatened or hemmed in, physically or psychologically. Psychiatric treatment settings are often crowded, and clients may find the physical press of other people and the lack of privacy overwhelming; similarly, they may feel confined and frustrated by the rules and restrictions. Some individuals use physical or verbal violence as a way of venting frustration, of letting off steam; often such people find it difficult to express themselves in words and have not developed any constructive channels for their feelings (e.g., sports, hobbies). Others use hostility and aggression self-protectively; by keeping others at a distance they make rejection impossible.

BOX 11-6

**PARANOIA: EXAMPLES OF APPROPRIATE ACTIVITIES**

*Wood, leather, or metal projects* constructed according to written instructions are sufficiently complex to challenge this type of individual. The project shown is a good example. Other possibilities include high-level clerical tasks (organizing files, using computerized data bases), design tasks, jewelry making, and puzzles.

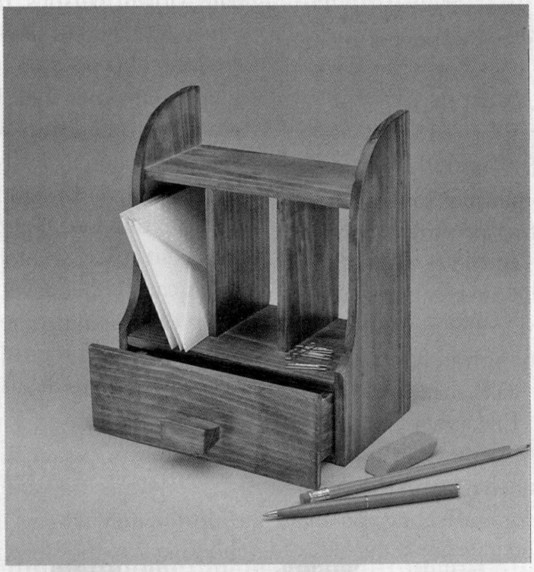

**Desk organizer.** This relatively complex kit involves the separate assembly of case and drawer (compare this to the simpler heart basket shown in Box 11-1). Many pieces are of similar size and shape. The kit requires organizational skills for orienting the pieces and ordering the assembly. This is a suitable project for someone with a high cognitive level and good attention span. Prior woodworking experience is helpful. (Photo courtesy of S&S Arts and Crafts, Colchester, CT.)

## Diagnoses in Which Anger, Hostility, or Aggression Is a Common Symptom

Some persons with psychotic disorders (paranoid schizophrenia, manic–depressive psychosis, psychotic depression, organic mental disorders) become hostile. Usually something has happened to provoke this response, but it is often hard to figure out exactly what. Substance abusers and persons with antisocial personality disorders may also show hostility. Some brain disorders are disinhibiting, meaning that the person no longer feels bound by customary social taboos. Finally, any person may become angry, hostile, and even violent if sufficiently provoked; anger can be a normal response to illness and disability (34, 44).

### Strategy for Therapeutic Use of Self

Staff should be sensitive to clients' feelings generally and alert to signs that a client is feeling tense, threatened, or suspicious. People's body language gives clues to their mental state. For example, stiffness or rigidity in the set of the mouth or the shoulders usually signifies anger or anxiety. Threatening gestures and the destruction of objects, no matter how small or insignificant, are other signs. The sooner the possibility of aggressiveness is recognized, the sooner it can be dealt with.

The general approach is to get these people to talk about what is bothering them and to help them use words to express their feelings rather than just acting them out. It is important not to respond in kind, no matter how insulting or provocative the person's behavior might be. If the person is very excited, it can help to say the same calming words several times (broken-record technique) (44).

Try to speak to the person privately, avoiding a public display that may make her feel more threatened or embarrassed. Encourage her to discuss her feelings. Tell her exactly what must be corrected about how she is behaving in the situation, explain that her behavior is affecting you and the other people present, and give her some alternatives for handling it. Avoid punishing or criticizing; these approaches are humiliating and tend to escalate aggressiveness.

It is important to be direct and clear about what is expected. Follow through by enforcing any limits you set. To illustrate, if you have told Mr. Jones that he will have to leave the group if he touches anyone again, you had better make sure you have other staff available who can remove him if this happens. Otherwise, Mr. Jones may continue to test your limits because you obviously cannot be taken at your word.

Be especially cautious with clients who say that you or another staff member or client remind them of someone they do not like. This should be considered a warning that the person may attack when psychotic and out of control. Violent acts are more likely in those who have a self-reported history of violence than in those without such a history (10).

### Strategy for Modifying the Environment

Because of the potential for violence, hostile individuals may have to be isolated from others who irritate them. While speaking to hostile or potentially violent persons, the OTA should stand 4 or 5 feet away and to the side, not facing the person directly. This position gives the person room and is not confrontational. It is not a good idea to be alone with someone who may become violent. Similarly, when in any room, be sure that the door is left open, and position yourself so that you are closer to the door than is the client. Do not touch the client. Even what you intend as a comforting touch can be perceived as an attack. Remove all sharp objects and other potential weapons from the area. Even brooms and mops have been used to beat people to death, so *think*.

### Strategy for Selecting Activities

Unfortunately, there is no handy formula for choosing activities for the angry, hostile, or aggressive person. Therapists who follow objects relations theory believe activities that encourage sublimation of aggressive feelings are best. These need not be openly aggressive activities. For example, symbolic activities like art and dance may permit the person to express feelings in a socially acceptable way; this seems especially useful for those with poor verbal skills. Activities that require large, forceful motions (e.g., wedging clay) can also express aggressiveness, but reports suggest that these increase anger and aggressiveness (34, 45). Avoid activities that require frustration tolerance and attention to detail. For obvious reasons, eliminate activities that involve sharp tools or small, heavy, throwable objects. Activities that use repetitive motions may help some people organize and control their feelings.

**BOX 11-7**

**ANGER, HOSTILITY, AND AGGRESSION: EXAMPLES OF APPROPRIATE ACTIVITIES**

- *Active sports* and other gross motor activities such as dance are useful for releasing tension.
- *Sanding a large wood project* involves repetitive gross motor movements and is mildly destructive; it is an example of an activity that might help reduce tension.
- *Peeling potatoes* is another activity that can serve the same purpose; the tool should be a potato peeler with a rounded point (not a knife). Activities that involve sharp or potentially dangerous tools (e.g., woodworking, metal hammering) should be used only when both therapist and patient feel comfortable that the patient can control himself or herself.
- *Anger management* (23, 24, 26, 45) and *conflict resolution training* (20) may benefit those who have problems managing, controlling, and expressing anger. Such training gives the person the skills of preplanning a response to angry feelings, identifying anger when it occurs, problem solving to handle anger, and empathizing with and forgiving the other party (24).
- *Assertiveness training* provides skills that use reason and verbal expression to meet needs.

Addressing the stress that is fueling the hostile, angry or aggressive state is another option. When angry, a person experiences a high level of physiological arousal (e.g., increased heart rate, respiration, energy) that interferes with rational thinking and problem solving. Aggressive people may not understand that this is happening or may not know that they can learn to monitor and control this arousal by relaxation and stress management techniques (19, 44). Furthermore, they may benefit from specific stress management strategies, such as learning to monitor and reduce demands and to increase resources to deal with situations. Training in assertiveness skills (learning to use words and reason) can replace the habit of expressing rage (Box 11-7).

## Seductive Behavior and Sexual Acting Out

*Seductive behavior is any behavior that would normally be seen as explicitly (openly) sexual or as provoking a sexual response from others.* Examples are highly varied. They may be as subtle as touching someone's shoulder or loosening a tie or collar or as blatant as making sexual remarks or asking a staff member for a date. Sexual acting out is openly sexual behavior in response to unconscious feelings. This includes engaging in sexual acts with other clients. Sometimes the phrase *sexual acting out* is used to describe extreme behaviors of people who have lost contact with reality while in a psychotic state. Such individuals may, for example, masturbate openly, disrobe in public, tuck their shirts into their panties and dance around, or fondle other patients.

Sexual needs do not disappear when a person becomes mentally ill; people with mental illnesses have the same needs as everyone else, but they sometimes have more difficulty gratifying their sexual needs. Inpatients who may have been used to daily sexual activity before hospitalization find that they can see their sexual partners only on weekend passes. To add to their frustration, the lack of privacy may make masturbation difficult or impossible. Individuals with severe and persistent mental disorders may not have developed sufficient social skills to be able to form close relationships in which sexual needs can be gratified. So it should not be surprising that some clients seem preoccupied with sex.

Sometimes what looks like seductive behavior is really a bid to get attention or to see how a staff member will react. Clients who can make staff members sufficiently uncomfortable can make sure that those staff members will never confront them about their real problems. Similarly, people who feel unattractive or insecure may set up a sexual confrontation so that a staff member will reject them, thus confirming their worst fears.

In addition, clients who are hallucinating may attempt to remove their clothes because they feel insects crawling on them or because they hear voices commanding them to do so. King (30) points out that sexual promiscuity may have its roots in "skin hunger," or a need for warmth and tactile input. So it is important to pinpoint the motivation behind the person's behavior before deciding what to do about it.

### Diagnoses in Which Sexual Acting Out or Seductiveness Is a Common Symptom

The most extreme forms of sexual acting out (disrobing, open masturbation) usually occur only in people who are psychotic. Less common, these behaviors are associated with psychosexual disorders (exhibitionism, sexual masochism). The other behaviors mentioned may be seen in any client (or indeed in anyone anywhere).

### Strategy for Therapeutic Use of Self

Clients who are behaving inappropriately should be told so in a calm, nonjudgmental manner. Such clients should be stopped from doing things that will later embarrass them. For example, if a woman will not stop her lewd dancing, she should be excused from the dance activity for the day. The rules of the particular setting should be strictly enforced (e.g., most inpatient settings forbid physical contact between patients).

Clients who try to involve staff in sexual relationships may be expressing needs that are not directly sexual. For example, an adolescent boy who fears that he is homosexual may behave seductively to a woman therapist to test his own sexual identity. Some clients may confuse the closeness of the therapeutic relationship with the intimacy of a sexual one (see Chapter 10). When a client behaves seductively toward a staff member, the staff member should carefully explain the nature of the therapeutic relationship and should discourage further overtures gently but firmly. The staff member should avoid *any* physical contact and should not allow the person to talk about the possibility of a sexual relationship between them. As a last resort, if the client is not able to stop, the OTA should arrange for another person to work with the client.

Notify staff and document all sexually preoccupied behavior and remarks to prevent incidents that may happen at night or when fewer staff are around. Encourage clients to tell on others who abuse or harass them sexually.

### Strategy for Modifying the Environment

Crowded situations, in which physical contact is almost unavoidable, are not a good idea. The client should have personal space and be protected from the sudden touch, smell, and warmth of others.

### Strategy for Selecting Activities

No one would dispute that sex is the best activity for gratifying sexual needs. If the person's religious beliefs permit and the assistant feels comfortable, masturbation can be suggested as an alternative. Also, it is possible to release a great deal of tension, sexual and otherwise, through forceful gross motor activities. Activities that involve other people, especially with physical contact, should be used cautiously, depending on the person's tolerance and self-control. Social skills

BOX 11-8

**SEDUCTIVE BEHAVIOR AND SEXUAL ACTING OUT: EXAMPLES OF APPROPRIATE ACTIVITIES**

- *Forceful gross motor activities* that can be done alone or without physical contact include, for example, exercise, running, wedging clay, and woodworking.
- *Activities involving others in nonsexual physical contact* are sports like volleyball, basketball, and touch football, and dance.
- *Swimming, cycling, weight training and aerobics,* and *yoga* are example of activities with limited or no physical contact that still permit physical release.

training and other activities that teach or reinforce appropriate social behavior are also recommended (Box 11-8).

## Cognitive Deficits: Confusion and Impaired Memory

*A cognitive deficit is an impairment or defect in one or more of the mental functions needed for thinking.* Some of these processes are orientation, alertness, concentration, attention span, memory, comprehension, judgment, and problem solving.

*Orientation* is knowledge of where one is, what time it is (hour, day, date, season), and who one is with. This is sometimes called orientation to time, place, and person and abbreviated as orientation 3 (meaning orientation in three spheres of information). Problems in this area are described as *disorientation* or *confusion.* Generally, disorientation to time alone is the least severe form; disorientation to place and time is more severe; and disorientation to person, place, and time is the most severe.

*Alertness* is awareness of the immediate environment. Problems in alertness may be described generally as *low arousal* (seemingly unaware of stimulation), *clouding of consciousness* (meaning literally that the person seems to be in a fog) or impairment of a specific aspect of alertness. Concentration and attention span are aspects of alertness.

*Concentration* is the ability to focus one's mental energies on the task at hand. The intensity of focus is the primary concern. *Attention span* is the length of time that concentration can be maintained. Impairment in attention span may be described *distractibility* (meaning a tendency to lose focus because another stimulus catches one's interest) or *inattention* (usually meaning the inability to pay attention even though no competing external stimulus is present). Responses to these symptoms are discussed in the next section.

*Memory* is the ability to recall past events and knowledge. Health professionals commonly distinguish between short-term memory and long-term memory to indicate the difference between memory of events from months or years ago (*long-term memory*) and memory of more recent events (*short-term memory*). Thus the ability to remember one's date of birth or the names of one's children reflects long-term memory, and the ability to remember whether one had lunch or where one's eyeglasses are reflects short-term memory. Experimental psychologists sometimes use short-term memory to mean memory of events that occurred within the past few seconds (sometimes called "working memory") rather than hours or days (48). Because this can cause confusion among treatment staff, make sure that you understand which kind of short-term memory is being described. Problems in remembering important information are *memory impairment.*

*Comprehension* is the ability to understand. Comprehension is composed of many skills, including the ability to recognize words, to identify objects, to place things in order by time or size or some other quality, to extract essential information from a spoken or written passage, and to classify or sort or group objects in a logical fashion.

Comprehension depends upon the development of concepts. We can think of concepts as containers for experiences—for example, our concept of *dog* includes many varieties and sizes of dog; when we see a four-legged animal, we compare it to other items in the concept *dog* to see if it belongs in this container. A person's ability to comprehend depends on the number of concepts available and the way they are organized. To illustrate, an unsophisticated concept of *muscle* might refer just to physical strength ("he's got muscles"). A student of physical medicine or anatomy has a more sophisticated concept—in fact a highly organized group of concepts—including, for example, striated muscle, voluntary muscle, antagonist, and deep hip flexor.

Trouble comprehending may have other than psychological causes. Language skills, prior education, and life experience all affect comprehension. Physiological changes from brain damage or chemicals in the body can also impair comprehension. Problems in comprehension are usually described as *inability to comprehend.*

*Judgment* is the ability to recognize and comply with established social norms and standard procedures. Like comprehension, judgment may reflect background and social class. Using foul language probably indicates bad judgment in an otherwise conservative businessman but may be the social norm for a dock worker. Problems in judgment are usually called *impaired judgment;* some examples are urinating on the street, making sexual innuendoes to co-workers, and sitting down on a bench marked with a sign that says "Wet Paint."

*Problem solving* is the ability to recognize, analyze, and ultimately figure out solutions for problems that arise in the course of everyday activity. Some examples of problems that most people have to solve are budgeting money and getting from place to place. Everyone but the very wealthy has to figure out how to pay for things like repair of the water heater or a new car. When the car breaks down or the train is delayed, an alternative way of transporting oneself has to be found. Living on one's own in the community depends on the ability to solve problems such as these. Because cognitive impairments have such a profound effect on a person's ability to function independently, they are discussed several times in this text (see Chapters 6, 22, and 23).

People who realize that their thinking is not as clear as it once was or that they have forgotten and left a pot burning on the stove (for the fourth time) may become very frightened and anxious. They may begin to check things many times over or engage in ritualistic actions. Or they may become anxious, agitated, or even belligerent. Commonly, long-term memory and recall of events from many years ago are excellent. Problems in short-term memory are deeply disturbing, and the person may make up stories to cover them up. This is called *confabulation.*

Many cognitively impaired individuals are also depressed; it is not always clear whether the depression is the cause of the cognitive problems or the result. Most people believe that the depression and the cognitive problems interact with each other in a negative way; the more such people have problems in thinking and remembering, the more depressed they become. Likewise, the more depressed they are, the more likely they are to forget things and have trouble concentrating. Thus the depression and the cognitive problems fuel each other, and these people may become more depressed and more impaired as time goes by. Furthermore, disturbed or insufficient sleep may contribute to cognitive deficits and depression; usually this is temporary, but it may require intervention in adhering to a daily schedule and learning strategies to improve continuity of sleep.

Some individuals with cognitive problems have very *labile* emotions. This means that they rapidly shift from being calm and comfortable to crying or laughing uncontrollably. For example, an elderly nursing home resident who remembers the death of a childhood pet may suddenly burst into tears.

People who are disoriented frequently get lost, especially in strange new environments, such as hospitals and nursing homes. They need help finding their rooms and their way to the bathroom.

Those with poor judgment usually do not recognize that their judgment is off; that they are doing something inappropriate, like washing their hair in the water fountain; or offensive, like fondling the assistant's derriere. They may try to laugh it off or prevent further criticism by arguing. Both of these behaviors can be considered defenses against the anxiety and pain that would result if they understood what they had done.

Problems in carrying out motor actions are often associated with cognitive deficits. These may be more or less severe and can be analyzed according to Allen's cognitive levels (see Chapters 3, 15, and 23). *Dressing apraxia* is a severe form in which the person has trouble carrying out the proper sequence of actions to get dressed and may, for example, put her socks on over her shoes or wear two skirts.

To summarize, cognitive deficits can seriously impair a person's ability to function. The person with cognitive deficits may have a wide range of emotional reactions in response to decreasing function. When working with cognitively impaired persons, it is important to consider their emotional response and to evaluate whatever cognitive skills are still intact.

## Diagnoses in Which Cognitive Deficits Are Common

Cognitive deficits occur to varying degrees in many psychiatric disorders. They are always found in organic mental disorders; in these disorders, which include Alzheimer's dementia, the impairment is usually severe and progressive, meaning that it gets worse over time. Cognitive deficits can also result from physical disease. Any disease that impairs circulation affects the brain because less blood and therefore less oxygen reaches it. Brain infections and trauma to the head can result in cognitive problems that may be permanent or transient. In planning interventions it is important to differentiate permanent disabilities from those that are temporary.

Drugs and alcohol affect brain chemistry and therefore can cause cognitive deficits. Phencyclidine (PCP) abuse often results in impaired alertness, concentration, and attention span. Prolonged or extensive alcohol abuse is associated with an organic mental disorder characterized by permanent impairment of intellectual abilities. Some prescription medications, including several used for treatment of psychiatric disorders, can cause temporary cognitive deficits that disappear when the medication is discontinued.

Finally, patients receiving electroconvulsive therapy (ECT) as a treatment for depression usually are disoriented and have short-term memory loss for several days after receiving treatments. With time, these mental functions usually recover, although the person may never be able to remember events that occurred around the time of the treatments.

## Strategy for Therapeutic Use of Self

General rules for approaching the person with cognitive deficits are difficult to prescribe. Various clients function at various levels; some forget only an occasional fact or today's date; others are so disoriented that they think Nixon is president or that they are in a factory rather than a nursing home. It is important to approach each person as an individual and to pitch your comments and directions to the person's present level of functioning. By doing this, you help the lower-functioning individual feel more secure and avoid insulting those who are higher functioning. Keeping this important precaution in mind, the following guidelines should be used.

Because being disoriented can be very frightening, be sure to remind these patients of where they are and who you are. For someone with severe memory impairment (this includes those receiving ECT) it may be necessary to repeat this information each time you see the person. Wearing a name tag with your name and title in large print can help. Keep in mind that disoriented clients may have trouble finding the bathroom; orient them to this and any other important aspects of the environment. Other information that patients may need to know includes the time of day, what is happening now, and what will be happening next.

Although people with cognitive impairment may do very inappropriate things because of poor judgment, the assistant should consistently show a warm and accepting attitude. Clients should not be punished or threatened no matter how inconvenient or unpleasant their behavior has been. Instead, the assistant should gently explain what is expected and then help clients behave appropriately. It is important to intervene immediately when clients do something wrong and to help them correct it then and there. Otherwise they may not know what you are talking about when you mention it later.

Whenever clients are given directions, whether on how to do an activity or how to get to the cafeteria, the directions should reflect the five Cs: *calm, clear, concise, concrete,* and *consistent.* Speak in a calm tone of voice, articulating the words clearly. You may have to speak more slowly than you do usually, but your tone of voice should be respectful, not patronizing or impatient. Whatever you have to say, make it brief; the person's attention span is short. Use common everyday language, not abstract or difficult words that are hard to understand. Finally, use the same words every time you give the directions. Incorporating the person's own words can be helpful. To illustrate, if a man asks where you put his "specs," use this word rather than *glasses* or *eyeglasses* when you tell him where to find them. If you expect the person to remember the directions and use them later, have him or her repeat them to you. Better yet, write them down or make sure that the client writes them down.

Finally, match your tempo to what the person seems able to handle. The cognitively impaired may take a while to respond; it just takes them longer to process ideas and information.

## Strategy for Modifying the Environment

Three main principles are used to modify the environment. First, control the environment to maximize safety. Second, use the environment to cue desired behavior. Third, avoid environmental cues that may trigger undesirable behavior (22).

Cognitively impaired persons, more than any other group of patients, need a consistent and well-designed environment. Good lighting will help keep the person oriented. Even at night, lighting should be kept fairly bright. Colored lines (whether tiled, taped, or painted) on the floor leading to the bathroom and other frequently used areas are also good orientation aids. Reflector tape is recommended.

Locations should be clearly marked with signs. Large print should be used. Pictographs or pictorial symbols may be more easily recognized than words; an example is a picture of a cup and saucer on the door of the cafeteria. Signs or symbols on patients' room doors may help them find their rooms; making the sign can be a good project. Persons with cognitive impairment may need to label, mark, or color code objects in their rooms to help them find them. In general, the environment should be simplified and all needed objects and locations should be clearly marked. Items that are often needed should be visible. Items that are rarely used or that may distract should be hidden (Fig. 11-1).

*External memory* aids such as a large clock, large calendar, and radio are valuable. These help

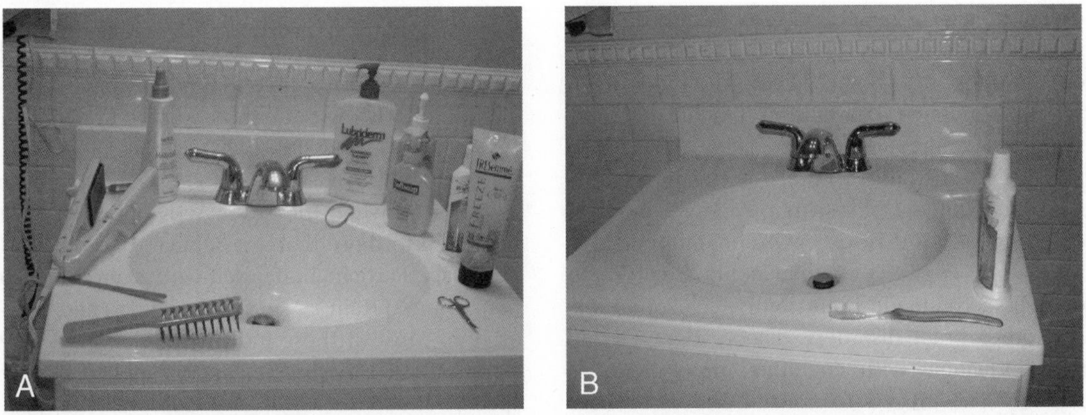


**Figure 11-1. A. Cluttered environment.** Though the toothpaste and brush are present, they are hard to find. The presence of other objects distracts from the task of tooth brushing. **B. Clarified environment.** This setup clarifies the task and cues the person by providing only the appropriate tools. *Note:* Persons with memory impairment may not recognize the upright dispenser or associate it with toothpaste. Those with weak grip strength will find a traditional tube of toothpaste easier to use than the upright dispenser shown here.

orient the patient to time and to current events. Patients who must remember to do things at a certain time can use *cuing devices* such as programmable alarm watches and timers. Many electronic devices store specific kinds of information; speed dialing on telephones is one example. Sometimes such devices are difficult for the patient to learn to use, in which case their value is questionable. We recommend that to stay current, clinicians make regular visits to electronics stores. Note, however, that devices that require new learning will require training and may be unsuccessful for the person with cognitive impairment.

Because people with cognitive impairments rely so much on structure and routine in the external environment to help them stay organized, they are very sensitive to any changes. Therefore, the environment should be kept the same from day to day; this is true of the occupational therapy clinic as well as the person's living area.

The question of how much stimulation should be available in the environment is fascinating and much debated. Research has shown that environments with low amounts of stimulation can impair cognition because they deprive the senses of necessary information. However, it is also true that too much stimulation can aggravate cognitive impairments because the person cannot process so much information at one time. Clinicians agree, however, that any stimulation presented should be clear and unambiguous. For example, when music is used, it should be played on a good stereo system rather than a cheap tape deck with poor sound quality.

Another factor to be considered in designing an environment for someone with cognitive impairments is its similarity or dissimilarity to the person's home environment. Ideally, the person should remain at home as long as possible, using compensatory devices and the support of other people. When entering the hospital or nursing home, not only are such patients often seriously ill and in psychological distress, but their distress is further exacerbated by the strangeness of the environment. Residents' discomfort can be lessened somewhat if they are allowed to keep mementos of home in the room. They should also be encouraged to set up their belongings in whatever way makes sense for them, as this will encourage carryover of dressing and hygiene and grooming routines. Finally, when someone is planning to return home or is to transfer to another facility, the future environment must be considered. Teaching of new skills or reinforcement of old skills should take place in an environment similar to this future one.

A large amount of research evidence and specific suggestions exist on environmental management for cognitive impairments related to dementia, traumatic brain injury, schizophrenia, and other brain disorders. The reader working with individual · with cognitive impairments is strongly encouraged to consult the references which give additional details on modifying the environment (4, 21, 22, 29, 40).

## Strategy for Selecting Activities

The person's prognosis must be considered when selecting activities. Some cognitive impairments are transitory and the person is expected to regain full function (e.g., post-ECT memory impairment). These patients should be given simple, structured, short-term activities that are relevant to their interests to help them maintain their abilities and confidence until they recover. Activities that can be finished in one day are preferable; the person may refuse to work on a project two days in a row if he or she does not remember it. Once cognitive functions begin to return to normal, the person should be quickly reintroduced to familiar activities and skills he or she needs in her occupational roles.

Other conditions (e.g., dementia associated with alcoholism) are permanent but stable; the condition will not get better, nor will it get worse. For these individuals, the specific cognitive deficits must be identified and analyzed in relation to previous occupational roles. Then the person can be taught ways to adapt to the disability within these roles or to find new occupational roles more appropriate to the present condition. The general approach is to simplify known activities rather than introduce new ones.

A third group of conditions, unfortunately, are permanent and progressive; the person will become less and less able to function and eventually will die. These patients need help to maintain for as long as possible whatever skills remain. They should be encouraged to be as independent as they can while they can. Activities should be restricted to those that are familiar, relevant, and necessary. Participation in self-care is important to help them retain a sense of dignity and self-esteem. Most of these individuals can learn new skills only by rote practice and as applied to very specific situations. Gitlin and Corcoran (21) provide specific suggestions to modify objects and tasks to improve performance. In general, the idea is to reduce complexity and make the task clear and doable.

Some general guidelines apply to all three groups. First, unfamiliar and complex activities should be avoided because they will add to confusion. Activities that require independent decision making may overwhelm someone with limited judgment; activities that involve simple choices (e.g., between two colors or two food items) can build confidence, however. The OTA should help these patients carry out activities they value.

Depending on individual need, the person may benefit from reality orientation. This approach, which aims to keep the person aware of what is going in the world, is described in Chapter 22. Touring around the halls and practicing travel within the treatment facility is appropriate for severely disoriented patients.

Some of those who have confusion or impaired memory find it helpful to write things down. They should be encouraged to carry a notebook with them at all times; designing and organizing the notebook can be an ongoing activity. Taking an excursion to town to select an appointment book at the stationery or office supply stores can be a way to assess travel and orientation skills (Box 11-9).

**BOX 11-9**

**COGNITIVE DEFICITS: EXAMPLES OF APPROPRIATE ACTIVITIES**

- *Current events discussion, patient government or resident council,* and *reality orientation* are designed to help the person stay oriented and involved.
- *Life tasks* should emphasize self-care and whatever other tasks may be needed for a particular individual (e.g., cooking, housework, laundry, shopping).
- *Familiar crafts and hobbies* can help bolster self-confidence when the ability to do more complex tasks has been lost.
- *Short walks or shopping excursions* provide variety, exercise, and a sense of added purpose.

## Attention Deficits and Disorganization

*Attention deficits are problems in directing attention to a task or in sustaining attention for a reasonable length of time. Disorganization is a lack of planning and order that interferes with successful completion of activities.* Attention deficits and disorganization are often associated with the other cognitive deficits already described. However, because the general management of these symptoms is different, they are discussed separately.

Clients may have trouble concentrating on a task or paying attention to it over time for several reasons. They may be distracted by hallucinations, memories, or other internally generated stimuli or by things around them in the external environment. Individuals with brain disorders may process information more slowly than other people; by the time they figure out what is happening, something else is going on, and they have trouble keeping up.

Clients who have trouble paying attention are likely to have trouble with organization as well. However, another possible cause of disorganization is overstimulation; they have difficulty focusing on one thing at a time because there is so much that catches their attention (this is common in mania). Still another is poor judgment, evidenced by trying to do too many things at one time. Also, someone may appear disorganized simply if he or she lacks the skills or knowledge to perform the activity. To illustrate, someone who has done little cooking will have trouble assembling the necessary ingredients and implements and carrying out the steps efficiently.

### Diagnoses in Which Attention Deficits and Disorganization Are Common

Both attention deficits and disorganization occur in organic mental disorders, in PCP and alcohol abuse, and in schizophrenia and affective psychoses. Persons with learning disabilities often have these problems. Normal individuals are likely to have impaired attention and to be disorganized when they are under stress or otherwise preoccupied.

### Strategy for Therapeutic Use of Self

It may be difficult to get the attention of someone with severe cognitive impairment. If so, say the person's name *loudly*. If necessary, shout; although this may feel uncomfortable to you at first, it is the only way to get the attention of severely regressed individuals. Those who do not respond to what you say to them *may* respond to being touched firmly but gently on the arm or shoulder.

Lonergan (31) describes therapeutic and benevolent touch as especially effective for persons with dementia.

Be alert to communication in nonverbal behavior. Gestures and grunts may indicate pain or interest. Body positioning, restlessness and facial expression may clues as to the person's mental and physical state.

Clients who are disorganized or having trouble paying attention to a task may simply not be capable of doing that particular task at this time; if so, their attention should be directed to another, simpler activity. The new activity should be introduced matter-of-factly, so as to avoid making the person feel incompetent (e.g., "I think that we should save this for another day; I need to work out some of the details. Try this instead.") The goal is to help the client feel comfortable and competent within the limits of his or her present abilities.

Glantz and Richman (22) point out that many behaviors that look like a problem or deficit can be seen as a strength if rephrased and looked at positively. For example, The person who has limited attention span may be able to attend to a task for 3 minutes. Similarly, the person who works in an unsafe manner may be able to work safely if a safe structured environment is provided. Therefore, speak positively to clients and confirm that they are able to do many things; this enhances independence.

### Strategy for Modifying the Environment

Distractions can be reduced by having the person work alone, facing a blank wall. Limit the tools and supplies to those needed for the immediate step or task. If the person is distracted by internally generated stimuli (e.g., hallucinations), vigorous stimulation may be necessary to get his or her attention.

Casby and Holm (8) report that classical and/or favorite music played in the background may reduce stereotypical and disruptive behaviors in persons with dementia. In using music, careful observation of the effects on clients' functional performance is essential, since it is also possible for music to be distracting and confusing.

### Strategy for Selecting Activities

Simple, well-delineated activities that have a definite sequence consisting of very few steps are recommended. The assistant may need to do the more difficult steps for the person. Activities that are creative or that have flexible standards or goals should be avoided; they will only increase disorganization.

For persons who have been evaluated with the Allen Cognitive Level Test or Allen Diagnostic Module, activities should be matched to cognitive level. Observation of performance will guide the OTA in determining whether to increase or to decrease the level of difficulty. Allen (3, 4) recommends that tasks be within the person's current ability; the practitioner should intervene rapidly to provide a less-demanding activity if the person shows signs of confusion, frustration, or discomfort.

For persons with dementia, adaptations and environmental modifications (e.g., enlarged telephone buttons, compartmentalized medicine boxes, posted signs) to enable performance of activities of daily living can be very helpful. In addition, the person can learn to rely on other people or on purchased services (takeout food, housekeeper or home attendant) to supplement for lost function (46).

Evaluation and intervention related to safety and emergency management are very important (Box 11-10).

## SELF-MONITORING FOR SELF-MASTERY OF SYMPTOMS

Major psychiatric disorders are lifelong chronic conditions. To have a good quality of life, consumers need to manage their illnesses. Proper diet and nutrition, medication maintenance, fitness and exercise, use of social support, and avoidance

**BOX 11-10**

## ATTENTION DEFICITS AND DISORGANIZATION: EXAMPLES OF APPROPRIATE ACTIVITIES

- *Simple craft projects* such as mosaic tile trivets (shown here), leather coin purses, plastic-dip flowers, sewing kits, and copper tooling can all be used, although some steps may have to be modified. For instance, oxidizing the copper might be skipped altogether or done by the assistant or a volunteer.

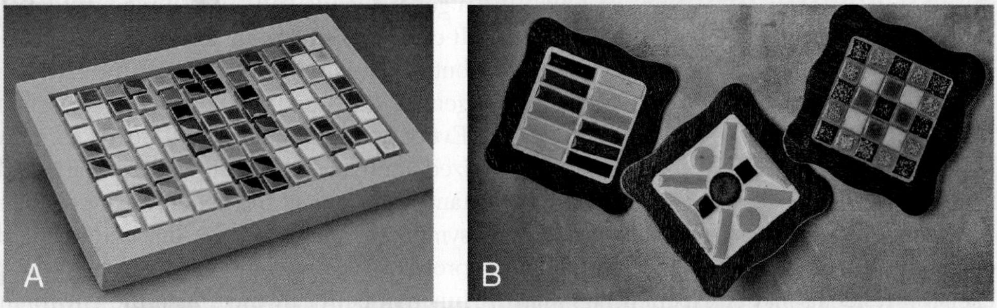


**A. Frame trivet. B. Wood coaster.** These projects use mosaic tile and offer options for grading the activity to accommodate different levels of energy and cognitive ability. The trivet requires a longer attention span to complete because it has a larger tiled surface. To finish the coaster, one must glue the backing to frame, which may be done by a volunteer or the OTA. (Photo courtesy of S&S Arts and Crafts, Colchester, CT.)

- *Self-care* and *life tasks needed in the person's occupational roles* are most important. Helping a housewife organize her kitchen or do the laundry more efficiently will probably be more important to her than learning copper tooling.
- *Training in safety and emergency procedures* may make the difference in allowing the person to remain in the community.
- *Coping skills and stress management* can be modified to the level of the person's understanding and control of anxiety and extreme emotional arousal which further interferes with cognition.
- *Computer games* that reinforce specific cognitive skills may also be used. Medalia and Revheim (35) recommend that the target deficits (e.g., linear sequencing, organization) be identified and that the client's interests and level of functioning be considered when selecting software. Nakano (37) reports that computer-based programs are effective only when therapists also encourage and support the client.

of triggers and situations that may cause distress are important skills and habits that enhance recovery. Copeland (11) reported on the Wellness Recovery Action Plan (WRAP), in which consumers create a "wellness toolbox" to recognize, reduce, and if possible eliminate troubling symptoms. The following elements are included:

- A daily maintenance list (of routines and activities that maintain health)
- A list of personal triggers (events or things that tend to provoke symptoms or relapse) and ways to respond to these
- A list of personal early warning signs and the best ways to respond

- Ways to recognize when symptoms are worsening and ways to respond to this
- A crisis plan or advance directive

Although intended originally for consumers with emotional symptoms, these strategies can be used by anyone for any kind of disruptive illness or situation. Detailed information is given in the article (11). Frese (19) also gives useful suggestions specific to schizophrenia.

## SUMMARY

Symptoms are the behavioral or reported subjective evidence of underlying psychological and physiological problems. They give us clues about what clients or residents may be experiencing, what they seem to be having trouble with, and what we can do to make them more comfortable. This chapter presents some ideas about how to respond to clients who exhibit specific behaviors or report specific internal experiences, such as hallucinations. The occupational therapy assistant's response is shaped around three variables: therapeutic use of self, modification of the environment, and selection of activities.

The information in this chapter is intended as a general guide and not as a rigid system of rules. It cannot substitute for a proper intervention plan but can be useful for refining the plan once the general goals and methods have been identified. Every person is unique and needs an individualized approach. Occupational therapists and assistants cannot treat the patient's symptoms because symptoms are caused by the underlying disease process. However, the OTA can help the person function better by modifying the environment so that he or she can manage it and by selecting and modifying activities that use his or her remaining capabilities.

## REVIEW QUESTIONS AND ACTIVITIES

1. Define *symptom*, and explain why symptoms are useful guides to understanding patient behavior and feelings.
2. Identify the three tools used by occupational therapy practitioners to help consumers experiencing psychiatric symptoms function as best they can and engage in occupation. Explain why we call these tools "response variables."
3. Describe the following symptoms: anxiety; depression; mania; hallucinations; delusions; paranoia; anger, hostility, and aggression; seductive behavior and sexual acting out; cognitive deficits; and attention deficits.
   - For each symptom, identify the diagnoses associated with it.
   - For each symptom, discuss how the OTA can use self, environment, and activity to facilitate better functioning for the patient.
   - Identify the characteristics of appropriate activities for a person experiencing each symptom.
   - For each symptom, describe one or more unsuitable activities and explain what makes them unsuitable.
4. Cognitive deficits may be temporary or permanent. How does this affect the interventions used and the goals for the person?
5. Discuss the role of the OTA in promoting wellness and consumer self-management of symptoms.
6. *Challenge activity:* Give a detailed description of how you would set up the work area for someone in a manic state to make the project shown in Box 11-3.
7. *Challenge activity:* Examine Figure 11-1. What safety problems are present in part A that have been removed in part B?
8. *Challenge activity:* Look at the figure in Box 11-10. Write an analysis of how you would use one or the other of these projects for persons with the different symptoms described in the chapter. How would you set up the work area? What adaptations or modifications would be appropriate? How can you make the activity easier or more difficult?
9. *Challenge activity:* Research the effectiveness of computer activities for persons with cognitive impairments. Discuss whether these are effective interventions, for whom, and under what conditions.
10. *Classroom activity:* Write each symptom described in this chapter on a separate piece of paper and put the papers in a container. Each of 10 students draws a slip of paper; and, taking turns, acts as a patent who has the symptom he or she drew. For each "patient," a second student acts as an OTA who is meeting the patient for the first time. The OTA student must use the three response variables to help the patient. The rest of the class helps guess the symptom and then discusses the therapeutic response. (Additional students can act as other patients or staff, as needed.)

## REFERENCES


1. Allen CK. Cognitive Disabilities: Part One: Measurement and Management [Workshop]. New York: Advanced Rehabilitation Institutes, 1985.
2. Allen CK. Occupational Therapy for Psychiatric Diseases: Measurement and Management of Cognitive Disabilities. Boston: Little, Brown, 1985.
3. Allen CK. Professional judgment. In: Allen CK, Earhardt CA, Blue T, eds. Treatment Goals for the Physically and Cognitively Disabled. Rockville, MD: American Occupational Therapy Association, 1992.
4. Allen CK, Blue T, Earhardt CA. Understanding cognitive performance modes. Ormond Beach FL: Allen Conferences, Inc., 1997.
5. American Psychiatric Association. Diagnostic and Statistical Manual of Mental Disorders. 4th ed. Text rev. Washington, DC: APA, 2000.
6. Beck AT. Cognitive Therapy and the Emotional Disorders. New York: International Universities, 1976.
7. Beck AT, Rector NA. Cognitive therapy for schizophrenic patients. Harv Ment Health Lett 1998;15(6)4–6.
8. Casby JA, Holm MB. The effect of music on repetitive disruptive vocalizations of persons with dementia. Am J Occup Ther 1994;48:883–889.
9. Champagne T. Expanding the role of sensory approaches in acute psychiatric settings. Am Occup Ther Assoc Ment Health Special Sect Q Newslett 2005;28(1):1–4.
10. Convit A, Jaeger J, Lin SP, et al. Predicting assaultiveness in psychiatric inpatients: A pilot study. Hosp Community Psychiatry 1988;39:429–438.
11. Copeland ME. Wellness recovery action plan: A system for monitoring, reducing and eliminating uncomfortable or dangerous physical symptoms and emotional feelings. Occup Ther Ment Health 2001;17(3–4):127–150.
12. Delusions and delusional disorders, part 1. Harv Ment Health Lett 1999;15(7)1–3.
13. Early MB. T.A.R. Introductory Course Workbook: Occupational Therapy: Psychosocial Dysfunction. Long Island City, NY: La Guardia Community College, 1981.
14. Ellis A. Humanistic Psychology: The Rational-Emotive Approach. New York: McGraw-Hill, 1974.
15. Engel JM. Bipolar disorders: The "moody blues." Am Occup Ther Assoc Ment Health Special Sect Q Newslett 1995; 18(4):1–3.
16. Engel JM. Evaluation and treatment of persons with major depressive disorder. Am Occup Ther Assoc Ment Health Special Sect Q Newslett 1995;18(3):1–3.
17. Falk-Kessler J, Froschauer KH. The soap opera: A dynamic group approach for psychiatric patients. Am J Occup Ther 1978;32:317–321.
18. Frese FJ. Schizophrenia: Surviving in the World of Normals [video]. Beachwood, OH: Wellness Reproductions, 1991.
19. Frese FJ. Twelve aspects of coping for persons with schizophrenia. Available at: homepage.powerup.com.au/~nmanser/frese1.html. Accessed Feb 2007.
20. Gibson D. Theory and strategies for resolving conflict. Occup Ther Ment Health 1986;5(4):47–62.
21. Gitlin LN, Corcoran MA. Appendix B: Examples of environmental strategies for targeted management areas. In: Gitlin LN, Corcoran MA. Occupational Therapy and Dementia Care: The Home Environmental Skill-Building Program for Individuals and Families. Bethesda MD: American Occupational Therapy Association Press, 2005.
22. Glantz C, Richman N. Occupation-based, ability-centered care for people with dementia. OT Practice 2007;12(2): 10–16.
23. Grogan G. Anger management: I. A perspective for occupational therapy. Occup Ther Ment Health 1991;11(2–3): 135–148.
24. Grogan G. Anger management: 2. Clinical applications for occupational therapy. Occup Ther Ment Health 1991; 11(2–3):149–171.
25. Gutman SA. Understanding suicide: What therapists should know. Occup Ther Ment Health 2005;21(2): 55–77.
26. Harborview Anger Management Program. Helping angry and violent people manage their emotions. Hosp Community Psychiatry 1987;38:1207–1210.
27. Jamison KR. An Unquiet Mind: A Memoir of Moods and Madness. New York: Vintage, 1995.
28. Janowsky DS, Leff M, Epstein RS. Playing the manic game: Interpersonal maneuvers of the acutely manic patient. Arch Gen Psychiatry 1970;22:252–261.
29. Katz N, ed. Cognition and Occupation across the Life Span. 2nd ed. Bethesda, MD: American Occupational Therapy Association Press, 2005.
30. King LJ. Sensory integration as a broad spectrum treatment approach. Philadelphia: Continuing Education Programs of America, 1978.
31. Lonergan E. Benevolent touch: Use for persons with Alzheimer's disease and related dementias. Am Occup Ther Assoc Ment Health Special Sect Q Newslett 1996;19(4):3, 6.
32. MacRae A. The model of functional deficits associated with hallucinations. Am J Occup Ther 1997;51:57–63.
33. MacRae A. An overview of theory and research on hallucinations: Implications for occupational therapy intervention. Occup Ther Ment Health 1991;11(4):41–60.
34. Managing and averting anger. Harv Ment Health Lett 2002;18(12)1–4.

35. Medalia A, Revheim N. Using computers in cognitive rehabilitation with psychiatric patients. Paper presented at Institute 08, the AOTA annual conference. Baltimore, MD, Apr 3, 1998.
36. Mu K, Gabriel L. Comprehensive behavior support—Strategies to cope with severe challenging behavior. OT Practice 2001;6(2);12–16.
37. Nakano M. Treatment approaches for attention deficits in schizophrenia. Occup Ther Ment Health 2004;17(2):35–47.
38. Neville A. The model of human occupation and depression. Am Occup Ther Assoc Ment Health Special Sect Q Newslett 1985;8(1):1–4.
39. Obsessive-compulsive disorder, part II. Harv Ment Health Lett 2005;22(5):1–4.
40. Painter J. Enhancing function for persons with Alzheimer's disease. OT Practice 1998;3(1):24–29.
41. Rihmer Z. Suicide risk in mood disorders. Curr Opin Psychiatry 2007;20(1):17–22.
42. Rosen S, Scott JB. Behavior management strategies for students with autism. OT Practice 2003;8(11):16–20.
43. Seligman ME. Helplessness: On Depression, Development and Death. San Francisco: Freeman, 1975.
44. Stancliff BL. Anger: How this emotion affects your patient, you, and the rehab process. OT Practice 1996;1(8):36–45.
45. Taylor E. Anger intervention. Am J Occup Ther 1988; 42:147–155.
46. Trace S, Howell T. Occupational therapy in geriatric mental health. Am J Occup Ther 1991;45:833–838.
47. Turner IM. The healing power of respect: A personal journey. Occup Ther Ment Health 1989;9(1):17–32.
48. Wilson BA, Moffat N, eds. Clinical Management of Memory Problems. Rockville, MD: Aspen Systems, 1984.
49. Working off depression. Harv Ment Health Lett 2005; 22(6):6–7.

## SUGGESTED READINGS

Copeland ME. Wellness recovery action plan: A system for monitoring, reducing and eliminating uncomfortable or dangerous physical symptoms and emotional feelings. Occup Ther Ment Health 2001;17(3–4):127–150.

Devereaux E, Carlson M. The role of occupational therapy in the management of depression. Am J Occup Ther 1992;46:175–180.

Engel JM. Bipolar disorders: The "moody blues." Am Occup Ther Assoc Ment Health Special Sect Q Newslett 1995; 18(4):1–3.

Engel JM. Evaluation and treatment of persons with major depressive disorder. Am Occup Ther Assoc Ment Health Special Sect Q Newslett 1995;18(3):1–3.

Frese FJ. Twelve aspects of coping for persons with schizophrenia. Available at: homepage.powerup.com.au/~nmanser/frese1.html. Accessed Feb 2007.

Gitlin LN, Corcoran MA. Appendix B: Examples of environmental strategies for targeted management areas. In: Gitlin LN, Corcoran MA. Occupational Therapy and Dementia Care: The Home Environmental Skill-Building Program for Individuals and Families. Bethesda MD: American Occupational Therapy Association Press, 2005.

Glantz C, Richman N. Occupation-based, ability-centered care for people with dementia. OT Practice 2007;12(2): 10–16.

Gutman SA. Understanding suicide: What therapists should know. Occup Ther Ment Health 2005;21(2):55–77.

Kautzmann LN. Schizophrenia, part 1. Am Occup Ther Assoc Ment Health Special Sect Q Newslett 1996; 19(1):1–4.

Kautzmann LN. Schizophrenia, part 2. Am Occup Ther Assoc Ment Health Special Sect Q Newslett 1996; 19(2):1–4.

Mace NL, Rabins PV. The 36-Hour Day: A Family Guide to Caring for Persons with Alzheimer's Disease, Related Dementing Illness, and Memory Loss in Later Life. 3rd ed. New York: Warner, 2006.

Managing and averting anger. Harv Ment Health Lett 2002;18:12:1–4.

Mu K, Gabriel L. Comprehensive behavior support—Strategies to cope with severe challenging behavior. OT Practice 2001;6(2):12–16.

Painter J. Enhancing function for persons with Alzheimer's disease. OT Practice 1998;3(1):24–29.

CHAPTER 12

# Safety Techniques

***The cautious seldom err.***

CONFUCIUS (4)

## CHAPTER OBJECTIVES

After studying this chapter, the reader will be able to:

1. Explain why safety must be considered in all interactions with consumers.
2. Explain the rationale (reasons) for universal precautions.
3. Wash hands using the protocol for universal precautions.
4. List recommendations for infection control in occupational therapy.
5. List and explain 15 recommendations for safety in the clinic.
6. Recognize the occupational therapy assistant's responsibility to maintain certification in first aid and cardiopulmonary resuscitation.
7. Discuss the psychiatric emergencies of suicide, elopement, and assault, and explain how to prevent and respond to these emergencies.
8. Describe the role of the occupational therapy assistant in teaching consumers about safety.
9. List home modifications that will increase safety for the cognitively impaired consumer.

Occupational therapy assistants (OTAs) must put safety first so that they can protect their patients and themselves. Some persons with psychiatric disorders are at risk for harming themselves, either by accident or on purpose. Some are suicidal; others have histories of violence; and others are just confused or careless and are likely to get lost, have accidents, or expose themselves to infection or environmental dangers.

Persons hospitalized for psychiatric reasons often require the protection of physical boundaries (locked doors) and attentive staff. Locked units restrict the use of sharps and other objects that can be used violently or self-destructively, and some have padded seclusion rooms for separating violent or out-of-control patients from others. When patients leave a locked unit to come to occupational therapy or when occupational therapy is conducted on the unit, special precautions are needed so that they do not harm themselves. Occupational therapy personnel are legally liable for negligence if a person under their care is injured because staff failed to follow proper procedures.

But consumers may also be seen in their own homes, in an outpatient clinic, or in a homeless shelter. Safety education and training in responding to emergencies can improve a consumer's functional independence in the community. No matter what the setting or service recipient, it makes sense to follow standard general safety, public health, and fire code regulations and to teach clients about them so that they can follow them at home.

This chapter presents guidelines for general safety in the occupational therapy department. This chapter is not meant to substitute for training in state-of-the-art disease prevention methods or basic first aid. The author assumes that the reader will maintain certification in first aid and cardiopulmonary resuscitation (CPR), including training for an automatic electronic defibrillator (AED). Universal precautions for the prevention of disease transmission will be addressed, however. Infection control and similar information can be found on the Centers for Disease Control and Prevention's website (www.cdc.gov).

The chapter also introduces special safety precautions for working in hospitals with clients who are at risk for elopement, suicide, or assault and discusses ways to teach consumers about safety.

## UNIVERSAL PRECAUTIONS

*Universal precautions* refers to the set of procedures recommended by various governmental and health agencies to prevent the spread of infection. The precautions particularly target infections that are caused by disease agents that may be found in blood and other bodily fluids. The human immunodeficiency virus (HIV), responsible for acquired immune deficiency syndrome (AIDS), and the hepatitis B virus are two examples.

Health care students and workers worry about the risk of contracting HIV from those in their care. For occupational therapists (OTs) and OTAs, the risk is much smaller than for members of some other professions, who are more likely to come in contact with bodily fluids. Even for members of these professions, the risk of catching HIV is insignificant compared with the risk of contracting a more infectious disease, such as hepatitis or tuberculosis. Many disease-causing agents can be transmitted from person to person. Remember that infection can travel both ways; the patient can contract a disease from the health care worker as well. For these reasons, it is important that health care workers observe basic infection control procedures and universal precautions with *all* other persons in the work environment.

Since 1992, employers (e.g., hospitals) have been required to have an exposure control plan and to provide adequate hand-washing facilities (including single-use towels or hot-air blowers) and protective barriers such as gloves for the use of employees who may come in contact with blood or other bodily fluids (16). Because many individuals are allergic to latex or to the talc used with some gloves, more than one type of glove should be available. Small community-based programs may not reliably provide these controls and supplies, so the obligation falls on the OTA to learn and to follow the current federal guidelines.

## Hand Washing

The first and most effective method of disease prevention is regular and thorough hand washing. Box 12-1 provides details about when and how hands should be washed. The times suggested are based on Marcil's (9) work with AIDS patients but can wisely be applied to other patient care situations.

The key points of any hand-washing sequence are to clean all hand surfaces and crevices, to use soap and reasonably hot water, to avoid recontamination from sink or faucets or other surfaces, and to use clean disposable towels or hot air to dry the hands.

## Protective Barriers

Because persons in the later stages of dementia may not have control over their bodily functions, because some patients have poor habits of personal

**BOX 12-1**

### HAND WASHING: THE FIRST DEFENSE AGAINST INFECTION

When to wash

- Before starting work
- Before and after treating patients or consumers if physical contact is involved
- Before donning and after removing gloves
- During performance of normal duties
- Before and after handling food
- After personal use of the toilet or toileting of a patient
- After sneezing, coughing, or contact with oral and nasal areas
- Before eating or preparing food
- Before leaving the room of a patient on isolation or precautions
- On completion of duty

How to wash (follow steps in order)

1. Bring at least three paper towels to the sink.
2. Remove hand jewelry, including watch.
3. Turn on water to good stream of tolerable but hot water.
4. Using soap, make a good lather.
5. Using one hand, wash the other up to and including the wrist, taking care to clean between fingers and under fingernails.
6. Repeat procedure for other hand.
7. Dry hands, using one towel and a patting motion. Follow with a second and, if needed, a third towel.
8. Use last towel to turn off faucets.
9. Use last towel to turn doorknob or open door of sink area.
10. Discard towels in trash container.
11. Apply hand lotion to prevent cracking of skin (a route for infection to enter).

hygiene, and because medications may cause vomiting, the occupational therapy worker may occasionally encounter a patient's bodily fluids. Thus protective barriers (primarily gloves) must be worn when cleaning areas that have been or *may have been* contaminated. Adhesive bandages should be used to cover tiny cuts and even hangnails *at all times* and should be changed whenever hands are washed.

### Infection Control in Common Areas

The occupational therapy clinic in mental health settings appears less medical than the physical disabilities clinic. A homelike appearance and informal atmosphere should not be taken as an excuse for ignoring proper infection control. Tables, counters, and other surfaces should be washed and disinfected daily and any time contamination is suspected. Adequate supplies of cleaning materials such as hand soap, paper towels, trash bin, a pail and mop, sponges, detergents, and disinfectants should be maintained. Disposable gloves, utility gloves, adhesive bandages, and a first aid kit should be kept in each occupational therapy area.

Linens used in homemaking groups should be replaced or laundered after each use. Cosmetics and personal hygiene items (combs, toothbrushes) should never be shared. For personal hygiene sessions, patients should bring their own supplies or the therapy assistant should provide brand new items for each person. Many cosmetic companies provide samples on request for this purpose.

By federal regulations, eating, drinking, smoking, applying cosmetics or lip balm, and handling contact lenses are prohibited when there is a likelihood of occupational exposure to blood or bodily fluids (16).

### Universal Means Universal

It is tempting to believe that certain clients, especially those similar to oneself or one's family and friends, could not possibly be a source of infection. With this feeling comes the impulse to relax and omit or tone down infection control procedures. It is not possible to tell whether someone is infected just by appearances. Using universal precautions *universally* limits the spread of infection from person to person. And if the precautions are *always* used, mental energy is not wasted on figuring out whether or not to use them. A habit of consistent, universal application of the procedures is the only responsible and ethical course of action for the health care worker.

## CONTROLLING THE ENVIRONMENT

Consumers often say that they enjoy coming to occupational therapy because the clinic has so many interesting things in it. Unfortunately, some of these "interesting things" are not very safe unless handled properly. The safety of clients and staff can largely be protected by organizing the occupational therapy clinic properly and by having all staff follow certain procedures.

1. *Keep track of your keys.* In some settings, occupational therapy staff attach their keys to their clothing with a metal or plastic clip, a leather thong, or a spiral cord. Do not set your keys down and turn around to do something else. Remember that even in community settings, staff have keys to areas from which consumers are restricted.
2. *Make sure restricted items are not taken onto inpatient wards.* Depending on the setting, patients may not be permitted to have certain objects on the ward. Some examples are razors, belts, anything in a glass container, hair lifts, hair picks or rattail combs, plastic bags that are head size or larger, wire hangers, and anything breakable (2). In practical terms, this means that a client may not be able to take some finished projects and supplies to his or her room. Examples are ceramic pieces, leather lace, yarn and cord, macramé, and cosmetics in glass containers.

Any questionable items should be discussed with nursing staff *before* they are brought onto the unit.

3. *Have everything ready before patients arrive in the clinic or treatment area.* The assistant who has to run around finding supplies and tools and getting people started cannot at the same time pay attention to where all the patients are and what they are doing. For the same reason, any tools or supplies that may be needed in the course of the group should be available in the same room, in neat and accessible storage. If staff is busy rummaging through the supply cabinet, patients have ample opportunity to get in trouble. *Never* leave patients from a locked ward alone and unattended.
4. *Use shatterproof mirrors.* This solves the problem of clients hurting themselves or another person with pieces of a broken mirror, but this precaution may not be needed in every setting, depending on the population.
5. *Use good judgment about who comes to occupational therapy.* Inpatients on suicidal or elopement observation may not be permitted to leave the unit. Even if they are allowed to come to occupational therapy, the assistant or therapist running the activity should carefully consider the risks before permitting the person to attend the group. Is this person going to take so much energy and attention that others will be neglected? Is this a safe activity for this particular person? Will other staff be close by in case there is a problem?
6. *Organize tool and supply cabinets to permit a fast, accurate count of all potentially dangerous items.* There are several ways to achieve this. Many clinics use a shadow board, in which every tool has a shadow or outline marking its place. Any tool that is missing can be identified immediately. The shadows can be cut out from brightly colored contact paper or painted on. Having consumers return tools to the rack at the end of the session helps them develop good work habits and feel responsible and in control (7). Allen (1) recommends using transparent plastic containers for small items; these containers are available as flat, compartmentalized boxes or as small standing chests of drawers. Knives and other sharp objects must be kept in locked storage.
7. *Alert consumers to potential dangers in activities.* You should inform them about any materials that may cause injury and teach them how to prevent it. For example, paper, foil, glazed ceramics, and even sandpaper may cut. A reed, dowel, or wire can cause eye injuries. Wood has splinters.
8. *Follow safety precautions for toxins.* Some of the substances used in occupational therapy activities can be harmful or fatal if ingested; a few have been classified as carcinogens. The OTA should read the label of every spray can and jar in the clinic and follow the precautions indicated. It is very harmful, for example, to breathe even small amounts of the mist from hair spray, silicone spray used on tiles, and spray paint or lacquer. The fumes from magic markers and plastic dipping from films and resins can cause dizziness. Some leather dyes and wood finishes are toxic. Exposure to wood dust can cause allergic reactions, and prolonged or repeated exposure is associated with increased incidence of nasal cancer.[1] Some glues and their vapors are toxic. Ceramic glazes that contain lead should not be used in occupational therapy, nor should any paint containing lead (e.g., flake white oil color) or cadmium (e.g., cadmium red). Anything that might irritate the eyes or lungs (e.g., grout) should be used cautiously. Provide adequate ventilation whenever solvents or aerosol sprays are used.

[1] A summary of the health effects of common wood finishes and solvents is presented in Mustoe (10).

All users, clients and staff alike, should wash their hands thoroughly after handling toxic materials; the room should be damp mopped rather than swept to avoid sending particles into the air (12). Do not transfer dangerous materials to unmarked containers. Keep them in their original containers wherever possible. If a small amount is poured out for patients to use, it should be put in an appropriate container, not paper, plastic, or foam plastic, and discarded after the session. ***Never** use any container that might be mistaken for a food or drink or medication container.* Place jars and containers of all liquids near the center of the table, where they are less likely to be knocked over. Because of the danger from accidental ingestion of toxins or carcinogens, eating, drinking, and smoking must be prohibited in areas where these supplies are used.

9. *Know and use proper safety equipment.*[2] Safety goggles, appropriate clothing, and sometimes dust masks should be worn by patients and staff using any power tool. Long hair and long sleeves should be fastened back so that they do not drop into tools, fluids, or heat sources. Neoprene gloves should be worn when handling alcohols and solvents. Vapor masks should be worn when solvents are used in large quantities or for a long time, as in furniture stripping and refinishing. Eyewash kits should be available.

   Staff who are in a hurry may be tempted to do without safety equipment "just this once." Just this once may be one time too many; we all pick up lots of carcinogens in other ways, and it is the cumulative effect that matters; every little bit just adds to it. Remember that toxin exposure (e.g., lead) can cause cognitive deficits. An important consideration is that some individuals may have allergies to foods, fibers (e.g., wool), and animals. The dust from plaster and clay can be very irritating to the lungs, skin, and eyes.

10. *Observe the local fire code.* Flammables should be kept in a separate cabinet designed for that purpose. Fire extinguishers and fire blankets should be mounted in easily accessible places wherever fire or flammables are used. The OTA should know how to use them.

   "No Smoking" and "No Eating and Drinking" signs and signs indicating the location of safety equipment should be clearly visible.[3] Doorways and fire exits should be kept clear, unlocked, and unobstructed. Fire drills should be scheduled regularly to acquaint staff and consumers with evacuation routes and procedures. Clients should not be permitted near the ceramic kiln when it is operating. The door to the kiln should be padlocked so that no one will open it while it is on.

11. *Pay attention to the condition of the floor.* Clean up spills immediately. Highly waxed floors are slippery and dangerous for shop and kitchen areas. It makes sense to sweep up sawdust and debris in the workshop fairly frequently; this means every half hour or even more often, depending on level of use.

12. *Eliminate electrical hazards.* Be sure that the current is sufficient for the demand; do not overload a circuit or use multiple-outlet plugs. Appliances with a three-prong plug have to be grounded; if there is no three-prong outlet available, do not use the appliance unless the green grounding wire is screwed into the switch plate. Make sure that electricity and water cannot come in contact with each other

[2] Safety equipment appropriate for shops in which solvents, carcinogens, and flammables are used can be obtained from Lab Safety Supply, Janesville, WI 53567–1368.

[3] These fire safety items are available from Lab Safety Supply, Janesville, WI 53567–1368.

in the clinic. Have electrical outlets near sinks or other water sources disconnected if necessary. Arrange for damaged cords, including cords that get hot, and plugs to be repaired or replaced immediately. Be sure that electrical equipment is unplugged or switched off before you leave the clinic. This is especially important for devices that have a heating element (irons and curling irons, copper enameling kilns, and coffee makers). It is often a good idea to have a central power cutoff installed for shop areas or kitchens.

13. *Observe food safety guidelines and fire safety precautions in the kitchen.* Because the occupational therapy kitchen is used by so many staff and clients, things can get out of hand fairly quickly unless all involved take responsibility for keeping it clean and safe. Generally one person is designated to have final responsibility, and this is often the OTA. The refrigerator and freezer should be kept at the proper temperatures. Leftover canned food should be transferred to another container and clearly marked, including the date. The refrigerator should be cleaned out once a week to discard items at risk for spoiling. The occupational therapy kitchen should be equipped with good, thick pot holders and mitts. The oven should be well insulated to prevent accidental burns. Consumers and staff must learn to tie back long hair and roll up their sleeves and wear aprons while working at the stove. Handles of pots should be turned so that they do not stick out past the edge of the stove.

    Consumers need to be observed closely; it is not at all unusual for a person with a mild cognitive impairment to try to pick up something hot with a bare hand or reach into boiling water. Because medication may cause poor co-ordination, have consumers set containers on a firm surface before liquids are poured into them. This is most important when the liquids are hot.

14. *Apply techniques for proper positioning, energy conservation, and work simplification, and teach these to consumers.* Occupational therapy assistants generally learn these techniques in relation to persons with physical disabilities, but they apply to everyone. Observe and correct the consumer's body and hand position to prevent repetitive strain injuries; teach the person about nondeforming postures. Provide rest breaks and explain their importance. Teach consumers how to be organized in their approach to a task. Refer to physical disabilities texts for particulars if you are unfamiliar with these ideas.

15. *Provide increased structure for those functioning at lower cognitive levels.* Be alert to varying functional levels, especially in persons undergoing changes in medications. A patient may approach a familiar task with confidence and yet be a danger to self because of a cognitive impairment. Trace and Howell (15) analyze the preparation of a cup of instant coffee, citing numerous risks for unsafe behavior.

## MEDICAL EMERGENCIES AND FIRST AID

Occupational therapy assistants need to know how to respond to medical emergencies whether they work in inpatient or outpatient settings. Fainting; seizures; and minor cuts, burns, and contusions are the most common medical emergencies. Serious burns and wounds, fractures, poisoning, choking, cardiac arrest, and strokes are less common but still occur. The outcome of these serious conditions depends heavily upon the ability of the person nearest the scene to respond quickly and correctly. The general rules for responding to a medical emergency are covered in any basic first aid course.

### Seizures

Some of the medications used to treat psychiatric disorders are associated with an increased likelihood of seizures. The OTA should know what a seizure looks like and what to do if a patient has one. The usual pattern in a seizure is for the person to become rigid and statue-like for a few seconds and then begin to move with an all-over jerking motion. The person may void urine or feces or stop breathing and will probably turn bluish. The procedure for responding if someone starts having a seizure is covered in first aid courses.

### Bleeding

Bleeding can range from relatively minor to quite serious and even fatal. Because sharp objects and power tools are used in occupational therapy, it is important for all staff to know how to respond to a bleeding emergency. The first goal is to stop the bleeding; it may be necessary to send someone else for help, and sometimes the only person available will be another patient. Be sure the person summoning help knows whom to contact and what to say. It is also important to avoid contaminating the wound. Again, basic first aid courses cover this information.

### Burns

Most of the burns that occur in occupational therapy are relatively minor first-degree burns and can be treated with basic first aid. Second- and third-degree burns require immediate medical attention. Because second- and third-degree burns are treated differently and it can be difficult to tell which is which unless you have seen them before, the occupational therapy assistant should summon help when the burn has any blistering or when skin is missing or charred.

Scalding with boiling water is a hazard in the kitchen. If boiling water is poured on the person's clothes, the first step is to remove the clothing. If boiling water has gotten into the shoes, remove them first.

### Sunburn

Photosensitivity, or increased sensitivity to the sun's rays, is a side effect of some medications used to treat psychiatric disorders and of some other common prescription medications (e.g., tetracycline). Because occupational therapy activities may be conducted out of doors, the OTA must know what medications patients are taking. Sunburn can be prevented by having the person wear an effective sun block, a hat, and (if necessary) long pants and long sleeves. Be sure the person applies sun block everywhere, especially to the shoulders, neck, ears, the top of the head (bald men), and the tops of the feet and backs of the hands if these are bare. Sunglasses are recommended because the eyes are also affected by the medications.

### Strains, Sprains, Bruises, and Contusions

Strains, sprains, bruises, and contusions are common types of soft-tissue damage; blood vessels under the skin are broken and bleed into surrounding areas, but there is no external bleeding. Pain, discoloration, and swelling result if these injuries are not treated promptly. The protocol is RICE (rest, ice, compression, elevation), which is explained in basic first aid courses.

## PSYCHIATRIC EMERGENCIES

Psychiatric emergencies can occur in any setting. We tend to associate them with inpatient environments because locked units and hospitalization suggest that the residents are more impaired. But with shorter hospital stays and more rigorous admissions criteria, seriously ill consumers are now seen in outpatient and community settings.

Furthermore, suicide is a risk even for persons who are seen in outpatient physical medicine settings and who have no acknowledged mental health problems. It is important for the OTA to be able to recognize and respond to the suicidal client.

## Suicide

Some of the basic precautions for dealing with the suicidal person are covered in the section on depression in Chapter 11. In inpatient settings the OTA must be alert to the possibility that the depressed and suicidal individual will try to elope from the treatment facility or to remove objects from the occupational therapy clinic to use them in a later suicide attempt.

Suicidal persons who succeed in eloping from a locked inpatient unit may try to commit suicide immediately by the first means possible (jumping in front of a moving car or train, off the roof, or out of a high window). Therefore, the OTA should take precautions to prevent the patient from eloping. The patient must be escorted from the unit to occupational therapy alone or in a small group; no one can be expected to keep track of more than four patients when any of them are on suicide observation. Depending on the setting and the complexity of the physical layout, it may be safe to escort only two or three patients at a time. Similarly, such patients should be excluded from community field trips. Occasionally, staff from other disciplines (e.g., psychiatrists) may put pressure on the occupational therapy staff to take suicidal patients on trips; this seems to occur more when the patient appears to be getting better. The occupational therapy practitioner should refuse to do this if he or she has any suspicion at all that the person may be suicidal.

The OTA needs to be especially alert to ways in which tools and supplies can be used in a suicide attempt. The list of dangers is extensive: toxins (leather dyes), flammables (turpentine), sharps (needles, pins, scissors, knives), matches, objects that can be used in hanging (belts, yarn, leather, lace), and so forth. The person who is intent on suicide will use anything at hand: break a mirror or a light bulb, stick a fork in an electrical socket, or try to drown in the toilet. The fact that suicide can be achieved with objects that appear to be harmless poses a real problem in occupational therapy. Inpatients who are grossly suicidal should not be permitted off the unit or admitted to the occupational therapy clinic. But because individuals may be more impulsive and suicidal than they appear, precautions should be taken with any person who has any history of suicidal ideation or actual suicide attempts. Consumers who are receiving antidepressant medications and who show an increase in activity level may be at risk, as explained in Chapter 8.

In inpatient settings, all supplies and tools should be kept under lock and key; tools (and needles, pins, matches, flammables and toxins, and items in glass containers) should be counted before patients enter the clinic and before any of them leave. When patients have to leave the room to go to the bathroom or get a drink of water, a staff member must accompany them; likewise, any sharps should be accounted for because with some wounds it takes only a few minutes to bleed to death.

In outpatient settings the OTA needs to be aware of the potential for suicide. Box 12-2, based on Rihmer (13) and Stoudemire (14), lists some of the factors that may increase the risk of suicide. The OTA, while not trained to assess suicidal intent, should be alert to possible signs (Box 12-3). The OTA must use good judgment, discretion, and speed in seeking psychiatric evaluation of any person who expresses suicidal intent or who shows other signs of planning suicide (5).

## Assault

Assaultive individuals should not be seen in occupational therapy until they are properly sedated with medications; there is simply no reason to risk the safety of others. However, occasionally a person

BOX 12-2

**RISK FACTORS FOR SUICIDE**

- Current axis I major mental disorders
- Past suicide attempts
- The more lethal the attempt (e.g., use of gun), the greater the risk
- The less likely the rescue, the greater the risk
- Comorbid axis II disorder
- Family history of suicide
- Adverse childhood experiences (loss of parents, abuse)
- Unemployment
- Poor physical health
- Alcoholism or drug abuse
- Cigarette smoking
- Sudden life changes
- Living alone
- Gender, race, age (older white men, adolescent males most likely)
- Psychosocial problems (family tension, school problems, breakup with girlfriend or boyfriend may affect children and adolescents significantly)

Data from Rihmer Z. Suicide risk in mood disorders. Curr Opin Psychiatry 2007;20(1):17–22; Stoudemire A. Clinical Psychiatry for Medical Students. 3rd ed. Philadelphia: Lippincott-Raven, 1998.

becomes assaultive while in occupational therapy. Often this is an escalation of general anger or hostility; sometimes the assaultiveness could have been contained if staff had noticed the situation and responded to it more quickly (see "Anger, Hostility, and Aggression," in Chapter 11). At other times, the assault occurs without warning, seemingly unprovoked, and the person may have no memory of the incident after it occurs; clients who have abused phencyclidine (PCP) are especially prone to this (1). If by any chance the situation does get out of control and the person strikes out or appears ready to do so, the OTA should take the following steps, in order:

BOX 12-3

**SIGNS OF SUICIDAL INTENT**

- Talking about killing oneself or wanting to die
- Recent acquisition of the means to die (e.g., stockpiling medication, buying a gun)
- Making a will or taking out life insurance
- Giving away personal belongings
- Seeking promises that someone else will take care of pets, children "if anything happens to me"
- Passive suicidal behavior (not eating, drinking too much, engaging in unsafe behaviors)

1. Call for more staff.
2. Remove other patients from the area.
3. Attempt to calm the patient.

If you need more staff, yell or scream if you must. Ask a higher-functioning consumer to telephone or go for help. Similarly, a relatively competent consumer can be in charge of escorting the others to a safe area.

Talking to the disturbed person in a calm, soothing tone may help him or her calm down; if you can get the person to talk, he or she will usually be more manageable. More staff will be needed to calm and subdue the person who actually gets out of control. Under no circumstances should the OTA attempt to overpower the person by physical force. Someone in a psychotic rage is extremely powerful; all energy is channeled into striking out. As many as six men may be required to restrain a small person during a violent episode. There are two exceptions to this general rule: The OTA may be able to restrain a child younger than 8 years of age; and the assistant may feel compelled to step in if others are in danger. In either case, the assistant should first call for more staff.

The use of restraint and force is a last resort; every attempt to calm the person by other means should be exhausted first. Because the correct use of restraint is more easily learned by demonstration and practice than by reading about it, it is not covered in this text. Students should expect to learn restraint techniques during their fieldwork, if such techniques are needed in the setting.

In an outpatient setting, incidents of personal violence usually require calling the police or ambulance service. Assaultive persons should not be allowed to remain in the community because they are likely to commit further violent acts. If a violent incident occurs, the assistant should follow the treatment setting's procedure for reporting and documenting such incidents. Once the incident is over and the person is calmed or removed from the scene, the OTA should encourage other consumers who may have been present to express their feelings about what has happened.

## Elopement

The psychiatric meaning of *elopement* is much less romantic than its everyday meaning. *Elopement* means "running away from an inpatient treatment facility" without being discharged in the customary way. Patients may elope because they just don't want to be there or because they don't want to receive treatment or because they have something specific they want to do, like commit suicide or hurt someone else.

Preventing elopement starts with securing doors and windows. Doors should be locked except when in use. Windows should be kept closed, or if opened, should have gates or window guards. Some circular lock fittings on screens or windows can be opened by using the lids of some magic markers; occupational therapy staff should be alert to this possibility when ordering supplies.

When escorting patients to and from a locked unit, the OTA should be especially careful; it is easy to lose a patient if your back is turned. Similarly, patients who want to escape from a locked unit may lurk by the door, waiting for an unsuspecting staff member to unlock it. Sometimes these patients are disoriented and confused and won't know where to go once they do escape; others have a definite plan. Always look behind you to see who is nearby when you are opening a locked door. And be sure to notify nursing staff when you take patients off the ward.

Trips from a locked ward into the community present special concerns.

Sometimes it is hard to determine in advance just who is likely to try to run away during a trip. Two staff members should always accompany patients from a locked unit if there are four or more patients in the group; it is best to have two staff members even with smaller groups because one can stay with the group if the other has to go after someone who is running away. If you are alone with a group and a patient elopes, return the other patients to the ward or to the care of a responsible staff member before going after the one who ran away.

## TEACHING CONSUMERS ABOUT SAFETY

Independent living in the community requires knowledge and application of household and personal safety precautions, personal hygiene, basic first aid, and emergency procedures. Helping consumers master these skills is a service the OTA can provide. Ogren (11) suggests that health and safety skills for community living should include knowledge of emergency phone numbers, simple first aid, household safety hazards, and how and where to obtain medical care. Kartin and Van Schroeder (6) advocate instruction in personal safety (use of locks, how to deal with strangers) and earthquake procedures in addition. They list sample activities for safety instruction, including making photographs or cartoons of common safety hazards, having guest speakers from fire or police departments or from the hospital or the Red Cross, and having consumers list emergency numbers on an index card to keep by the telephone. Because people with low cognitive levels lack knowledge and judgment, education about safe sex techniques is also important. Reproducible activity sheets for reinforcing safety precautions can be found in Korb and associates (8).

We cannot anticipate every emergency or bizarre situation that someone may encounter in the community. Rote learning of specific safety procedures is not sufficient preparation for safe independent living (17). Safety instruction must also incorporate activities that require the person to identify problems and generate alternative responses. The OTA should develop the habit of clipping newspaper articles and collecting stories and anecdotes about health and safety situations a consumer might encounter. These can be turned into a file of paper and pencil activities or discussion topics.

## MODIFYING ENVIRONMENTS TO ENHANCE SAFETY

Particularly with increased age, consumers are at risk from unsafe conditions in their homes and communities. Barrows (3) notes that medication-related obesity and diabetes, smoking, and cardiac conditions increase risks. Some consumers have cognitive impairments, some have vision impairments, and some have mobility and strength impairments that further compromise their safety. Consumers may be resistant to changes in their home environments. As with any other intervention, home safety modifications should represent a collaboration between therapy practitioner and consumer. Recommended home modifications, mostly from Barrows, are shown in Box 12-4.

## SUMMARY

All occupational therapy staff have a legal and professional obligation to ensure the health and safety of their patients and clients, their co-workers, and themselves. Because life is not always predictable, the OTA needs a habitual attitude of alertness, attention, and common sense. The goal of occupational therapy is to help people enjoy and master the activities and skills they need to function in their lives. We need to teach consumers that pleasure, comfort, and satisfaction in performing many everyday activities rely on reducing the potential for injury and infection by using appropriate safety measures.

**BOX 12-4**

### RECOMMENDED HOME MODIFICATIONS FOR CONSUMER SAFETY

- Provide railings for balance.
- Remove tripping hazards such as throw rugs.
- Arrange furniture for easy movement.
- Reduce clutter.
- Change multiple locks to single key.
- Replace switched lights in public areas with motion-sensitive lighting.
- Provide task lighting under cabinets and other dark spots.
- Organize storage and match to consumer's cognitive level.
- Use transparent storage boxes if consumer can tolerate this much stimulation.
- Clear nonessential items from areas next to cooktops and sinks.
- Install ground fault interrupter (GFI) switches for all outlets near water
- Install temperature guard for tub, shower, and water heater.
- Replace oven-top tea kettle with electric version with automatic shut-off.
- Purchase auto shut-off versions of other appliances such as electric irons.
- Replace batteries on smoke alarms and carbon monoxide detectors twice yearly; have these checked regularly by someone other than the consumer if cognitive deficits are a problem.
- Check that consumer has sufficient strength and mobility to use bathroom appliances, small tools, and other items in the home; if indicated, replace with modified versions.
- Provide adequate storage space so that consumers do not store items on the back of the toilet (where they may fall in).
- Provide grab bars for clients who may otherwise reach for a less sturdy support like a towel rod.
- Insulate exposed pipes.
- Label liquids clearly to avoid misuse (e.g., drain cleaner and cleaning products versus shampoo and personal hygiene products).

## REVIEW QUESTIONS AND ACTIVITIES

1. Why is safety a particular concern when working with persons with mental disorders?
2. What are the reasons for universal precautions?
3. Practice washing your hands using universal precautions for infection control. Then teach this to someone else.
4. How can one prevent infections from spreading in the occupational therapy clinic?
5. Write each of the 15 recommendations for safety in the clinic on an index card. Use the cards to test yourself on your ability to describe these recommendations in detail.
6. Why is it important for the OTA to maintain certification in first aid and CPR?
7. What are some of the signs of possible suicide? What precautions should the OTA take?
8. How should one respond if a patient seems to be more agitated than usual? What should the OTA do if the patient becomes assaultive?
9. Define *elopement* as the term is used in mental health settings. Identify specific strategies staff can use to prevent elopement.
10. Why is it important for consumers to know about safety?
11. Why are persons with psychiatric disorders possibly at risk for injury in their homes?
12. List home modifications that will increase safety for the cognitively impaired consumer.

## REFERENCES


1. Allen CK. Cognitive Disabilities: Part One: Measurement and Management [Workshop]. New York: Advanced Rehabilitation Institutes, 1985.
2. Bailey DS, Cooper SO, Bailey DR. Therapeutic Approaches to the Care of the Mentally Ill. 2nd ed. Philadelphia: Davis, 1984.
3. Barrows C. Home adaptations—Creating safe environments for individuals with psychiatric disabilities. OT Practice 2006;11(18):12–16.
4. Confucius. The Confucian Analects, 4:23. In: Bartlett J, ed. Familiar Quotations. 15th ed. Boston: Little, Brown, 1980.
5. Gutman SA. Understanding suicide: What therapists should know. Occup Ther Ment Health 2005;21(2):55–77.
6. Kartin NJ, Van Schroeder C. Adult Psychiatric Living Skills Manual. Kailua, HI: Schroeder, 1982.
7. Kidner TB. The hospital pre-industrial shop. Occup Ther Ment Health 1982;2(4):63–69.
8. Korb KL, Azok AD, Leutenberg EA. Life Management Skills. 2: Reproducible Activity Handouts Created for Facilitators. Beachwood, OH: Wellness Reproductions, 1991.
9. Marcil WM. AIDS facts and implications for occupational therapy. In: Marcil WM, Tigges KN, eds. The Person with AIDS: A Personal and Professional Perspective. Thorofare, NJ: Slack, 1992.
10. Mustoe G. Respiratory hazards: Choosing the right protection. Fine Woodworking 1983;41:36–39.
11. Ogren K. A living skills program in an acute psychiatric setting. Am Occup Ther Assoc Ment Health Special Sect Q Newslett 1983;6(4):1–2.
12. Reid C. Craft activity precautions. OT Practice 1996;1(8):48–49.
13. Rihmer Z. Suicide risk in mood disorders. Curr Opin Psychiatry 2007;20(1):17–22.
14. Stoudemire A. Clinical Psychiatry for Medical Students. 3rd ed. Philadelphia: Lippincott-Raven, 1998.
15. Trace S, Howell T. Occupational therapy in geriatric mental health. Am J Occup Ther 1991;45:833–837.
16. U.S. Department of Labor. Universal precautions: Department of Labor final rule on bloodborne pathogens. Washington, DC: USDL, 1992.
17. Willson M. Occupational Therapy in Long-Term Psychiatry. Edinburgh, UK: Churchill Livingstone, 1983.


## SUGGESTED READINGS


American Red Cross. American Red Cross First Aid: Responding to Emergencies. San Bruno, CA: StayWell, 2005.

Bertorelli P. Keeping ten fingers: Injury survey pinpoints hazards in the shop. Fine Woodworking 1983;42:76–78.

McCann M. Health Hazards Manual for Artists. 5th rev. New York: Lyons, 2003.

National Ag Safety Database. Basic First Aid: Script. Available at: www.cdc.gov/nasd/docs/d000101-d000200/d000105/d000105.html. Accessed Mar 2007.

CHAPTER 13

# Group Concepts and Techniques

***Our humanity rests upon a series of learned behaviors, woven together into patterns that are infinitely fragile and never directly inherited.***

MARGARET MEAD (16, P. 29)

## CHAPTER OBJECTIVES

After studying this chapter, the reader will be able to:

1. Describe the advantages of using groups in occupational therapy.
2. Differentiate treatment groups from other groups that may occur naturally.
3. Recognize cohesiveness and other qualities that increase group effectiveness.
4. Identify and describe roles that members may take within a group.
5. Classify group skills according to Mosey's developmental levels of group skills.
6. Discuss the role of the leader in a therapy group.
7. Outline the responsibilities of the leader in preparing for the group, beginning the group, maintaining the group, and ending the group session.
8. Recognize a group protocol and differentiate the elements of the protocol.
9. Describe the five-stage group and the situations in which this group is appropriate.
10. Relate program evaluation to assessment of outcomes of therapy groups.
11. Learn and apply vocabulary pertinent to therapy groups.

Much of occupational therapy (OT) treatment for persons with mental health problems is carried out in groups. A 1983 survey showed that all occupational therapists working in psychiatric hospitals and community mental health centers at that time used groups with their patients and that groups were applied across a wide variety of settings for the physically disabled and for geriatric patients (7). The study was repeated in 1993, and findings were that groups were still used extensively in psychiatric and other settings; furthermore, the authors suggested that insurers and reimbursement sources may pressure OT practitioners to increase their use of groups because of the cost savings of group treatment as compared with one-on-one treatment (6).

This chapter explains why and how group treatment is conducted in OT in mental health settings. Although some review of group dynamics is included, we assume that the reader already has a basic knowledge of groups and how people behave in them. People live and work in groups; relating to others effectively is essential for everyday functioning. Because persons with mental disorders may have trouble relating to others, both individually and in groups, it is important to consider how people generally develop these skills.

The ability to lead groups effectively is one of the most valuable skills the occupational therapy assistant (OTA) can bring to psychiatric work. An understanding of how therapy groups differ from other kinds of groups and of the role of the leader in the group is essential. These topics, as well as a procedure for designing group session plans and a protocol for new group, are covered in some detail. The chapter includes a discussion of how to analyze, intervene in, and create group environments so as to maximize the individual's ability to relate to others. As with so many other clinical skills, however, the ability to run a group increases with practice and studious self-examination. The material presented in this chapter should prepare the reader to *begin* this process.

## DEFINITION AND PURPOSE OF GROUP TREATMENT

What is a *group?* We all participate in groups in work, school, social, and family situations. A group is three or more people who are together for some period to accomplish a common goal or share a common purpose. If this seems a little vague, it is only because the definition must include many kinds of groups. One important point, however, is that a group, in our definition, is not just a collection of people; it is a collection of people who have *a shared purpose in being together.* This makes a group different from other collections of people, such as those waiting in line in supermarkets or riding in an elevator or subway car (although groups may arise spontaneously in these situations).

What, then, is *group treatment?* A previous chapter states that treatment is a planned process for creating change so that the person can carry out his or her chosen daily life activities as independently and comfortably as possible. If we add this concept to our definition of a group, we come up with the following: *Group treatment is a planned process for creating changes in individuals by bringing them together for this purpose.*

Treating people in groups means that several individuals can receive treatment simultaneously. This is usually less expensive than having the therapist treat each person individually, one at a time. Therefore, group treatment is considered *cost effective.* However, cost-effectiveness alone is not a good enough reason for choosing a group treatment; it must also meet the needs of the individual. In most cases group treatment offers more opportunities for learning, and, therefore, for change, than does one-on-one therapy. The reason should be obvious: In a group there are more people from whom to learn. Furthermore, peer learning (learning from those one perceives as equals rather than from those one perceives as authorities) feels comfortable to many people. There are possibilities for different kinds of interactions, greater potential for problem solving and creativity, and more opportunities for reality testing, trying out new roles, and so on. Consumers who could benefit from the advantages offered by a group and who have adequate trust in other human beings are good candidates for group treatment.

## GROUP DYNAMICS: REVIEW OF BASIC CONCEPTS

We have all participated in groups that worked well, that reached their goals through the combined efforts of all the members, in a way that was relatively satisfying to the members. Likewise, we have all known groups that never seemed to get off the ground, that failed to reach their goals because the members could not work together; such groups are dreary for all concerned. What accounts for the difference between these two kinds of groups? Why do some groups succeed where others fail? What ingredients are necessary for a group to be successful?

### Cohesiveness and Other Therapeutic Factors

*Group cohesiveness* is the sense of solidarity the members feel toward each other and the group; it is based on a sense of closeness and identification with each other or with the group itself. Cohesiveness serves the same purpose in a group that trust and rapport serve in the individual patient–therapist relationship; it ties people to each other with a sense of "we-ness" or belonging together. Group members feel accepted by each other and accepting toward each other.

Cohesiveness gives a group strength to face its tasks. Individual members feel safe trying out new and unfamiliar roles because they trust that the group will not reject them if they fail. Similarly, people find it easier to share feelings and concerns in a cohesive atmosphere. Members of cohesive groups are willing to be influenced by the group and willing to take the risk of trying something new or disagreeing with the group (30). Because many people will not take risks in situations they perceive to be uncertain, the OTA must consider the cohesiveness of a particular group before implementing any treatment activities that require self-disclosure or performance of unfamiliar tasks. Cohesiveness is considered a prerequisite for work in any group (30). *Questions to consider:* Do the group members seem to trust one another? Do they work together? Do they support and encourage each other? How much do they reveal about themselves to the other members?

Although cohesiveness occurs spontaneously in many groups, it often must be facilitated. Cohesiveness can be encouraged by adjusting the length and frequency of meetings and by enhancing perceptions of intermember similarity. *Length* refers to the amount of time group meetings run, and *frequency* refers to how often they occur. The more hours a group spends together, the more cohesive it is likely to be; you can verify this by thinking about the amount of time you spend with other OT students and how you feel about this group as differentiated from the rest of the students in your school. *Intermember similarity* is the degree to which group members believe they are like each other or share a sense of purpose or reason for being together in the group. The more similar to others in the group the members feel, the more cohesive the group will be. Again, you can verify this from your own experience. In therapeutic groups the leader may have to point out to the members the ways in which they are like each other; similarities may be based on cultural background, common experiences, shared interests, shared goals, or other factors. A study by Banning and Nelson (2) suggests that activities that elicit humor and laughter may also promote cohesiveness through the shared experience of pleasure.

A study by Falk-Kessler and associates (10) examined the therapeutic factors in OT groups through a survey of patients in day treatment centers affiliated with a state hospital. According to the survey, the factors rated most helpful by patients were group cohesiveness, interpersonal learning-output, instillation of hope, and universality. These factors were previously identified and analyzed by Yalom (30, 31) in relation to verbal therapy groups. *Group cohesiveness,* which was rated by patients as the single most important factor, has already been discussed. *Interpersonal learning-output* refers to learning successful ways to relate to others. *Instillation of hope* is based on an increased sense of hopefulness from seeing that other group members improve. *Universality* provides a shared experience as the person learns that others are in the same boat.

Other factors seen as important by those responding to this survey included *guidance* (accepting advice), *family reenactment* (experiencing the group as similar to the family in which the person grew up), and *altruism* (giving to others). In a 1992 study by Webster and Schwartzberg (28), consumers ranked altruism as the third most valued factor in therapy groups, suggesting that the opportunity to give to others is very important to them.

## Group Goals and Norms

*Group goals* are the purposes for which the group meets. They establish a commonality that supports cohesiveness. Examples range from neighbors who organize to fight crime in their area to clients who come together to learn money management or cooking. Without clear goals and a good reason for being together, many groups fall apart. In treatment groups the participants need to know why they are meeting and what they can expect to accomplish. Activities should be chosen for their potential to meet the declared goals of the group; these goals must have meaning to the members.

*Group norms* are the rules or standards for behavior that are expected in the group. They define the limits of permissible and acceptable behavior. Group norms are to a group what laws and etiquette are to a society; they enable social interaction to proceed safely because the range of things that can happen is predictable. New members may not be aware of the norms; if so, the rest of the group will teach or tell the new member what kind of behavior is expected. This process, called *socialization,* may take some time; usually the new member is permitted a grace period to learn the ropes. To preserve their own integrity, groups, like societies, enforce their norms by punishing members who violate them. This punishment, often called a *sanction,* may be as severe as expulsion from the group or as mild as a verbal chastisement.

In therapeutic groups, the leader has the major responsibility for enforcing norms, although group members should do so wherever possible. It is a good idea to choose norms for the group that reflect the social norms of its community counterpart. For example, in a work group, paying attention to the task rather than to one's emotional needs and those of the other group members is a norm that mirrors work behavior expected on the job.

The clarity of norms and goals affects cohesiveness. If they are unclear or inconsistent or not honored by all of the members, cohesiveness suffers. On the other hand, if all of the members of the group know why they are in the group and what behavior is expected of them, they are likely to work together and feel cohesive with the rest of the group. Many people have been in a class in which the instructor failed to provide written objectives or assignments or grading criteria and did not communicate what or how students were expected to learn or a class in which some students were allowed to do extra assignments and take makeup examinations and others were not, for no apparent reason. Boredom, anxiety, and rebelliousness are typical reactions to such situations. This illustrates what can happen when the goals and norms are not clearly stated and consistently enforced. Making sure that the goals and norms are clear to all the group members and that they are enforced in a consistent and fair manner is the responsibility of the group leader; when new members enter the group, the leader must restate or reclarify the goals and norms. Sometimes group members with strong group interaction skills do this.

## Functional Roles within a Group

If you watch any small group interact for an hour or so, you will see that the individuals in the group behave in very different ways. For example, five students may be studying together for a biology examination. Angie suggests that they ask each other questions; Robert says it would be better to go over the notes. After a few minutes Tanya asks if they can settle this dispute by going over the notes and then asking questions. Meanwhile, Mario has gotten coffee for everyone and Sandra is not really paying much attention because she has been copying Angie's notes from a class she missed. Each student is playing a different role in the group. As the study group progresses, they may switch roles or take on new ones; for instance, when the group gets cranky and tired, Angie may suggest taking a break to get something to eat, or Sandra may give a pep talk about how important this test is.

Whenever people interact in groups, individual members take on different functional roles (3). These roles, which help the group work toward its goals and satisfy the needs of its members, are spelled out in Table 13-1. Examples illustrate how an individual may act in each role. The examples are based on interactions within a student group that is planning a fund-raiser. The roles fall into three categories: task roles, group maintenance roles, and antigroup or egocentric roles. *Task roles* develop in relationship to the group's goals and the problems it must solve to reach them. *Group maintenance roles* are needed to promote and maintain cohesiveness and closeness among group members; the leader is likely to take on several of these roles, depending on the changing needs of the group. For example, the leader may act as gatekeeper and encourager to get the group started and the participants talking to each other and later perform the roles of harmonizer and group observer.

Not all roles taken by members of groups are beneficial to the functioning of the group. *Antigroup* or *egocentric roles* serve the needs of individuals but interfere with the group's progress. Some individuals adopt these destructive roles in almost any group, and they need support and training to develop more positive group behaviors. But even people with the ability to take on productive group roles sometimes enact these destructive and negative roles. This may happen if a group is given a task that is not relevant or at the right skill level or if the leader is too dominant or too permissive. For instance, men may take on antigroup roles if they are given a task that they perceive as feminine or childish (e.g., fabric collage).

The OTA helps group members gain awareness and group skill by analyzing with them the functional group roles they habitually take and supporting them in their exploration of new roles. The central purpose of OT groups is to help the person succeed in personally valued occupational roles (worker, student, and so on). To do this, the OTA identifies which functional group roles are needed for the person's occupational role. For example, a superintendent of a large staff in an apartment building must use the roles of orienter and energizer. The OTA analyzes which of the essential roles the person is able to assume and which ones the person needs to develop further. The OTA then designs and assigns roles in groups that enable the person to practice and become skilled at the targeted functional roles. In addition, the OTA, like any group leader, must be able to recognize what functional roles he or she may have to assume or

**TABLE 13-1 ROLES OF GROUP MEMBERS**

| ROLE | EXAMPLE |
|---|---|
| **Task roles** | |
| **Initiator-contributor:** Suggests new ideas or new ways of looking at a problem | Ralph suggests manufacturing and selling silk-screened T-shirts |
| **Information seeker:** Asks for facts and further explanation of them | Ginny asks Ralph to explain what's involved in silk-screening |
| **Opinion seeker:** Asks for opinions and feelings about issues under discussion | Nick asks the others whether they think the T-shirts would sell |
| **Information giver:** Provides facts or information from own experience | Marco says he saw silk-screened T-shirts at a street fair sell very well at a good price |
| **Opinion giver:** Expresses feelings or beliefs not necessarily based on facts | Nick says he believes the T-shirt fad is past; no one wants to wear shirts with slogans on them. He suggests a bake sale |
| **Elaborator:** Spells out suggestions by giving examples or developing scenarios of how it might work out | Ralph says maybe the group could come up with a few designs and show them to other students. Based on their reactions, the group could decide whether the T-shirt idea is a good risk |
| **Coordinator:** Pulls ideas together by showing relationship among different ideas expressed | Ginny says it should be easy to tell if the T-shirt fad is past by the students' reactions. The bake sale is a good backup idea |
| **Orienter:** Focuses group on its goals, keeps discu-ssion from wandering off the point, and so on | Michelle reminds the group that they have to decide soon because the funds are needed in 10 weeks |
| **Evaluator-critic:** Assesses accomplishments of group in relation to some standard | Michelle reminds the group that they have to decide soon because the funds are needed in 10 weeks |
| **Energizer:** Prods or arouses group to act; stimulates and boosts morale | Jergen says all of the ideas sound good to him and this group seems more harmonious than other student clubs he's been in |
| **Energizer:** Prods or arouses group to act; stimulates and boosts morale | Marcia says, "We can pull this off if we all work together, so let's get with it." |
| **Procedural technician:** Performs routine tasks that help group accomplish its task | Gertrude arranged for enough chairs for the meeting, started the coffee, and got a portable chalkboard and chalk |
| **Recorder:** Writes down main points of discussion; records group decisions | Sharon keeps minutes of the meeting and reads her notes to the group at the end |
| **Group maintenance roles** | |
| **Encourager:** Praises, accepts, supports others in group; encourages different points of view | Rick says that Ralph has a good idea, and that maybe everyone should think about it seriously |
| **Harmonizer:** Settles differences between other members by reconciling disputes or relieves tension by joking | After a violent debate between Jergen and Ralph about what to charge for the T-shirts, Valerie jokes, "This ain't no fancy boutique, guys." |

**TABLE 13-1 ROLES OF GROUP MEMBERS *(Continued)***

| ROLE | EXAMPLE |
|---|---|
| **Compromiser:** Gives in to a dispute and changes his or her position to preserve group harmony | Jergen admits that maybe people can't afford to pay $20 for a T-shirt; he's willing to compromise at $12 |
| **Gatekeeper:** Keeps communication going; this may mean asking others to speak or suggesting ways to give everyone a chance to talk | Gertrude says some people haven't spoken yet and she wonders what they think about the T-shirt prices |
| **Standard setter:** Expresses norms or standards for group | Valerie says it will be easier to work together if people listen to each other and stop shouting |
| **Group observer:** Records communication of group; offers this record to group for its comment and interpretation; provides interpretations when needed | Angela notes that Jergen has snapped at Ralph several times today (this is a role the therapist may play) |
| **Follower:** Goes along with the general mood and decisions of the group | The student group included 18 people, but not all participated in the discussion; the rest listened and voted by a show of hands on the final plan |
| **Antigroup (egocentric) roles** | |
| **Aggressor:** Belittles or attacks group members, group, or its purpose; shows disapproval or tries to take credit for actions of others | Tricia says she'd be happy to listen to Ralph's ideas, but because he never follows through on them, she thinks it's a waste of time |
| **Blocker:** Prevents group from progressing, by resisting change, opposing decisions, rehashing dead issues, and so on | Lenore says she wants to know why the group always has to get involved with "these hare-brained schemes" |
| **Recognition seeker:** Calls attention to self by boasting, talking about own talents, insisting on having a powerful position, and so on | John says he has a first-class collection of T-shirts that he'll bring in for the next meeting |
| **Self-confessor:** Expresses personal problems, political ideology, or other concerns to captive audience of group | Gilberto says he is completely bummed out by the F he got on the anatomy quiz and wants to know if anyone else failed |
| **Playboy:** Isn't involved with group; shows disinterest by clowning around, being cynical, and so on | Wanda flirts openly with Marco and Nick, ignoring everyone else |
| **Dominator:** Tries to take control by manipulating group or members; tactics may include interrupting, bossiness, flattery, seduction | Frank interrupts Ralph repeatedly, telling him to "get on with it" and "leave out the boring details" |
| **Help seeker:** Tries to get sympathy of group by acting helpless, victimized, or insecure | Leslie says she isn't sure she can really contribute too much because she's dyslexic |
| **Special-interest pleader:** Pretends to speak on behalf of a particular group but really is using group to express own biases | John says the group has to make sure all the money is accounted for because "some people here aren't too responsible" |

Adapted with permission from Benne KD, Sheats P. Functional roles of group members. J Social Issues 1948;4(2):42–47.

delegate when group members do not have the skill to do so. Getting new groups started may also necessitate the leader's taking a more active role.

Which functional roles are taken by individuals depends on the roles that are necessary for the group to accomplish its goals; not every situation calls for every possible role. Groups in the early stages of development may crumble if severe standards are set, but more mature groups can use the same standards as a spur for growth. The roles that individuals undertake in a group depend also on their experience. Someone who is used to the role of procedural technician and who has taken on other group roles may feel threatened and overwhelmed if pushed into a leadership position. The highest level of group skill is flexibility and responsiveness in taking on any task role and group maintenance role as the situation demands (18).

### Group Process

Many relationships develop within a group; these relationships shift and change in response to many factors. The term *group dynamics* expresses the constantly evolving, never static quality of groups. What factors contribute to this dynamism?

One factor is the individual member. Personality, experience, and the current emotional state of the member interact with the group process. For example, sibling rivalry (shown by competition with other group members for the leader's attention and approval) and other transferential reactions[1] have their origins in past family relationships. A second factor is the reactions of the participants to each other; complementary or mutually destructive patterns can develop. Subgroups form as members make alliances with each other; these subgroups may exclude others or reinforce the status of their members or compete with other subgroups. Sometimes the entire group gangs up against one member, blaming that person for the group's failure to achieve its goals; this is called *scapegoating*.

The following questions may help an observer discover the relationships within the group: Who talks to whom? Who arrives and leaves together? Who seems left out? Do the members talk to each other or only to the leader? Who talks the most? Who sits where? Which people always sit together? Which people never sit together?

Accurate assessment of group process requires sophisticated analysis based on extensive knowledge and experience of group therapy and group dynamics. Entry-level OTAs are not expected to possess this skill but may develop it through continuing education and supervised clinical practice.

## DEVELOPMENT OF GROUP SKILLS

Everyone knows one or two people who are exquisitely skillful in group situations; these rare individuals circulate gracefully at parties, bring strangers together, and make lonely people feel comfortable. On the job or in community groups such as the Parent-Teachers Association (PTA), they can get people organized, give them motivation and direction, take care of uninteresting details, and then step back to let others shine. These people are worth emulating; they have a high level of group skill. If you look around you, it is very likely you will find different degrees of group skill among otherwise mature individuals such as your colleagues, classmates, and peers.

How do human beings develop this ability to interact effectively with others? Anne Mosey (17-19), an occupational therapist, analyzed the development of *group interaction skill*. Mosey defines group interaction skill as

> the ability to be a productive member of a variety of primary groups. Through acquisition of the various group interaction subskills, the individual learns to take appropriate group membership roles, engage in decision making, communicate effectively, recognize group norms and interact in accordance with these norms, contribute to goal attainment, work toward group cohesiveness, and assist in resolving group conflict (19, p. 201).

[1] Discussed as transference and countertransference in Chapter 10.

Recognizing that we are not just born with these skills and that people with mental disorders may need help to develop them, Mosey identified five levels of group interaction skill: parallel, project, egocentric-cooperative, cooperative, and mature. She described the subskills learned at each level and estimated the age at which most people learn these skills. She also described what a group leader or parent or teacher may do to help people at each level acquire the subskills needed for the next level. The following sections summarize Mosey's ideas regarding group interaction skills.

## Parallel Level

The skill needed at the *parallel level* is the ability to work and play in the presence of others, comfortably and with an awareness of their presence. This skill is usually learned between the ages of 18 months and 2 years, when the child becomes gradually more comfortable playing around other children. Most of the play is solitary, although the children interact briefly from time to time—for example, to show one another something. For this parallel play to continue for long, however, there must be at least one adult available to give each of the children support, encouragement, and attention when they need it. Problems such as taking toys from the other child or throwing a temper tantrum because one cannot immediately have one's own way are common but must be discouraged if the child is to progress to the next level.

## Project Level

The skill learned at the *project level* is the ability to share a short-term task with one or two other people. This skill develops somewhere between ages 2 and 4 years. The child is interested in the task or the game and recognizes that he or she needs other people to do it; therefore, the child is willing to take turns, to share materials, to cooperate, to ask for help, and to give it. Children in this stage are not so much interested in the other people as in the task. The activities shared at this level last for only a short time, usually not more than half an hour, and the child may engage in a number of activities in succession; each may have different participants. A parent, teacher, or other adult is needed to provide individual attention and to intervene when children have difficulty sharing.

## Egocentric-Cooperative Level

The skill at the *egocentric-cooperative level* is awareness of the group's goals and norms and willingness to abide by them. This skill is based on sensitivity to the rules of the group and the rights of self and others in the group. Because children at this stage feel a sense of belonging to and being accepted by the group, they can carry out long-term activities that allow them to experiment with different roles and levels of participation. Differences among group members become apparent as each tries on functional *task* roles needed for the achievement of the various stages of activities (Table 13-1); this provides an opportunity to recognize and reward the achievement of others and to seek recognition for oneself. In theory, these skills are normally acquired somewhere between 5 and 7 years of age. Supervising adults still must provide support and encouragement to meet the esteem needs of group members.

## Cooperative Level

The skill at the *cooperative level* is the ability to express feelings within a group and to be aware of and respond to the feelings of others. Thus individuals at this level can assume group maintenance roles, which support the emotional well-being of the group. This skill usually develops between ages 9 and 12, through participation in groups whose members are of the same sex and approximate age. Adults are usually excluded from these groups, which seem to function better on their own. Groups may form spontaneously, with members selected on the basis of their similarity to each

provides feedback @ this stage

other. The group's activities or tasks are not viewed as important; instead the feelings, both positive and negative, of each member on a variety of subjects are the main agenda.

### Mature Level

The skill at the *mature level* is the ability to take on a variety of group roles, both task roles and group maintenance roles, as needed in response to changing conditions in a group. This skill is synonymous with the upper end of the continuum of group interaction skill as defined by Mosey earlier in this chapter. Mosey believes that this skill is learned between ages 15 and 18 years, as the adolescent participates in various clubs and groups whose members are of both sexes, come from different backgrounds, and have different interests and skills. It must be acknowledged, however, that exposure to this experience does not in itself guarantee that the adolescent will develop a mature level of group interaction skill; there are many adults whose behavior in groups is restricted to the few membership roles with which they feel comfortable. The development of group interaction skill may continue into middle and even late adulthood, provided the individual is willing to risk trying out new roles.

Mosey shows us that skill in interacting within a group develops gradually throughout childhood and adolescence. Some people with psychiatric problems function at a level of group interaction skill that is lower than one would expect for someone their age. It is not clear exactly why this is so; one can speculate that the mental disorder interfered with the acquisition of these skills during childhood and adolescence. Donohue and Lieberman (5), in a report of a study of social competence among persons with major mental disorders (bipolar affective disorder and schizophrenia), suggest that persons with schizophrenia (in particular) may need help developing sociability (interest and enjoyment in being with others) and social presence (tolerance and ability to assert oneself effectively). They further suggest that sociability is learned in parallel- and project-level experiences and that social presence is acquired in project, egocentric-cooperative, and cooperative group experiences.

When encountering the person with weak or poorly developed group skills, it is wisest to assume that such an individual is doing the best he or she can and that the person will not be able to cope with demands for higher level group interaction. The OTA can structure groups to meet the needs of people at various levels by changing the tasks and by delegating or assuming functional group roles. In this way, the OT practitioner can provide a learning environment for both high- and low-functioning members.

## HOW THERAPY GROUPS ARE DIFFERENT FROM OTHER GROUPS

We have just discussed the developmental process by which people learn to interact effectively in group situations. Daily life presents many opportunities for practicing group interaction skills; work, family, school, and social life all involve participation in groups. To lead a therapy group successfully the OTA needs to understand the difference between a therapy group and other groups that occur naturally.

First of all, therapy groups are artificial situations designed to help patients acquire new skills or practice old ones. Second, the group leader is responsible for making sure that learning occurs. In a sense, this makes the therapy group similar to a class in school. Another important difference is that regardless of the specific activity used or skills taught, the group also acknowledges the emotional experience of each member. In other words, each person's feelings about what he or she is doing and what is going on in the group are considered important. For example, in a work group the focus is on acquiring work skills. Therefore, behaviors that would not be acceptable on the job are discouraged. Although discussion of feelings is frowned on during the work activity, time for such discussion is set aside at the end of each session. In this way someone, who feels that she is always given dull and boring jobs, can air her feelings and the group can help her explore them.

## ROLE OF THE LEADER IN AN ACTIVITY GROUP

Activity groups differ from other therapy groups in that *doing*, or activity, is the medium through which the group members achieve their goals. Thus activity groups become laboratories designed so that members can experiment with the occupational roles relevant to their daily lives. In this model, the most important function of the group leader is to assign members specific tasks and roles similar to those they may have to assume in real life. For example, in a newspaper group, the leader may assign members to roles as chief editor, copy assistant, and reporter. Role assignment for each member takes into account the job responsibility of the person's real-life occupational role; assigned roles should be similar to these.

The leader is also responsible for making sure that group members feel safe during the group's activities and that the group focuses its energies on its goals. The group leader may take a very active role, selecting tasks for individual members and intervening in disputes, or the more distant and observing role of a consultant, or the leader may participate as an equal member in the group—this depends on the group interaction skills of individual members and the purpose for which the group is designed.

The leader must assume only the roles that members are not able to assume because of insufficient group interaction skill and must delegate to members the roles they are able to assume. In addition, the leader must recognize and delegate the role functions that members need to develop to increase their group interaction skill to the next level. For example, if one of the goals of the group is to help members learn to make decisions on their own, the leader cannot assign tasks and responsibilities, as this defeats the entire purpose. On the other hand, patients with very poor attention spans and only parallel level group skills cannot be expected to carry on a discussion of what activity they should choose.

The relationship between a member's level of group skill and the role of the therapist or group leader is depicted in Table 13-2, which lists the things a therapist or group leader should do to help members develop group skills at each level. It is unusual to find a group whose members are all at a single level. Sometimes, for example in acute short-term settings, there may be individuals at all five levels within the same group. Even in such situations, the information in the table can guide you to help individuals relate to each other and the group. You, as the leader, may step into various roles to meet the needs of the members.

When working with individuals of any diagnosis, including in settings other than psychiatry, it is important to know each person's level of group skill and to understand what it means in terms of his or her abilities with group situations. For example, it is pointless to ask a person who has only parallel-level group skills to take a leadership role in community meetings; on the other hand, it *is* reasonable to ask the person to remain in the meeting and not be disruptive.

### Leader Behavior

In addition to understanding the relationship between the members' group skill levels and the therapist's behavior, there are several other factors to which the group leader should be sensitive. As indicated in the section on cohesiveness (earlier in this chapter), an atmosphere in which the

## TABLE 13-2 ROLE OF THE THERAPIST IN DEVELOPMENTAL GROUPS

| LEVEL OF GROUP SKILLS[a] | INDICATORS OF NEED TO DEVELOP SPECIFIED ROLE OF THE THERAPIST |
|---|---|
| **Parallel group:** Members have limited attention span and may be quite unaware of others; unless encouraged to notice others, they may ignore them and isolate themselves | 1. Explain purpose and activities of group to member<br>2. Help person feel accepted, safe, valued<br>3. Support and encourage minimal interaction, such as eye contact, casual conversation<br>4. Set limits on disruptive behavior<br>5. Help person select simple, short-term activities that are not self-isolating |
| **Project group:** Members express anxiety about working with others, fearing that they will be unable to complete a task or that other person will take over; issue is whether to trust another person enough to share a task with him or her | 1. Explain purpose and activities of group to member<br>2. Help person feel accepted, safe, valued<br>3. Support and encourage sharing of tasks, cooperation, giving and seeking assistance, and so on<br>4. Help members select simple, short-term tasks that can be shared by two or more people<br>5. Encourage experimentation with different ways of sharing, members taking different roles |
| **Egocentric-cooperative group:** Members have trouble engaging in long-term tasks with others; problems may include concern with competition, indifference to the rights of others, and inability to ask for and receive recognition | 1. Take on group membership roles only as required by needs of group<br>2. Encourage group to function as independently as it can, stepping in only when group cannot proceed without help<br>3. Model appropriate expression of needs<br>4. Assist development and discussion of norms<br>5. Help members feel accepted, safe, valued |
| **Cooperative group:** While able to carry out long-term group tasks, people at this level need to expand their ability to express their feelings and be aware of feelings of others | 1. Participate in group or provide advice from sidelines; not an authority figure<br>2. May help group develop initially<br>3. May intervene to promote cohesiveness |
| **Mature group:** People at this level need to learn to step into roles as needed and to maintain balance between achieving group task and meeting emotional needs of group members | 1. Participate as a member<br>2. When necessary, demonstrate group membership roles<br>3. Select members to achieve variety and balance in backgrounds, interests, skills, and so on |

[a]Groups are designed to help members acquire the named level of group interaction skill—e.g., those in the project-level group do not have project-level skills but are trying to develop them.

Adapted with permission from Mosey AC. Activities Therapy. New York: Raven, 1973.

members feel accepted and valued is essential if people are to risk themselves by trying new things. New learning is unlikely unless such an atmosphere exists. Leaders can promote cohesiveness and create a climate that encourages learning and risk taking by orienting the group to its goals and activities, by spelling out the norms, and by paying attention to their own behavior. Behaviors of the leader with respect to consistency, autonomy, nurturing, and interpersonal learning have particularly strong effects on the group.

### Consistency

The first of the behaviors of the leader, *consistency*, is the foundation of successful groups. The leader must show the same degree of respect, interest, and authority toward every group member. Also, the leader should try as much as possible to behave similarly in each meeting of the group. In other words, the leader's behavior should be dependable. The group members should know what to expect from the leader. Some aspects of leader behavior that appear quite subtle can have a profound influence on the group. For example, if the leader one day is preoccupied with personal problems and is thus more subdued than usual, group members may wonder why or feel uneasy, as though the leader were a different person. If the leader shows favoritism toward one member, others may feel wronged. The leader who wears jeans one day and a business suit the next should not be surprised if members respond to the change in appearance and message, and so on.

### Autonomy

The second aspect of leader behavior to consider is the *degree of autonomy* the leader permits among the members. In other words, how much opportunity for independence and decision making does the leader give the group? As a general rule, members should be given as much independence as they can handle and no more. One way to figure out how much independence is appropriate is to observe. If members seem confused and unable to act, they may have been given too much responsibility, too much independence. If, on the other hand, they refuse to act responsibly or repeatedly argue with the group leader or seem not to work to capacity, they probably are not being given enough responsibility. Determining the appropriate level is sometimes a problem for new group leaders and is an area in which a supervisor who is experienced in working with therapy groups can help. A good supervisor will also be able to help the new group leader learn how to analyze and respond to problems within the group process (interaction among members). The entry-level practitioner cannot be expected to be able to do this independently but should be able to develop skills in analyzing group process after several years of supervised group leadership experience.

### Nurturing

The third aspect of leader behavior that affects the group is *nurturing behavior*, defined here as any behavior by the leader that supports and promotes the growth of the individual members. Encouragement and praise are the most common examples, but nurturing can take many other forms. It should always be matched to the maturity of the group or its members. A young mother who is highly skilled at housework but who is depressed for other reasons will probably not be convinced or encouraged by the group leader praising her homemaking skills. It may be more nurturing for the leader to help her find a way to teach these skills to others. This also activates *altruism*, one of the most valued elements of the therapy group.

### Interpersonal Learning

The fourth important aspect of leader behavior is the leader's skill at promoting *interpersonal learning*. Interpersonal learning consists of all of the processes or relationships among individuals that result in a change in behavior, knowledge, or attitude on the part of any one or more of the people involved. In simpler words, interpersonal learning includes everything a person learns from interactions with other people. Examples of this are learning how one is perceived by others, taking on unfamiliar group membership roles, asking for and receiving attention, becoming more aware of how others feel, and learning new skills from another person.

The leader should be able to use the resources of the group to help each member learn more about himself or herself and about the others. The *resources of the group* are all of the possibilities for different kinds of interactions and learning among group members, each of whom has different knowledge, skills, feelings, and beliefs to share with the others. The leader cannot assume, however, that these resources will be shared automatically; often the leader has to take charge of the communication process in the group to encourage each member to interact with every other member.

*Interactive groups* are those in which every member communicates with every other member and with the group leader. By contrast, in *leader-mediated groups* members communicate only with or through the group leader (30). Opportunities for interpersonal learning are greatest with a pattern of interactive communication. However, in groups that include persons at lower levels of group interaction skill (parallel or project), the members cannot be expected to interact so freely. Instead, the leader mediates the conversation, asking members for their feelings or for a reaction to what another member has said, for example. Box 13-1 shows some techniques that leaders use to stimulate members to interact.

At higher-level groups (egocentric-cooperative and above), the pattern and direction of communication should be monitored. Novice group leaders tend to fall into the pattern of addressing one member, who then responds; then the leader

**BOX 13-1**

**TECHNIQUES TO PROMOTE INTERACTION IN A GROUP**

Environmental

- Arrange the group in a circle so that all the participants (including leader) are at same level and can see each other.
- Position talkative members so that they are next to less-verbal members.
- Consider sitting sit next to members who tend to monopolize or who act out and explains privately to those members that you will help them with this.

Leader behaviors

- Tolerate silence; let time work for you.
- Avoid responding directly to a member question or comment; instead, *redirect* the question to the group or another group member.
- When a member is talking for a while, break eye contact and scan the group; this leads the talker to make eye contact with others and encourages other members to respond.

Specific questions or comments leader can use

- "James, what did you think about what Brenda just said?"
- "Iliana, do you agree with what Mira said?"
- "Hmmmn, I wonder if anyone else has something to share on that topic."
- "Helen, you've had a lot to say. It's time to give someone else a turn."

addresses another, who responds again to the leader; and the pattern repeats itself, with members responding to the leader rather than to each other (Fig. 13-1*A*). This pattern results in a series of dialogues between the leader and individual members. To encourage members to respond to each other, the leader must refrain from answering the member's comments, instead redirecting the question to the group or a specific member. This may be done verbally ("Vinh, what do you think of that?") or nonverbally (looking at another member, raising eyebrows and widening eyes or nodding to prompt a response). This leads quickly to a pattern of member-to-member communication, with only occasional mediation from the leader (Fig. 13-1*B*).

The pattern of communication within the group is only one factor in interpersonal learning, which also depends on each member's learning style, or preferred way of learning. The leader facilitates whatever method of learning is most effective for each person. Some of the learning methods that can be used are feedback, reinforcement, trial and error, and imitation or role modeling. These methods are discussed in Chapters 2 and 3. Typically, several methods are used simultaneously. For example, one person imitates the behavior of another. Other members give feedback about how well this worked. If the behavior worked well, they also reinforce it. The group leader facilitates this process by asking what the group thinks of the way John is dressed today or what they think about how Ann is dealing with her shyness.

In summary, the group leader should promote interaction and interpersonal learning among the group members. The group interaction skills of each of the members will define how much interpersonal learning is possible or practical. It is often difficult for students and new therapists to put these elementary principles into practice while running a group. There is always a strong temptation to step in and give one's own opinion or provide information or show someone how to

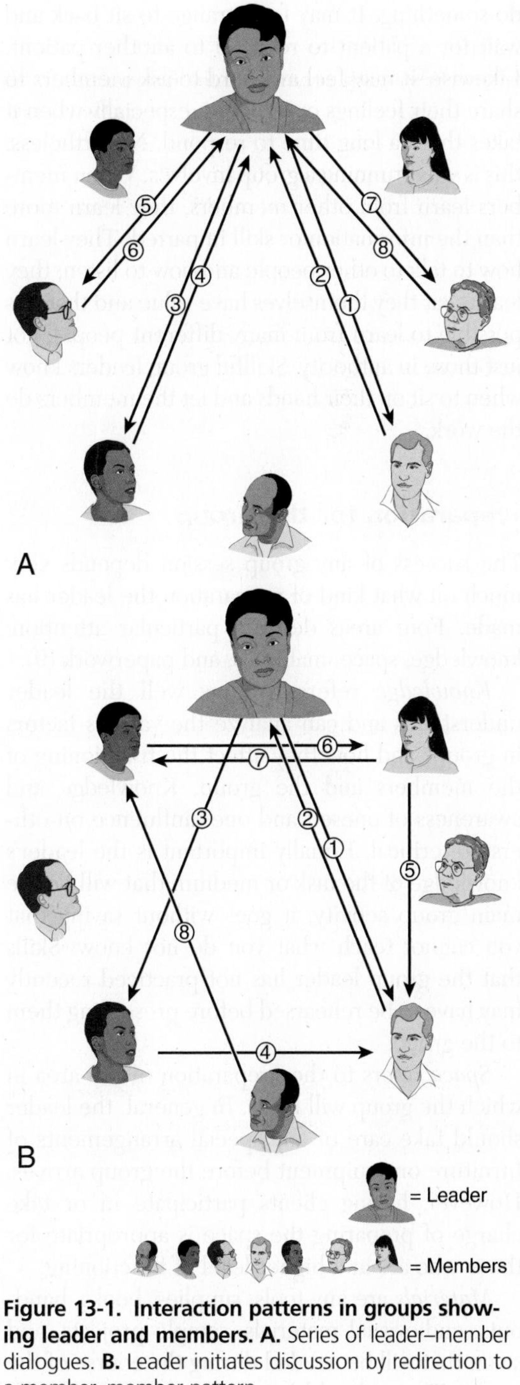


**Figure 13-1. Interaction patterns in groups showing leader and members. A.** Series of leader–member dialogues. **B.** Leader initiates discussion by redirection to a member–member pattern.

do something. It may feel strange to sit back and wait for a patient to respond to another patient. Likewise, it may feel awkward to ask members to share their feelings or opinions, especially when it takes them a long time to respond. Nevertheless, this is what running a group involves. When members learn from other members, they learn more than the information or skill imparted. They learn how to talk to other people and how to listen; they learn that they themselves have value and that it is possible to learn from many different people, not just those in authority. Skillful group leaders know when to sit on their hands and let the members do the work.

## Preparation for the Group

The success of any group session depends very much on what kind of preparation the leader has made. Four areas demand particular attention: knowledge, space, materials, and paperwork (9).

*Knowledge* refers to how well the leader understands and can analyze the various factors in groups and how they affect the functioning of the members and the group. Knowledge and awareness of oneself and one's influence on others are critical. Equally important is the leader's knowledge of the task or medium that will be the main group activity; it goes without saying that you cannot teach what you do not know. Skills that the group leader has not practiced recently may have to be rehearsed before presenting them to the group.

*Space* refers to the preparation of the area in which the group will meet. In general, the leader should take care of any special arrangements of furniture or equipment before the group arrives. However, having clients participate in or take charge of preparing the space is appropriate for those who are at a higher level of functioning.

*Materials* are any tools, supplies, books, handouts, audiovisual materials, sample projects, and so on that will be needed during the course of the group. These should be prepared in advance by the group leader or someone else, perhaps a volunteer or a higher-functioning member. The specific requirements depend on the type of group and the functional level of the participants. For example, with lower-functioning groups it is necessary to prepare separate materials for each person and to set these up so that each has a separate and defined work area, although several people may sit at one table. In higher-functioning groups it may make sense to have the members take out their own projects and obtain and return tools as they need them.

*Paperwork* is the final item; it consists of attendance sheets, the group protocol and session plan, the group leader's notebook, and any other forms or documents that the leader may need during the group. With the exception of taking attendance, the leader should avoid writing during the group session but should do so as soon as it is over. Having a notebook handy in which the behavior of each group member can be briefly noted makes it easy to keep track of patients' progress.

Even with all of this preparation things can still go awry, but the leader will find it easier to cope with a minor crisis when everything else has been prepared. The situation to be avoided is the members arriving at the same time as the group leader, who then must unlock cabinets, hunt for missing items, take attendance, and so forth, all at once.

Writing a session plan for each group meeting helps the leader be prepared. A sample plan is shown in Box 13-2. At a minimum such a plan should include the following:

- A clear statement of the goals for the session
- A list of needed materials and supplies
- Mention of environment or setting for session
- A plan for introducing the group meeting (e.g., leader, members, purpose)
- A plan for conducting the activity (can be point by point and may include exact wording of your statement)
- A plan for ending the group with a discussion and summary

**BOX 13-2**

### SAMPLE GROUP SESSION PLAN: GROCERY SHOPPING

**Goals**

Members will learn to:

- Use coupons and advertising circulars
- Compare prices
- Compose a shopping list based on a menu

**Supplies**

- Menu from yesterday's group meeting
- Newspapers
- Advertising circulars
- Paper
- Pencils
- Calculator

**Environment**

- For this session, meet in the kitchen.
- Have one member write the menu on flip chart using large letters so all members can see.

**Introduction**

- Reintroduce self and the name of the group.
- Explain why the group is meeting (e.g., "You all want to live independently and this is part of community living.")
- Remind members that yesterday they planned a menu for Friday's lunch, which they will be cooking.
- As needed, introduce new members to the group.
- As needed, restate the rules.

**Activities**

1. "Friday this group will prepare a lunch for staff and members of the club. There will be 35 people. The budget is $_____. The menu you developed yesterday is posted. Today we need to plan our shopping. How do you think we should go about this?"
2. Call on members as needed to get discussion going. Focus on member experiences. Then have members list needed ingredients and calculate quantities.
3. "This is a lot of groceries when we have only $_____. What shall we do?" Get members to discuss. Get them to think about prices, coupons, in-store specials, and so on.
4. Explain the concept of comparison shopping (ideally, get a member to do this). Distribute newspapers and advertising circulars.
5. Help members develop a plan for when to shop (Thursday) and what to buy at each store.
6. When this is done, ask members to clean up the papers in preparation for discussion.

Processing and Discussion

- Get the members to talk about what they have learned.
- Preview the next group meeting.
- Ask members to consider how what they did here might be of use in their own lives.
- As needed, focus on behaviors of the members (emphasize positive).
- Remind members to bring their bus passes for Thursday because the group will be going shopping.

## Beginning and Ending a Group Session

The leader can increase the therapeutic value of a group by paying particular attention to the beginning and end of each session. The beginning of the session prepares participants for what is to follow. New group members should be introduced or all members should introduce themselves again; this is especially important when the members do not know each other or the group meets infrequently. The leader should state the purpose of the group or ask a member to do so and describe the activity for the day; this may not be necessary in long-running groups whose activities are continuous. The leader may also suggest what the members might get out of the group experience; setting expectations in advance helps members meet them.

At the end of the group, after participants have enjoyed themselves or have been involved with an activity and with each other, they need time to reflect on the experience before moving on to the next thing on their schedules. Having members clean up the room and put things away gives them time to chat informally with each other about what has occurred. A discussion at the end allows them to reflect on what has taken place, share their feelings, and consider how what has been learned in the group may be applied elsewhere in "real life." The leader may summarize the day's activities and ask participants to reflect on them and share their thoughts. Alternatively, the leader may ask a member (in a higher functioning group) to lead the discussion. In groups whose members have lower levels of group skills, the leader takes more responsibility for summarizing and ending the group. Peloquin (21, p. 780), working with patients who had cognitive problems, used the following four-step approach:

1. Remind members of the purpose of the group.
2. Set the stage for discussion. Give members time to think about their experience before asking them to speak.
3. Help members discuss the skills they have used. Be sure to link the tasks or activities performed by the patients to their individual treatment goals.
4. Summarize what was accomplished and encourage members to return for the next session.

At the very end of the session, the leader reminds members of the time and day of the next meeting and briefly describes the activity and goals for that session. This establishes a flow between sessions. It takes time to carry out these steps at the beginning and end of the group, but it is time well spent.

## Record Keeping

As mentioned earlier, it is important to keep track of how members are progressing in the group; keeping a notebook is one way to do so. A very small notebook or a few pages in one used for other purposes will do. Some observations that should be noted are any progress toward goals, changes in interactions with others, new problems or behaviors seen, and possible side effects of medication. Even though there may be only a few minutes between the end of the group and the next meeting or group that the leader must attend, it is very important to note observations while they are fresh. Writing one or two words about each group member takes little time, but reviewing several days of such notes can yield valuable insights into the process of the group and the progress of its members (27) (Box 13-3).

**BOX 13-3**

### SAMPLE NOTES FROM A PROJECT-LEVEL GROUP

**Clerical Group 11/1**

*Clark, Angela:* Stuffed envelopes together, set up task and worked well, chatting, much progress!!!!

*Marshall, Lamar:* Collating, took 15 minutes to decide how; a lot of laughing about this

*Martin:* new member; took papers off to the side to fold them; wouldn't join partner (Margaret); finally did so but continued to work as if she weren't there

*Margaret:* Cried, said Martin didn't trust her; wants to work with Angela and Clark; I worked with Martin and Margaret as a team of three. Martin still solitary. Does he belong in this group?

## PROGRAM DEVELOPMENT

Starting up a new OT program for persons with mental health problems requires knowledge, skill, and experience. Therefore, program development is typically the responsibility of the OT, generally one with several years' experience in mental health and administration; mature and experienced OTAs may also find tremendous satisfaction in program development. The entry-level assistant can collaborate in program development by planning individual activity groups, which become part of the overall program.

### Planning an Activity Group

One of the biggest challenges new group leaders encounter in their clinical work is planning and running a new activity group (9). There seem to be so many possibilities that it is hard to focus on just one. Fortunately, there is a logical, step-by-step way of approaching this:

1. Identify the patients or consumers who need a group.
2. Assess their specific needs and general level of group skills.
3. Identify rules and resources in your setting.
4. Narrow the focus and outline the main goals.
5. Write a group protocol.

#### Members

The first step in developing a new group is to identify some people who seem to need one. This involves thinking about the people you are servicing and the kind of groups that already exist. You may notice individuals who are not in any OT groups or who have gaps in their schedules. Or you may perceive that a particular need is not being met by existing groups—for example, patients on a locked ward may not be able to attend sports and exercise groups off the ward and may benefit from a yoga or calisthenics group. Or in an outpatient rehabilitation setting, patients with arthritis may find a group on body mechanics and energy conservation helpful. A supervisor or co-worker may identify a particular need or suggest individuals for you to work with.

#### Needs and Skill Level

The second step is to assess the specific needs and general level of group skills of the prospective participants. You may have already begun this during the first step. In other words, you may have noticed a particular need (e.g., exercise, nutrition, wellness). But what if you have identified some individuals who seem to need a group, but you don't know what kind of group they need? In a mental health setting it may be helpful to think about the general goals of psychiatric OT, as delineated in Chapter 16; this may give you some ideas. For example, you may have decided that the consumers who really need a group are the ones who sit around all day and do not function well enough to participate in task groups or current events and other verbal groups. You observe that they have marginal grooming and hygiene and show little interest in anything but television. From these observations you may guess that they could benefit from a group focusing on self-care or leisure skills. Another way to identify their needs is to review the results of the evaluations of each potential member.

Besides identifying the needs of prospective members, you need to learn how well they can function within a group. Because of other demands it is not always possible to set up a separate evaluation session for this, and you can instead observe each person informally or interview other staff who know the person well. Figure 13-2 presents a checklist developed by Mosey. It lists behaviors for each of the five developmental levels of group interaction skill. The observer checks off any behaviors the person shows. The level that has the most behaviors checked is probably that individual's current level, although it is common for a person to exhibit a few behaviors at the next higher

**Group Interaction Skills Survey**

*Level of Group Interaction Skill*

*Parallel level*

Engages in some activity but acts as if it is an individual task as opposed to a group activity.
Aware of others in the group.
Some verbal or nonverbal interaction with others.
Appears to be relatively comfortable in this situation.

*Project level*

Occasionally engages in the group activity, moving in and out according to own whim.
Seeks some assistance from others.
Gives some assistance when directly asked to do so.

*Egocentric-cooperative level*

Aware of group's goal relative to the task.
Aware of group norms.
Acts as if belongs in the group.
Willing to participate.
Meets esteem needs of others.
Able to get others to meet own esteem needs.
Recognizes rights of others.
Not overly competitive.

*Cooperative level*

Makes own wishes, desires, and needs known.
Participates in group activity but seems concerned primarily with own needs and needs of others.
Able to meet needs other than esteem needs.
Tends to be most responsive to group members who are similar to self in some way.

*Mature level*

Responsive to all group members.
Takes on a variety of task roles.
Takes on a variety of social and emotional roles.
Able to share leadership.
Promotes a good balance between task accomplishment and satisfaction of group members' needs.

**Figure 13-2. Group interaction skills survey.** (Adapted with permission from Mosey AC. Activities Therapy. New York: Raven, 1973.)

level. Assessing group interaction skill informs you as to what each person will be capable of—for example, those at the project level of skill are not capable of mutual problem solving through discussion and will find it easier to learn from short-term, concrete activities in pairs or small subgroups.

Other factors that should be considered in addition to group interaction skills include the participants' cognitive skills, in particular their attention span, memory, and capacity for new learning. If these skills are deficient, you will have to conduct the group and structure the activities in a way that compensates for the deficiencies (analyzing and adapting activities are covered in Chapter 23).

## Rules and Resources

The third step is to identify the rules and resources of your setting. These determine what is possible. Included are the equipment and materials available, the rooms or other environments that can be used as settings for groups, the role of OT in the setting, and the rules of the particular facility or agency.

If you want to run a group that needs special equipment or materials, you must allow sufficient time to budget money for it and order and receive what you need. You may have to work in a room that does not suit your purposes, simply because it is the only room available. The roles of OT, other activities therapies, and other professional disciplines in your setting may also constrain what kinds of groups you can run. For example, there may be a recreation therapy department that provides all sports and exercise.

Finally, you will have to observe the rules of the agency; there may be rules about what patients can and cannot do and other rules governing staff. For instance, two staff members may be required to accompany inpatients on field trips. If you are planning field trips, you will have to make sure another staff member can come. You should, therefore, think about these things before you design the group, to save yourself time and duplication of effort later on. In general, you will have to work within these boundaries; if you decide that certain rules are unreasonable and should be changed (and you may be right), remember that changing them can consume time and energy and so prepare yourself for what may be a long (and not necessarily victorious) struggle.

## Focus and Goals

The fourth step is to narrow the focus of the group and outline your main goals for it. You may feel that the patients have needs in several areas, and you may have a number of ideas for activities. You will now have a choose a focus from among these tantalizing choices. This is perhaps the most difficult decision in designing a group. The new leader may be tempted to try to meet several different needs in one group, thinking that the group could have 15 minutes of self-care activities, followed by 15 minutes of leisure activities, followed by a 30-minute work activity. Or perhaps the group do a different activity every time it meets. These examples are rather absurd, but they illustrate that trying to meet too many needs at the same time results in a confusing blur of unrelated and, therefore, meaningless activities. It is best to address only one area at a time, although incidental learning in other areas may occur simultaneously; for example, self-care groups may provide opportunities for some socialization and learning of communication skills.

Once you have chosen the focus of the group, you can begin to outline the goals. These goals should be developed from the evaluation results and individual treatment goals of the participants in the group. They should express in general behavioral terms what you hope they will achieve, goals that these individuals feel are important and that are possible for them to reach. Table 13-3 presents an example of how the OTA may follow the first four steps in developing a new group. The fifth step is to write a group protocol.

# Writing a Group Protocol

A group protocol is a written plan that describes the goals of a group and the methods by which these goals will be achieved. It is an outline of what will be happening in the group. It is, practically speaking, a treatment plan for the group.

## Purpose

Writing a group protocol has several purposes. The first is to communicate with other staff who may refer members to the group. By reading the

**TABLE 13-3 IDENTIFYING A FOCUS FOR THE GROUP**

| STEPS | EXAMPLE |
|---|---|
| 1. Identify patients who need a group | There are eight patients who sit around watching TV all day and don't attend any groups. |
| 2. Identify specific needs . . . | Review of evaluation results and treatment plans and informal observation of patients reveal very poor hygiene and grooming.<br>None seems to be able to relate to other people except when he or she wants a cigarette.<br>They never get any exercise and seem to have no interests or skills. |
| . . . and general level of group skills | It's unlikely that these patients will interact with anyone unless leader structures group so that they are forced to.<br>All have very short attention spans (less than 15 minutes).<br>I can't imagine them giving feedback to each other or even noticing others. |
| 3. Identify institutional parameters | This is a large state hospital.<br>The wards in this building are locked. |
| • Space available | Some activities are held in activities center in a separate building.<br>Most groups are on ward and can be held either in day room or in a small (8- by 10-foot) OT room. |
| • Equipment and materials available | There are tables, chairs, and a few craft supplies.<br>A lot of therapists use donations of scraps from factories for craft groups.<br>I have to be inventive. |
| • Role of OT | In this hospital OT staff aren't allowed to lead discussion groups.<br>Psychiatric director says they don't have necessary training.<br>They are supposed to do only activity groups. |
| • Rules of institution | Students are not allowed to take groups off grounds or to lead groups by themselves in activity center, although they can do so on ward. |
| 4. Narrow focus and outline main goals | Focus of this group will be mainly self-care, with minimal opportunities for socialization.<br>Goals for patients:<br>• To brush teeth, bathe, comb hair, and shave daily<br>• To change clothes daily<br>• To wash hands before each meal and after using toilet<br>• To wash hair at least once a week |

*OT*, occupational therapy.

Modified with permission from Early MB. T.A.R. Introductory Course Workbook: Occupational Therapy: Psychosocial Dysfunction. Long Island City, NY: LaGuardia Community College; 1981.

group protocol, staff can decide whether or not a particular person is suited for, or may benefit from, the group.

The second purpose is to define the type of individual who may benefit from the group. This gives you some control over who the members will be and helps screen out those whose needs and level of group skill are too limited or too advanced for the group.

The third purpose is to clarify your goals, your methods, and your own role as leader of the group. Thinking these issues through on paper before you actually start the group helps you be clearer and more effective in your leadership once the group actually begins.

A fourth purpose of writing the group protocol is that it helps you identify how you will know when a group member has achieved the goals you have set. In other words, it helps you describe how someone will act when he or she is ready to graduate from the group.

## Format

Many formats are used for writing group protocols, but most contain similar information. The elements typically written into a group protocol are shown in Figure 13-3. These elements may be combined and may have different titles, depending on the style of the treatment center, but all of

**Typical Elements of the Group Protocol**

| | |
|---|---|
| Name | Should convey therapeutic purpose if possible |
| Description | Brief, clear, conveying purpose, accurate sense of what happens in group |
| Structure | Time, place, size, leader's characteristics |
| Goals or behavioral objectives | May be multiple and extensive; should be clear, behavioral, as specific as possible |
| Referral criteria | Describes kind of patient who might benefit from group; may include intake procedure |
| Methodology | Includes both medium (activity) and method (how the activity or medium is used); includes detail on flow of activities during group meeting |
| Curriculum or agenda | For groups with an educational or topical focus; gives detail on specific items of instruction to be covered in a series of sessions |
| Leader's roles | States what leader will and will not do in group; addresses functional roles to be taken by group leader |
| Evaluation | Indicates how achievement of group goals will be assessed (e.g., patient survey, therapist observation, peer supervision) |

**Figure 13-3. Typical elements of a group protocol.**

the information is generally included. The *name of the group* should reflect the main goals of the group. Alternatively, it may reflect the task or activity and general level of the group. However, naming the group after the activity may have undesirable consequences. If the group is named after the activity (e.g., basic woodworking group), people may think of the group as "arts and crafts." However, the therapist running the group may actually be teaching work skills and habits. It is usually easier for staff and patients to understand the purpose of the group if the name reflects its goals rather than the task or activity. Examples of names for groups that reflect the goals are independent living skills group and community socialization group. Earhart (8), however, contends that patients are concerned about what they will be doing in the group and that including the task content or the name of the activity in the title meets this need.

The *description* of the group should include its purpose and a brief and clearly written statement of what happens in the group. Technical language should be avoided unless essential to the description. Acronyms and abbreviations should be avoided because they may not be understood by everyone who reads the protocol.

The section on the *structure* of the group is used to convey information about the time, place, and size of the group. For example, a meal-planning group may include four to six members and meet four mornings a week for 1.5 hours in the community room. The qualifications (e.g., OTA) or professional or social characteristics (a male staff member) of the group leader can be stated in this section.

The *goals* or *behavioral objectives* of the group should be stated behaviorally and with as much specificity as possible. They should be relevant to the members' needs and should be set at a level that they can achieve. Some examples of behavioral objectives that meet these requirements are the following:

- To tolerate the presence of others while working on a task as evidenced by staying in the room and refraining from disruptive behavior or disrespectful speech
- To initiate social conversation with others
- To perform simple assembly tasks accurately using written or demonstrated two-step instructions
- To learn basic house-cleaning skills

Some groups have goals that involve changes in awareness or attitudes or values; such goals are very difficult to state in behavioral terms because they focus not on behavior but on internal psychological or cognitive states. Nevertheless, if these are among the main purposes of the group, they should be included. Examples of such goals are the following:

- To increase awareness of one's own safety and that of others, as evidenced by following shop rules and reminding others to do so
- To develop a feeling of personal competence, as evidenced by spontaneous or elicited comments about one's achievements or skills
- To improve awareness of one's effect on others, as evidenced by cooperation in cleanup and sharing of space

*Referral criteria* describe what kind of person should be referred to the group. The description may include specific skill deficits and prerequisite behaviors. Skill deficits identify the kinds of problems that will be addressed (e.g., poor hygiene and grooming). Prerequisite behaviors state minimum skills or behaviors needed to participate successfully in the group (e.g., able to tolerate the presence of others or not actively assaultive or suicidal). Other entrance criteria may restrict the group by age, sex, cultural background, or special interest; this is appropriate in most grooming groups and in groups that focus on cultural identity (e.g., Caribbean cooking group) or special interest. In some settings and for some groups, each person should be interviewed before entering the group. This may be done by the group leader or by the occupational therapist or assistant who is managing the person's OT program. These intake procedures can help determine how well the individual meets the referral criteria and at the same time provide an opportunity to introduce the purpose of the group and to engage the person's commitment or interest. The referral criteria should spell out the intake procedure if one is required.

Often, several referral criteria are used to define the population for which a group is designed. Writing clear criteria allows you to define the limits of the group. The following is an example of how such criteria may be written for a low-level task skills group:

- Males and females
- Ages 17 to 65+
- Able to attend to a task for 5 to 15 minutes
- Have task skill deficits (e.g., poor concentration, inattention to detail, poor rate of production)
- Are not actively assaultive or suicidal

A potential member must meet all of the stated criteria to join the group. This ensures that all of the group members have similar problems and skill levels, which generally makes the group easier to run.

The *methodology* section is one of the most important sections, giving detail on how the time of the group will be used to achieve the stated objectives. Within this section are commonly included both the media (activities) and method (how the activity or medium is used). *Media* refers to the activities or tasks that will be used to help the members meet their goals within the group. Sometimes only one activity, or medium, is used. For our purposes, *medium* means the same thing as *activity*. Almost any activity can be used in groups (e.g., gardening, collating papers, shopping for clothes for work). The theoretical approach or frame of reference will be part of this section, if appropriate (e.g., cognitive-behavioral).

*Method* describes how the medium or media will be used to work toward the goals. The method includes the general plan of what will happen in the group. The following excerpt illustrates one way the method section for a low-level task skills group may be written:

> The group will be making small leather projects. The therapist will assign a specific job to each member. Jobs will be graded from simple to complex, depending upon the individual's current level of functioning or need for challenge. Members will be encouraged to move from completing a simple task to completing a more complex one.
>
> Members will relate primarily to the therapist. Interaction with other group members may also occur. This, however, is not the primary focus of the group. The therapist will be supportive and set standards for each member.
>
> When a member is able to work consistently, maintain set work standards, and show some initiative and minimal interaction with peers, he or she will be referred to another group.

Some groups, such as independent living skills or men's sexual identity group, lend themselves to multiple topics or units of instruction. Independent living skills may include the use of public transportation, basic cooking and nutrition, care of clothing, and so on. Men's sexual identity may include topics such as men's roles in society, sexual orientation and homosexuality, meeting and dating women, developing nonsexual relationships with women, and so on. A section on *curriculum* or *agenda and topics* for such groups can elaborate the specific items of instruction to be covered in each of a number of successive sessions.

It is also a good idea to develop *session plans*, which spell out in detail what will happen in each meeting of the group. A session plan identifies the goals for the session (Box 13-2), the sequence of activities, and the materials needed. Several books give such session plans (also called lesson plans or modules of instruction) for consecutive group meetings. These can help the group leader set the sequence of instruction in (for example) independent living skills (14) or work skills (15).

The *role of the leader* may be stated within the method section or separately. Wherever it is addressed, the role of the leader should spell out the functional group roles (task roles and group maintenance roles, as detailed in Table 13-1) that the leader will undertake to support the group. This section may be brief or highly detailed, depending on the nature of the group. Two examples follow:

- *For a parallel level task group:* The therapist will assign specific tasks to each patient. The therapist will support and encourage task completion and will set standards for each patient.
- *For a community safety discussion group:* The therapist will open the discussion and will facilitate participation by members. The therapist will not offer opinions but will encourage members to reach their own.

Defining the role of the leader in the group protocol helps the OT practitioner analyze how to relate to the members of the group. People at different levels of group interaction skill require different levels of involvement from the group leader. Members at the parallel and project levels need much more assistance and supervision than do those at higher levels. Table 13-2 gives more detail on this point.

The *evaluation* section is not always included but should be. This section provides for measuring the achievement of the stated purposes of the group. To what extent does it "improve self-esteem" or "increase consistent application of safety procedures"? The choice of evaluation procedure depends on the content of the group, the skills of the members, and the overall quality management plan of the facility or of the OT department. Evaluation may be done by surveying the participants' satisfaction with the group or by having a peer therapist make independent ratings of members' behavior. See "Program Evaluation," later in this chapter, for more detail on this element of the group protocol.

Sections not listed in Figure 13-3 but occasionally included in a group protocol are exit criteria, reasons for discontinuation, and resources and references.

*Exit criteria* describe the demonstrated behaviors or skills of a person who has achieved the goals of the group. These should be quite specific and stated in behavioral terms. In fact, the exit criteria actually restate the goals of the group in an observable or measurable form. The exit criteria should be so clear that any observer could determine whether or not a particular person has met them. Possible exit criteria for a low-level task skills group are the following:

- The person works consistently for 40 minutes.
- The person works at an acceptable rate.
- The person maintains given work standards.
- The person shows minimal initiative by asking the therapist questions and spontaneously interacting with peers.

*Reasons for discontinuation* are the various factors that may cause the leader to discharge a member from the group before he or she has achieved the goals set in the exit criteria. There are many reasons a particular person may be eliminated from a group; for example:

- The person has been discharged from the treatment setting.
- The person displays uncontrollable assaultive or suicidal behavior.
- The person fails to attend the group on a regular basis.

*Resources and references* refer to items that may be used to help the group reach its goals (these may alternately be listed under materials for the group, as in Box 13-2). For example, if the main purpose of the group is to teach safe sex practices, resources may include condom samples, videos on acquired immune deficiency syndrome

(AIDS) and other sexually transmitted diseases (STDs), and a list of guest speakers. References may include written material to be used as background information by the group leader and for distribution to group members. Materials in the first language of the members (if other than English) should be included. Listing the resources and references in some detail makes it easy for another staff member to take over the group in the absence of the original leader.

In summary, writing the group protocol is the final step in designing a group. The protocol describes the goals of the group and the methods by which these goals will be achieved. Figure 13-4 illustrates how the elements of the group protocol can be combined into a clear description of a group. It describes a self-care group for male inpatients on a locked ward in a state hospital; it is a continuation of the example begun in Figure 13-3. A protocol for a group to educate and support caregivers of persons with dementia is shown in Figure 13-5. Other group protocols can be found in Appendix B.

There are several other group protocol formats in addition to the one used here; the reader may wish to look at other examples in Arbesman and associates (1) and Gibson and co-workers (11). Some of the elements in the group protocol can be combined so that a protocol may include, at a minimum, name, goals, methods, and referral information. In a sense, however, writing the group protocol is only the beginning; getting the group off to a good start and keeping it running are the real challenges.

## STARTING A NEW GROUP

Getting a new group started can be more difficult than picking up a group that has already been running for some time. The first problem is that all of the members are new to the group. They may not know each other; and, if so, several sessions may be needed just to help them feel comfortable. They are not in the habit of coming to the group, so the leader may have to round them up and remind or encourage them to attend.

The second problem is that because the group is new, its goals and activities have not been tested; only the experience of trying the activities with the group will reveal whether the goals are achievable and whether the activities and method are effective. The group leader must keep objective records of what happens in each group, and analyze these observations thoughtfully.

## ADAPTATIONS OF GROUPS FOR VERY REGRESSED INDIVIDUALS

Occupational therapists and assistants provide treatment to a range of individuals, some of whom have very severe psychiatric disabilities. These severely regressed individuals may be mute, sit for long hours in one position, have postural and sensory-integrative deficits (described in Chapter 3), and appear unresponsive to most efforts of staff. Attempting to treat these patients in the kinds of groups described thus far in this chapter would be an exercise in futility.

Ross and Burdick (24) developed a group approach for patients who have significant cognitive impairment owing to mental illness or neurological conditions, based on principles from sensory integration. A central assumption is that cognitively impaired persons can learn by receiving, processing, and responding to sensory stimulation. Their approach uses a system of five stages or components that are included in every treatment session. These stages and some sample activities for each stage are presented in Table 13-4.

Because of their limited attention spans, very regressed individuals can tolerate a group situation for only half an hour or so. Therefore, the group leader must be very active and provide the momentum to move the group through the five stages. In addition, the leader must use touch, eye contact, voice control, and sometimes hand-over-hand techniques to get individuals with low arousal to

**Men's Unit: Self-Care Group**

*Description:* Self-care group for male patients who require assistance with personal hygiene.

*Structure:* The group will meet every weekday for 45 minutes from 8:30 to 9:15 A.M. The group will meet on the ward using bathrooms, day room, and patients' rooms. The group is limited to six patients at one time. A male staff member (COTA, OT aide, or member of nursing staff) will lead the group.

*Goals:* Through participation in this group, patients will learn to:

1. Brush teeth, bathe, comb hair, and shave daily
2. Change clothes daily
3. Wash hands before each meal and after using toilet
4. Wash hair at least once a week

*Referral criteria:* To be considered for admission to the group, a patient must meet all of the following criteria:

1. Male
2. Aged 19 to 65+
3. Deficient in self-care skills as evidenced by body odor and so on
4. Able to tolerate presence of others

*Methodology:* Activities will include grooming and hygiene activities, such as bathing, shaving, hair care, tooth care. The therapist will teach self-care skills to the group and individual patients. Patients will be encouraged to carry out tasks on their own. In general, one task at a time will be taught. Once some patients have mastered that task, another will be introduced, but the therapist will continue to teach the first task until all patients have learned it.

The therapist will set individual goals for each patient and will reinforce performance by giving patients praise or tangible rewards when they reach them. The therapist will provide feedback to individuals and will encourage independent performance of self-care tasks.

Once a patient demonstrates consistent self-initiated performance of the skills taught in this group, he will be referred to other groups. Some patients with chronic illness may have to remain in the group indefinitely.

*Role of the leader:* The therapist will select and teach skills and will provide feedback and reinforcement during performance of tasks. The therapist will encourage and support the gradual development of independent self-care habits and will help patients prepare to leave the group upon completion of goals.

*Evaluation:* The treatment team will regularly evaluate the goals and prognosis of each patient. Patient satisfaction surveys are administered at intervals determined by the continuous quality improvement (CQI) leader.

**Figure 13-4. Sample group protocol: self-care group.**

**Dementia Caregivers' Education and Support Group**

*Description:* This is a support and education group for people caring for loved ones with Alzheimer's disease and other dementias.

*Structure:* The group will meet on Tuesday afternoon during the respite care program, from 2:00 to 3:00 P.M. in the small lounge. Membership is open. Self-referral is encouraged.

*Goals:* Through participation in this group, members will learn:

1. The course and nature of dementia
2. How to manage problem behaviors by altering the environment
3. How to make it possible for the person with dementia to participate in household activities, such as meal preparation and gardening
4. How to compensate for a person's diminishing memory and abilities
5. How to make the home safe for the person with cognitive deficits

*Referral criteria:* Any person with partial or total responsibility for care of a person with dementia may join the group. Self-referral and referral by word of mouth are encouraged.

*Materials and resources:* AOTA film, *A Part of Daily Life;* copies for each member of consumer guide from AOTA; *Understanding the ABCs of Alzheimer's Disease*, task analysis worksheets, cue cards, markers, flip chart.

*Methodology:* Group will provide emotional support to members, giving opportunities for discussion and sharing of feelings about caring for the person with dementia. Educational content will include a series of brief lectures on the course of dementia. Group will also teach members about task breakdown, environmental management, behavioral management, safety techniques, and so on, using written and audiovisual materials. Video segments will be used to demonstrate how to break down tasks, provide cuing, use hand-over-hand instruction, and so on. Members will practice in skills in pairs and trios and develop cue cards for enacting management methods at home. Flip chart will be used to work through the breakdown of a task; members will be helped to develop cue cards for themselves. As appropriate, members will engage in role-play to resolve problem situations in caregiving.

*Role of the leader:* The OT practitioner will select activities and focus for sessions based on needs expressed by members. Leader will provide information in short lectures with accompanying handouts; will teach skills via video; demonstration; and practice; and will encourage members to share tips and skills with each other. Leader will manage flow of the group so that all members feel supported and validated.

*Evaluation:* Pretest and post-test to evaluate mastery of information. Member satisfaction surveys administered at 6-month intervals.

**Figure 13-5. Sample group protocol: dementia.**

**TABLE 13-4 FIVE-STAGE GROUP—SENSORY INTEGRATIVE MODEL**

| STAGES | REPRESENTATIVE ACTIVITIES |
|---|---|
| **Stage 1:** Opening of session and is designed to welcome members and to stimulate as many senses as possible | Say hello by touching feet or elbows<br>Pass bell or other unusual object<br>Show and assist members to handle a manipulative toy<br>Offer scented items |
| **Stage 2:** Movement is used to increase nonverbal communication, expression of feelings; use simple, basic movements; match movements to task abilities of members | Shake hands<br>Clapping<br>Group in a circle to raise and lower parachute<br>Movement with scarves or ropes<br>ROM dance |
| **Stage 3:** Visual-motor perceptual activities are presented to increase demands on members to respond more thoughtfully, less automatically; promotes integration between sensory stimulation, movement, and cognition | Games such as Simon Says<br>Large floor dominoes<br>Relay races<br>Pantomime games (e.g., pretend to do the laundry or garden)<br>Texture matching with eyes occluded |
| **Stage 4:** Verbal or symbolic activities are used to enhance cognitive functioning | Make fruit salad (each member contributes)<br>Memory games<br>Build a tower of cardboard bricks<br>Read a poem together<br>Counting and matching games |
| **Stage 5:** Closing program provides opportunities to emphasize positive qualities of experience; familiar and relaxing activities are used | Repeat activities from stage 1<br>Shake hands or hold hands<br>Pass out candy or refreshments<br>Say good-bye to each person |

ROM, range of motion.
Data from Ross M. Integrative Group Therapy-Mobilizing Coping Abilities with the Five-Stage Group. Bethesda, MD: American Occupational Therapy Association, 1997.

respond. Not all the stages need be of equal length—for example, the leader may need to spend half of the session in stage 1 to arouse some patients.

The *five-stage group* is appropriate for people who function at lower cognitive levels. These individuals may be nonverbal, have developmental disabilities or cognitive deficits, and may be unable to express themselves or to demonstrate appropriate social behavior. Interested readers are referred to Ross (23).

Kaplan (12, 13) advocates the use of *directive groups* with people who are severely functionally impaired. These individuals cannot generally be scheduled into existing groups, as they are disruptive to the other members and obtain little benefit themselves. The purpose of the directive group is to prepare them to function in other groups that are more readily available but that require a higher level of task and social functioning than the person can demonstrate. The "directive" aspect of the group refers to the group leaders' active involvement in nurturing, supporting, and facilitating behaviors that lead to understanding the purpose of the group, attending the group for 45 minutes, concentrating enough to participate, and tolerating the presence of others. The protocols and procedures for such directive groups have been well outlined by Kaplan (12).

## OTHER MODELS FOR GROUPS

Occupational therapy practitioners use groups as a treatment method across all practice settings, with families (20), with persons young and old, with those who have physical disabilities (26), and with those who have mental health disorders. Groups may follow a specific practice model or frame of reference, such as cognitive-behavioral (29), sensory-integrative (23), or biomechanical, or psychoeducational. When leading a group that is designed for a specific practice model, the protocol should reflect this. The role of the leader, the interventions used, the choice of activities, and other aspects would correspond to the practice model.

For example, a group using a cognitive-behavioral model would emphasize identifying and disputing unreasonable beliefs that impair the ability to engage in occupations and achieve satisfaction in occupational roles. The leader would, therefore, ask group members to dispute a member's self-defeating ideas and provide another perspective. Feedback from one's peers is more likely to be accepted than that of the leader. For example, in a cooking group, if a member begins to criticize her own cooking, the leader may ask other members to give their opinions (29).

Groups using the sensory-integrative model have already been discussed (see "Adaptations of Groups for Very Regressed Individuals," earlier in this chapter). Scott (25) describes a contract-based wellness group along a behavioral model. Perrins-Margalis et al. (22) report on a horticulture (gardening) group in a clubhouse setting. Olson (20) describes a variety of groups designed for children, adolescents, parents, and families using developmental and cognitive-behavioral concepts. Cole (4) provides an introduction to the use of groups within several practice models.

## PROGRAM EVALUATION

Program evaluation is a procedure for measuring whether a program is achieving its objectives. Program evaluation is part of the total quality management (TQM) approach, which includes quality assurance (QA) and continuous quality improvement (CQI), discussed elsewhere in the text. Although program evaluation may be applied to any part of the OT program, it is discussed here because the assistant may encounter it in the context of measuring the effectiveness of a given group. In the case of a therapy group, evaluation focuses on whether the members' participation in the group has resulted in the behavioral changes specified in the goals. Designing or selecting appropriate program evaluation instruments requires knowledge of evaluation procedures and methodology and is, therefore, the responsibility of the OT. However, the assistant who is the group leader may administer or participate in the selection and development of the evaluations and should thus understand their purpose.

Program evaluation is designed to examine the effect of a treatment regimen on those who received it. One way of doing this is to collect evaluation data before patients receive the treatment and then repeat the evaluation after they have received treatment for some time. This is called a *pretest–posttest design;* for this design to be meaningful, the particular evaluation must be free of practice effects, meaning that it should not be possible for someone to perform better the second time because of having done it the first time. Evaluations used in physical medicine (e.g., measures of hand strength or range of motion) are usually free of practice effects, but this is not always true of evaluations of social interaction and psychological factors.

Another method of program evaluation is the *post-test design.* Participants are evaluated after they have received treatment, and the results are compared with what normally might have been expected without treatment. Another method is to collect data from hospital records. For example, in an outpatient program the criterion may be length of time between hospitalizations or total number of days without hospitalization per year. Other measures used to evaluate the effectiveness of OT groups include surveys of patients' satisfaction (what patients say about what they got out of the group) and evaluation checklists in which patients' performance can be rated by the leader or preferably a staff member not directly involved with the group.

A significant problem with all program evaluation in mental health is that it is often difficult to demonstrate conclusively that the improvement in a person's condition is the result of the treatment program or therapy group and not some other factor. These other factors, known as *intervening variables,* may include medication, other therapies, and other life experiences.

Program evaluation and the publication of the results in the form of outcome data are absolutely essential if OT is to retain its position in the mental health field. It is certainly much more difficult to show that a patient's behavior has been changed by an OT group than it is to prove that the same patient has improved because of a particular medication. Nevertheless, if we as a profession cannot do this, there is no reason anyone should continue to pay for our services. Our immediate and pressing challenge is to design and carry out careful program evaluations that demonstrate the effectiveness of our interventions.

## SUMMARY

This chapter provides the entry-level OTA or student with the basic concepts and methods for developing a new group or leading one that has already been developed. Groups are used in OT not only because they are cost effective but also because they provide more varied and extensive learning opportunities than are available in individual treatment. Effective group leadership consists of being able to identify and help members make use of the opportunities available in the group.

## REVIEW QUESTIONS AND ACTIVITIES

1. Why are groups used in occupational therapy for persons with mental disorders?
2. State several ways in which treatment groups are different from other groups that may occur naturally.
3. State ways in which the leader can improve group cohesiveness. Why is this important?
4. What other therapeutic factors are important in groups?
5. What is the difference between group goals and group norms? How are norms enforced by a group?
6. Name and describe each of the task roles, group maintenance roles, and antigroup roles (Table 13-1).
7. List in order and then describe each of Mosey's five developmental levels of group skills.
8. To develop a higher level of group skill, the person must be placed in a group operating one level above his or her present level of skill. Why?
9. Discuss the role of the leader in a therapy group. Write a short essay about the various roles the leader may fill.
10. How can a leader get members to interact more? Give specific examples.
11. Outline the responsibilities of the leader in preparing for the group, beginning the group, maintaining the group, and ending the group session.
12. How can you remember what happened in a group so that you can report on it later?
13. Outline steps in planning a new group.
14. What is a group protocol? What elements would be included?
15. What kind of group is appropriate for cognitively impaired individuals who have very low arousal?
16. List the stages of the five-stage group and name activities appropriate for each stage.
17. In some settings using a specific practice model, the groups may be designed to agree with the model. Why would this matter?
18. What is the relationship between program evaluation and pretest–post-test or other methods of assessing outcomes of groups?
19. *Study activity:* Make flash cards of all the italicized terms in this chapter; place the term on one side and the definition on the reverse side. Use the cards when studying.
20. *Study and exam review activity:* Write multiple-choice test questions based on information from this chapter. Use vocabulary and examples within the text as sources. (As an incentive, the instructor may decide to include student-authored questions on a real exam.)
21. *Classroom activity:* List all roles in Table 13-1 on separate slips of paper and place them in a container. Each student should draw one or two pieces of paper. Act out scenarios in which members of the class take on different task, group maintenance, and antigroup roles. The rest of the class can name the roles and discuss them.
22. *Clinical or lab activity:* Write a session plan for a real or simulated group and then carry it out. Compare what actually happens to what you planned.
23. *Clinical or lab activity:* Write a protocol for a new group.

## REFERENCES


1. Arbesman F, Armacost P, Hays C, et al., eds. Occupational Therapy: Protocols in Mental Health. Baltimore, MD: Cox Associates, 1984.
2. Banning MR, Nelson DL. The effects of activity-elicited humor and group structure on group cohesion and affective responses. Am J Occup Ther 1987;41:510–514.
3. Benne KD, Sheats P. Functional roles of group members. J Social Issues 1948;4(2):42–47.
4. Cole MB. Group Dynamics in Occupational Therapy: The Theoretical Basis and Practice Application of Group Treatment. 3rd ed. Thorofare, NJ: Slack, 2005.
5. Donohue MV, Lieberman H. Social competence of male and female psychiatric patients: Sociability, social presence, socialization and age of onset of psychosis. Occup Ther Ment Health 1992;12(1):25–46.
6. Duncombe LW, Howe MC. Group treatment: Goals, tasks and economic implications. Am J Occup Ther 1995; 49:199–205.
7. Duncombe LW, Howe MC. Group work in occupational therapy: A survey of practice. Am J Occup Ther 1985;39: 163–170.
8. Earhart CA. Occupational therapy groups. In: Allen CA, ed. Occupational Therapy for Psychiatric Diseases: Measurement and Management of Cognitive Disabilities. Boston: Little, Brown, 1985.
9. Early MB. T.A.R. Introductory Course Workbook: Occupational Therapy: Psychosocial Dysfunction. Long Island City, NY: LaGuardia Community College, 1981.
10. Falk-Kessler J, Momich C, Perel S. Therapeutic factors in occupational therapy groups. Am J Occup Ther 1991;45:59–66.
11. Gibson D (editor). Group protocols: A psychosocial compendium. Occup Ther Mental Health 1990;9(4):15–136.
12. Kaplan KL. Directive Group Therapy. Thorofare, NJ: Slack, 1988.
13. Kaplan KL. The directive group: Short-term treatment for psychiatric patients with a minimal level of functioning. Am J Occup Ther 1986;40:474–481.
14. Kartin NJ, Van Schroeder C. Adult Psychiatric Life Skills Manual. Kailua, HI: Schroeder, 1982.
15. Kramer LW. SCORE: Solving community obstacles and restoring employment. Occup Ther Ment Health 1984;4(1): 1–135.
16. Mead M. Male and female. In: Maggio R, compiler. The Beacon Book of Quotations by Women. Boston: Beacon, 1992.
17. Mosey AC. Activities Therapy. New York: Raven, 1973.
18. Mosey AC. The concept and use of developmental groups. Am J Occup Ther 1970;24:272–275.
19. Mosey AC. Three Frames of Reference for Mental Health. Thorofare, NJ: Slack, 1970.
20. Olson L. Activity groups in family-centered treatment: Psychiatric occupational therapy approaches for parents and children. Occup Ther Ment Health 2006;22(3–4):1–156.
21. Peloquin SM. Linking purpose to procedure during interactions with patients. Am J Occup Ther 1988;42:775–781.
22. Perrins-Margalis NM, Rugletic J, Schepis NM, et al. The immediate effects of a group-based horticulture experience on the quality of life of persons with chronic mental illness. Occup Ther Ment Health 2000;16(1):15–32.
23. Ross M. Integrative Group Therapy: Mobilizing Coping Abilities with the Five-Stage Group. Bethesda, MD: American Occupational Therapy Association, 1997.
24. Ross M, Burdick D. Sensory Integration: A Training Manual for Therapists and Teachers for Regressed Psychiatric and Geriatric Patient Groups. Thorofare, NJ: Slack, 1981.
25. Scott AH. Wellness works: Community service health promotion groups led by occupational therapy students. Am J Occup Ther 1999;53(6):566–574.
26. Sladyk K. Traumatic brain injury, behavioral disorder, and group treatment. Am J Occup Ther 1992;46:267–269.
27. Ward JD. The nature of clinical reasoning with groups: A phenomenological study of an occupational therapist in community mental health. Occup Ther Ment Health 2003;57(6):625–634.
28. Webster D, Schwartzberg SL. Patients' perception of curative factors in occupational therapy groups. Occup Ther Ment Health 1992;12(1):3–24.
29. Yakobina S, Yakobina S, Tallant BK. I came, I thought, I conquered: Cognitive behavior approach applied in occupational therapy for the treatment of depressed (dysthymic) females. Occup Ther Ment Health 1997;13(4):59–73.
30. Yalom ID. The Theory and Practice of Group Psychotherapy. New York: Basic Books, 1970.
31. Yalom I. The Theory and Practice of Group Psychotherapy. 3rd ed. New York: Basic Books, 1985.


## SUGGESTED READINGS


Borg B, Bruce MA. The Group System: The Therapeutic Activity Group in Occupational Therapy. Thorofare, NJ: Slack, 1991.

Brown T, Harwood K, Heckman J, Short JE, eds. Mental Health Protocols for Occupational Therapy. Baltimore, MD: Chess, 1989.

Cole MB. Group Dynamics in Occupational Therapy: The Theoretical Basis and Practice Application of Group Treatment. 3rd ed. Thorofare, NJ: Slack, 2005.

Fidler GS. The task-oriented group as a context for treatment. Am J Occup Ther 1969;23:43–48.

Gibson D, ed. Group Process and Structure in Psychosocial Occupational Therapy. Binghamton, NY: Haworth, 1988.

Gibson D, ed. Group Protocols: A Psychosocial Compendium. Binghamton, NY: Haworth, 1989.

Hasselkus BR. The meaning of activity: Day care for persons with Alzheimer's disease. Am J Occup Ther 1992;46: 199–206.

Howe MC, Schwartzberg SL. A Functional Approach to Group Work in Occupational Therapy. 3rd ed. Philadelphia: Lippincott Williams & Wilkins 2001.

Kaplan KL. Directive Group Therapy: Innovative Mental Health Treatment. Thorofare, NJ: Slack, 1988.

Posthuma BW. Small Groups in Therapy Settings: Process and Leadership. Austin, TX: Pro-Ed, 1988.

Remocker AJ, Sherwood ET. Action Speaks Louder: A Handbook of Nonverbal Group Techniques. 6th ed. Edinburgh, UK: Churchill Livingstone, 1998.

Ross M. Integrative Group Therapy: Mobilizing Coping Abilities with the Five-Stage Group. Bethesda, MD: American Occupational Therapy Association, 1997.

Yalom ID. Inpatient Group Psychotherapy. New York: Basic, 1983.

SECTION IV

# Occupational Therapy Process

CHAPTER 14

# Overview of the Intervention Process

***You want to know what has been helpful? When they sit down and talk with my mom about working with me and make sure everything is working good. When people are all telling you the same thing. . . . I want to be included in the plans that are made for me.***

MARY ANN FAHL QUOTING A PATIENT, KEVIN (11)

## CHAPTER OBJECTIVES

After studying this chapter, the reader will be able to:

1. Describe the occupational therapy process as holistic and dynamic.
2. Name and describe the function of each stage in the occupational therapy process.
3. Discuss the role of the occupational therapy assistant in each stage of the process.
4. Define *outcomes* and discuss how outcomes are identified and reviewed.
5. Understand the influence of theory and practice models on the process of intervention.
6. Explain what is meant by *clinical reasoning* and name several aspects or types.
7. Appreciate the influence of evidence-based practice on the occupational therapy process.

The purpose of occupational therapy (OT) is to help people do the things they want and need to do despite a disability. From the moment the occupational therapy practitioner is first notified that the person needs service, every action should be directed toward this end. Throughout the intervention process, the patient (client or consumer) needs to know what is being done and why; effective therapy practitioners thus begin with the client's point of view. This is the best way to ensure that occupational therapy interventions will have a lasting, positive, and meaningful effect.

This chapter begins with an overview of the important points of the process section of the *Occupational Therapy Practice Framework: Domain and Process* (*OTPF*) (3). The chapter next provides a brief overview of the intervention process, with discussion of the eight classical stages. Each stage is described and related to the others. Different clinical environments are analyzed for their effects on the way each stage is enacted. The role of the occupational therapy assistant (OTA) is addressed.

The chapter also considers clinical reasoning, the complex cognitive (thinking) and affective (feeling) process by which the therapist analyzes the patient's situation and generates ideas for intervention. Although the occupational therapist (OT) is responsible for controlling and documenting the intervention process, the assistant, even at entry level, may be delegated some of this responsibility. In addition, because the OTA has frequent contact with the client, the OTA contributes invaluable insights for determining treatment goals and direction. Occupational therapy assistants with advanced service competencies and long experience might expect to undertake more of the occupational therapy process.

## OCCUPATIONAL THERAPY PRACTICE FRAMEWORK: PROCESS

The *OTPF* (3) has two main sections: domain and process. The domain section was discussed in Chapter 4. The process section is considered here. It begins with five main ideas that are to be considered throughout intervention. These important points are presented in Box 14-1. The first point is that *the occupational therapy process is dynamic and evolving*. Although the steps or stages discussed later appear to proceed in a logical order, in the clinic the stages merge and mix. For example, a thorough evaluation may be deferred so that immediate medical needs can be addressed (15).

**BOX 14-1**

### THE FIVE IMPORTANT POINTS OF THE *OCCUPATIONAL THERAPY PRACTICE FRAMEWORK* PROCESS

- The process is dynamic and evolving.
- Context is embedded in our understanding of intervention.
- Clients are individuals, whether they receive services as individuals or as members of groups or populations.
- The client must be an active participant (client-centered process).
- The outcome is engagement in occupation.

Modified from American Occupational Therapy Association. Occupational therapy practice framework: Domain and process. Am J Occup Ther 2002;56:609–639.

And, at any point during the delivery of treatment, the need for a new evaluation may be recognized.

The second idea is that *context is embedded in our understanding of intervention.* Contexts, both physical environments and the other contexts of the *OTPF,* affect occupational performance. Therefore, the therapists working with the client keep in mind the contexts to which the client will be going after treatment. If the client is returning to a family home with good social support and traditions of helping, then perhaps independent function is not the priority it might be for a client going to a single-room occupancy hotel. Contexts also affect the delivery of services. Consider, for example, the difference between a clubhouse setting and a large state hospital (see Chapters 7 and 9).

A third point is that *clients are individuals, whether they receive services as individuals or as members of groups or populations.* As discussed elsewhere in this text (see Box 7-1), the person who receives occupational therapy services may be designated by a variety of names, depending on the context of care. Whether a resident or inmate, consumer or patient, the service recipient is considered a client and a collaborator in the intervention process. When OT practitioners provide services to groups and larger populations, we understand the members of these larger entities as individuals.

The fourth idea is that *the client must be an active participant, engaged in a client-centered process.* To engage in occupation requires internal motivation that comes from the person. Even when the person appears unable to communicate desires and interests, therapy practitioners must use other information to make a best guess as to what the person wants. At every point in the process, the client is considered a leading partner in decision making.

The fifth and final point is that *the outcome of occupational therapy intervention is engagement in occupation.* Occupational therapy practitioners provide many different interventions using a variety of methods. Some of these affect body functions and structures or otherwise aim to improve the person's underlying abilities. Examples of these methods are range of motion exercises, sensory integration modalities, and anger management training. Use of these methods alone does not constitute occupational therapy. Therapists must connect clients to an ability to engage in occupation. Thus anger management training must be applied to functioning on the job or in other occupations (e.g., a club or hobby).

## EIGHT STAGES IN THE INTERVENTION PROCESS

The occupational therapy intervention process as outlined in the *OTPF* (3) differs slightly from what is described in this chapter, which follows the *Standards of Practice for Occupational Therapy* (5). The OTPF names three major stages: evaluation, intervention, and outcomes. This is helpful for seeing more clearly the relationships among finding out what one needs to know (evaluation), providing services to bring about desired changes (intervention), and determining what changes were achieved (outcomes). *Outcomes* are the measurable goals that the intervention aims to achieve. For a worker with depression expressed as irritability, a possible outcome might be working a full shift daily for 2 weeks without having an angry outburst. Outcomes are first identified during evaluation and intervention planning. Assessment of outcomes (to what extent they have been achieved) occurs formally during intervention review and also periodically throughout intervention implementation.

In clinical practice, the OTA is likely to notice more than the three stages named in the *OTPF.* Hinojosa et al. (17) point out that screening occurs routinely in many settings and should be included. Similarly, the assessment of outcomes is not the end of the relationship between the occupational therapy staff and the patient. Therefore, the eight stages we consider here begin with the referral and end with discharge of the person from occupational therapy service. The stages themselves are as follows:

1. Referral
2. Screening
3. Evaluation
4. Intervention planning
5. Intervention implementation
6. Intervention review
7. Transition planning
8. Discontinuation of service.

The stages are summarized in Box 14-2, described briefly in the sections that follow, and discussed in more detail in later chapters.

## Referral

The process begins with the *referral,* which is a request for service. However, in many states occupational therapy services can be reimbursed

BOX 14-2

### EIGHT STAGES IN THE OCCUPATIONAL THERAPY PROCESS

1. **Referral.** The physician or other referring professional requests OT service for an identified patient. The OTA may relay the referral to the supervising OT but should not accept the referral independently. The OT documents receipt of referral in compliance with state laws and other regulations.
2. **Screening.** The purpose is to determine whether the patient needs further OT evaluation and treatment. OT practitioners observe and briefly interview the patient and/or collect information from the medical record. The OT is responsible for screening and may direct the OTA to collect specific data.
3. **Evaluation.** The purpose is to find out more about the client, what he or she wants and needs to do, and the obstacles to occupational engagement. The *occupational profile* (the client's occupational history and goals) and the *analysis of occupational performance* (a study of how the client performs to determine his or her limitations and strengths) are the two major parts of evaluation. Information is collected from the patient and other sources. The OT determines what information is needed and how to obtain it and may assign the OTA to carry out structured interviews, distribute and collect questionnaires, search the medical record, and administer structured evaluations—provided the OTA has demonstrated service competency. The OT is responsible for synthesizing, analyzing, and documenting the entire evaluation.
4. **Intervention planning.** Based on the results of evaluation, a plan is developed in keeping with the patient's goals. Specific outcomes are identified, and approaches and methods for achieving these are identified. Working with the patient, the OT and/or OTA (depending on the focus of treatment) determine short- and long-term goals based on the identified problems. Consideration is given to time frames, applicable standards, and other guidelines. The OT practitioner selects the methods and specific treatment activities to be used to work toward these goals.
5. **Intervention implementation.** The treatment plan is carried out. In many settings, the OTA is responsible for this aspect of the treatment process, involving the patient in activities to support participation in occupation. Intervention may be directed at modifications of the task or the environment. Documentation of intervention is essential and follows state laws and other guidelines.
6. **Intervention review.** At regular intervals or continuously (depending on treatment setting), the OT practitioners consider whether the intervention plan is working, what progress has been made, and what changes might be appropriate. The plan is modified as needed. Additional referrals or evaluations may be ordered.

*(continued)*

**BOX 14-2** ***(Continued)***

7. **Transition planning.** OT practitioners work with the client, the family when appropriate, and the rest of the treatment team to make sure that the patient will be able to function optimally after leaving the treatment setting. Transition plans may include living arrangements, transition from school to work, employment and leisure, and/or continuing treatment, depending on the consumer's need. All OT practitioners who have worked with the patient should contribute to the transition plan.
8. **Discontinuation of service.** The patient is discharged from the program. Achievements in the program and plans are discussed. A final note is written by the OT with contributions from the OTA, documenting changes in the client's status from the initial evaluation to the final service intervention. Any follow-up plans are also documented. Outcomes are documented in a manner consistent with local guidelines and program evaluation priorities.

Data from American Occupational Therapy Association. Guidelines for supervision, roles, and responsibilities during the delivery of occupational therapy services. Am J Occup Ther 2004;58:663–667; American Occupational Therapy Association. Occupational therapy practice framework: Domain and process. Am J Occup Ther 2002;56:609–639; American Occupational Therapy Association. Roles and responsibilities of the occupational therapist and the occupational therapy assistant during the delivery of occupational therapy services. OT Practice 2002;7(15):9–10; American Occupational Therapy Association. Standards of practice for occupational therapy. Am J Occup Ther 2005;59:663–665; Gutman SA, Mortera MH, Hinojosa J, Kramer P. Revision of the occupational therapy practice framework [The Issue Is]. Am J Occup Ther 2007;62:119–126; Hinojosa J, Kramer P, Crist P. Evaluation: Obtaining and Interpreting Data. 2nd ed. Bethesda MD: American Occupational Therapy Association Press, 2005.

only if they are initiated by an order or referral signed by a physician. In other words, federal and state medical care programs and private insurance companies will pay for occupational therapy services only if a physician (or other qualified professional) has requested the service in writing. This may apply in outpatient as well as inpatient settings, even in free-standing agencies such as psychosocial clubs.

The OT is responsible for the referral process (5). This requires attention to the practice model or models that apply to the setting, which should be clearly evident in the referral forms. The OT aims to do the following:

- Facilitate appropriate referrals (i.e., of clients who can benefit from the available services)
- Reduce or discourage inappropriate referrals (e.g., of clients who are unable to benefit because they have extreme symptoms or for services that are not reimbursable)
- Teach the staff, in particular physicians and other referral sources, about the goals, methods, and services of occupational therapy in the particular setting.

A predetermined list of reasons for referral might be provided to physicians and other potential sources of referrals. This might be a list of phrases that can be written into the order or (more time saving) a checklist form that can be used as the referral document (Fig. 14-1). Periodic quality review allows the occupational therapy staff to monitor the effectiveness and ease of referrals; at intervals, referring staff are invited to give their opinions about the referral form and process. Figure 14-2 provides a sample quality review survey of referrals.

**COMMUNITY CLINIC**

**REQUEST FOR OCCUPATIONAL THERAPY SERVICES**

Date of request ____________________

Patient name ______________________ Sex _____ Age _____ ID Number __________

Diagnosis ________________________________________________

Precautions and restrictions ________________________________________

________________________________________________

Referral problem: Problem in activities of daily living (specify) ____________________

________________________________________________

Vocational or educational problem (specify) ____________________

________________________________________________

Leisure problem (specify) ____________________

________________________________________________

Possible cognitive disability ____________________

________________________________________________

Social, interpersonal, or role problem (specify) ____________________

________________________________________________

Other (specify) ____________________

________________________________________________

Specify services requested (screening, evaluation, consultation, etc.) ____________________

________________________________________________

________________________________________________

________________________________________________

Requested by ____________________

**Figure 14-1. Sample request for occupational therapy services.**

Only the OT may accept referrals to occupational therapy (5). The OTA promptly notifies the OT supervisor of any referral request directed to the OTA. The supervisor can then decide what role the assistant will take in the person's screening, evaluation, and treatment. It is also possible for an OT or OTA to initiate the referral by speaking with the doctor or other referring professional about the person's need for treatment. Regardless of who initiates the referral, it must always be documented in the chart.

**OCCUPATIONAL THERAPY REFERRAL SURVEY**

Dear Staff: Your opinion matters to us. Please help us improve the occupational therapy referral procedure by taking a minute or two to complete this form.

| **REFERRAL FORM** | **excellent** | | **satisfactory** | | **needs work** |
|---|---|---|---|---|---|
| Ease of completion | 1 | 2 | 3 | 4 | 5 |
| Usefulness of categories | 1 | 2 | 3 | 4 | 5 |
| Match to patient needs | 1 | 2 | 3 | 4 | 5 |
| Availability of forms | 1 | 2 | 3 | 4 | 5 |

Comments/suggestions ______________________________

______________________________

| **RESPONSE TO REFERRALS** | **excellent** | | **satisfactory** | | **needs work** |
|---|---|---|---|---|---|
| Speed of response | 1 | 2 | 3 | 4 | 5 |
| Specificity of response | 1 | 2 | 3 | 4 | 5 |
| Usefulness of response | 1 | 2 | 3 | 4 | 5 |

Comments/suggestions ______________________________

______________________________

**PLEASE DROP COMPLETED SURVEY IN THE SURVEY BOX ON THE DESK.**

**THANK YOU!**

**Figure 14-2. Sample occupational therapy referral survey.**

## Screening

The purpose of *screening* is to determine whether a person needs occupational therapy evaluation or intervention. If you have ever been to a hospital emergency room, you were probably screened by the emergency room nurse. This process is sometimes called *triage;* the nurse decides how serious your problem is and sends you home with a clinic appointment for another day or tells you to take a seat and wait or admits you immediately if your condition is serious. Screening in occupational therapy is similar. You can think of screening as a filter through which a person must pass before receiving occupational therapy services. Not every potential client needs occupational therapy, and some of those who need it may be too ill to attend until after their medication begins working.

Screening is designed to answer the following questions: Does this person have any problems functioning in daily life activities and occupational roles? Are these problems treatable by occupational therapy? Does the person demonstrate readiness to attend occupational therapy and benefit from it? If not, should the person be evaluated for occupational therapy after medication begins to take effect or the person is medically stable?

Screening is usually done by interview or observation or by review of the person's history and medical record. The OT performs the screening independently or as a member of the interdisciplinary team. The OT decides what information is needed and may direct the OTA to collect some of it by interviewing the client or family, reviewing the medical record, or observing performance in an activity and recording behavior on a structured form, such as a checklist or rating sheet. The assistant then reports the information to the therapist, who makes the final decision about whether to admit the person to occupational therapy.

Sometimes screening is done before the referral has been received; this is most common in short-term settings with a high turnover rate and large numbers of clients but not enough occupational therapy staff to serve all of them. The supervising occupational therapist decides who can benefit most or who needs the service most and obtains a documented referral if required by state or federal guidelines.

In some psychiatric settings, all clients are routinely referred to occupational therapy; in such cases there is no formal screening. In acute inpatient settings the patients are often too symptomatic to attend occupational therapy, but the occupational therapist must still see them and document that they cannot be evaluated further until their symptoms subside.

## Evaluation

*Evaluation* begins once it has been determined, with or without a formal screening, that a person needs occupational therapy services. The purpose of evaluation is to find out enough about the person to determine the direction of intervention. The OT, who is responsible for this process, decides what data are needed (2, 4, 5). The *OTPF* (3) suggests that evaluation should begin with the occupational profile and the analysis of occupational performance. The *occupational profile* describes the person's occupational history and interests, what is currently important to the person, and other information relevant to the person's experiences and goals related to engagement in occupation. Information may be obtained through formal interview or casual conversation (3). The *analysis of occupational performance* is a study of the person's ability to engage in the desired occupations. Observing the client's performance is the foundation of the analysis, which also may use tests and other assessments. The therapist studies the person's performance, considers possible reasons for problems, and speculates about possible interventions that may be helpful. The therapist chooses and uses an appropriate practice model or frame of reference to structure this mental process.

In making decisions about evaluation, the OT weighs the cost in time and personnel resources of the assessments used, the patient's immediate needs, the projected length of stay of the patient, the projected plan for continuity of care in other settings, and the frame of reference of the treatment setting. In some situations, the development of the occupational profile and performing the analysis of occupational performance are deferred so that assessments of client factors may occur (17). The OT may direct the OTA to interview the patient, observe the person in activities, or administer structured assessments and tests. Information is gathered from multiple sources—the medical record, the patient, the family or employer, other treatment settings, mental health professionals who have worked with the person in the past. The OT performs any assessments that require special expertise and analyzes and consolidates the information.

Assessments (e.g., tests and observations) are used to measure the person's current level of functioning and to identify skills and talents and interests that if developed more, might improve function. Skills that are lacking and that require environmental compensation (e.g., help from others) may also be identified. Results of the assessments are recorded in the patient's chart.

During the evaluation process, the client and OT practitioners identify possible outcome areas . Outcomes are the measurable and observable results of an intervention. (6). All occupational therapy outcomes should be focused on engagement in occupation. As an example, a young man with paranoid schizophrenia may say that he wants to complete college but that he has dropped out. His current problems with college are an inability to concentrate owing to hallucinations and some suspiciousness of classmates and professors. Outcomes could be phrased in terms of whether he can complete a course, or attend school for a given number of days, or be able to take notes and pass the course despite the hallucinations, or be able to socialize with classmates and meet with the professor despite his suspiciousness. In a client-centered process, the client and the therapist jointly determine the outcomes.

Client involvement in identification of outcomes is essential. Babiss (6) and others (16, 20) note that different stakeholders value different outcomes. Stakeholders are people or groups that have a stake (an interest) in the outcome of intervention; these may be the client, the family, the insurance company, health care providers, government agencies, and others. For example, health insurers may value reduced length of stay or increased length of time between suicide attempts or return of body weight to a normal range (for someone with anorexia). Government agencies may value the return to work of someone who is disabled. However, the client may value other outcomes more, such as personal satisfaction or feelings of competence. Outcomes will be discussed again later in the chapter.

The person's current level of functioning is sometimes called the *baseline.* Treatment effectiveness can be measured by comparing the outcomes with this baseline level. This is possible only when the same thing is measured using the same test both times. It is always preferable to include assessments that yield quantifiable baseline data and measurable outcomes so that change can be documented. Data collection and evaluation are covered in detail in Chapter 15.

## Intervention Planning

*Intervention planning* is based on the results of the evaluation and the outcomes of interest tentatively identified by the client and the therapist. Planning entails identifying the client's problems, choosing outcomes, and selecting reasonable goals and methods to achieve them. The person's *prognosis,* or the degree to which we can predict recovery from disability and the ability to resume a normal life, is considered. In mental disorders, it is often difficult to judge whether a particular person with a given diagnosis and history is likely to achieve a specific intervention goal. Similarly, it is difficult to estimate time frames for goal achievement, particularly in short-term settings.

Some higher-functioning clients with good prognoses will be able to develop new skills or improve their present ones and return to a reasonably independent life in the community. Other clients may be able to succeed in the community only if their environment and responsibilities are modified to compensate for their disabilities and if they have family or treatment personnel to whom they can turn for support. Some function less and less well as time goes by but can maintain their abilities longer if occupational therapy is provided.

The client's problems are identified by analyzing the information gathered from interviews, medical records, and evaluations. The occupational therapist tries to evaluate the person's potential to benefit from intervention on the basis of prognosis and history. This evaluation is the basis for determining the general direction of intervention and for setting intervention goals. Intervention may be directed toward *prevention* of predicted future disability; an example is teaching a potential child abuser nonabusive methods of controlling a child. A second possible approach is *rehabilitation,* or the development of necessary life skills and the underlying functions, such as cognitive skills, that support them. The client's development of activities of daily living or work skills is an example of rehabilitation. The third major approach is *maintenance,* or helping the person continue functioning as well as possible despite disability, even though functioning is likely to remain the same or deteriorate over time. Alternately, intervention may be directed toward health promotion and wellness, or compensation and modification of the environment to improve engagement in occupation.

Once the approach to intervention has been determined, the specific focus and goals are selected in collaboration with the client and/or family. Intervention may focus on performance skills, performance patterns, activity demands, client factors, and/or the context. While working with the client to define the goals, occupational therapy practitioners can begin thinking about the most effective methods to reach them; this can be a joint effort between OT and OTA. Knowledge of what treatment groups, activities, and other resources are available in the treatment setting and the surrounding community contributes to this planning process. The therapist can then make recommendations and suggest alternative plans to the client and family.

The therapist must estimate how long it will take the person to achieve a treatment goal. Those that will take a long time are long-term goals; the therapist breaks these down into smaller steps, or short-term goals, so that the person sees achievement even though the final target may be far off. Some goals do not have to be divided into steps because they are inherently short term.

The OTA who has participated in the client's evaluation will often also assist the OT in developing treatment goals (2, 4, 5). The assistant has considerable expertise in independent daily living skills and therapeutic activities and may work effectively in selecting and adapting the intervention methods. The OTA may also be assigned to explain the intervention plan to other staff and to the client and family.

The approach, focus, and extent of intervention planning depends significantly on treatment setting, length of time available for treatment, and other resources. Therapy practitioners in a short-term setting will be more concerned with evaluation and with helping the person make a transition to the next level of care than with long-term planning. Careful intervention planning is crucial to the ultimate outcome of treatment and will be covered in greater detail in Chapter 16.

## Intervention Implementation

*Intervention implementation* is the actual performance of the methods and activities outlined in the intervention plan. The OT has overall responsibility for implementation (2, 4, 5). With increasing pressures to reduce costs and use the least expensive personnel, the OTA is often responsible for much of the actual intervention, which may be done individually or in groups and which may use a wide variety of therapeutic media and other resources. Proper supervision must be provided by the OT (2, 4). Students and new therapists tend to be more involved in carrying out intervention than are experienced or supervising therapists, whose tasks are primarily evaluation and management. Pelland (30) notes that students or novice therapists occasionally fail to use the documented plan and may have difficulty determining which of the documented goals should be pursued first. Lack of experience with timing and with the clinical environment may also cause confusion and poor implementation. Supervision and working with experienced colleagues are essential at this stage.

Regardless of the specific activity or approach employed, intervention should be executed thoughtfully, with careful attention to the client's interest in and understanding of the intervention.

The OTA must be certain that the person is aware of the purpose of the intervention and must help him or her understand why it is important. Sometimes client with cognitive impairments or serious mental disorders forget why therapy is important. Peloquin (31) gives suggestions for how to help the patient link the activities used with their purposes:

1. Explain the purpose of the group or activity.
2. Encourage the patient to think about the purpose and ask him or her to share this view.
3. Discuss the skills used and link them to the activities or tasks performed.
4. Summarize what has transpired.

This four-step process ensures that the clinician has verbalized the purposes to the patient and has engaged the patient in understanding the purpose of the occupational therapy intervention.

Several chapters in this text are devoted to describing specific intervention approaches and activities, so only the most general aspects of intervention implementation are discussed here. See Chapters 17 through 23 for more detailed information.

## Intervention Review

*Intervention review,* usually performed after some of the intervention has occurred, is a process for determining the effectiveness of the plan (3). The client is involved in the review process, as possible depending on cognitive level. Review may lead to modification of the plan, to discontinuation of the plan, or to discharge of the patient from treatment. The OT has overall responsibility for the review (2, 4, 5).

Reevaluation may be a part of the review. The OTA follows the direction of the OT in carrying out reevaluation, which in all respects, except timing, is identical to the initial evaluation. As stated earlier, use of standardized assessments that yield quantifiable data help to document effectiveness of therapy. Data can help in decisions about upgrading or downgrading goals and activities in response to the client's changed level of functioning. Furthermore, the data obtained through reevaluation also provide information about the person's readiness for transition to the next level of care.

## Transition Planning

*Transition planning* is the stage in which the next care setting is identified and arrangements are made. Ideally, planning for transition to the next care setting begins at first meeting the client. The questions to be addressed include these: Where will the person live, and with whom, after this intervention context? What activities will structure his or her day—work, leisure, self-care, organized day treatment, or a combination? Will the person need additional services to carry out daily life activities? If so, what are they? What is the best place for this person to receive continuing treatment, an aftercare service of the hospital, a community mental health center, a home health agency? Transition of adolescents with mental disorders from the school setting to the work setting is part of this stage in the intervention process.

Accurate assessment of the client's ability to function and identification of the conditions under which he or she is likely to function best are the foundation on which good transition planning is built. The occupational therapist and assistant may be the only members of the treatment staff in a position to observe regularly how the person performs routine tasks and deals with problems that arise. This information is crucial for predicting ability to function in the community and for identifying the degree and kind of supports needed by the individual.

When the social worker often has final responsibility for transition planning, as is the case in many mental health inpatient settings, occupational therapy staff should communicate their observations and recommendations to the social worker. The OTA, who is likely to have firsthand knowledge of the client's abilities, interests, and preferences, should share this knowledge with the OT and others responsible for transition planning. Depending on circumstances, experience, and expertise, the OT may ask the OTA to take a lead role in planning for transition. Overall, the OT has ultimate responsibility for occupational therapy's contribution to the transition plan (2, 4, 5).

Unfortunately, transition from acute care units may be performed in a slipshod fashion because of time pressures and limitations on how long persons with psychiatric diagnoses are allowed to remain in inpatient settings. Inadequacy of community resources to meet needs and underfunding of mental health services in general make planning quite challenging. Unfortunately, some patients are discharged to the street, with only a clinic appointment for follow-up. This is a tragic situation that should shame us all; occupational therapy practitioners can help by advocating in political and social venues for adequate funding, supported housing, and appropriate care for persons with chronic mental illness.

### Discontinuation of Service

*Discontinuation of service* is the final step in the intervention process. As discussed in Chapter 10, this is an opportunity for the client and the occupational therapy staff to review what has transpired over the course of the intervention process. The client should be helped to identify and assess accomplishments and to formulate goals for the future. Occupational therapy staff should double-check any arrangements for continuing treatment to make sure the person will be able to follow through on them. Finally, a discontinuation note in the client's chart must document the evaluation findings, intervention goals, and outcomes of intervention, including recommendations for continuing treatment elsewhere. The OT manages this process with contributions from the OTA (2, 4, 5).

Depending on the setting, some stages in the intervention process may be eliminated or deferred. Restrictions on the length of inpatient hospitalization may collapse the stages of the intervention process. For example, if the patient will not be allowed to stay in the hospital for more than 7 days, it is not possible to do anything but evaluate him or her and work out a good discharge plan, leaving the intervention planning and implementation to the staff of the outpatient treatment facility. Chapter 7 describes different kinds of treatment settings and the types of services the occupational therapist and assistant might provide in each of them.

## A HOLISTIC PERSPECTIVE—A DYNAMIC PROCESS

The stages in the intervention process form a unified whole. Though discussed separately here, in the mind of the experienced therapist they often merge. From the moment the referral is received, the therapist accepts the client or patient as a partner in therapy and begins to sort and analyze information and ideas and to weigh alternative plans for treatment and continuity of care. For example, a therapist in an acute care setting will consider transition options on first meeting the patient, simply because patients' stays are so short in such settings. The patient will be concerned about whether and when he or she can return home. Thus screening and evaluation will focus on transition planning rather than on intervention. In some settings evaluation may be ongoing; the therapist in a long-term setting may identify a need for further evaluation of a patient as new information comes to light or as the patient's health status changes in response to intervention or deteriorates as a result of the disease process.

Students and new assistants may wish to consider each stage separately at first to learn what happens and what to do at each stage. While learning the stages, they should try to see the connections between them and to understand them as a fluid and flexible continuum. Occupational therapy staff who comprehend the continuity of the entire process will be able to persuade consumers, other professionals, and reimbursers of the importance of each step in intervention.

To review, occupational therapy intervention is a client-centered, occupation-centered, and outcome-oriented process.

### Client Centered

The patient or client should be involved at every step; involving the client demonstrates respect for the person's priorities and values. Recognizing the client as a partner in the intervention process, the therapy practitioner uses collaborative communication skills to invite maximum client participation. The client contributes valuable information and should be encouraged to ask questions and give opinions.

### Occupation Centered

The purpose of occupational therapy intervention is for the client to achieve maximum engagement in occupation, in accordance with goals the client values. The "client's occupational needs, problems and concerns" (3, p. 125) focus the evaluation, plan, and interventions on situations that are important to the client's occupational life. Therapy practitioners use actual occupations and occupational tasks, and therapeutic activities, to develop the client's ability to engage in occupations. While some methods that are not activities or occupations may be used, these are always connected to occupational functioning and goals.

### Outcome Oriented

Outcomes are the results of interventions. The most important result or outcome is improved ability to engage in occupation, but many other outcomes can be stated under this main idea. Remember that intervention may target an individual, a group, or a population. Some sample outcomes include reduced fatigue in persons with multiple sclerosis (as a result of energy conservation techniques), increased time on task for a child with attention deficit-hyperactivity disorder (ADHD; as a result of sensory training), and increased number of job placements in supported employment for persons with serious mental disorders as well as increased tenure in employment for these patients.

Outcomes may be used in many ways and for this reason the wording should be carefully considered. Some of the uses of outcomes are as follows:

- To compare some aspect of the client's occupational functioning before intervention and after intervention
- To communicate to the client the achievements in therapy
- To establish an understandable and measurable desired result
- As a basis for program evaluation
- To provide evidence for research
- To document effectiveness to ensure reimbursement

The OTA assists the OT in the development of outcomes and the collection of outcomes data. Use of a single valid and reliable evaluation measure before intervention and during intervention review ensures that results are measurable and comparable. Data from many clients can be considered together if the same evaluation measures are used. This collected data become more powerful and useful the larger the number of cases that are included. Collection of outcomes data and outcomes research contribute to the body of evidence that supports our profession.

## THEORY AND THE OCCUPATIONAL THERAPY PROCESS

Theory (discussed in Chapters 2 and 3) can be the key to unlocking the mystery of the patient's situation, even when the situation seems more straightforward than mysterious. For example, the person with very poor hygiene and grooming at first glance seems to need an activities of daily living (ADLs) evaluation followed by some sort of intervention in ADLs. The wise occupational therapy practitioner will want to know, however, *why* this person's ADL are so poor. Is it the result of dementia or part of a lifelong mental illness? Has there been a sudden and abrupt decompensation after a lifetime of normal functioning? Is this a sign of rapid deterioration into an advanced state of substance abuse? Is the person unconsciously using this behavior to avoid a situation that feels psychologically overwhelming? Each of these possibilities suggests a different theoretical model, and each model in turn suggests a line of inquiry and a focus of evaluation and intervention. The therapist will be conversant with several models appropriate to the setting and the population. Then, on meeting the client or reviewing the medical record, the therapist can rapidly formulate hypotheses and sort and discard potential courses of action before determining where to start. As the process continues and the client becomes better known, the therapist may change course, using a model that better fits the person's new direction. Sizing up the person's situation and selecting useful theories is central to the process of clinical reasoning.

## CLINICAL REASONING

Faced with the task of developing an evaluation and intervention plan that the client will find meaningful and empowering, the occupational therapist needs a logical approach to gathering information and using it to generate intervention goals and methods. Although many approaches to organizing data and planning intervention have been presented over the years in the occupational therapy literature, until the 1990s little had been written about how experienced and skillful clinicians approach the problem of planning treatment. How does the therapist know which practice model to select, which evaluations to administer, which problems to target, and which approaches to use?

### Asking the Right Questions

The beginning of this chapter described clinical reasoning as a complex cognitive and affective process—in other words, a process of analysis using thinking and feeling. The therapist, educated in many theories and practice models and trained in various techniques, must consider and select theories and methods that best apply to the situation. At the same time, the therapist must feel for the patient and the patient's dilemma—that is, the therapist must step back from the role of therapist and into the patient's story. The therapist must come to understand how the person's life looks from the inside. In her Eleanor Clarke Slagle lecture in 1983, Rogers (32) identified three crucial questions on which the therapist should focus (Box 14-3). These questions form the core concerns of the clinical reasoning process and current today.

The first question, What is the person's status?, is evaluative. Before the therapist begins to think about intervention goals and outcomes and methods, he or she must develop an understanding of who the patient is, what the patient's problems and strengths are, and how strongly motivated for treatment the patient is. The therapist considers the person's engagement in the areas of occupation, his or her performance skills and performance patterns, the contexts in which the occupation occur, and any pertinent client factors that may be obstacles or supports. The therapist manages and coordinates data gathering and evaluation to create an occupational profile and obtain information to answer questions about the client's occupational performance. This is not a random process; the therapist selects from among the many assessments available the ones most likely to yield useful results. The selection is based in part

**BOX 14-3**

### THE FOCUS OF CLINICAL INQUIRY

First question: What is the patient's status?
- What is the patient's occupational role status?
- What problems does he or she have?
- What strengths does he or she possess?
- What is he or she motivated to try?

Second question: What are the available options?
- What approaches are available?
- What outcomes are predicted for each of these? What results can we expect?
- How much time is needed to reach the objectives using each of these approaches?

Third question: What ought to be done?
- Which options are consistent with this patient's values?
- Has the patient been informed of the consequences of different treatment options and been allowed to choose among them?

Adapted with permission from Rogers JC. Clinical reasoning: The ethics, science, and art [Eleanor Clarke Slagle Lecture]. Am J Occup Ther 1983;37:601–616.

upon facts about the person's age, sex, diagnosis, history, and current and past occupational roles. The therapist knows instantly, for example, that a successful 33-year-old lawyer admitted with a diagnosis of manic episode is not likely to need an ADLs evaluation but that a 33-year-old homeless person with a 15-year history of schizophrenia probably will. The more coherent and organized the therapist's knowledge of occupational therapy theory and methods and the more experience he or she has with psychiatric patients in general and with this type of patient in particular, the more efficient and focused the evaluation is likely to be.

To arrive at an answer to the second question, What are the available options?, the therapist must search his or her memory for knowledge and experience that relates in any way to the patient's problem. This includes thoughts about occupational therapy theory and techniques acquired through basic or continuing education or in clinical practice or through reading journal articles or talking with or observing other professionals. The therapist thinks about previous patients who were similar to this one, considers the outcome of the treatment they received, and tries to imagine how that treatment might work with this person. The therapist also takes into account the person's environmental context. What supports are available? How might they help or hinder the person's ability to function? Ultimately the therapist generates a mental list of all possible treatments that might address this patient's problems.

The third question, What ought to be done?, focuses on the ethical aspects of treatment. As Rogers (32) states, "Simply because a goal appears technically feasible for the patient does not mean that it should be set as a goal". The patient has a right to self-determination, a right to design his or her own life as he or she deems best.

The notion that through human occupation each person becomes what he or she does and by doing shapes his or her own identity has always been at the core of occupational therapy (12). In other words, the patient should select his or her own treatment goals, and these may conflict with those the therapist would choose. Ultimately, the patient has a right to refuse treatment. Professional ethics oblige the therapist to try to persuade the patient to accept a treatment that the therapist knows or suspects will improve the person's condition or without which the patient's condition will deteriorate. This does not mean that the patient will accept the plan or can be made to do so. Whatever we may feel about society's obligation to persons with mental illness, legal and constitutional protections guarantee them the right to refuse treatment when they are not an immediate danger to themselves or others.

## Using Multiple Reasoning Tracks

Several studies have attempted to specify and examine in detail the reasoning processes of experienced occupational therapists (9, 10, 13, 14, 18, 19, 23–29, 33, 35, 36, 38). Fleming (14) suggests that experienced therapists shift easily among three reasoning tracks: procedural, interactive, and conditional. *Procedural reasoning* applies to the disability and the treatment options. For example, thoughts about the patient's diagnosis of schizophrenia, its long-term implications of diminished functioning, and the possible treatment interventions (e.g., sensory integration, psychosocial club) are considered procedural.

*Interactive reasoning* applies to understanding and relating to the patient as an individual. This reasoning track focuses on the relationship with the patient, with communicating receptivity, and with acceptance for his or her needs and concerns.

*Conditional reasoning* includes the larger context, the "what if" brainstorming of events that might change the current conditions and the need for the patient to participate. This involves the use of imagination to create mental scenarios of what might happen if a given approach were tried, to create a picture of what the patient's life might have been like before the onset of illness, and to see a future vision of what is possible for the patient.

Creating a vision includes sharing the vision. Hope motivates patients, and part of the therapist's job is to cultivate hope. Mattingly (23) describes the use of *narrative reasoning*, which involves telling a story that will capture interest and spark confidence in the patient. This may require the creation of a context in which boring and repetitive tasks can be put into a meaningful context in terms of a life story, for example. Another way to nurture optimism and motivation is to link the present task specifically and concretely to a future vision of the person's life.

And there are other aspects of clinical reasoning. Schell and Cervero (35) described *pragmatic reasoning*, which is about getting things done, thinking through problems that might arise and finding efficient strategies to take care of details. An example is the OTA keeping a pad of sticky notes in her pocket so that she can leave a note on the mirror in a resident's room to advise morning nursing staff that the resident should be encouraged to dress herself (22).

Clinical reasoning is a continual process. The therapist is constantly generating ideas about what should be assessed and how, what intervention methods are possible, and which ones to choose. This continues from the moment the person is first referred until discharge (and often longer in the therapist's mind). The occupational therapy assistant collaborates with the therapist in this process of clinical inquiry by helping to gather data, generate intervention alternatives, and recommend intervention choices based on knowledge of the person's needs and values. The depth and breadth of clinical reasoning expands when OT and OTA collaborate. Although not ultimately responsible for the intervention plan, the assistant attempts, like the therapist, to observe the patient carefully and objectively, to formulate questions and hypotheses, and to develop intervention options.

### Role of the OT Assistant

The role of the occupational therapy assistant in the clinical reasoning process has only recently been addressed in the literature (22). In a single case report on the activities of an occupational therapy assistant with 16 years in mental health practice, the authors found that the OTA engaged in exactly the same kinds of reasoning just described: procedural, interactive, conditional, narrative, and pragmatic. The assistant is close to the patient in the treatment situation and for this reason often has access to information not available to staff who spend less time with the patient. The assistant is most likely to have a different, perhaps more complete, version of the patient's story based on numerous meetings and much time spent together. Often the assistant is viewed by the patient as less threatening and on a more nearly equal level in contrast to the authoritative position accorded other staff. This perceived equalization of status may engage the patient to share information he or she might withhold (intentionally or not) from the therapist, doctor, or social worker. For the same reason, suggestions made by the assistant are taken a little differently by the patient and may be more easily accepted and enacted. Occupational therapy assistants should recognize, cultivate, and tap their power to clarify and contribute to the clinical reasoning process.

## EVIDENCE-BASED PRACTICE

Related to clinical reasoning is the concept of *evidence-based practice,* the reasoned and judicious use of the best evidence to select interventions to meet specific clinical needs (34). This is a professional effort to provide the most authoritative answers to the questions that every patient and therapist asks: What is the best treatment? How can I decide between different treatment approaches? What can I expect to get from this treatment? And what are the risks and benefits? Evidence comes in many forms, from large reviews of the literature on a topic, to recommendations of a senior therapist based on years of experience.

The highest level of evidence comes from meta-analyses and systematic reviews. A meta-analysis combines data from several similar research studies to analyze the results with larger groups of people. A systematic review is a presentation of information from many studies of a topic done according to the randomized controlled trial standard.

The next level of evidence is the randomized controlled trial (RCT). In an RCT, the participants of a study are assigned randomly to either the experimental group (that receives the target intervention) or the control group (that receives some other intervention or none at all). Random assignment reduces bias in interpreting results and also prevents selection bias. Selection bias occurs when the researcher assigns participants to groups according to how well they are likely to do.

The fourth level of evidence consists of research studies that do not meet the standard of an RCT. Such studies may suggest directions for further research but are considered weak evidence because of possible bias.

The lowest level of evidence is expert opinion. Expert opinion is plentiful in a field such as occupational therapy, in which many methods are traditional and based on past practice and the recommendations of generations of past therapists. In the absence of other higher level evidence, expert opinion is still deemed useful and authoritative.

However, many occupational therapy scholars have been working diligently since the 1990s to put together resources for occupational therapy practitioners to locate and skillfully use higher levels evidence (1, 7, 8, 21). A group of occupational therapists in Australia have developed a database to catalog studies relevant to occupational therapy that provide evidence of effectiveness. The database, known as OTseeker (Occupational Therapy Systematic Evaluation of Evidence) is available on the Web at www.OTseeker.com and gives occupational therapy practitioners access to a range of studies that may be useful in choosing or recommending various approaches (7). A Web-based tutorial explains how to conduct a search. By looking on OTseeker, the OTA may be able to find answers to clinical questions. Using research evidence can inform practice decisions for all aspects of patient care, even the therapeutic relationship (37).

Finally, OTs and OTAs can provide evidence of the effectiveness of interventions by documenting outcomes carefully, by publishing reports on their work (including single case reports), by combining their efforts with other therapists to enlarge the number of participants, and by engaging in systematic research.

## SUMMARY

This chapter presents the intervention process as sequential, with eight discrete stages. In practice these stages overlap at times, as the therapist and assistant explore various options for understanding and helping the patient. Using clinical reasoning, we try to understand the person's problems from his or her point of view. We try to learn how he or she sees things and to envision the world as the patient would like to have it, even if he or she is not ready to see it clearly. We mentally review the various possibilities for treatment approaches and try to imagine how the patient might react. This requires a back-and-forth process of gathering new data even while we are proceeding with interventions planned on the basis of data previously collected. In this sense, intervention is not so much like a path with a clear-cut beginning and end but more like an expanding network of possibilities that we explore together with the patient. When possible, we seek and use the best research evidence to inform our decisions and to communicate options to the patient.

## REVIEW QUESTIONS AND ACTIVITIES

1. Briefly state the purpose of occupational therapy.
2. State the five big ideas of the process section of the *Occupational Therapy Practice Framework (OTPF)*. Explain each.
3. List the eight stages in the occupational therapy process.
   - Describe what happens in each stage.
   - Overall, what are the responsibilities of the OT and the OTA in the process?
4. What is the purpose of screening?
5. What are the two main aspects of evaluation? And how does the OTA contribute to evaluation?
6. Define these terms: *outcome, baseline,* and *prognosis.*
7. Describe three different approaches for occupational therapy intervention and describe how they differ.
8. How are short-term goals and long-term goals related to each other? How are they related to outcomes?
9. Describe the role of the OTA in planning intervention.
10. Why is it important for the patient to understand the purpose of treatment? How can the OTA help a patient remember the purposes of treatment?
11. Explain what is meant by a *client-centered, occupation-centered, outcome-oriented process?*
12. State some of the purposes or uses of outcomes data.
13. How does the therapist relate theory and practice model to intervention?
14. What three questions does Rogers believe are at the center of the clinical reasoning process?
15. Contrast the following types of clinical reasoning: procedural, interactive, conditional, narrative, and pragmatic.
16. What is evidence-based practice?
17. What are some sources of evidence and how are they ranked?
18. What is OTseeker?
19. *Computer activity:* go to www. OTseeker. com and complete the tutorial. Then, with a small group of classmates (two to four students in a group) formulate a question. Each student then uses OTseeker to locate articles of interest. Group members compare notes on what they have learned and each group reports back to the class.

## REFERENCES


1. Abreu BC, Chang P. Getting started in evidence-based practice. OT Practice 2002;8(19):CE–8.
2. American Occupational Therapy Association. Guidelines for supervision, roles, and responsibilities during the delivery of occupational therapy services. Am J Occup Ther 2004;58: 663–667.
3. American Occupational Therapy Association. Occupational therapy practice framework: Domain and process. Am J Occup Ther 2002;56:609–639.
4. American Occupational Therapy Association. Roles and responsibilities of the occupational therapist and the occupational therapy assistant during the delivery of occupational therapy services. OT Practice 2002;7(15):9–10.
5. American Occupational Therapy Association. Standards of practice for occupational therapy. Am J Occup Ther 2005;59:663–665.
6. Babiss F. An ethnographic study of mental health treatment and outcomes: Doing what works. Occup Ther Ment Health 2002;18(3–4):1–146.
7. Bennett S, Hoffmann T, McCluckey A, et al. Introducing OTseeker (Occupational Therapy Systematic Evaluation of Evidence): A new evidence database for occupational therapists. Am J Occup Ther 2003;57:635–638.
8. Chiu T. Evidence-based practice forum—Learning from evidence: Service outcomes and client satisfaction with occupational therapy home-based services. Am J Occup Ther 2002;56:217–220.
9. Cohn ES. Clinical reasoning: Explicating complexity. Am J Occup Ther 1991;45:969–971.
10. Crepeau EB. Achieving intersubjective understanding: Examples from an occupational therapy treatment session. Am J Occup Ther 1991;45:1016–1025.
11. Fahl MA. Mental illness and family involvement. Am Occup Ther Assoc Ment Health Special Sect Q Newslett 1996;10(3):1–2.
12. Fidler GS, Fidler JW. Doing and becoming: Purposeful action and self-actualization. Am J Occup Ther 1978; 32:305–310.
13. Fleming MH. Clinical reasoning in medicine compared with clinical reasoning in occupational therapy. Am J Occup Ther 1991;45:988–996.
14. Fleming MH. The therapist with the three-track mind. Am J Occup Ther 1991;45:1007–1014.
15. Gutman SA, Mortera MH, Hinojosa J, Kramer P. Revision of the occupational therapy practice framework [The Issue Is]. Am J Occup Ther 2007;62:119–126.
16. Heard CP, Greaves M, Doe J. Living the process in psychiatric vocational assessment: A consumer outcome perspective. Occup Ther Ment Health 2000;17(2):20–34.
17. Hinojosa J, Kramer P, Crist P. Evaluation: Obtaining and Interpreting Data. 2nd ed. Bethesda MD: American Occupational Therapy Association Press, 2005.
18. Hooper B. The relationship between pretheoretical assumptions and clinical reasoning. Am J Occup Ther 1997;51: 328–338.
19. Kautzmann LN. Linking patient and family stories to caregivers' use of clinical reasoning. Am J Occup Ther 1993;47: 169–173.
20. Kielhofner G, Hammel J, Finlayson M, et al. Documenting outcomes of occupational therapy: The center for outcomes research and education. Am J Occup Ther 2004;58:15–23.
21. Law M. (ed) Evidence-Based Rehabilitation—A Guide to Practice. Thorofare, NJ: Slack, 2002.
22. Lyons KD, Crepeau EB. The clinical reasoning of an occupational therapy assistant [Case Report]. Am J Occup Ther 2001;55:577–581.
23. Mattingly C. The narrative nature of clinical reasoning. Am J Occup Ther 1991;45:998–1005.
24. Mattingly C. What is clinical reasoning? Am J Occup Ther 1991;45:979–986.
25. Mattingly C, Gillette N. Anthropology, occupational therapy, and action research. Am J Occup Ther 1991; 45: 972–978.
26. Neistadt ME. The classroom as clinic: Applications for a method of teaching clinical reasoning. Am J Occup Ther 1992;46:814–819.
27. Neistadt ME. Teaching clinical reasoning as a thinking frame. Am J Occup Ther 1998;52:221–229.
28. Neistadt ME. Teaching strategies for the development of clinical reasoning. Am J Occup Ther 1996;50: 676–684.
29. Neistadt ME, Wight J, Mulligan SE. Clinical reasoning case studies as teaching tools. Am J Occup Ther 1998;52: 125–132.
30. Pelland MJ. A conceptual model for the instruction and supervision of treatment planning. Am J Occup Ther 1987; 41:351–359.
31. Peloquin SM. Linking purpose to procedure during interactions with patients. Am J Occup Ther 1988;42: 775–781.
32. Rogers JC. Clinical reasoning: The ethics, science, and art [Eleanor Clarke Slagle Lecture]. Am J Occup Ther 1983; 37:601–616.
33. Rogers JC, Holm MB. Occupational therapy diagnostic reasoning: A component of clinical reasoning. Am J Occup Ther 1991;45:1045–1053.
34. Sackett DL, Straus SE, Richardson WS, et al. Evidence-based Medicine—How to Teach and Practice EBM. Edinburgh, UK: Churchill Livingstone, 2000.

35. Schell BA, Cervero RM. Clinical reasoning in occupational therapy: An integrative view. Am J Occup Ther 1993;47: 605–610.
36. Schwartz KB. Clinical reasoning and new ideas on intelligence: Implications for teaching and learning. Am J Occup Ther 1991;45:1033–1037.
37. Tickle-Degnen L. Client-centered practice, therapeutic relationship, and the use of research evidence. Am J Occup Ther 2002;56:470–474.
38. Ward JD. The nature of clinical reasoning with groups: A phenomenological study of an occupational therapist in community mental health. Am J Occup Ther 2003;57:625–635.

CHAPTER 15

# Evaluation and Data Collection

***It is not only by the questions we have answered that progress may be measured, but also by those we are still asking. The passionate controversies of one era are viewed as sterile preoccupations by another, for knowledge alters what we seek as well as what we find.***

FRIEDA ADLER (1)

## CHAPTER OBJECTIVES

After studying this chapter, the reader will be able to:

1. State the purpose of evaluation and explain why skillful and accurate evaluation is important.
2. Define *asset* and *deficit* in relation to occupational functioning.
3. Relate context and pattern to evaluation of occupational performance.
4. Relate the process of evaluation to the client's expected environment.
5. Recognize the responsibilities of the occupational therapist and occupational therapy assistant in evaluation.
6. Describe ways in which information for the occupational profile and the analysis of occupational performance can be obtained.
7. Describe appropriate practices when obtaining information from the medical record and when administering interviews, observations, and assessments.
8. Differentiate between observation and interpretation.
9. Define important concepts related to measurement and standardization.
10. Discuss how one might determine what is an appropriate environment for conducting an assessment or observation.

Evaluation is the foundation of intervention; it supplies the information on which the plan is built. Occupational therapy (OT) practitioners evaluate factors related to occupational performance. They are concerned with how clients are functioning now and how they have functioned in the past. Only when we know the answers to these questions can we begin to consider how we might help them function better in the future. We strive to identify and understand the problems our clients are facing, the goals they envision for themselves, and the resources they possess that might help them. We also consider the contexts of their occupational lives and the constraints and opportunities afforded by these contexts. Our clients are our partners in intervention; by conveying respect and interest, we involve them in all aspects of the process.

This chapter describes the kinds of information occupational therapists (OTs) and occupational therapy assistants (OTAs) collect about persons with mental health problems. The purpose of evaluation and the concepts used to select and organize information will be explored. The roles of the professional practitioner (OT) and technical practitioner (OTA) are outlined and contrasted, with special consideration given to the development of competencies beyond the entry level for the OTA. This chapter explains how to collect data by looking at medical records, observing patients, administering assessments, and interviewing clients and family members. Methods for recording and reporting information are also discussed. Selected occupational therapy interviews and assessments are described in detail, including the purpose of each assessment and how to administer it. Some standardized tests and other less commonly used assessments a OTA might be asked to administer are also described.

## DEFINITION AND PURPOSE OF EVALUATION

Evaluation is the planned process of collecting, interpreting, and documenting information needed to plan intervention (5). This may include observation, interview, review of medical records, and testing. The word *assessment* is used to identify specific tests, instruments, interviews, and other measures used in evaluation (5).

The main purpose of evaluation in psychiatric occupational therapy is to identify clients' goals (what they want to be able to do) and their abilities within the relevant performance contexts. Evaluation aims to identify clients' functional skills in activities of daily living, education, work, play, leisure, and social participation. If they cannot do the things they need and want to do, the occupational therapist wants to know why not; furthermore, the therapist hopes to identify changes or interventions that might make doing possible. Although procedures vary with the setting, the kinds of diagnoses treated, and other factors, in general evaluation seeks to answer the following questions:

- What activities and occupational roles does the person identify as important?
- What is interfering with the client's engagement in these activities and roles?
- What skills and habits are needed to carry out these activities and roles?
- Which of these skills and habits does the person have already?
- Which skills and habits were evident in the past?
- Which skills and habits has the person never developed?
- What are this person's interests? What does this person find motivating?
- To what extent is it possible for this person to develop new skills or redevelop past skills?
- In what contexts will this person live and work and play?
- What aspects of the environment facilitate or interfere with the person's ability to function?
- What environmental modifications, resources, or supports can improve this person's ability to function?
- What has been the effect of the person's illness on functional abilities? What is the person's view of the illness and the medications as they affect ability to function? What is the prognosis?

We could go on listing questions for several more pages, but these summarize the main points. It may be helpful to return to this list later, when you actually participate in an evaluation.

## ASSETS AND DEFICITS

An important purpose of data collection and evaluation is to find out how the person has functioned in the past and is functioning now. We consider what skills the person needs to engage in occupations and to carry out chosen and valued occupational roles. Our understanding of what the person needs and wants to be able to do is the starting point of our evaluation.

To appreciate this point, look at the following descriptions of behavior. Try to decide whether each is an asset (strength) or a deficit (problem behavior). An *asset* is a useful, adaptive behavior, one that helps the client get what he or she needs and carry out daily life activities. A *deficit* is a behavior that interferes with meeting the client's needs and doing the things he or she needs and wants to do.

1. He didn't listen to the directions. He just went ahead on his own.
2. She stared out the window during the lecture.
3. She always wears tailored suits to work.
4. He praised each child who finished the block design puzzles.

How did you classify these behaviors, as assets or as deficits? Do you see them as strengths? Or as problem behaviors? At first consideration, many people would say that the first two are deficits and the second two are assets. But is this always true?

In the first example the man may have already known the directions; in that case, didn't it show initiative for him to proceed on his own? In the second example, isn't it possible that the woman already knew the information in the lecture or that she was thinking over a point the lecturer had made? A woman who wears tailored suits (the third example) would be appropriately dressed for many jobs. That is the way a lawyer, banker, or sales executive is expected to dress. However, dressing this way would make doing the job difficult for a special education teacher or an occupational therapy assistant working with children with multiple handicaps. Similarly, praising a child who has done something well (the fourth example) encourages him or her to keep trying and to do new things and is a useful behavior in a teacher or therapist. However, when testing a child's intelligence, a psychologist is supposed to follow the test instructions exactly and should not add to them or alter them. Praising the child may change the results of the test.

As all of these examples illustrate, a given behavior may be an asset or a deficit, depending upon a person's life situation and occupational and social roles. Of course, some behaviors are almost always deficits, regardless of context. Very poor hygiene and grooming can only interfere with getting along with other people socially and on the job. Other behaviors are almost always assets—for example, cooperating with others. In general, however, we need additional information about the person before we decide which behaviors are deficits and which are assets.

Some facts that can help us understand whether a behavior is an asset or a deficit are the person's age, sex, family situation, education, occupation, work history, leisure habits and history, self-care habits, social relationships, and cultural background. Information about the patient's interests, goals, and values clarifies what is important to that person. Diagnosis, prognosis, and prescribed medications must also be known, because they may affect future abilities.

## CONCEPTS CENTRAL TO THE EVALUATION PROCESS

All of the information we have listed so far consists of many small and interrelated facts, which are sometimes better understood and organized by applying our understanding of aspects of occupational performance identified in the *Occupational Therapy Practice Framework* (*OTPF*) (7): contexts, and patterns. We will begin with contexts.

## Contexts

*Context* or *contexts* describes the conditions that surround and give meaning to occupational functioning (7). Seven aspects of context are recognized: cultural, physical, social, personal, spiritual, temporal, and virtual. The reader's familiarity with these is assumed; readers who require more information should consult the *OTPF* (7).

### Definitions of Contexts

The *cultural context* derives from the larger groups with which a person identifies him or herself. This includes cultural identifiers such as race and ethnicity, family background, beliefs and values, customs, rituals, and traditions. Even when the person self-identifies as a member of a minority group, the cultural context will also include the customs and expectations of the larger society in which the person participates. This might include economic and legal factors (e.g., laws governing public assistance, patients' rights) as well as the general social expectations for individuals to behave in a way that respects the rights and property of others.

The *physical context* includes nonhuman aspects of the environment, such as objects, buildings, structures, natural features, the geography, and the sensory elements of the environment. Examples of elements of the physical context are pets and plants, furniture, tools, housing, public and private transportation, urban or rural aspects, noise, pollution, and natural beauty.

The *social context* concerns other people, groups and organizations with which the person interacts. Obvious examples are relatives, friends, caregivers, and employers. Social groups of which the person may be a member are also included (e.g., exercise class, church, parent–teacher organization). Especially relevant for persons with mental disorders is the *social support* available. Social support is the way in which and the extent to which relationships with other people help the person meet needs and carry out daily activities. For example, the person with chronic schizophrenia who lives with his or her parents in a ranch house in a middle-class suburb has a very different social support system from a person with the same diagnosis who lives in a single-room occupancy hotel in a big city and has no contact with his or her family.

The *personal context* includes such features as age, gender, education, and socioeconomic status. Some aspects of personal context are related to cultural context, in that economic conditions and educational opportunities are associated to some extent with culture.

A person's *spiritual context* includes those things that the person believes give life higher meaning and purpose. This may be a traditional relationship with a personal God through organized religion. Alternately, it may be a dedication to social justice, or a love of fine art and music, or a feeling of communion with nature.

The *temporal context* locates the performance of occupation in time, whether by time of day, time of life, the season, or other time orientation. Included in temporal context are the notions of duration (for how long) and frequency (how often). Also important are life events and crises, such as starting school, leaving home, marriage, death of a spouse (life cycle events). Considering the temporal context helps us appreciate the past, present, and future as the person might envision them. It helps us place the present moment in relation to the person's past and future goals. The person newly diagnosed with major depression and taking antidepressant medication for the first time may see the diagnosis in a very different light from another person who has been depressed for years and has tried a number of different medications.

Some activities and occupations occur within a *virtual context.* Rather than a real-life, here-and-now experience, these activities are performed in association with technology and occur without physical contact. Simulated environments; simulated occupational experiences (such as with a driving simulator); and the use of computers, text messaging, and other forms of telecommunication all represent virtual context experiences.

## Understanding and Applying Contexts

While the seven named contexts have been described as discrete and separate from each other, in reality they overlap and intermix. All aspects of the person's context(s) and their psychological message(s) are considered. This includes *all* of the environments the person passes through or is exposed to in daily life activities.

- Where does the person live? In the city or the country, alone or with other people, in a house or an apartment?
- On a psychological level, is the neighborhood clean, safe, and pleasant or dirty, dangerous, noisy, and frightening?
- Are parks and recreation facilities nearby?
- Does the person live near friends and family or in isolation?
- How much of the neighborhood does the person know and use?
- If the person has a job, what is the work environment like?
- What kinds of environments does the person pass through on the way to and from work?
- Does the person spend a large part of the day in a virtual context (either at work or in leisure hours)?
- How accessible is a spiritual context that is meaningful to that person?

It is important to know the individual's cultural group, because each group has its own values and heritage of "normal" behavior affecting engagement in occupation. For example, a 28-year-old mother of two may be expected to behave differently depending on whether her background is Cuban, Jamaican, Italian, Norwegian, Jewish, or Hindu. Her cultural group membership may dictate whether it is acceptable for her to have a career outside the home, to wear pants, or to go shopping on Saturdays or Sundays. An individual's interests and values may reflect the cultural group or conflict with it. Sometimes the person's family or cultural group pressures him or her into abandoning personal interests and values. We saw this in the case of David (Chapter 2), whose childhood interest in sports and games was discouraged by his parents.

We consider how contexts affect functional performance in terms of the opportunities they provide *and* the demands or constraints they place on the person. For example, a family caregiver may help the person function by setting up a cold meal to be eaten at midday or may interfere by limiting opportunities for the person to perform independently. Legal, political, and economic factors can constrain a person's efforts to function if, for example, eligibility for public medical benefits ends after the person has worked for a while.

The effects of context on ability to function cannot be overstated. One way to understand this is to consider how your life would be different if your contexts changed. What if you moved your home to a different location? How would you travel to school? What would you do in your spare time, with whom and where? How far would you have to walk to the grocery store, dry-cleaner, handball court, swimming pool, park, museum, or church? Would you be able to keep in touch with your old friends? Where and how would you meet new ones?

Context influences what you are able to do and what you *have* to do. For example, some people who live in cities prefer not to own automobiles, arguing that cars use energy, emit air pollution, and contribute to global warming. But if they lived elsewhere, they might have to buy a car just to get around. If the nearest supermarket is 8 miles away and there is no public transportation, there really is not much choice. Valuing the environment so much that you refuse to drive a car would be a deficit. Many behaviors that are assets in one situation are deficits in another, and vice versa.

Watanabe (67) points out that occupational therapy practitioners should consider the extent to which the person makes use of available opportunities. For example, the person who stays indoors, watching television and playing computer games most of the time and venturing out only to do routine and predictable chores, is using very little of the available contexts. The person's world becomes small; nearby social and recreational opportunities are ignored. Similarly, someone who has a computer but does not learn to use it will miss the chance to have real-time online video chat with grandchildren in a distant state.

## Patterns

Along with the performance context, we also need to know about the person's *performance patterns.* What are the person's habits, routines, and roles? How does the person budget time among different activities? How much does he or she sleep or watch television? Does he or she schedule time for leisure and play activities? How much time does he or she spend on self-care and home-making? The way time is allocated among activities is only one aspect of patterns. How and why the person pursues each activity are equally important, as the following example illustrates:

**CASE EXAMPLE**

Ms. F., an architect, is at the top of her field. Her designs have won top honors in major competitions. Ms. F.'s major leisure interest is tennis. She is an excellent player and frequently wins local tournaments. She follows a daily exercise program to train and develop her muscles for tennis. She says she wishes she could see more of her friends and family but her schedule won't permit it.

Ms. F. seems to work as hard in her "leisure" as she does in her job. Both are highly competitive and stressful. She seems to thrive on this, and Ms. F.'s drive and discipline are assets to her in both areas. There isn't much variety in her activities, however. Everything seems to revolve around work and tennis. Ms. F. would probably feel a failure in either area very deeply, because she has nothing to balance them. Consider, for example, how Ms. F. might react to an automobile injury that leaves her dominant side partially paralyzed.

Remember that habits can be classified as useful, impoverished, or dominating. Persons with severe chronic mental illness generally have some habits that are impoverished, often in the areas of routine activities of daily living (ADLs) and time use. Poor housing and limited finances contribute to impoverishment of habits. But, in Ms. F's case, her use of tennis might be seen as a dominating habit because it interferes with other aspects of daily life, such as seeing friends.

## Expected Environment

In addition to general background information, occupational roles, performance context, social support, and performance patterns, it is very important to know where an inpatient will be going after discharge. This is sometimes called the *expected environment* (54). Only a few inpatients are transferred to another inpatient facility. Others go home or to halfway houses, board and care homes, single-room occupancy hotels, community residences, or supervised apartments. When the expected environment is different from the previous environment, the contexts for performance change. For this reason, the person may need to develop new skills or refine or modify the way everyday activities are done. Someone who will be living independently for the first time, even in a supervised apartment, will need to be able to care for clothing, budget money, and manage other self-care tasks.

To summarize, the main purpose of evaluation is to assess to what extent the person is able to carry out daily life activities and occupational roles with a sense of purpose, pleasure, and competence. Which of the present behaviors are assets and which are deficits can be determined only when the individual's contexts, social support, patterns, and expected environment are considered.

## AREAS FOR DATA COLLECTION

Whether using an interview, an observation, or a specific assessment instrument, the occupational therapy assistant will collect information with a specific focus, as directed by the OT. Any one area (or several areas) may be the focus. Here is a brief overview of the possibilities:

Areas of occupation

- Activities of daily living (hygiene, grooming, eating, dressing, functional mobility)
- Instrumental activities of daily living (care of children or family member, managing finances, community mobility, health and safety routines, homemaking and household management, preparing and cleaning up after meals)
- Educational activities (performing activities related to school, such as taking notes and doing homework, exploring educational options)
- Work activities (looking for work, and performing adequately on the job in aspects such as neatness, attention to detail, rate of performance; also, planning for retirement and making the transition to retirement)
- Play and/or leisure activities (exploring and participating, knowing what is available and making use of available resources)
- Social participation (interacting with others in the community, in the family, in peer relationships)

Performance skills

- Process skills (being aware and paying attention to what is happening, staying organized in time, staying organized in space, adapting to change)
- Communication and interaction skills (relating to other people, exchanging information, using and interpreting nonverbal behavior consistent with the social group)
- Motor skills (maintaining posture appropriate to tasks; moving self and objects; demonstrating sufficient strength, coordination, and energy)

Performance patterns

- Habits (degree to which behavior has become automatic, and whether the pattern is useful, impoverished, or dominating)
- Routines
- Roles

Contexts

- Cultural, physical, social, personal, spiritual, temporal, and virtual contexts
- How the context(s) support or interfere with the person's occupational goals

Client factors

- Global and specific mental functions (orientation, energy, memory, logic)
- Emotional functions (self-control, range of feelings expressed, coping strategies)
- Psychosocial and psychological skills (self-expression, self-control, ability to relate to others individually or in a group)
- Emotional functions and experience of self (self-control, range of feelings expressed, coping strategies, body image, self-esteem)
- Sensory functions (hearing, seeing)
- Other client factors (movement related, cardiovascular, respiratory, skin)

## ROLES OF THE OT AND THE OTA

The roles of the OT and the OTA during evaluation are interrelated and complementary. The OT initiates, manages, guides, and documents the evaluation and has final responsibility for obtaining and interpreting the information needed to plan treatment. The OT decides what information is needed and how to obtain it (9). The OTA contributes to the evaluation under the OT's supervision.

## The OT is the Manager of Evaluation

The OT starts the evaluation and identifies the areas to be evaluated (9). Although the *OTPF* (7) suggests that evaluation should begin with the *occupational profile* and the *analysis of occupational performance,* in many situations the OT will begin elsewhere. Several occupational therapy scholars have argued that a bottom-up or environment-first evaluation is appropriate in many situations (28, 35, 68). This is in contrast to the occupational profile and analysis of occupational performance, which are top-down. What do these terms mean?

*Top-down evaluation* begins with the client's goals. No other data are collected until the client's perspective is understood. The occupational profile is a clear example of this.

*Bottom-up evaluation* begins with the factors that appear to impede occupational engagement. An example in a burn unit is the assessment of wounds and the need for specific splinting to prevent contractures. Clearly in this case, the medical necessity cannot wait for an interview to learn the client's goals. In a psychiatric setting, the assessment of cognitive level would represent a bottom-up evaluation.

*Environment-first evaluation* is appropriate when safety is a factor, as for example when assessing the home environment for an elderly client to reduce risk of falls.

The therapist using a top-down approach will first obtain information to complete the *occupational profile.* Interviews, questionnaires, and casual conversation can provide background on the person's occupational history and interests, experiences, and goals. The *analysis of occupational performance* would be done once the therapist has a sense of the person's goals and problems. Analysis of occupational performance may require the therapist to use one or more assessments or other measures to, for example, identify the performance problems related to housework, homemaking, and cooking or dressing, hygiene, and ADLs. Problems with occupational performance may be present in any of the areas: activities of daily living, work, education, play, leisure, and social participation.

If warranted, the top-down approach would then proceed to assessment of performance skills, patterns, and contexts as well as client factors. Some performance skills that are particularly relevant in psychiatric practice are process skills and communication skills. Motor skills may be impaired by adverse effects of medications. In some cases, the therapist would look at client factors related to mental processes (e.g., attention span, memory, sequencing) and emotional controls (e.g., social conduct, values, coping skills). Other areas may be assessed, depending on the theory or practice model the therapist is following. For example, in the model of human occupation, more than 60 different assessments are available to examine factors as diverse as the person's locus of control (sense of self-control versus control by others or by fate) and environmental press (degree and kind of stimulation and demands from the environment). Individuals who have, or who are suspected to have, physical limitations should be evaluated in these areas too.

Another factor that affects the way in which the OT approaches evaluation is the constant change in regulations from regulators and insurers. For example, Transmittal 63 from the Centers for Medicare and Medicaid Services (CMS) requires that the evaluator use one of four specified performance measures (none of which is specific to occupational therapy) or another functional assessment measure that has been published in the peer-reviewed literature, or another documented method to define the patient's functional status. This information is required so that progress toward goals can be measured, specifically in relation to the environment the person will be going to after this episode of care (4). OTs and OTAs must stay current as regulations change, in order to optimize the quality of patient care and maintain reimbursement of services.

The OT chooses the methods to be used in evaluation and explains the evaluation plan to the client, to the family (when relevant), and to other health professionals involved with the client. The OT may conduct functional assessments that require special training, such as the *Assessment of Motor and Process Skills* (*AMPS*), which measures a person's motor skills and organizational abilities as revealed in familiar household tasks (27).

The OT may perform all of the assessments or may assign some to the OTA. Before assigning any part of the evaluation to the OTA, the therapist must feel confident that the OTA is skilled in the particular assessment and would obtain the same or very similar results to what the OT would obtain with that instrument. This is known as *establishing service competency* (6, 8). Service competency can be established by using standardized or criterion-referenced tests and comparing the results obtained by the OTA with those obtained by the OT. (A criterion-referenced test provides clear descriptions of performance for each rating.) Another way to establish service competency is to have raters view and rate the same videotaped performance. The OT is responsible for the evaluation and for assisting the OTA to develop service competency in areas that will be delegated. The OTA is responsible for acquiring service competency in a given instrument before undertaking independent use of the instrument. The OTA may help the OT to identify instruments for which he or she could easily develop service competency, given sufficient training.

When the evaluation is completed, the OT organizes, analyzes, and interprets the information. Summarizing the person's occupational performance problems and goals and making note of particular assets (strengths) and deficits (problems), the OT writes an initial evaluation note, which becomes part of the medical record. Because the evaluation is the foundation of intervention planning, it is extremely important that it be accurate and complete. In inpatient settings, very short lengths of stay limit the time available for evaluation; more thorough evaluation may be possible in outpatient settings, where consumers may be seen over a longer period.

### The OTA Assists in Evaluation

The OTA collects data as directed by the OT (6, 8, 9). The OT determines the methods and procedures to be used. Experienced OTAs with established service competency may be given more responsibility for selecting evaluation methods and specific assessments in some areas, such as activities of daily living. Assessments administered by the OTA should be structured; each should have a definite procedure and be performed the same way each time it is administered. The OTA collects information, administers assessments and interviews, and records observations and results. The OTA then organizes this information and reports it to the OT, who is responsible for analyzing and interpreting the information. The report may be oral or written, depending on the requirements of the setting. Finally, the OTA may be assigned to record this information in the medical chart or report it to other professionals working with the client.

## THE OTA'S METHODS OF DATA COLLECTION

The OTA may obtain information by review of medical records, by interview, by administering checklists or questionnaires, by observation or by administering tests and assessments.

### Review of Medical Records

The OTA may be asked to collect some or all of the following information about a person: age, gender, family situation, education, occupation, work history, leisure habits and history, self-care habits, social relationships, cultural background, diagnosis, medical history, psychiatric history, current medications, and medication history. Looking in the medical record is one quick and reasonably accurate way to obtain this information. In inpatient settings, the chart is kept at the nursing station. Many people use the charts, and so they are not always available, especially in short-term settings. The OTA also has to cooperate in sharing charts with other staff. Charts should not be removed from the nursing station unless specific permission is given by the nurse in charge.

Many medical charts are divided into sections; this aids in locating facts because the reader can review just the pertinent sections. The information an assistant is assigned to collect is often found in the admitting note and the social worker's history. Written by the person who admits the patient to the hospital or outpatient clinic, the admitting note summarizes the details about why the person was admitted, his or her behavior and symptoms at the time of admission; the tentative diagnosis; any known medical or psychiatric history; and age, sex, occupation, and family background. The social worker's history will include more details about the patient's family and occupation, education, cultural background, financial situation, and habits. In inpatient and residential care settings, the nurses' notes over the past few days give information about how the person has functioned and adjusted (such as whether the patient is sleeping, eating, and socializing with others). The doctor's notes may indicate changes in diagnosis or medication. Records from past treatments, including hospitalizations, if available, often yield more detail about the person's history and the success of various previous treatments. Reports on psychological and neurological testing, if available, can be valuable also; often these are read by the therapist rather than the assistant. Any occupational therapy notes or goals or evaluation information from previous admissions may provide details that will prevent needless repetition of past procedures.

The OT who assigns the assistant to gather data from the patient's chart will specify what information is needed. For example, the OT might want to know only the education, work history, and previous living situation. In general, when assigned to find specific information, the assistant should ignore everything else, regardless of how interesting it is (e.g., that the patient believes he is a CIA agent). However, the OTA should stay alert for information that might help the OT with the patient's evaluation and treatment plan (e.g., that the patient's four most recent admissions occurred after he ran out of his medication). Any information about precautions (dietary, medical, suicide, or elopement risk) should always be noted.

## Interviewing

Besides looking in the medical record, the other way to collect information is to interview the patient or a family member or other person who is close to the patient. An interview is a conversation whose purpose is to find out more about the patient. Various types of information may be sought, including the person's self-care habits and skills, academic history, vocational history, play history, social skills, interpersonal relationships, occupational roles, and leisure interests and experiences.

Interviewing cannot be learned by reading a book. The best ways to learn interviewing are to watch someone who is good at it, analyze the process, and try it yourself. It helps to practice in school with classmates and friends, to listen to feedback from others, and to have yourself videotaped so that you can see how you come across. Some concepts of communication in the therapeutic relationship were discussed in Chapter 10. These are meant to be a foundation for all phases of the treatment process, starting with screening and evaluation. It will help to review these concepts before attempting your first interview.

specific time of day?



All of the interviews the assistant will be assigned to conduct are structured or semistructured. Both types of interviews consist of sets of questions to be asked in a given order. In a structured interview, the interviewer is supposed to ask questions in the exact order they are given. In a semistructured interview, the questions may be rephrased and more questions added. The purpose of this is to get more details and more information. During the training phase in which you establish service competency, you will learn whether you can change the wording or add or skip questions.

You may be asked to give the interview to someone other than the patient (e.g., the operator of the community residence where the patient lives). Some consumers may not give accurate information, may not be able to assess their own behavior objectively, may not remember necessary facts, or may not be willing to tell the truth. Someone else may be a more reliable informant. A *reliable informant* is someone who knows the situation, can think and communicate, and is willing to talk. It makes sense to get the information from someone who is willing and able to give it.

## Preparing for the Interview

Prepare for the interview by selecting a comfortable environment. The room should be private, quiet, and well ventilated; have comfortable seating; and be free of distracting stimuli. Be sure to consider general safety precautions about being alone with clients and having help available. The interviewer should have the interview form, pencils or pens, and a watch or clock and should set aside enough time to cover the information in the interview. The amount of time needed depends on the number of questions and the attention span of the person being interviewed. The interviewer should review the medical record to find any facts that pertain to the interview. The person should not be asked to provide the same information twice unless there is a good reason for it.

## Making the Client Comfortable

The interviewer should pay attention to what the person is saying; the interviewer's behavior and body language should communicate this listening attitude. The interviewer who is physically relaxed, seated comfortably, and able to move freely will be more comfortable and thus more receptive to the interviewee. Making eye contact with the person and leaning forward to show interest also convey receptivity. Eye contact should be varied, and one should avoid staring. The OTA should make an effort to understand cultural preferences and meanings of nonverbal behavior. For example, some people are made uncomfortable by direct face-to-face orientation and are more at ease when the interviewer is seated at an angle or at the side. Similarly, sustained eye contact may be viewed as intrusive, rude, or disrespectful. And, in some cultures, having members of the extended family present is important.

One of the hardest interviewing skills to develop is knowing when to comment and what to say. It helps to think of the client as telling a story that really interests you. Then your comments and questions will flow naturally. Try not to change the subject or interrupt while the person is speaking. Remember that periods of silence may help the client collect his or her thoughts.

Being aware of yourself helps you be a better interviewer. Try to be in touch with what you are communicating and what you are feeling about the client. Any prejudices you have about the person will impair your ability to listen. If, for example, you believe that the person is unmotivated and annoying, you may not be open to focusing on the person's strengths. Or if you think the client is too smart or too rich or too good looking to have any problems, you may miss some real problems that interfere with functioning.

## Beginning the Interview

Start any interview by saying hello and introducing yourself if you do not already know the person.

* sometimes private rooms aren't available

Always explain the purpose of the interview. Think of it from the interviewee's point of view. It is hard to share painful or shameful or difficult things. Make the person comfortable before you start asking questions. Shaw (64) presents the following contrasting situations at the beginning of an interview:

- The client enters the office; you remain seated, waving the client to a chair. You then begin to question him about his work history.
- The client is waiting in the clinic; the therapist approaches and introduces himself. The therapist invites the client into the office and suggests that he might be comfortable in a particular chair. The therapist opens by explaining the purpose of the interview (64, p. 28).

Obviously, the second situation is more likely to make people comfortable and help them talk. Imagining yourself in the client's position can help you figure out what to do.

### Obtaining and Remembering Information

The next stage in the interview is to ask for specific information. This part of the interview is most successful if the interviewer embodies the techniques and qualities described in Chapter 10. One should be especially observant of the client's behavior, facial expression, tone of voice, and body language. More detail on what and how to observe is given later in this chapter.

During the interview, you will need to take notes; try to keep them to a minimum, jotting down only key facts and phrases. Allot some time for yourself after the interview to go back and fill in the missing information; be sure to complete the information as soon as possible after the interview so that details are not forgotten. Discuss with the client the fact that you have to take notes to be accurate about important details.

Peloquin (60) recommends that the interviewer use part of the time to help the patient develop a *therapy set,* an understanding of occupational therapy generally and how it will benefit the patient specifically. For example, the depressed homemaker who has had difficulty getting things done might be told that the activity program in the hospital will help her become accustomed to a routine and give her opportunities to learn new ways of doing things or to practice old ones. The OTA should follow the direction of the therapist in regard to helping patients develop a therapy set.

### Ending the Interview

End the interview by indicating that the time is up or that the interview is complete; this is easiest if you prepare the person at the beginning of the interview by explaining how long the interview will take. It is not always easy to bring an interview to a close; the person may keep talking and you don't want to be rude and interrupt. Let the person know that you appreciate the information that has been provided. Encourage the person to ask you questions and try to answer them. Do not try to interpret or analyze the interview; tell the person that you and the OT need time to review the information. Set a time for your next meeting, if there is to be one, or inform the person about what will happen next (the patient will see the OT or attend an evaluation group, for example).

## Questionnaires and Checklists

Another type of structured assessment is a questionnaire or checklist that the client completes independently and later discusses with the therapist. The OTA is often assigned to give out questionnaires and collect completed ones. The assistant should treat questionnaires just like any other structured assessment and should not add to or change the directions or help the client interpret them, unless this is part of the standard procedure.

## Observation

Observation is a method of collecting information by watching what a person does. It goes on throughout the intervention process; we are constantly watching and listening to the client, from the moment we first meet him or her. Of all of the skills the OTA needs, observation is perhaps the most critical. We base our ideas and plans on what we observe; therefore, we must learn to observe accurately and uncritically.

To observe clearly, one must distinguish between observation and interpretation or inference. *Observation* is the process of taking note of behavior or anything else we can take in through our senses. We *see* what the client does, we *hear* what he or she says; these are observations. *Interpretation* or *inference* is the process of giving meaning to what we have observed. Why the client did something, how what the client said relates to other things we know about him or her—these are inferences and interpretations.

One quick way to differentiate between an observation and an inference or interpretation is to examine the words that are used. Observations usually include action words (verbs) that describe what the person did. Inferences and interpretations usually contain opinion or value words. Keeping this distinction in mind, identify whether the following descriptions are observations:

- She traced the pattern after lifting it up several times and looking underneath.
- She was hostile to the patient who passed her the glue.
- She didn't want to finish the project.

If you paid attention to the words, you probably realized that only the first is an observation; it describes what the patient did. Another person watching the patient would be able to agree that this is what happened. The second description contains an opinion word: *hostile.* We cannot tell from this description what the patient actually did. Did she glare, clench her teeth, or snatch the bottle away? Can we be sure that the patient was indeed hostile? Or was she perhaps indifferent, frightened, or suspicious? Can you think of specific behaviors that would be conclusive evidence of hostility?

You can probably recognize what is wrong with the third "observation"; it presumes that we can see inside the person's mind. How do we know she did not want to finish the project? Did she say so? If so, this behavior should be part of the description. "The patient said she didn't want to finish the project" *is* an observation, because it reports behavior without interpreting it. It is also perfectly accurate to state as an observation that the patient did not finish the project, if that is the case.

Beginners frequently find observation difficult because there is so much to observe and they do not know what to focus on. This feeling is even more overwhelming when the observation is supposed to be *unstructured* or *naturalistic;* this means that the client is observed while doing something that he or she would be doing anyway—that is, the person is not asked to do something in particular. Box 15-1 provides some categories, descriptive words, and group roles (15) to help guide such unstructured observations. The list is by no means comprehensive or exhaustive. The careful reader will note that opinion words occur on the list; these should be used cautiously, only when the observer is certain they are valid.

Whether to take notes while observing has been debated countless times; notes can capture details that might otherwise be forgotten, but other details may be missed while the observer is writing. The role of the observer during an observation is to observe: to watch, listen, and sense what is going on. Preparation, paperwork, and note taking should be done before or after the observation, not during it. It is impossible to observe well when your attention is elsewhere.

It is wise to write brief notes for yourself as soon as the observation is over. These notes need not be grammatical or even make sense to anyone but you; their purpose is to jog your memory when you record or report them formally later on.

BOX 15-1

## GUIDE TO OBSERVING AND DESCRIBING BEHAVIOR

General Appearance
- Clean, neat, appropriately dressed
- Fastidious, meticulous
- Dramatic, theatrical
- Looks younger than stated age
- Bizarre dress or makeup
- Inappropriate dress
- Disheveled, stained clothing
- Noticeable body odor

Physical Behaviors
- Relaxed, at ease
- Restless, overactive
- Agitated
- Slow, listless, inactive
- Formal, stiff, reserved
- Appears tense or uncomfortable
- Shuffling gait
- Hesitating or uneven gait
- Grimaces or has facial tics
- Postures
- Drools
- Expectorates (spits)
- Incontinent
- Masturbates
- Smokes incessantly
- Rocks self
- Scratches or rubs self
- Makes repetitive movements
- Makes odd movements
- Bites nails
- Chain smokes
- Always drinking coffee

Attitude toward OTA
- Seeks assistance when appropriate
- Seeks approval
- Rejects attention from assistant
- Ignores therapy assistant
- Does not follow instructions
- Ingratiates self
- Combative, argumentative
- Tests limits
- Relates to therapist but not peers
- Relates to peers but not therapist

Described Sensations
- Has odd sensations
- Feels familiar things to be new
- Feels new things to be familiar
- Does not feel like self
- Surroundings don't look real
- Feels numb all over
- Reports distorted sense of time
- Reports body seems strange to self
- Reports hearing things not there
- Reports seeing things not there
- Reports strange odors

Attitude
- Helpful, cooperative
- Seems pleasant but obstructs
- Demands attention or praise
- Makes excuses for own actions
- Blames others for problems
- Contemptuous
- Rigid, not flexible
- Seems self-centered
- Appears indifferent
- Antagonistic
- Appears bored
- Appears resentful
- Seems suspicious
- Makes negative remarks
- Appears timid
- Seems fearful or apprehensive

Communication
- Logical, clear
- Speaks slowly, hesitantly
- Speaks rapidly, speech seems pressured

**BOX 15-1** ***(Continued)***

- Initiates conversation
- Repetitive, perseverative
- Rambles
- Uses vulgar language
- Swears, curses
- Uses words oddly
- Makes up words (neologisms)
- Rhymes
- Speaks in low tone of voice
- Mute
- Speaks only when others initiate
- Loud, boisterous, shouts

Expressed Thoughts

- Dwells on illness or symptoms
- Focuses on here and now
- Dwells on past
- Expresses few thoughts
- Can't make up mind
- Things are hopeless; person is no good
- People are unfair, out to get him or her
- Reports intrusive, unwanted thoughts

Cognitive Behaviors

- Alert, responsive, concentrates well
- Bewildered, confused
- Forgetful
- Seems not to pay attention
- Learns new steps with difficulty
- Easily distracted
- Repeats errors
- Concentrates on details but misses the main point
- Shows good judgment (example?)
- Shows poor judgment (example?)
- Plans actions before acting
- Skips from topic to topic
- Seems dull, slow to respond

Mood and General Disposition

- Difficult to ascertain
- Enthusiastic, excited
- Smooth, even disposition
- Easily upset, irritable
- Tearful
- Shows little reaction or emotion
- Seems ill at ease
- Independent, appears aloof
- Positive attitude (toward . . . ?)
- Negative attitude (toward . . . ?)
- Excessively cheerful, euphoric
- Sad
- Angry
- Anxious, worried
- Constricted, restrained
- Gloomy, pessimistic
- Appears preoccupied
- Mood doesn't fit situation
- Manic

Behavior toward Others

- Polite, well-mannered
- Rude, inconsiderate
- Outgoing, enthusiastic
- Isolates self, withdrawn
- Avoids opposite sex
- Seeks opposite sex exclusively
- Teases
- Behaves seductively
- Monopolizes one person's attention
- Hangs back, seems timid
- Is a member of a clique

Skills

- Good eye–hand coordination
- Clumsy, awkward
- Artistically creative
- Good verbal skills
- Skilled with machine or tool (specify)
- Good with spatial relations
- Good social skills
- Good vocabulary
- Good gross motor coordination
- Mechanically skillful

*(continued)*

**BOX 15-1 *(Continued)***

Participation
- Attends regularly
- Often absent
- Arrives late, early
- Remains only a short time
- Leaves and then returns
- Socializes but does not participate in activity
- Observes only
- Participates infrequently

Work Behaviors
- Shows initiative; sees work and does it
- Needs explicit instructions on all steps
- Works best alone
- Works directly with others
- Works with one other person
- Accepts criticism
- Rejects criticism
- Seeks out direct supervision
- Seldom completes projects
- Impatient with detail
- Meticulous with detail
- Has realistic view of own efforts and abilities
- Underestimates efforts and abilities
- Overestimates efforts and abilities
- Tenacious, persistent
- Consistent, reliable
- Work shows planning

Roles Patient Assumes in a Group
- Leader
- Follower
- Initiator/contributor
- Information seeker
- Information giver
- Opinion seeker
- Opinion giver
- Evaluator/critic
- Coordinator
- Orienter
- Compromiser
- Harmonizer
- Blocker
- Aggressor
- Observer

List adapted with permission from Buffalo Psychiatric Center, Buffalo, NY. Roles based on Benne KD, Sheats P. Functional roles of group members. J Social Issues 1948;4(2):42–47.

## Tests and Assessments

Many tests and assessments are used throughout occupational therapy practice, and some examples will be highlighted later in the chapter. In general, each test will include a procedural manual with a detailed guide as to how the test is to be administered. Frequently, the test also includes materials, scoring sheets, and other items. The OTA should study the test well in advance of using it and work with someone experienced, so that service competency is ensured. Also, before each use of an assessment, it's prudent to check that no parts are missing, and that all forms and other items are ready to use.

Have everything prepared before the client arrives; this allows for better use of your time with the client and prevents upsetting the client with the delay or raising concerns about your competence, either of which might prejudice the results. Make sure you have recorded all necessary identifying information (e.g., time and date) and that you or the client fill out any required information (e.g., age, sex, medical records number).

Be careful to work within the guidelines of the governmental and other authorities that regulate occupational therapy practice. While many assessments are appropriate for OTA administration, this does not mean in all settings and all situations. The individual OTA should take on only those tasks in which he or she is service competent and that fall within the scope of OTA practice in the particular setting. If you have questions about whether a certain assessment should be an OTA responsibility, be sure to get clarification before proceeding.

## CONCEPTS RELATED TO ASSESSMENT AND MEASUREMENT

The purpose of assessment is to measure. When using assessments, one should know what the assessment is measuring and how well it does so. In this section, we will look briefly at some measurement-related factors. The first regards standardization.

*Standardization* is a way of ensuring accuracy and consistency. In regard to assessments, standardization is generally achieved in relation to normative data or to criteria. Normative data are a collection of data from many administrations of the test or assessment. This means that many people, patients and nonpatients, have been given the assessment and their scores recorded. Working from the scores of this large group, the developers of the assessment predict what the normal range of scores is like. Once the normal range has been identified, the score of a particular individual can be compared with it. An assessment that is *norm referenced* will provide tables of normative data. These data are sometimes skewed by cultural or other bias—for example, if the test has been given only in English or only to literate persons. Normative populations that are dissimilar to the person being assessed may be a poor standard against which to compare that person's results.

The other common method of standardization is by *criteria.* A criterion (singular form of *criteria*) is a standard against which an individual's performance is measured. Tests of reading level, for example, are *criterion referenced.* To appreciate the differences between norm-referenced and criterion-referenced measures, the reader might consider the way grades are awarded in a course. If the course is graded on a curve, then the professor has used a norm-referenced standard, aiming to distribute the scores in a normal distribution. If the professor grades students on their achievement of specific competencies, this is a criterion-referenced standard.

Perhaps the two most important concepts in measurement are reliability and validity. *Reliability* represents the consistency of the results when the test is repeated. *Test–retest reliability* shows the degree of sameness of scores when a test is repeated. *Interrater reliability* shows the degree to which two people giving the test will obtain similar results. Both kinds of validity are useful. Test–etest reliability shows that the test is stable, that what it is measuring and the way in which it is measuring can be trusted to some extent. Interrater reliability allows different evaluators to use the same test and compare results, combine data, and so on.

*Validity* shows the degree to which the test measures what it says it is measuring. Some tests have fairly obvious validity, known as *face validity*—for example, a test of range of motion seems to be a valid measure of the degree to which motion occurs at different joints in an individual. Other tests, such as the Allen Cognitive Level (ACL) test, discussed later in the chapter, claim to measure something that is not so obvious. The ACL test measures cognitive level through performance of leather-lacing tasks. The face validity of the ACL tests raises questions: It doesn't "look like" a test of cognitive level. Nonetheless, research suggests that it is a valid measure of some construct related to cognition or to a particular form of cognition that also involves motor behavior and spatial relations (20, 63).

The OTA assigned to administer standardized assessments and tests must take care to follow directions and adhere to the procedures set forth in the manual. Such assessments and tests are designed to be given in a highly specific way; the instructions are spelled out, and the person administering the assessment is expected to follow them exactly. When directions are not consistently followed, the person's score cannot reliably be compared to the norms or criteria. A simple analogy illustrates this point: An oral thermometer does not give an accurate reading when the person has been outside, or exercising, or had anything to eat or drink within the past half hour. A reading of 101°F obtained immediately after the subject drinks a cup of tea is meaningless.

The reader who is interested in learning more about measurement theory as applied in occupational therapy is encouraged to consult evaluation references (10, 35).

## SOME ASSESSMENTS SUITABLE FOR OTA ADMINISTRATION

The following discussion focuses on assessments that are appropriate for the OTA to administer, at entry level.

### Interviews

As discussed earlier in the chapter, interviewing is a skill that develops over time, with practice. The entry-level OTA will find that the following interview instruments provide a good foundation.

#### Occupational Performance History Interview

One of the semistructured interviews the assistant might be asked to conduct is the *Occupational Performance History Interview*, Version 2.0, known as the *OPHI-II* (40). It is used to obtain an occupational history, determine how well the person is functioning in occupational roles, and estimate the balance between occupational and leisure activities. The *OPHI-II* has three parts: a semistructured interview about the client's occupational history, rating scales, and a life history narrative (33, 40). The interview itself has five sections: Occupational Roles, Daily Routine, Occupational Settings, Activity/Occupational Choices, and Critical Life Events (40). The questions that make up the Occupational Roles section are presented in Figure 15-1. The Daily Routine section asks about how the person uses time. The Occupational Settings section asks about the kinds of environments in which occupations occur. The Activity/Occupational Choices section asks about how a person chose the occupations he or she now does and looks at the person's sense of control and volition regarding occupation. The Critical Life Events section asks about turning points that may have changed the person's life's direction.

The *OPHI-II* is highly flexible, allowing the interviewer to rephrase questions and probe for more information to obtain sufficiently detailed answers. Flowcharts in the manual guide the interviewer to move to different sections or questions, depending on how the person answered a previous question. For example, if the person says that he has never worked, the questions about work are skipped, and the interviewer asks "Why do you think it is that you have not worked?" (40). After completing the interview, the therapist uses a 4-point rating system to rate the person's occupational functioning. Three separate scales are used: Occupational Identity, Occupational Competence, and Occupational Settings. The reader is referred to the *OPHI-II* manual for the rest of the interview questions, the rating system, and other components (40).

The *OPHI-II* is a well-developed assessment with strong research evidence and a large and readable manual (39). Kielhofner (39) has stated that the *OPHI-II* could be administered by an OTA with established service competency. With careful study of the manual and supervised training with someone experienced with the *OPHI-II*, the motivated OTA can master this useful interview.

## Occupational Roles

The Occupational Roles section is made up of questions that explore the occupational roles that make up the person's lifestyle.

### Worker, student, caretaker roles

- **Tell me a little about yourself.**
  Do you currently work?
  Are you currently in school?
  Are you responsible for the care of children, a partner, or __________?
  ***[Or]***
  **I understand that you are a worker/student/responsible for your __________?**
  ***[pursue line of questioning for all current student/worker/caretaker roles]***
- **How did you come to [have this job/choose this line of work or study/have responsibilities for your __________]?**
- **What do(es) your work/studies/caretaking involve?**
  ***[Or]***
- **What kind of [responsibilities do you have/things do you have to do] as a __________?**
  How well do you handle these responsibilities/taks?
  Do you like doing them?
- **What would you say is the main thing you get out of your work/studies?**
  ***[Or]***
  **What is the main reason that you do this?**
- **What kind of worker/student/caretaker would you say you are?**
  Can you give me an example of something that shows how this is so?
  ***[Or]***
  Tell me something that happened recently that would show what kind of worker/parent/partner/son/daughter you are.
  ***[Or]***
  Tell me something that you did recently as a worker/parent/partner/son/daughter that you are really proud of.
  ***[If not currently a student or worker]***
- **Have you worked in the past?**
  [If Yes] **How did you come to [have this job/choose this line of work or study]?**
  ***[And/or]***
  What kind of worker would you say you were?
  How much of your time/energy did your work take?
  Was work difficult for you?
  What would you say is the main thing you got out of your work?
  Why did you quit [working/this line of work/this job]?
  How has your illness/injury/disability affected your work?
  [If No] **Why do you think it is that you have not worked?**
- **What about your past student experiences?**
  What kind of a student would you say you were?
  How much of your time/energy did your studies take?
  Was school difficult for you?
  What would you say is the main thing you got out of your studies?
  How far did you go in school?
  How has your illness/injury/disability affected your studies?

**Figure 15-1. Occupational Performance History Interview version 2.0.** Occupational Roles section. (Reprinted with permission from Kielhofner G, Mallinson T, Crawford C, et al. The User's Manual for The Occupational Performance History Interview. Version 2.0. Chicago: MOHO Clearinghouse, University of Illinois at Chicago, 2004. Used with permission of the Model of Human Occupation Clearinghouse.)

**Friend, volunteer, amateur, hobbyist and other roles**

- **In addition to your work/studies/other responsibilities is there anything else that takes up a lot of your time and energy that is really important to you?**
  ***[Or]***
  **Is there any special thing that you do a lot?**
  ***[Or]***
- **It seems like your role at _________ (referring to the setting or the group) is to _________ (referring to some special informal role such as being a leader, helping others, being the one who cheers everyone up, and so on).**

**Home-maintenance role (if not currently a student or worker)**

- **Do you live in an apartment/home/dormitory/nursing home/other?**
  Who else do you live with?
  What kind of responsibilities do you have to keep up your home/apartment/room?
  ***[Or]***
  **How do you divide up the responsibilities to keep up your home/apartment/room?**

**Religious/organization participation**

- **Do you actively participate in any organizations or in church/temple groups?**
  Tell me about it.
  What kinds of things do you do?
  How did you get started?
- **Why do you do this?**
  Is it just for fun or more serious?

**Figure 15-1.** ***(Continued)***

## The Role Checklist

The *Role Checklist,* developed by Oakley (56) and Oakley and co-workers (57) and described by Barris and associates (11), also provides information on occupational roles as perceived by the client. The *Role Checklist* is a short written inventory that can be completed by people who have basic literacy and intact cognition. It lists 10 major life roles and an unspecified eleventh that can be added by the client. The client is asked to indicate which roles have been performed in the past, are performed in the present, or will be performed in the future. In the second part of the checklist, the client is asked to rate the value attached to each role. Service competency for administration of the *Role Checklist* can easily be developed because the directions are simple and most of the task is completed by the client. This checklist is valuable for quickly assessing roles important to the client so that priorities for treatment can be established. This assessment has been subject to a large number of studies, which verify its quality (38).

## The Canadian Occupational Performance Measure

The *Canadian Occupational Performance Measure* (*COPM*) is a structured interview that measures a client's own perceptions about his or her own occupational performance (47). This is an excellent foundation for establishing treatment priorities because it elicits from the client the goals that the client deems most important. In most cases, the OT administers the *COPM,* but the advanced technical-level practitioner might find the *COPM* useful in case management in the community. Use of the *COPM* by the OTA should not be undertaken independently; it requires establishment of service competency and supervision by an OT.

### Model of Human Occupation Screening Test

A new interview under development is the *Model of Human Occupation Screening Tool* (*MOHOST*) (59). This is a 24-item brief assessment covering areas related to occupational participation. Information can be collected by interview, review of medical records, casual conversation, consultation with members of the team, and other methods. It is a way of organizing information that may have been gathered from multiple sources. The *MOHOST* is currently under research review and validation.

There are many other structured and semistructured interviews. Some are used only for research; others are used only in certain types of hospitals or parts of the country. Regardless of the particular interview instruments, the OTA will have many opportunities to practice and develop interviewing skills. Students and new graduates may find that some of their first interviews go badly or that clients refuse to give them certain information. Usually, there is a discernible reason for this; by thinking about the attitudes you expressed and the questions you asked and how you asked them, you can become more sensitive to the needs and feelings of the person and more skillful at interviewing. With attention and practice it is easy to become a competent interviewer.

## Observation Checklists

Sometimes a checklist or other structured format is used to record observations. Of these, the *Comprehensive Occupational Therapy Evaluation* (*COTE*) scale (19, 45) is perhaps the most widely used. The *COTE* scale may be used for a single observation or a series of observations of a client performing a task (Fig. 15-2). It lists 25 behaviors and provides a scale for rating them. Behaviors are divided into three areas: General Behavior (7 items), Interpersonal Behavior (6 items), and Task Behaviors (12 items). Each can be rated on a scale of 0 (normal) to 4 (extreme or grossly abnormal). Some items, activity level (1C) for example, have two rating scales, reflecting the possibility of abnormal behaviors in either direction. The observer chooses either hyperactive (overactive) or hypoactive (underactive), depending on the client's behavior. Figure 15-3 presents the definitions used in rating the 25 behaviors.

The *COTE* scale contains 15 columns, so that the client's behavior during up to 15 sessions can be noted on the same page; this is helpful in measuring progress and documenting effects of medication and electroconvulsive therapy (ECT). Some therapists use the 15 columns in a different way, to rate several clients during the same group session; each person is rated in a different column. The ratings can then be transferred to each client's individual form.

Whether the *COTE* or another observational scale is used, when observing a client for purposes of evaluation, the assistant must remain an observer and not interfere with what the client is doing. The OTA must not give help, advice, or encouragement; recommend that the client try a different technique; or even smile approvingly. All of these behaviors may change what the person does, and what then ends up on the rating form is how the client performs with advice and support rather than how he or she performs independently. Administering an assessment and providing treatment are different tasks that require different behaviors from the occupational therapist or assistant.

## Assessments of Daily Living Skills

Several structured assessments are designed to assess self-care and independent living skills (10, 30, 53). Persons with severe chronic psychiatric disorders may have problems with such areas

## Comprehensive Occupational Therapy Evaluation Scale

| DATE | | | | | | | | | | | | | | | |
|---|---|---|---|---|---|---|---|---|---|---|---|---|---|---|---|
| I. GENERAL BEHAVIOR | 1 | 2 | 3 | 4 | 5 | 6 | 7 | 8 | 9 | 10 | 11 | 12 | 13 | 14 | 15 |
| A APPEARANCE | | | | | | | | | | | | | | | |
| B NONPRODUCTIVE BEHAVIOR | | | | | | | | | | | | | | | |
| C ACTIVITY LEVEL (a or b) | | | | | | | | | | | | | | | |
| D EXPRESSION | | | | | | | | | | | | | | | |
| E RESPONSIBILITY | | | | | | | | | | | | | | | |
| F PUNCTUALITY | | | | | | | | | | | | | | | |
| G REALITY ORIENTATION | | | | | | | | | | | | | | | |
| SUB-TOTAL | | | | | | | | | | | | | | | |
| II. INTERPERSONAL BEHAVIOR | 1 | 2 | 3 | 4 | 5 | 6 | 7 | 8 | 9 | 10 | 11 | 12 | 13 | 14 | 15 |
| A INDEPENDENCE | | | | | | | | | | | | | | | |
| B COOPERATION | | | | | | | | | | | | | | | |
| C SELF-ASSERTION (a or b) | | | | | | | | | | | | | | | |
| D SOCIABILITY | | | | | | | | | | | | | | | |
| E ATTENTION-GETTING BEHAVIOR | | | | | | | | | | | | | | | |
| F NEGATIVE RESPONSE FROM OTHERS | | | | | | | | | | | | | | | |
| SUB-TOTAL | | | | | | | | | | | | | | | |
| III. TASK BEHAVIOR | 1 | 2 | 3 | 4 | 5 | 6 | 7 | 8 | 9 | 10 | 11 | 12 | 13 | 14 | 15 |
| A ENGAGEMENT | | | | | | | | | | | | | | | |
| B CONCENTRATION | | | | | | | | | | | | | | | |
| C COORDINATION | | | | | | | | | | | | | | | |
| D FOLLOW DIRECTIONS | | | | | | | | | | | | | | | |
| E ACTIVITY NEATNESS OR ATTENTION TO DETAIL | | | | | | | | | | | | | | | |
| F PROBLEM SOLVING | | | | | | | | | | | | | | | |
| G COMPLEXITY AND ORGANIZATION OF TASK | | | | | | | | | | | | | | | |
| H INITIAL LEARNING | | | | | | | | | | | | | | | |
| I INTEREST IN ACTIVITY | | | | | | | | | | | | | | | |
| J INTEREST IN ACCOMPLISHMENT | | | | | | | | | | | | | | | |
| K DECISION MAKING | | | | | | | | | | | | | | | |
| L FRUSTRATION TOLERANCE | | | | | | | | | | | | | | | |
| SUB-TOTAL | | | | | | | | | | | | | | | |
| TOTAL | | | | | | | | | | | | | | | |

SCALE 0-NORMAL, 1-MINIMAL, 2-MILD, 3-MODERATE, 4-SEVERE

COMMENTS

(THERAPIST'S SIGNATURE)

**Figure 15-2. Comprehensive Occupational Therapy Evaluation Scale.** (Reprinted with permission from Brayman SJ, Kirby TF, Misenheimer AM, Short MJ. Comprehensive occupational therapy evaluation scale. Am J Occup Ther 1976;30:94–100. Copyright © 1976 by the American Occupational Therapy Association, Inc.)

## PART I. GENERAL BEHAVIOR

**A. APPEARANCE**

The following six factors are involved: (1) clean skin, (2) clean hair, (3) hair combed, (4) clean clothes, (5) clothes ironed, and (6) clothes suitable for the occasion.

0—No problems in any area.
1—Problems in 1 areas.
2—Problems in 2 areas.
3—Problems in 3 or 4 areas.
4—Problems in 5 or 6 areas.

**B. NONPRODUCTIVE BEHAVIOR**

(Rocking, playing with hands, repetitive statements, appears to be talking to self, preoccupied with own thoughts, etc.)

0—No nonproductive behavior during session.
1—Nonproductive behavior occasionally during session.
2—Nonproductive behavior for half of session.
3—Nonproductive behavior for three-fourths of session.
4—Nonproductive behavior for the entire session.

**C. ACTIVITY LEVEL (a or b)**

**(a)** 0—No hypoactivity.
1—Occasional hypoactivity.
2—Hypoactivity attracts the attention of other patients and therapists but participates.
3—Hypoactivity level such that can participate but with great difficulty.
4—So hypoactive that patient cannot participate in activity.

**(b)** 0—No hyperactivity.
1—Occasional spurts of hyperactivity.
2—Hyperactivity attracts the attention of other patients and therapists but participates.
3—Hyperactivity level such that can participate but with great difficulty.
4.—So hyperactive that patient cannot participate in activity.

**D. EXPRESSION**

0—Expression consistent with situation and setting.
1—Communicates with expression, occasionally inappropriate.
2—Shows inappropriate expression several times during session.
3—Show of expression but inconsistent with situation.
4—Extremes of expression-bizarre, uncontrolled or no expression.

**E. RESPONSIBILITY**

0—Takes responsibility for own actions.
1—Denies responsibility for 1 or 2 actions.
2—Denies responsibility for several actions.
3—Denies responsibility for most actions.
4—Denial of all responsibility—messes up project and blames therapist or others.

**F. PUNCTUALITY**

0—On time.
1—5–10 minutes late.
2—10–20 minutes late.
3—20–30 minutes late.
4—30 minutes or more late.

**G. REALITY ORIENTATION**

0—Complete awareness of person, place, time, and situation.
1—General awareness but inconsistency in one area.
2—Awareness of 2 areas.
3—Awareness of 1 area.
4—Lack of awareness of person, place, time, and situation (who, where, what, and why).

**Figure 15-3. Definitions for the Comprehensive Occupational Therapy Evaluation Scale.** (Reprinted with permission from Brayman SJ, Kirby TF, Misenheimer AM, Short MJ. Comprehensive occupational therapy evaluation scale. Am J Occup Ther 1976;30:94–100. Copyright © 1976 by the American Occupational Therapy Association, Inc.)

**PART II. INTERPERSONAL**

**A. INDEPENDENCE**
0—Independent functioning.
1—Only 1 or 2 dependent actions.
2—Half independent and half dependent actions.
3—Only 1 or 2 independent actions.
4—No independent actions.

**B. COOPERATION**
0—Cooperates with program.
1—Follows most directions, opposes less than one half.
2—Follows half, opposes half.
3—Opposes three-fourths of directions.
4—Opposes all directions and suggestions.

**C. SELF-ASSERTION (a or b)**
**(a)** 0—Assertive when necessary.
1—Compliant less than half of the session.
2—Compliant half of the session.
3—Compliant three-fourths of the session.
4—Totally passive and compliant.
**(b)** 0—Assertive when necessary.
1—Dominant less than half of the session.
2—Dominant half of the session.
3—Dominant three-fourths of the session.
4—Totally dominates the session.

**D. SOCIABILITY**
0—Socializes with staff and patients.
1—Socializes with staff and occasionally with other patients or vice versa.
2—Socializes only with staff or with patients.
3—Socializes only if approached.
4—Does not join others in activities, unable to carry on casual conversation even if approached.

**E. ATTENTION-GETTING BEHAVIOR**
0—No unreasonable attention-getting behavior.
1—Less than one-half time spent in attention-getting behavior.
2—Half time spent in attention-getting behavior.
3—Three-fourths of time spent in attention-getting behavior.
4—Verbally or nonverbally demands constant attention.

**F. NEGATIVE RESPONSE FROM OTHERS**
0—Evokes no negative responses.
1—Evokes 1 negative response.
2—Evokes 2 negative responses.
3—Evokes 3 or more negative responses during session.
4—Evokes numerous negative responses from others and therapist must take some action.

**PART III. TASK BEHAVIOR**

**A. ENGAGEMENT**
0—Needs no encouragement to begin task.
1—Encourage once to begin activity.
2—Encourage 2 or 3 times to engage in activity.
3—Engages in activity only after much encouragement.
4—Does not engage in activity.

**B. CONCENTRATION**
0—No difficulty concentrating during full session.
1—Off task less than one-fourth time.
2—Off task half the time.
3—Off task three-fourths time.
4—Loses concentration on task in less than 1 minute.

**C. COORDINATION**
0—No problems with coordination.
1—Occasionally has trouble with fine detail, manipulating tools or materials.
2—Occasional trouble manipulating tools and materials but has frequent trouble with fine detail.
3—Some difficulty in gross movement—unable to manipulate some tools and materials.
4—Great difficulty in movement (gross motor); virtually unable to manipulate tools and materials (fine motor).

**D. FOLLOW DIRECTIONS**
0—Carries out directions without problems.
1—Occasional trouble with more than 3 step directions.
2—Carries out simple directions—has trouble with 2.
3—Can carry out only very simple one step directions (demonstrated, written, or oral).
4—Unable to carry out any directions.

**Figure 15-3.** ***(Continued)***

***E. ACTIVITY NEATNESS**

0—Activity neatly done.
1—Occasionally ignores fine detail.
2—Often ignores fine detail and materials are scattered.
3—Ignores fine detail and work habits disturbing to those around.
4—Unaware of fine detail, so sloppy that therapist has to intervene.

***F. ATTENTION TO DETAIL**

0—Pays attention to detail appropriately.
1—Occasionally too concise.
2—More attention to several details than is required.
3—So concise that project will take twice as long as expected.
4—So concerned that project will never get finished.

**G. PROBLEM SOLVING**

0—Solves problems without assistance.
1—Solves problems after assistance given once.
2—Can solve only after repeated instructions.
3—Recognizes a problem but cannot solve it.
4—Unable to recognize or solve a problem.

**H. COMPLEXITY AND ORGANIZATION OF TASK**

0—Organizes and performs all tasks given.
1—Occasionally has trouble with organization of complex activities that should be able to do.
2—Can organize simple but not complex activities.
3—Can do only very simple activities with organization imposed by therapists.
4—Unable to organize or carry out an activity when all tools, materials, and directions are available.

**I. INITIAL LEARNING**

0—Learns a new activity quickly and without difficulty.
1—Occasionally has difficulty learning a complex activity.
2—Has frequent difficulty learning a complex activity, but can learn a simple activity.
3—Unable to learn complex activities; occasional difficulty learning simple activities.
4—Unable to learn a new activity.

**J. INTEREST IN ACTIVITIES**

0—Interested in a variety of activities.
1—Occasionally not interested in new activity.
2—Shows occasional interest in a part of an activity.
3—Engages in activities but shows no interest.
4—Does not participate.

**K. INTEREST IN ACCOMPLISHMENT**

0—Interested in finishing activities.
1—Occasional lack of interest or pleasure in finishing a long-term activity.
2—Interest or pleasure in accomplishment of a short-term activity—lack of interest in a long-term activity.
3—Only occasional interest in finishing any activity.
4—No interest or pleasure in finishing an activity.

**L. DECISION MAKING**

0—Makes own decisions.
1—Makes decisions but occasionally seeks therapist approval.
2—Makes decisions but often seeks therapist approval.
3—Makes decision when given only 2 choices.
4—Cannot make any decisions or refuses to make a decision.

**M. FRUSTRATION TOLERANCE**

0—Handles all tasks without becoming over frustrated.
1—Occasionally becomes frustrated with more complex tasks; can handle simple tasks.
2—Often becomes frustrated with more complex tasks but is able to handle simple tasks.
3—Often becomes frustrated with any tasks but attempts to continue.
4—Becomes so frustrated with tasks that he or she refuses or is unable to function.

*Rate either Activity Neatness or Attention to Detail, not both.

**Figure 15-3.** ***(Continued)***

as hygiene and grooming, housekeeping, money management, and other skills basic to independent community living. Because OTAs are often given major responsibility for assessing the self-care and daily living skills of such individuals, several assessments for this area are discussed.

### Milwaukee Evaluation of Daily Living Skills

The *Milwaukee Evaluation of Daily Living Skills* (*MEDLS*) (30) is a standardized assessment. A screening form is used to determine which areas of 21 subtests should be tested. The assessment is administered individually, using equipment that may be provided by the client; this creates a context in which the person's performance is most likely to approximate his or her natural performance.

### The Kohlman Evaluation of Living Skills

The *Kohlman Evaluation of Living Skills* (*KELS*) (53, 66) assesses several skills in the areas of personal care, safety and health, money management, transportation, use of the telephone, and work and leisure. The client must perform a task or respond to questions from the evaluator. As an example, for the task on making change, the evaluator presents the client with an item (magazine or bar of soap) marked with a price. The client must pretend to purchase the item with play money and is scored on whether he or she is able to identify whether the evaluator has given the correct change. The client is rated as "independent" or "needs assistance." There is a brief reading and writing test intended to supplement the rest of the assessment. The *KELS* is appropriate for screening; it does not measure skills in natural environment and thus may not accurately indicate the person's ability to function in the community (22, 25). A videotape that demonstrates how the *KELS* is administered is available (37).

## Assessment of Time Use

Engagement in occupation uses time. Details about time use provide insights into occupational preferences and patterns, the balance of life activities, and other aspects of occupational functioning.

### Occupational Questionnaire

The *Occupational Questionnaire* (65) is one of several assessments that seek information about how an individual spends time. The person is asked to fill out a grid of time blocks for each 30-minute period from 5:00 A.M. to 11:30 P.M., and to list the major activity for each time period for a typical weekday. After listing the activities, the person then answers four questions about each activity:

1. I consider this activity to be work, daily living work, recreation, rest.
2. I think that I do this very well, well, about average, poorly, very poorly.
3. For me this activity is extremely important, important, take it or leave it, rather not do it, total waste of time.
4. How much do you enjoy this activity? like it very much, like it, neither like it nor dislike it, dislike it, strongly dislike it.

One drawback of this and similar written questionnaires is that the person completing it must be able to read and write. Many persons with psychiatric disorders cannot read and write well enough to complete this kind of form (16, 24).

### Barth Time Construction

The *Barth Time Construction* (*BTC*) (12, 13) is an instrument that is less dependent on reading skill. The chart is divided into 24 rows, representing the hours of the day. Color-coded paper is used to represent 12 categories of activities (e.g., blue for sleeping, black for watching television, pink for grooming and dressing). The paper is precut to the width of the column, so the client need only cut it to size and glue it in the appropriate place. The client selects each color in turn and continues to cut and paste until the entire chart is filled. The evaluator uses the *BTC Summary Form* to record any unsolicited comments made by the client and afterward totals the hours spent in each of the 12 categories. These totals are converted to percentages of time per week spent in each activity.

Instructions and materials for the *BTC* are quite specific—for example, cylindrical glue bottles were selected so that persons with weak grasp would be able to use them easily. The *BTC* can be administered to as many as four clients at a time. The 12 categories include several in which some clients spend many hours but that they might not spontaneously record: shopping, television, meetings and groups, and drinking and drugs. The instructions are very brief, simply worded, and presented in large print. The person does not have to write a single word; therefore, the instrument can be used with persons who are less literate, Finally, the end product, the colored chart, depicts the person's use of time so vividly that the client can see it clearly; the chart is easily understood by other staff for the same reason.

## Assessment of Process Skills and Mental Functions

Process skills and mental functions are the cognitive, affective, and perceptual skills and abilities that allow people to manage complex information and goals. These skills and functions will typically be assessed by the OT. However, the OTA may be asked to administer certain select instruments such as the *Bay Area Functional Performance Evaluation* and the Allen tests.

### The Bay Area Functional Performance Evaluation

The *Bay Area Functional Performance Evaluation*, 2nd edition (*BaFPE*) (17, 36, 43) is a standardized instrument that assesses some of the general skills needed for independent functioning. It begins with a brief interview to orient the person to the purpose of the assessment and to collect basic information. This is followed by a task-oriented assessment (TOA) consisting of five tasks: sorting shells, a money and marketing task, drawing a house floor plan, constructing nine block designs from memory, and drawing a person. The evaluator rates the person's performance of these tasks using a rating guide included in the assessment; decision making, motivation, and organization of time and materials are some of the items rated. The evaluator also observes and records perceptual motor behaviors such as use of both hands in sorting shells. Finally, the way the client relates to other people is rated on a separate social interaction scale (SIS).

Normative data are available for the *BaFPE*, and research seems to show that it is reliable (gives comparable results every time it is given) and has construct validity (measures what it says it measures). An abbreviated form of the *BaFPE* is available (51).

### Allen Cognitive Level Test

In situations where the Allen Cognitive Level model is used, the OTA may be asked to administer the Allen Cognitive Level (ACL) test (2, 3, 20, 26, 34, 63) (Fig. 15-4). The OTA should practice to achieve proficiency and service competency before administering the ACL. Directions for materials, administration, and scoring of the ACL are given in Allen and associates (3).

The ACL uses the client's performance of progressively more difficult leather-lacing stitches to assess cognitive level. The test includes the running stitch, the whip stitch, and the single cordovan stitch. Allen (2) believes it is possible that women may do better than men on the test because of experience with sewing; the running stitch and the whip stitch are used in sewing, and

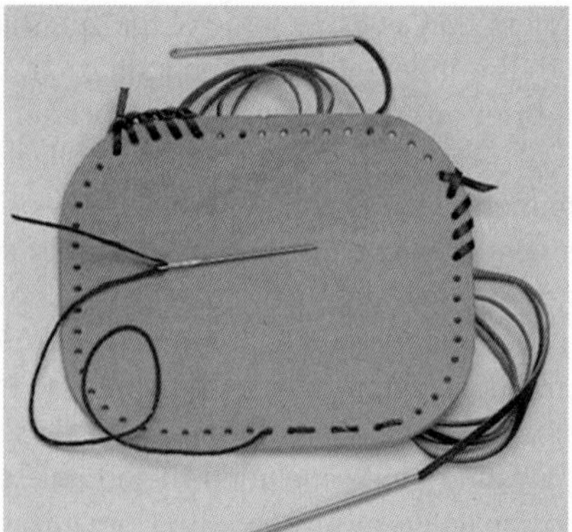

**Figure 15-4. The Allen Cognitive Level screening test** (Courtesy S&S Worldwide, Colchester CT.)

the single cordovan is similar to the blanket stitch. She also warns that visual problems, blurred vision as a side effect of medication, and hand impairment or motor incoordination can result in a score that is lower than the person's real cognitive abilities. On the other hand, experience doing leather lacing may falsely raise a person's score.

Allen recommends that the leather-lacing material be replaced after several administrations of the test because it twists more easily as it becomes worn. It is important not to add to or change the directions; telling the client to stop and think may falsely raise a level 5 to a level 6, for example.

## Assessments of Psychological Functions

Another very different kind of structured assessment the OTA might be asked to administer is the human figure drawing. Occupational therapists and psychologists have been using this kind of assessment for decades. Figure drawings may be interpreted as measures of mental maturity or as indicators of physical and/or sensory integrative dysfunction (42). Figure drawings may be interpreted also in relation to feelings about the self, one's ability to affect the environment, and one's relationship with one's family. Interpretation of figure drawings is the responsibility of the OT. A variant that is often used is the *House-Tree-Person Test* (10).

## Assessments of Sensory Functions

The *Adolescent/Adult Sensory Profile* is a paper and pencil form that asks the client to indicate his or her reaction to a range of sensory statements, such as "I'm afraid of heights" and "I dislike having my back rubbed" (21, 23). The results are then coded onto a scoring sheet and transferred to a profile page. The profile shows the degree to which the person is similar to "most people" in four aspects of sensory functioning. The results are shared with the client. The manual gives useful suggestions to help clients manage sensory reactions by modifying the environment, changing activities, and getting support from others.

## Assessments of Leisure Interests and Social Participation

For a range of clients who have mental disorders, engagement with others (social participation) and use of leisure time can be challenging and problematic. Persons in recovery from substance-abuse disorders, individuals with chronic schizophrenia and other persistent mental illnesses, and people experiencing depression are just a few of the groups for whom evaluation and assessment of leisure time and social participation is appropriate.

### The NPI Interest Checklist

The Neuropsychiatric Institute (NPI) Interest Checklist (52, 61, 62) is an example of a questionnaire the client can complete independently. It lists 80 activities; the client is asked to check off whether his or her interest in each activity is casual, strong, or nonexistent. The 80 activities are sorted into categories of manual skills, physical sports, social recreation, activities of daily living, and cultural and educational pursuits. Matsutsuyu (52) suggested that the therapist could infer the client's interests from the distribution of his or her scores in these five categories. Rogers and associates (62) showed, however, that individuals' scores in these categories did not always accurately reflect their interests. They suggested that the number of categories may have to be expanded, for example to separate activities that reflect traditional sexual roles. Further research suggested that therapists should use caution in their interpretations of the results (44). The original checklist, developed in 1969, listed many activities that are no longer in vogue. And it does not include some activities that are popular now. For this reason, the assistant will encounter other versions of the Interest Checklist in the clinic; Hemphill (31) indicates that "there are almost as many interest checklists as there are therapists." Despite these problems, the Interest Checklist (or a variation of it) is used effectively by many occupational therapy practitioners, often as a starting point for a discussion of how the person spends leisure time, how much enjoyment leisure provides, and what past activities might be renewed or new ones developed.

### Modified Interest Checklist

The version that seems to have the most research support at present is based on the original NPI version and is now modified to include information about participation and future interest in the activities. The Modified Interest Checklist (41) is shown in Figure 15-5. The advantage of using this version is that several studies have already been published demonstrating its usefulness with different populations, including adolescent males, adults with alcoholism, new mothers, and persons recovering from stroke (38).

### Adolescent Leisure Interest Profile

Henry (32) developed an assessment of adolescents' interest in, participation in, and feelings about leisure. The Adolescent Leisure Interest Profile (ALIP) is a questionnaire that contains 86 activity items in a checklist format. There are additional questions about degree of interest, frequency of participation, satisfaction, perceptions of competency, and social involvement during the activity.

To summarize, structured assessments are designed to be administered according to the directions given, using the same tools, materials, setup, and directions each time. Obviously, because of space limitations, not all of the structured assessments used by psychiatric occupational therapists across the country are presented here. We have selected some that the OTA is likely to encounter and have emphasized those for which the OTA might be asked at entry level to develop service competency in administration and scoring.

## Nonstandardized Assessments

Many *nonstandardized assessment instruments* have been and continue to be used in mental health clinics. Some of these involve tasks like constructing a mosaic tile ashtray or a paper mobile or a collage (48); some are paper and pencil tasks that require measuring or following directions; still others are questionnaires about the client's occupational history and interests. The OTA may expect to encounter others in the clinic and to observe the OT administering still others. Wherever an assessment lacks a set procedure for administration and scoring, the clinician must think carefully about the results. What does the assessment measure? Would another evaluator agree with the results? Or obtain the same results? If the client were tested again, would the results be similar? If not, does this indicate a change in the client or a weakness in the test? How can service competency be developed and ensured?

The use of nonstandardized assessments has been criticized as a waste of time and perhaps a misleading and unethical practice (18, 29). From a practical point of view, it is far preferable to use

## INTEREST CHECKLIST

| Activity | What has been your level of interest | | | | | | Do you currently participate in this activity? | | Would you like to pursue this in the future? | |
|---|---|---|---|---|---|---|---|---|---|---|
| | In the past ten years | | | In the past year | | | | | | |
| | Strong | Some | No | Strong | Some | No | Yes | No | Yes | No |
| Gardening Yardwork | | | | | | | | | | |
| Sewing/needle work | | | | | | | | | | |
| Playing cards | | | | | | | | | | |
| Foreign languages | | | | | | | | | | |
| Church activities | | | | | | | | | | |
| Radio | | | | | | | | | | |
| Walking | | | | | | | | | | |
| Car repair | | | | | | | | | | |
| Writing | | | | | | | | | | |
| Dancing | | | | | | | | | | |
| Golf | | | | | | | | | | |
| Football | | | | | | | | | | |
| Listening to popular music | | | | | | | | | | |
| Puzzles | | | | | | | | | | |
| Holiday Activities | | | | | | | | | | |
| Pets/livestock | | | | | | | | | | |
| Movies | | | | | | | | | | |
| Listening to classical music | | | | | | | | | | |
| Speeches/lectures | | | | | | | | | | |
| Swimming | | | | | | | | | | |
| Bowling | | | | | | | | | | |
| Visiting | | | | | | | | | | |
| Mending | | | | | | | | | | |
| Checkers/Chess | | | | | | | | | | |
| Barbecues | | | | | | | | | | |
| Reading | | | | | | | | | | |
| Traveling | | | | | | | | | | |
| Parties | | | | | | | | | | |
| Wrestling | | | | | | | | | | |
| Housecleaning | | | | | | | | | | |
| Model building | | | | | | | | | | |
| Television | | | | | | | | | | |
| Concerts | | | | | | | | | | |
| Pottery | | | | | | | | | | |

**Figure 15-5. The Modified Interest Checklist.** (Reprinted with permission from Kielhofner G, Neville A. The Modified Interest Checklist. Available at: www.moho.uic.edu/mohorelatedrsrcs.html#OtherInstrumentsBasedonMOHO. Accessed Aug 2007. Used with permission of the Model of Human Occupation Clearinghouse.)

## INTEREST CHECKLIST

| Activity | What has been your level of interest | | | | | | Do you currently participate in this activity? | | Would you like to pursue this in the future? | |
|---|---|---|---|---|---|---|---|---|---|---|
| | In the past ten years | | | In the past year | | | | | | |
| | Strong | Some | No | Strong | Some | No | Yes | No | Yes | No |
| Camping | | | | | | | | | | |
| Laundry/Ironing | | | | | | | | | | |
| Politics | | | | | | | | | | |
| Table games | | | | | | | | | | |
| Home decorating | | | | | | | | | | |
| Clubs/Lodge | | | | | | | | | | |
| Singing | | | | | | | | | | |
| Scouting | | | | | | | | | | |
| Clothes | | | | | | | | | | |
| Handicrafts | | | | | | | | | | |
| Hairstyling | | | | | | | | | | |
| Cycling | | | | | | | | | | |
| Attending plays | | | | | | | | | | |
| Bird watching | | | | | | | | | | |
| Dating | | | | | | | | | | |
| Auto-racing | | | | | | | | | | |
| Home repairs | | | | | | | | | | |
| Exercise | | | | | | | | | | |
| Hunting | | | | | | | | | | |
| Woodworking | | | | | | | | | | |
| Pool | | | | | | | | | | |
| Driving | | | | | | | | | | |
| Child care | | | | | | | | | | |
| Tennis | | | | | | | | | | |
| Cooking/Baking | | | | | | | | | | |
| Basketball | | | | | | | | | | |
| History | | | | | | | | | | |
| Collecting | | | | | | | | | | |
| Fishing | | | | | | | | | | |
| Science | | | | | | | | | | |
| Leatherwork | | | | | | | | | | |
| Shopping | | | | | | | | | | |
| Photography | | | | | | | | | | |
| Painting/Drawing | | | | | | | | | | |

**Figure 15-5.** ***(Continued)***

instruments that yield data that can be used to document effective functional outcomes. So why use nonstandardized assessments at all? Luebben and Royeen (50) point out that every standardized test started out as nonstandardized. Only after repeat administration, analysis, and refinement can any assessment be developed to a standardized form. Furthermore, standardized assessments may be a poor fit when evaluating the occupational performance of an individual in a specific situation. Nonstandardized assessments can be tailored to the situation and the individual and may give more valid results for the particular person than will a standardized assessment—and at less expense and in a shorter period of time. For example, a secretary or administrative assistant could be given a battery of standardized tests to aid in determining readiness to return to work after a major depressive episode and ECT. Or the OT could use a simple filing task of putting envelopes in order by ZIP code or file folders in alphabetical order. The informal assessment can be made specific to the person's job (such as the use of colored tab stickers in a medical office).

## THE PERFORMANCE CONTEXT FOR EVALUATION

We have suggested but not specifically addressed the question of the appropriate environment in which to evaluate or measure a person's ability to function. When meeting the client or consumer in the treatment or rehabilitation setting, the occupational therapy practitioner must recognize that the person's occupational life occurs in a range of settings that are quite different from the clinic. When assessing a person's ability to perform a task that is customarily performed at home or at work, it makes sense to administer the assessment in the actual performance environment rather than in the treatment setting. This is supported by many research studies and scholarly reports (22, 25, 46, 49, 55, 58).

As an example, the *Kitchen Task Assessment* (*KTA*) (14), an assessment of planning and organizational skills for persons with dementia, might best be conducted in the person's kitchen at home. The *KTA* requires the person to prepare pudding from a mix. The utensils and materials are specified, as is the setup. The person is expected to wash hands, to light the stove, and so on. Findings from the *KTA* are used to predict the person's level of functional independence and the need for caregiver assistance. When the *KTA* is conducted in the clinic environment, the consumer may be flustered by the unfamiliarity of the specific appliances and room layout. Alternatively, the person may find the task easier because the room is less cluttered or laid out more logically than the kitchen at home. Thus unreliable results may occur. In contrast, at home, the consumer is more likely to perform the tasks in a manner similar to that which would naturally occur (i.e., with no observer present).

We recommend strongly that the occupational therapy practitioner arrange for assessments to be done in the customary naturalistic environment of the individual. This is especially important when the assessment attempts to measure or predict a person's ability to function in the community.

## DOCUMENTATION AND COMMUNICATION OF EVALUATION DATA

Once the assistant has observed or assessed the client, there yet remains a final step in the data gathering and evaluation process: that of reporting the information to those who need to know it. This may be done in two ways, by writing in the medical record or by making an oral report. The two processes are discussed separately.

An evaluation note is written into the chart, generally by the OT. The OTA may contribute written or oral information, which the OT incorporates. Detailed suggestions for writing evaluation and observation data into note form are given in Chapter 17, along with sample notes.

The OTA should also be prepared to present observations orally to the OT supervisor, to other members of the occupational therapy department, and to other staff. Sometimes the presentation happens spontaneously, in the hallway or the nursing station. These presentations are casual and informal but must respect patients' confidentiality; the OTA must seek privacy when discussing any information that would be considered confidential. Other more formal presentations are made in team meetings, rounds, and department meetings. Regardless of the context, standard English and correct pronunciation should always be used. Furthermore, the OTA defers to the OT in reporting and does not interpret data unless directed and trained to do so.

Watching and listening to another occupational therapy staff member make a presentation is a good way to learn what is expected. Oral presentations should be loud enough to be heard by everyone present (try directing your speech to the person farthest away). Try to make eye contact with people you are comfortable with. It may be helpful to rehearse your presentation in advance, perhaps using a tape recorder.

The most important thing to consider when making any presentation is one's audience. Who are these people? What do they want to hear about? Doctors, for example, may want to know about how the medication is affecting the person. What terminology and vocabulary do they understand? As discussed previously, occupational therapy jargon, although appropriate for department meetings, will probably not be understood by other staff. Choose words that your audience will understand.

Students and new graduates often suffer perfectly normal fears about speaking in large groups. Their fears are legion: Will I say the wrong thing? Will they think I'm stupid? Will they notice I'm nervous? What if my voice cracks? What if I forget what to say? It may not help to hear that almost everyone has these fears in the beginning, but whether or not it helps, it *is* true. Public speaking, like many other professional skills (e.g., interviewing), is mastered only by doing. Practice helps.

## SUMMARY

Data gathering and evaluation are the foundation of the treatment process, providing essential information about who clients are, what their lives are like, the kinds of things they want and need to do, and the problems that stand in their way. The OTA works under the direction and management of the OT in regard to data collection and evaluation. The OTA contributes by collecting information from medical records and interviews and by performing observations and structured assessments as directed by the OT. The assistant also records and reports observations to the therapist and to other professionals working with the client.

The ability to observe dispassionately, free from personal bias or preconceived ideas, is essential. The observations and assessments performed by the assistant and others form the foundation of the treatment plan. For this reason, service competency must be established before the OTA evaluates the client. Wherever possible, assessment should be done in the environment that is customary for the individual. Being involved in any part of a client's evaluation is a serious responsibility but also a wonderful opportunity to explore and better understand the unique and sometimes perplexing world of another human being.

## REVIEW QUESTIONS AND ACTIVITIES

1. Why is good evaluation important to the occupational therapy process?
2. State the purpose of evaluation.
3. What is meant by *asset* and *deficit* in relation to occupational functioning?
4. In what ways is context important in evaluation of a client's occupational performance and goals?
5. Name the seven contexts recognized by the *OTPF*.
   - Describe each one.
   - Are the different kinds of contexts separate? Or do they overlap? Explain.
6. What is *social support*? Is it important? Why?
7. Patterns consist of habits, routines, and roles. Explain each of these concepts.
8. What is meant by an *impoverished habit*? A *dominating habit*?
9. What is an *expected environment* and why should it be considered?
10. What are the roles and responsibilities of the OT and the OTA during evaluation?
11. Contrast the top-down, bottom-up, and environment-first approaches to evaluation.
12. How can the information for the occupational profile be obtained?
13. How can the information for the analysis of occupational performance be obtained?
14. Give an example of a government or insurance regulation that affects the way occupational therapy practitioners evaluate patients. Explain.
15. What is *service competency*? How does the OTA establish service competency?
16. Describe the kinds of information relevant to occupational therapy that the OTA might find in the medical record. In what sections of the chart can information important for OT be located?
17. What is the purpose of interviewing the client or consumer?
18. What is meant by the term *reliable informant*?
19. How should one prepare for an interview?
20. What is the difference between *interpretation* and *observation*? Give an example.
21. Describe how the OTA should prepare to administer an unfamiliar assessment.
22. Define and give examples to illustrate the following terms: *standardization, norm-referenced, criterion-referenced, reliability,* and *validity.*
23. Why should standardized assessments be administered according to the procedures in the manual?
24. What is the best environment for assessment.
   - Does it matter? Why?
   - Give an example.
25. *Review activity:* After you have studied the extensive list of areas for data collection, what areas do you have questions about? How can you learn more?
26. *Review and study activity:* Make flash cards with the names (and acronyms) of assessments/interviews on one side and a description on the other.
27. *Clinical lab activity:* Take turns interviewing and being interviewed by classmates. (If available, videotape each other.) Give and receive feedback about interviewing skills.
28. *Clinical lab activity:* With classmates, taking turns as test administrators and simulated clients, practice administering available assessments and interviews. Write up the results of an interview or assessment in a form suitable for an oral report or a note in the chart.
29. *Computer activity:* Visit the website of the Centers for Medicare and Medicaid Services (CMS) and search for the most current regulations affecting occupational therapy evaluation. Share this information in an oral or written report.

## REFERENCES


1. Adler F. Sisters in crime. In: Maggio R, compiler. The Beacon Book of Quotations by Women. Boston: Beacon, 1992.
2. Allen CK. Occupational Therapy for Psychiatric Diseases: Measurement and Management of Cognitive Disabilities. Boston: Little, Brown, 1985.
3. Allen CK, Earhart CA, Blue T. Occupational Therapy Treatment Goals for the Physically and Cognitively Disabled. Rockville, MD: American Occupational Therapy Association, 1992.
4. American Occupational Therapy Association. AOTA's 1-Minute Update. Available at: www.aota.org/members/area19/links/031207.asp?PLACE=/members/area19/links/031207.asp. Accessed Mar 2007.
5. American Occupational Therapy Association. The Association: Clarification for the use of the terms assessment and evaluation. Am J Occup Ther 1995;49:1072–1073.
6. American Occupational Therapy Association. Guidelines for supervision, roles, and responsibilities during the delivery of occupational therapy services. Am J Occup Ther 2004;58:663–667.
7. American Occupational Therapy Association. Occupational therapy practice framework: Domain and process. Am J Occup Ther 2002;56:609–639.
8. American Occupational Therapy Association. Roles and responsibilities of the occupational therapist and the occupational therapy assistant during the delivery of occupational therapy services. OT Practice 2002;7(15):9–10.
9. American Occupational Therapy Association. Standards of practice for occupational therapy. Am J Occup Ther 2005;59:663–665.
10. Asher IE. Occupational Therapy Assessment Tools: An Annotated Index. 3rd ed. Bethesda, MD: American Occupational Therapy Association, 2007.
11. Barris R, Oakley F, Kielhofner G. The Role Checklist. In: Hemphill BJ, ed. Mental Health Assessment in Occupational Therapy: An Integrative Approach to the Evaluative Process. Thorofare, NJ: Slack, 1988.
12. Barth T. Barth Time Construction. In: Hemphill BJ, ed. Mental Health Assessment in Occupational Therapy: An Integrative Approach to the Evaluative Process. Thorofare, NJ: Slack, 1988.
13. Barth T. A new variation on an old theme: the Barth time construction. Am Occup Ther Assoc Ment Health Special Sect Q Newslett 1986;9(1):4.
14. Baum C, Edwards DF. Cognitive performance in senile dementia of the Alzheimers type: The Kitchen Task Assessment. Am J Occup Ther 1993;47:431–436.
15. Benne KD, Sheats P. Functional roles of group members. J Social Issues 1948;4(2):42–47.
16. Berg A, Hammitt KB. Assessing the psychiatric patient's ability to meet the literacy demands of hospitalization. Hosp Commun Psychiatry 1980;31:266–268.
17. Bloomer J, Williams S. The Bay Area Functional Performance Evaluation. In: Hemphill BJ, ed. The Eval-uation Process in Psychiatric Occupational Therapy. Thorofare, NJ: Slack, 1982.
18. Bonder BR. Issues in assessment of psychosocial com-ponents of function. Am J Occup Ther 1993;47:211–216.
19. Brayman SJ, Kirby TF, Misenheimer AM, Short MJ. Comprehensive Occupational Therapy Evaluation scale. Am J Occup Ther 1976;30:94–100.
20. Brown C. Clinical interpretation of "A comparison of the Allen Cognitive Level test and the Wisconsin Card Sorting test in adults with schizophrenia." An J Occup Ther 2000;54:134–136.
21. Brown C, Dunn W. Adolescent/Adult Sensory Profile. San Antonio, TX Psychological Corporation, 2002.
22. Brown C, Moore WP, Hemman D, Yunek A. Influence of instrumental activities of daily living assessment method on judgments of independence. Am J Occup Ther 1996;50:202–206.
23. Brown C, Tollefson N, Dunn W, Cromwell R, Filion D. The adult sensory profile: measuring patterns of sensory processing. Am J Occup Ther 2001;55:75–82.
24. Coles GS, Roth L, Pollack IW. Literacy skills of long-term hospitalized mental patients. Hosp Commun Psychiatry 1978;29:512–516.
25. Davis J, Kutter CJ. Independent living skills and posttraumatic stress disorder in women who are homeless: Implications for future practice. Am J Occup Ther 1998;52:39–44.
26. Decker MC. Evaluating the client with dementia. Am Occup Ther Assoc Ment Health Special Sect Q Newslett 1996;19(4):1–2.
27. Fisher AG. Assessment of Motor and Process Skills. Fort Collins, CO: Three Star, 1995.
28. Gutman SA, Mortera MH, Hinojosa J, Kramer P. Revision of the Occupational Therapy Practice Framework [The Issue Is]. Am J Occup Ther 2007;62:119–126.
29. Haertlein CAL. Ethics in evaluation in occupational therapy. Am J Occup Ther 1992;46:950–953.
30. Haertlein CL. The Milwaukee Evaluation of Daily Living Skills (MEDLS). In: Hemphill-Pearson BJ, ed. Assessments in Occupational Therapy Mental Health—An Integrative Approach. Thorofare, NJ: Slack, 1999.
31. Hemphill BJ. The evaluative process. In: Hemphill BJ, ed. The Evaluative Process in Psychiatric Occupational Therapy. Thorofare, NJ: Slack, 1982.
32. Henry AD. Development of a measure of adolescent leisure interests. Am J Occup Ther 1998;52:531–539.

33. Henry AD, Mallinson T. The Occupational Performance History Interview. In: Hemphill-Pearson BJ, ed. Assessments in Occupational Therapy Mental Health—An Integrative Approach. Thorofare NJ: Slack, 1999.
34. Henry AD, Moore K, Quinlivan M, Triggs M. The relationship of the Allen Cognitive Level test to demographics, diagnosis, and disposition among psychiatric patients. Am J Occup Ther 1998;52:638–643.
35. Hinojosa J, Kramer P, Crist P. Evaluation: Obtaining and Interpreting Data. 2nd ed. Bethesda MD: American Occupational Therapy Association Press, 2005.
36. Houston D, Williams SL, Bloomer J, Mann WC. The Bay Area Functional Performance Evaluation: Development and standardization. Am J Occup Ther 1989;43:170–183.
37. Kanny EM, Kohlman L. An occupational therapist evaluating functional living skills in psychiatry [video]. Seattle: University of Washington Health Sciences Center of Educational Resources, 1978.
38. Kielhofner G, ed. A Model of Human Occupation: Theory and Application. 4th ed. Baltimore: Lippincott Williams & Wilkins, in press.
39. Kielhofner G. Personal communication. Mar 14, 2007.
40. Kielhofner G, Mallinson T, Crawford C, et al. The User's Manual for The Occupational Performance History Interview. Version 2.0. Chicago: MOHO Clearinghouse, University of Illinois at Chicago, 2004.
41. Kielhofner G, Neville A. The Modified Interest Checklist. Available at: www.moho.uic.edu/mohorelatedrsrcs.html#OtherInstrumentsBasedonMOHO. Accessed Aug 2007.
42. King LJ. The person symbol as an assessment tool. In: Hemphill BJ, ed. The Evaluative Process in Psychiatric Occupational Therapy. Thorofare, NJ: Slack, 1982.
43. Klyczek JP. The Bay Area Functional Performance Evaluation. In: Hemphill-Pearson BJ, ed. Assessments in Occupational Therapy Mental Health—An Integrative Approach. Thorofare, NJ: Slack, 1999.
44. Klyczek JP, Bauer-Yox N, Fiedler RC. The Interest Checklist: A factor analysis. Am J Occup Ther 1997;51:815–823.
45. Kunz KR, Brayman SJ. The comprehensive occupational therapy evaluation. In: Hemphill-Pearson BJ, ed. Assessments in Occupational Therapy Mental Health—An Integrative Approach. Thorofare, NJ: Slack, 1999.
46. Law M. Evaluating activities of daily living: Directions for the future. Am J Occup Ther 1993;47:233–237.
47. Law M, Baptiste S, Carswell A, et al. Canadian Occupational Performance Measure. 2nd ed. Toronto: Canadian Association of Occupational Therapists, 1994.
48. Lerner C. The magazine picture collage. In: Hemphill BJ, ed. The Evaluative Process in Psychiatric Occupational Therapy. Thorofare, NJ: SLACK, 1982.
49. Letts L, Law M, Rigby P, et al. Person-environment assessments in occupational therapy. Am J Occup Ther 1994; 48:608–618.
50. Luebben AJ, Royeen CB. Nonstandardized testing. In: Hinojosa J, Kramer P, Crist P, eds. Evaluation: Obtaining and Interpreting Data. 2nd ed. Bethesda, MD: American Occupational Therapy Association Press, 2005.
51. Mann WC, Huselid R. An abbreviated task-oriented assessment (Bay Area Functional Performance Evaluation). Am J Occup Ther 1993;47:111–118.
52. Matsutsuyu JS. The Interest Checklist. Am J Occup Ther 1969;23:323–328.
53. McGourty LK. Kohlman Evaluation of Living Skills. Seattle: KELS Research, 1979.
54. Mosey AC. Three Frames of Reference for Mental Health. Thorofare, NJ: Slack, 1970.
55. Nygård L, Bernspang B, Fisher AG, Winblad B. Comparing motor and process ability of persons with suspected dementia in home and clinic settings. Am J Occup Ther 1994;48: 689–696.
56. Oakley F. Role Checklist, parts 1 and 2. In: Hemphill BJ, ed. Mental Health Assessment in Occupational Therapy: An Integrative Approach to the Evaluative Process. Thorofare, NJ: Slack, 1988.
57. Oakley F, Kielhofner G, Barris R, Klinger Reichler R. The Role Checklist: Development and empirical assessment of reliability. Occup Ther J Res 1986;6(3):157–170.
58. Park S, Fisher AG, Velozo CA. Using the assessment of motor and process skills to compare occupational performance between clinic and home settings. Am J Occup Ther 1994;48:697–709.
59. Parkinson S, Forstyth K, Kielhofner G. The Model of Human Occupation Screening Tool (MOHOST). Version 2.0. Chicago: MOHO Clearinghouse, University of Illinois at Chicago, 2006.
60. Peloquin SM. The development of an occupational therapy interview/therapy set procedure. Am J Occup Ther 1983; 37:457–461.
61. Rogers JC. The NPI Interest Checklist. In: Hemphill BJ, ed. Mental Health Assessment in Occupational Therapy: An Integrative Approach to the Evaluative Process. Thorofare, NJ: Slack, 1988.
62. Rogers JC, Weinstein JM, Figone JJ. The Interest Check List: An empirical assessment. Am J Occup Ther 1978;32: 628–630.
63. Secrest L, Wood AE, Tapp A. A comparison of the Allen Cognitive Level test and the Wisconsin Card Sorting test in adults with schizophrenia. Am J Occup Ther 2000;54: 129–133.
64. Shaw C. The interview process. In: Hemphill BJ, ed. The Evaluative Process in Psychiatric Occupational Therapy. Thorofare, NJ: Slack, 1982.
65. Smith NR, Kielhofner G, Watts JH. The Occupational Questionnaire. Available at: www.moho.uic.edu/mohorelatedrsrcs.html#OtherInstrumentsBasedonMOHO. Accessed Mar 2007.

66. Thomson LK. Kohlman Evaluation of Living Skills (KELS). In: Hemphill-Pearson BJ, ed. Assessments in Occupational Therapy Mental Health—An Integrative Approach. Thorofare, NJ: Slack, 1999.
67. Watanabe S. Four concepts basic to the occupational therapy process. Am J Occup Ther 1968;23:439–445.
68. Weinstock-Zlotnick G, Hinojosa J. Bottom-up or top-down evaluation: Is one better than the other? [The Issue Is]. Am J Occup Ther 2004;58:594–599.

## SUGGESTED READINGS

Asher IE. Occupational therapy assessment tools: An annotated index. 3rd ed. Bethesda, MD: American Occupational Therapy Association, 2007.

Bonder BR. Issues in assessment of psychosocial components of function. Am J Occup Ther 1993;47:211–216.

Haertlein CAL. Ethics in evaluation in occupational therapy. Am J Occup Ther 1992;46:950–953.

Hemphill-Pearson BJ, ed. Assessments in Occupational Therapy Mental Health—An Integrative Approach. Thorofare, NJ: Slack, 1999.

Hinojosa J, Kramer P. Evaluation: Obtaining and Interpreting Data. Bethesda, MD: American Occupational Therapy Association, 1998.

Kielhofner G, Henry AH. Use of an occupational history interview in occupational therapy. In: Hemphill BJ, ed. Mental Health Assessment in Occupational Therapy: An Integrative Approach to the Evaluative Process. Thorofare, NJ: Slack, 1988.

Model of Human Occupation Clearinghouse, University of Illinois at Chicago, 2006. Several instruments and checklists are available for purchase and download at www.moho.uic.edu.

Shaw C. The interviewing process in occupational therapy. In: Hemphill BJ, ed. Mental Health Assessment in Occupational Therapy: An Integrative Approach to the Evaluative Process. Thorofare, NJ: Slack, 1988.

CHAPTER 16

# Treatment and Intervention Planning

***The art of practice includes the ability to establish rapport, to empathize, and to facilitate choices about occupational and human potential within a community of others. Engaging in the art of practice commits the therapist to an encounter with an individual who is a collaborator in his or her plan for treatment.***

SUZANNE M. PELOQUIN (19)

## CHAPTER OBJECTIVES

After studying this chapter, the reader will be able to:

1. Identify and discuss the complementary roles of the occupational therapist (OT) and occupational therapy assistant (OTA) in intervention planning, implementation, review, modification, and outcome assessment.
2. Differentiate among different programs of intervention, such as rehabilitation and prevention.
3. Relate the development of outcomes to the intervention planning process.
4. Identify appropriate goal statements for problems related to mental disorders.
5. Identify the qualities of an effective goal statement.
6. Identify the components of an effective goal statement.
7. Relate long-term goals and short-term goals to each other, giving examples.
8. Discuss the value of quality assurance and continuous quality improvement for the intervention process.

Occupational therapy intervention or treatment[1] is a planned process for creating change so that the client will be able to carry out chosen daily life activities as independently and comfortably as possible. The client is the final authority as to which goals are most important. Occupational therapy practitioners have at their disposal a variety of methods that can be used to create change in the direction of the goal, but the methods must be chosen carefully, according to the person's needs. By its nature, treatment is individual and must be planned so that it meets the needs of the particular client.

The occupational therapist (OT) is responsible for the intervention plan (2, 4, 5). The occupational therapy assistant (OTA) may provide input to the therapist regarding the plan and may implement the plan and contribute to decisions about which methods to employ (4, 5). With experience, the assistant may become more practiced and make significant contributions, but the final responsibility for intervention planning and management still rests with the OT. In practice, this most often means that the therapist will determine a general intervention goal and the major steps within it and will make the final decision about the intervention methods. The assistant contributes to the plan as it is being developed by sharing observations of the client, making suggestions about what the person needs and is capable of, and suggesting intervention methods.

This chapter presents an overview of the intervention planning process. It starts by discussing some of the problems occupational therapy practitioners encounter in planning intervention for clients with psychiatric disorders that they do not encounter as often in planning intervention for patients with other kinds of problems. It considers the role of clinical reasoning in intervention planning and examines strategies for involving the client or consumer in developing the plan. The chapter analyzes how a goal is selected and considers several ways to go about writing a goal. Because OTAs work directly with patients and clients, carrying out intervention, this chapter explains how methods and activities are selected (how we determine what to do to move toward the goal) and how to carry plans over into the next setting. Finally, it describes how to monitor the success of intervention and when and how to modify the plan.

## TREATMENT PLANNING IN PSYCHIATRY

Planning treatment (or intervention) for a person with a psychiatric disorder is like trying to assemble a complex puzzle without having all of the pieces. Our scientific and clinical understanding of mental illness is not yet well enough developed for us to be certain of the real cause of the person's problems, and because of this it is hard to identify the best solution. To appreciate what a serious obstacle this can be, let us look first at the situation of someone with a *physical* disability.

**CASE EXAMPLE**

Mark is an 18-year-old high school senior who sustained a severe crushing injury to his right (dominant) hand as a result of a motorcycle accident. His index, middle, and ring, fingers were amputated just distal to the proximal interphalangeal (PIP) joint. When the cast was removed, it was noted that all motions of the thumb and fingers were severely limited. There is severe pain on movement. Mark has a girlfriend and several close friends. He belongs to the math and science club, the computer club, and the track team. Before the accident, he planned to attend college and major in computer science.

[1] Although the most recent standards of the American Occupational Therapy Association (5) use the term *intervention,* we will here and in subsequent chapters often use the more traditional term *treatment.*

We know enough about this patient to think about what might be an appropriate plan. First, we can anticipate that because of his injury, he will have problems performing bilateral (two-handed) activities such as dressing, grooming, and using a computer keyboard. We know that the immediate causes of Mark's difficulty are limited motion, weakness, and pain, and we know what caused them: a crushing injury. We can see the effects of the injury physically by examining the patient and looking at his radiographs. We know treatment methods that will increase range of motion and strength in the hand, and we know ways to reduce pain. We can suggest adaptive equipment and adapted methods for performing activities. In short, we know that once Mark tells us what goals are most important to him, occupational therapy can help him learn new ways to do the things he needs to do. We have ways to help him regain his physical functions and previous level of activity.

Contrast Mark's situation with the following case of someone of similar age and background who has a psychiatric disorder:

**CASE EXAMPLE**

Drew is a 19-year-old college freshman who has been living at home with his parents while attending school. During Thanksgiving weekend his parents found his room empty one morning and Drew could not be reached on his cell phone; after 24 hours, his parents notified the police. He was found 2 days later wandering on the street, wearing only his underwear. He had not eaten since he left home. His parents reported that he had been growing more isolated over the past 18 months, staying in his room for days at a time and refusing to come downstairs even for meals. He had been a good student, receiving As and Bs in his courses for the first 3 years of high school, but his grades fell to Cs and Ds in his senior year. He says he needs to be left alone because voices tell him that he "ruins other people's lives." Drew's diagnosis is schizophrenia, type unknown.

What exactly do we know about Drew? We know he has schizophrenia and has been having increasing difficulty functioning in his role as a student over the past year and a half. His grooming and hygiene skills have deteriorated; his ability to obtain a proper diet seems questionable; he is socially isolated. What can we do to help him? Where should we begin? Unlike physical disabilities, the causes of which can be seen on radiographs, physical examinations, and laboratory tests, the causes of the psychiatric disability associated with schizophrenia elude us. Brain research using sophisticated imaging equipment has identified abnormalities in the brains of individuals with schizophrenia but not the source of these anomalies. Psychiatrists know some medications that help relieve the symptoms for some consumers, but they are still trying to understand why and how these medications work.

In the meantime, however, how are we to help Drew? It is not clear what his immediate and long-term goals might be, although we can identify areas that will likely need attention: self-care, other independent daily living skills, nutrition, academic and study skills, leisure and social skills. But which one shall we tackle first, and why?

Once the goals are chosen, how shall we address them? As occupational therapy practitioners we are proficient in analyzing, teaching, and adapting activities of daily living and a wide range of work, education, leisure, and social interaction activities. We know how to break new learning into manageable small steps so that a person can master a complex skill one step at a time. We have many techniques and methods at our disposal. But how shall we choose which ones to use?

Part of our uncertainty about how to answer all of these questions stems from our ignorance of exactly how schizophrenia works to undermine a person's ability to function in daily life. Another source of uncertainty for beginners (students and new therapists) is inexperience with clients such as this one and the lack of a mental file of intervention attempts and outcomes.

When therapists plan intervention, they are taking patients' lives in their hands. Therapy practitioners do not have the same life-or-death responsibility as the surgeon at the operating table, but the decisions they make *will* affect the patient's life. People with severe psychiatric disabilities have fewer choices and in some senses less freedom than the rest of us; their disabilities limit what they can do and even how they can think about what they can do; social and economic pressures limit them still further. Therapists and other professionals are asked to make recommendations about where clients should live, what they should do during the day, how much supervision they should receive, and so forth. Clinical reasoning can help in making these decisions.

## USING PRACTICE MODELS TO APPLY CLINICAL REASONING IN PLANNING

In planning interventions, a practice model organizes our thinking. Let's look at the questions the occupational therapist might derive from the model of human occupation. Figure 16-1 shows assessment questions to be considered (11). The questions are determined by the elements and subsystems within the model. Using the diagram, OTAs can appreciate the multiple perspectives considered in an overall plan designed by the OT under the model of human occupation. Practitioners using other practice models follow a similar process to generate assessment questions based on the design of the chosen model. For example, the OT and OTA using the cognitive disabilities model ask questions such as these:

- Which sensory cues are disregarded by the person? To which sensory cues does he or she attend?
- Is the client able to follow a two-step direction?

The answers, according to the cognitive disabilities model, guide the construction of a intervention plan to adapt the client's life situation and to bring the task demands within the person's range of ability.

In the cognitive-behavioral model, to take a different example, some of the questions might be these:

- What are this person's beliefs and assumptions about life?
- What does this person say are the causes of any life problems?
- What errors in thinking are behind the client's beliefs?

The answers to these questions would guide development of a intervention plan to challenge and refute the erroneous thinking. Thus, using a specific practice model or frame of reference is invaluable in generating assessment questions and obtaining data on which to base the plan.

## STEPS IN INTERVENTION PLANNING

Let us break down this clinical reasoning process into discrete steps. Using these steps, the OTA can help formulate intervention plans in areas such as independent daily living skills. Box 16-1 highlights the steps in intervention planning.

The first step, reviewing the results of the evaluation or evaluations, should be executed with an open mind but with a clear idea of what kinds of information one is seeking. The OTA might be assigned a specific area of occupation in which to plan intervention; basic and instrumental daily living skills are examples. Obviously, evaluation results that relate directly to the area in question would be the most important, but other information may also be valuable. For example, the client's relationship with other family members in the household may give some clues about why he or she shows deficits in independent living skills. It is important not to confine your investigation to what

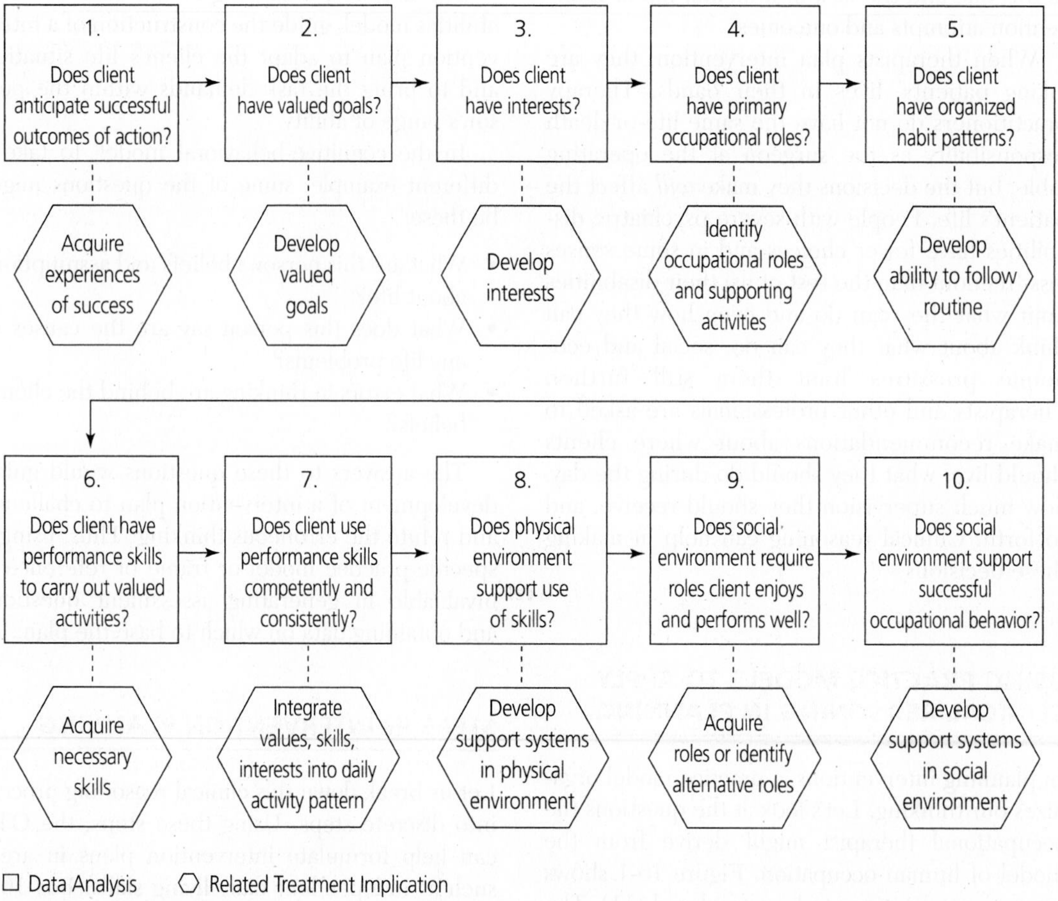


**Figure 16-1. Reasoning with the model of human occupation.** (Adapted with permission from Kielhofner G, ed. A Model of Human Occupation: Theory and Application. 3rd ed. Baltimore: Lippincott Williams & Wilkins; 2002.)

**BOX 16-1**

**STEPS IN PLANNING INTERVENTION**

1. Review the results of the individual assessment(s) and the evaluation and discuss them with the client.
2. Identify problems and, if possible, their causes.
3. Identify the person's strengths and assess/estimate the person's readiness and motivation for intervention.
4. Collaborate with the client to set goals (long and short term, in order of priority).
5. Identify intervention principles using the practice model.
6. Select methods appropriate to the practice model.

you expect to find and to maintain a curious and alert perspective. Try not to be too strongly influenced by the person's diagnosis or by the opinions of other staff. Deliberate ongoing openness to the person as an individual is the surest route to learning the client's strengths and potential.

The purpose of reviewing the evaluation is to obtain the answers to the second and third steps, to learn as much as you can about the client's problems (deficits), strengths (assets), and readiness or motivation for change. This requires combining information from many sources; you cannot expect to find the answers in one place, and you may have to combine what you know to come up with an answer. Try to define as clearly as you can the causes of the client's problems as well as the problems themselves. An understanding of the causes is often the key to the most effective approach to intervention.

For example, a patient may have very poor hygiene–as evidenced by greasy hair, stained teeth, and body odor-for a variety of reasons: He or she may never have developed good hygiene skills, he or she may have gotten out of the habit of using those skills, or his or her usual environment may make it difficult to perform hygiene and grooming tasks (e.g., because of homelessness). There may be cultural reasons: Daily bathing and frequent shampooing are Western values; personal hygiene standards elsewhere vary. There may be reasons that derive from the disease process: The person may not remember to bathe and care for his or her body, the sense of time may be distorted, or the person may be so frightened of other people that he or she ignores hygiene to drive others away. You can see that these various causes for the person's poor hygiene will lead to very different ideas about what kind of intervention is needed and where it should begin. Thinking through the causes in this way may lead you to consider whether you are using a practice model that is appropriate to the client's situation.

## PARTNERSHIP WITH THE CLIENT OR CONSUMER

A relationship with the consumer or client should be established before the therapist begins to plan intervention. Assessments such as the *Canadian Occupational Performance Measure (COPM)* (14), discussed in Chapter 15, or the *Community Adaptive Planning Assessment (CAPA)* (21) provide a clear picture of the goals valued by the client and suggest areas for intervention. If the evaluation phase has gone well, the OT and OTA should be able to use information from the interview and from assessments of the client's goals and interests to make a tentative plan for work on specific goals. The therapist (usually the OT) then discusses these with the client to verify their importance. The therapist continues to adjust the plan as the relationships of the OTA and OT with the client develop and the client's goals become better known. Thus clinical reasoning is continually focused and refined by the client's contributions.

The client can often tell you what is wrong and help define the problem. Involving the client in planning intervention to the extent the person is capable ensures that the client understands and agrees with the plan, a first step in securing motivation to work on goals. Even clients who have limited ability to verbalize their concerns can be guided to participate. In such cases the clinician may have to present limited choices from which the client can make a selection. For example, the client might choose which goal or area to tackle first (18).

The person's strengths must also be considered. Although the main focus of our energies will be on finding solutions to the client's problems, we need to appreciate and acknowledge the person's endurance, persistence, and courage in carrying on with life despite disability. The skills and habits the client has developed and maintained and the client's resolve to work hard and succeed can only be strengthened by our recognition and support.

Furthermore, we should consider the supports and resources present in the environment, such as helpful family members and the social support of friends.

Questions sometimes arise about a client's motivation for change. The person who fails to work toward goals that the therapist considers appropriate and necessary may be labeled as unmotivated. This may indicate that the goals do not reflect the person's real concerns. An example is the 27-year-old legal secretary with a diagnosis of paranoid schizophrenia who says she would rather collect public assistance and stay home and watch television than go back to work. Rather than force acceptance of a work adjustment training program, the occupational therapy practitioner might do better to explore the thinking behind this decision. The intervention cannot succeed unless the client is actively involved.

Any disagreements between the client and the staff about the best course must be discussed. If the staff has identified problems that they believe the client should address, they must explain them so that the client understands them. They must listen and respond to the client's questions, concerns, and preferences. In presenting recommendations, the staff stresses the tangible benefits that will result. If the client cannot accept the staff's recommendations, the staff must modify its expectations and work with the client to reach agreement about what should be done.

However, in inpatient settings with acutely ill persons it is not always possible to obtain the patient's cooperation and participation in planning intervention. It is very difficult to engage the attention or even the awareness of someone who is psychotic and out of touch with reality; therefore, in acute care settings, the staff may develop a intervention plan on behalf of the patient, sometimes in consultation with members of the patient's family.

Once the staff and the client or family have agreed on a general direction for intervention, the next step is to set specific goals. A goal is a statement about what the client will achieve. Goals can be classified as long term or short term. A *long-term goal* states the functional outcome or destination of the intervention. This is the ultimate aim; examples are "to get a job" and "to have my own apartment."

*Short-term goals* can be understood as small steps to achieve a long-term goal. A short-term goal considers the length of time available for treatment as well as the client's sense of time and ability to visualize the future; short-term goals are those that can be accomplished in a few weeks or less. Breaking down long-term goals into a series of short-term goals can make it easier for the client to tackle them. It has become common, particularly in settings that use the psychiatric rehabilitation model, to use the term *objective* when referring to short-term goals (13, 17). Thus we advise the reader that the terms *short-term goal* and *objective* for all practical purposes may be synonymous.

Goals should be organized in order of priority. *Priority* means the importance or urgency of the goal. In many cases, especially with persons who have severe and persistent mental illness, it is possible to come up with a list of 5 or 6 long-term goals and 20 or more short-term goals (or objectives). Not all of them will be equally important, however, and the therapist must decide which ones are to be tackled first. Some goals by their nature must be achieved before others; for example, someone who needs to learn basic cooking to live independently must first learn elementary kitchen safety. Usually only a few (not more than 3 or 4) goals are attempted at one time; sometimes only 1 goal is selected at first. Decisions about how many goals to choose should be based on the client's ability to divide his or her energies effectively among the different goals and on the amount of effort needed to reach a particular goal.

Regardless of which short-term goals are chosen first, there should be an overall plan that describes the long-term goals of the client's program. Although it may take months or years to reach these long-term goals, having a clear final aim helps unify the smaller goals. Otherwise the program is likely to be fragmented and the purpose obscured. In other words, short-term goals, such as "learning to follow a schedule" or "arriving on time for activity groups," should be part of a larger plan, the ultimate goal of which might be, for example, "to get a job and be financially independent."

These first steps in intervention planning (identification of problems, strengths, and motivation and setting of intervention priorities) should be done in consultation with other clinical personnel who are working with the client. If the other staff do not agree with the occupational therapy practitioner's assessment of the client's problems, they are not likely to support the plan. Plans that the client, the family, and the staff agree on have the best chance of success, because everyone will work toward them.

## GENERAL GOALS OF PSYCHIATRIC OCCUPATIONAL THERAPY

Let us start with the understanding that the overall aim of occupational therapy, regardless of area of specialization, is to help individuals engage in occupation, to function as independently as possible within the limits of their disabilities, in the contexts of their choice. Thus whether the OTA is helping the person who has arthritis learn to use energy conservation and joint protection techniques in cooking or the OT is providing tactile stimulation to the tactilely defensive child, the final purpose is the same; to make it possible for that person to function optimally within his or her chosen activities and occupational roles. Thus all goals should address functional occupation-centered outcomes.

### Categories of Intervention

It is traditional to classify occupational therapy intervention as fitting into one of four broad categories: treatment (sometimes called functional restoration), maintenance of function, rehabilitation, and prevention (24). The focus of intervention differs with the category.

*Treatment* or *functional restoration* aims to alter the underlying disease process; the principles and techniques of sensory integration fit into this category. It is not clear whether occupational therapy interventions, even those of sensory integration, really affect the underlying disease process in most psychiatric disorders. We do not yet know enough about the underlying disease process to say one way or the other.

*Maintenance of function* is aimed at assisting the person to use his or her remaining capabilities. This is often the focus of programs for individuals with chronic or progressive disorders, such as schizophrenia and organic mental disorders. In this approach, the occupational therapy practitioner works at creating an environment that supports and encourages individuals to care for their own needs and to take charge of their own lives in whatever way they can for as long as possible. Despite the best efforts of client and therapist, the long-term outlook in some cases is that the person will function less and less well as time goes by. Without occupational therapy, however, the person will more rapidly lose the ability to function.

*Rehabilitation* focuses on restoring the person's ability to function after the disease process has been medically treated. The client has lost the ability to function as a result of the disease; this loss of function is termed a *residual disability*. Even though the disease process has been cured (or more typically in psychiatry, stabilized with medication), the person still may not perform daily activities and carry out valued occupational roles with the same level of efficiency or success as before the illness. The word *habilitation* is used to distinguish intervention for clients who never developed these functional abilities because they became ill at a young age. Rehabilitation and habilitation are a major focus of psychiatric occupational therapy. However, this approach is appropriate only for persons who are able to change their habits and learn new skills. This is difficult to judge because some people resist changing for many months (perhaps because they are frightened of the responsibility this might imply) but then suddenly seem to begin applying themselves to their own rehabilitation. Cognitive level should be considered here. Persons functioning at level 4 and lower are not likely to learn new skills, even with great motivation and effort.

*Prevention* aims to intervene before dysfunction occurs. It is usually applied when a dysfunction is predicted. A supportive activity group for children of alcoholic parents is one example. Prevention overlaps with the other areas already discussed—for instance, maintenance of function is in some sense a form of prevention because it aims to prevent a deterioration that is otherwise inevitable.

### Matching Goal Statements to the Category of Intervention

Keeping these important categories in mind, look at the skills listed in Table 16-1. The skills are derived from the *Occupational Therapy Practice Framework: Domain and Process (OTPF)* (3), Mosey's adaptive skills, and other practice models. Several goals are listed for some skill areas; each goal may be phrased in such a way as to focus on rehabilitation or habilitation, maintenance of function, or prevention. Beginning the goal statement with verbs such as *to develop, to restore,* and *to improve* indicates an emphasis on rehabilitation or habilitation. Maintenance of function is the indicated focus of goals that begin with the words *to maintain ability to,* and prevention is the focus of goals that begin with the words *to prevent dysfunction of ability to.*

The reader may observe some overlap among groupings in the table. For example, some mental functions related to communication could easily have been listed under the communication/interaction performance skills. This reflects the current organization of the *OTPF,* which will no doubt be revised after the publication of this text.

The list in Table 16-1 is by no means exhaustive, and the reader should remember three important cautions in using this list. First, not every possible goal is listed; do not be discouraged if a goal you think is important is missing from the list. Second, other occupational therapy goals, such as those that relate to movement functions, may have to be addressed even for clients whose primary diagnosis is psychiatric—for example, the person who has depression and is recovering from a tendon repair following a wrist slashing will need physical restoration as well. Third, many of the listed goals themselves depend on smaller goals or subskills. The needs of the individual must be considered because, for many, the place to begin is with the subskills or underlying factors. The goals listed in Table 16-1 are an overview of the general objectives of psychiatric occupational therapy; they are only a reference point and are not meant to substitute for the highly specific goals that are developed for each client. Writing more specific, individualized, and measurable goals derived from these general goals is the subject of the next section.

## HOW TO WRITE AN INTERVENTION GOAL

Goals in an intervention plan should be written so that they describe very clearly what the person will do. Goals should follow logically from problems that have been identified by assessment and selected by the client and staff as important. The more specific the description of the problem, the easier it is to write the corresponding goal. Consider the following:

- Mr. Peters has low self-esteem.
- Ms. Danford has poor reality testing.

These problem statements are confusing because they describe not the person's behavior or indeed anything measurable or observable but rather some unverifiable internal state. Each could be converted into a statement of a specific

**TABLE 16-1 SOME GENERAL GOALS OF PSYCHIATRIC OCCUPATIONAL THERAPY**

| FOCUS OF INTERVENTION | GOALS (TO ESTABLISH, RESTORE, IMPROVE, OR MAINTAIN ABILITY TO . . .) |
|---|---|
| ADLs | Initiate and effectively perform to a socially acceptable level such activities as grooming, oral hygiene, bathing or showering, toilet hygiene, personal device care, dressing, feeding and eating, functional mobility, sexual expression |
| IADLs: community mobility | Travel within community on foot and by mechanical transport (car, bus) |
| IADLs: financial management | Use money and other forms of payment<br>Budget within one's means<br>Plan for financial goals |
| IADLs: health management | Develop and maintain physical and psychological health by health and wellness routines, adhering to medication schedule, decreasing health risk behaviors |
| IADLs: shopping | Prepare lists<br>Locate and select items<br>Use payment methods such as cash or other<br>Apply arithmetical knowledge to money transactions |
| IADLs: meal preparation and cleanup | Plan nutritious meals within budget<br>Prepare food<br>Cook<br>Clean up |
| IADLs: emergency response | Recognize unsafe situations and respond with effective measures (remedy dangerous condition, call 911, remove self and others from danger) |
| IADLs: home management | Organize and carry out tasks related to clothing care, cleaning, household maintenance, safety procedures |
| IADLs: care of others, childrearing | Provide physical care, nurturance, and appropriate activities for children and others under one's care |
| Education | Plan and carry out tasks related to schooling, such as homework, study, preparation for tests, extracurricular activities |
| Work: employment interests and pursuits | Identify aptitudes and interests, identify and pursue vocational training suited to one's aptitude, interests, skills |
| Work: employment seeking | Search, identify, and select work opportunities<br>Carry out application and interview process<br>Evaluate results of application and interview process |
| Work: job performance | Follow directions<br>Perform job tasks effectively within the context<br>Work neatly and with reasonable attention to detail<br>Follow a schedule, maintain attendance, adhere to time standards of the job<br>Demonstrate appropriate behaviors in grooming, interpersonal communication, safety |

*(continued)*

**TABLE 16-1 SOME GENERAL GOALS OF PSYCHIATRIC OCCUPATIONAL THERAPY *(Continued)***

| FOCUS OF INTERVENTION | GOALS (TO ESTABLISH, RESTORE, IMPROVE, OR MAINTAIN ABILITY TO . . .) |
|---|---|
| Work: retirement planning | Determine valued goals and interests and pursue them |
| Work: volunteer participation | Perform unpaid activities to benefit others |
| Play and leisure: exploration | Identify interests and skills and find appropriate opportunities to pursue them |
| Play and leisure: performance | Schedule time and follow through on using leisure to pursue interests |
| Social participation | Interact in ways that are socially appropriate to culture and context<br>Interact successfully with peers, family members, community |
| Motor performance skills | Move in environment effectively to accomplish task<br>Use objects<br>Engage in desired occupations |
| Process performance skills | Manage and modify actions to accomplish desired tasks and occupations<br>Use pacing to conserve energy<br>Obtain and use knowledge to execute tasks; organize tasks in time by initiating, continuing, sequencing, and completing actions effectively<br>Organize space and objects for effective task completion<br>Demonstrate flexibility in adapting to changes in tasks and environment<br>Adjust self to complete occupational tasks |
| Communication and interaction performance skills | Coordinate behavior so as to effectively convey and receive information in relation to others<br>Use gestures, eye contact, physical distance and personal space in ways that are socially appropriate and effective for communication<br>Give and receive information<br>Speak, ask, respond, modulate communication in a manner conducive to task completion<br>Interact comfortably with one other person and within a group<br>Relate to others with respect<br>Collaborate with groups and partners, and conform to groups as needed<br>Compromise, negotiate, cooperate, and compete with others<br>Use facial and bodily gestures, voice tone and volume to express feelings and ideas<br>Assert self |
| Performance patterns: habits | Demonstrate useful habits to support occupational engagement<br>Abstain from or diminish involvement in nonproductive or dominating habits |
| Performance patterns: routines | Demonstrate effective routines related to occupational engagement |

*(continued)*

## TABLE 16-1 SOME GENERAL GOALS OF PSYCHIATRIC OCCUPATIONAL THERAPY *(Continued)*

| FOCUS OF INTERVENTION | GOALS (TO ESTABLISH, RESTORE, IMPROVE, OR MAINTAIN ABILITY TO . . .) |
|---|---|
| Performance patterns: roles | Engage effectively in desired and necessary occupational roles<br>Identify, value, and carry out roles within a social context (e.g., worker, student, neighbor) |
| Sensory functions (pertaining to occupational engagement) | Attend to sensory stimuli<br>Correctly interpret sensory stimuli<br>Organize information received through senses<br>Integrate body parts in reaction to sensory stimuli |
| Mental functions (pertaining to occupational engagement) | Demonstrate alertness and responsiveness to situations in environment<br>Locate self in regard to time, place, and person<br>Recognize familiar faces<br>Concentrate and attend to a task long enough to complete it<br>Remember important information and skills<br>Place information, steps, concepts in order<br>Generalize learning to new situations<br>Make decisions<br>Solve problems as they arise<br>Initiate and maintain performance and attention in an activity<br>Cease an activity when it is appropriate or desirable to do so |
| Mental functions: experience of self (pertaining to occupational engagement) | Identify and enact ideas and beliefs important to the self<br>Perceive, understand, accept, and enact direction of self<br>Identify and pursue activities that bring pleasure to self |
| Mental functions: self-concept (pertaining to occupational engagement) | Accept and embrace self as having value<br>Identify one's assets and limitations |
| Mental functions: coping (pertaining to occupational engagement) | Identify stress, stress reaction, stressors<br>Identify, select, and apply stress management strategies |
| Mental functions: sense and use of time (pertaining to occupational engagement) | Sequence motor actions in time.<br>Maintain time orientation<br>Budget and schedule use of time |
| Mental functions: self-control (pertaining to occupational engagement) | Recognize one's own behavior and its internal and external causes<br>Control feelings and impulses<br>Take responsibility for one's own behavior<br>Modify one's behavior as appropriate for situation |

*ADLs,* activities of daily living; *IADLs,* instrumental activities of daily living.
Terms based on American Occupational Therapy Association. Occupational therapy practice framework: Domain and process. Am J Occup Ther 2002;56:609–639.

behavioral problem by the addition of some observable evidence. For example, "Mr. Peters demonstrates behaviors suggesting poor self-esteem, as evidenced by greasy hair, rumpled clothing, and stained teeth" is a specific observation of behavior. However, one is left with questions about whether these behaviors reflect poor self-esteem or perhaps something else. Therefore, problem statements that contain observable behaviors are preferred to those that refer to intrapsychic phenomena or other intangibles. Here are some problem statements that meet this criterion:

- Ms. Flint exhibits poor hygiene as evidenced by greasy hair, stained teeth, and body odor.
- Mr. Mills reports no regular leisure interests except watching television and drinking.
- Ms. Woolworth has been fired from many jobs as a result of arguments with supervisors.

Once the problems have been adequately described, the goals that correspond to them can be written. Goals also must be phrased in terms of how the client will behave or what the client will do once the goal is reached. Examples of goals for these three problems are as follows:

- Ms. Flint will wash her hair twice a week, bathe daily, and brush her teeth twice every day.
- Mr. Mills will attend the activity center two evenings a week and will have dinner with a friend once a week.
- For 3 weeks, Ms. Woolworth will not argue with the therapists and group leaders in her activity programs.

These goals have been written in behavioral terms so that all concerned, therapist, client, and other staff, will know when the goal has been reached. By contrast, it is impossible to agree on when or whether a goal such as "Mr. Peters will have increased self-esteem" has been reached; there is no way to measure success.

## RUMBA

Some therapists use the mnemonic RUMBA to evaluate the goal statements they write. RUMBA stands for these points:

Relevant
Understandable
Measurable
Behavioral
Achievable

A goal is *relevant* if it reflects the individual's life situation and future goals. As discussed previously, both client and therapist should agree that the goal is important; and other team members such as the social worker, the psychiatrist, and the nurse should support these goals. Making sure that everyone involved agrees that the goals are relevant helps prevent conflicts. For example, a 24-year-old man may describe his main goal as having a girlfriend. The therapist or assistant might explain that socialization groups at the day treatment center will help the person learn how to meet people and develop relationships with them.

A goal is *understandable* when it is stated in plain language and observable terms. Professional jargon is to be avoided, and the goal should be phrased so that the client and the family can understand it.

A goal is *measurable* when it contains one or more criteria for success. It is best if each criterion is stated in quantifiable terms (numbers) rather than qualitative ones. For example, "bathing once a day" is more easily measured than "having adequate hygiene." Similarly, it is important to include an estimated date of completion, a time by which the goal should be reached. Thus the measurable criteria should include any of the *measures* shown in Box 16-2 as well as a *time frame,* or time limit, by which the goal is to be achieved.

A goal is *behavioral* when it focuses on what the client must *do* to accomplish the goal. It is

**BOX 16-2**

## MAKING GOALS MEASURABLE AND TIME LIMITED

Measure
- Frequency, or *how often* (e.g., twice daily)
- Duration, or *how long* (e.g., for 30 minutes)
- Level of accuracy (e.g., with 50% accuracy)
- Number of times (e.g., 6 times)
- Level of assistance needed (e.g., with standby assistance)

Time frame
- By specific date (e.g., by March 27, 2008)
- By end of specific unit of time (e.g., by 30 days)
- After a specified number of sessions (e.g., after five sessions)
- By a known milestone (e.g., by discharge)

*achievable* when it is something that the person is likely to be able to accomplish within a reasonably short period as defined by the client and the therapist together. For instance, assume the client is a very isolated 24-year-old man who has always lived with his parents and who has never held a job. Getting a job and moving into his own apartment *might* be future goals but certainly not immediate ones; *achievable* goals with which to begin might be limited to traveling back and forth to the day treatment center on his own and arriving on time.

The following are some goals, developed from those in Table 16-1, using the RUMBA criteria:

Performance patterns: roles
- The client will identify the primary functions and tasks of her role as mother of a preschooler by the end of 3 weeks.
- The client will identify at least two ways in which her disability interferes with her functioning effectively in the role of mother of a preschooler and will identify ways to compensate within 3 weeks.
- The client will go with her child to a play date at a another parent's home, twice within the next 2 weeks.

Play and leisure: exploration
- The member will identify and discuss at least three interests that are important to him by the end of 2 weeks.
- The client will identify at least three ways to pursue his interest in watercolor painting by the end of the next session.

Instrumental activities of daily living (IADLs): health management
- The client will use the Yellow Pages to locate the telephone number and address of a pharmacy near her home by the end of the next session.
- The client will visit the pharmacy near her home and locate the prescription counter within the next week.
- The client will drop off and pick up her prescription medication at a pharmacy near her home, within 2 days of receiving the prescription.

Communication and interaction performance skills (physicality)
- The member will consistently stand *no closer than 3 feet* from another person when engaged in a work-related conversation by the end of 4 weeks.

- The member will maintain eye contact with the waitress for at least 3 seconds while ordering coffee at the local cafe.

## How to Write About Goals That Seem Unmeasureable

Despite application of the RUMBA criteria, the therapist or assistant may find that some goals appropriate for persons with psychiatric disabilities are difficult to measure. Abilities such as self-assertion, self-control, and independence (unlike range of motion or muscle strength) cannot be physically measured and quantified. There are at least two ways around this problem. The first is to include behavioral indicators of the desired goal in the criteria (17). For example, in the case of self-control:

- The client's family will report no violent behaviors during a visit of the client with her family for a meal over the weekend.
- The client will describe at least one constructive way in which she coped with her feelings during the visit with her family over the weekend.

The second way is to develop a rating scale for each goal. Goal attainment scaling (GAS) (9, 12, 16) identifies five levels of achievement for a goal. Two of the levels are higher than what is expected, two are lower than what is expected, and the middle level defines the expected outcome. Table 16-2

**TABLE 16-2 GOAL ATTAINMENT SCALE FOR TWO GOALS**

| | | GOALS | |
|---|---|---|---|
| PREDICTED ATTAINMENT | SCORE | SOCIAL INTERACTIONS | WEIGHT LOSS (HEALTH MAINTENANCE) |
| Most unfavorable outcome | −2 | Speaks to no one except therapist during 3-hour session | Gains 5 pounds within 1 month |
| Less than expected outcome | −1 | Says hello or other greeting to fellow workers during 3-hour training session | Maintains weight over 1 month |
| Expected level of outcome | −0 | Holds sustained, interactive conversation of 200 words or 10 minutes with one other worker during 3-hour session | Loses 5 pounds within 1 month |
| Greater than expected outcome | +1 | Holds interactive conversation of more than 200 words or 10 minutes with two or more workers independently or simultaneously during 3-hour session | Loses 10 pounds within 1 month |
| Most favorable outcome likely | +2 | Holds interactive conversation of 500 words or 20 minutes with three or more workers during 3-hour session | Loses 15 pounds within 1 month |

Modified with permission from Ottenbacher KJ, Cusick A. Goal attainment scaling as a method of clinical service evaluation. Am J Occup Ther 1990;44:519–525. Copyright ©1990 by American Occupational Therapy Association, Inc.

gives two examples of how this might be done. GAS provides the consumer, the team, and the reimburser with a clear understanding of what the person is expected to achieve.

Scott and Haggerty (20) used GAS concepts in a partial hospitalization (outpatient) setting to help clients set their own goals and define their own criteria for success in meeting them. With the use of a paper and pencil form, the client was asked to select a goal based on problems identified through evaluation. Next, the client was encouraged to explore and discuss why he or she chose that particular goal and how it related to the client's immediate and future concerns. Then the client was asked to state what outcome he or she would *expect* to achieve. (Scott and Haggerty give the example of a person who is chronically 15 minutes late; the expected outcome is that the person will be 10 minutes late.) Working from this expected outcome, the person then describes a least-favorable outcome and a most-favorable one. Finally, outcomes intermediate between the expected one and the extreme ones are described (less favorable, more favorable). Of course, it is not necessary to identify five different points on the rating scale; three points (expected, more than expected, and less than expected) are sufficient.

### Involving Clients in Setting Their Own Goals

Involving clients directly in selecting goals and measuring success can help them feel and become more independent and assertive; it can also give staff and clients some sense of how clients see their needs and what kinds of goals they believe are possible. Scott and Haggerty (20) point out that not all clients are capable of generating their own goals and attainment scales and that persons with organic disorders and cognitive disabilities need assistance from the therapist. Those who are acutely ill seem to have more difficulty monitoring themselves once they have set up the attainment scales, and this may be owing to their fluctuating symptoms; the approach seems to work better with those who are chronically ill.

To summarize, goals may be written by the OT or the supervised OTA in collaboration with the client and family. A particular client's involvement in selecting and refining goals may be limited to varying degrees by cognitive impairments or psychotic symptoms. Nonetheless, occupational therapy staff must try to involve the person as much as possible. Goals must address functional outcomes. Goals should be relevant to the client's needs and values and stated in terms that the client can understand. Goals should contain some criterion against which success can be measured, and they must indicate the behavior the person is to demonstrate. They must include a time frame that is reasonable and that corresponds to the reimbursement guidelines applicable to the situation. Finally, they must be achievable—that is, realistic for this person at this time in his or her life.

## SELECTING APPROPRIATE INTERVENTION PRINCIPLES

Once the goals are written, the next task is to figure out how to reach them. At the beginning of this chapter, we emphasized the importance of identifying the causes of the client's problems as well as the problems themselves. In other words, occupational therapy practitioners try to choose a theory or principle or a practice model that best explains the client's problems, to guide in selecting methods of intervention. To return to our example, a person may have poor hygiene for any of many reasons. It makes a difference whether the reason is that the client never learned the necessary hygiene and grooming routines or just forgets or does not wash because his or her skin feels funny when he or she touches it. Or perhaps the person is afraid of washing away part of his or her body. Each of these reasons leads to different notions about how to approach the problem.

If the reason for the person's poor hygiene is that he or she never learned proper grooming and hygiene, the most logical approach would be to teach the client the skills; but we must first determine whether there are any sociocultural or personal reasons that might interfere with the desire to learn. Use of the development of adaptive skills model would be appropriate in this case.

If the reason is that he or she forgets, we need to know more about why (organic memory loss, disorganization, depression and lack of focus, having too many things to do, or lack of a reinforcing environment are just a few possible reasons), and then we can figure out a way to help the person remember. Perhaps memory aids or the assistance of another person is necessary. The therapist might apply the cognitive disabilities model in such a situation.

If the reason is that the client's skin "feels funny," then we might suspect a sensory processing problem, and we might ask the OT whether this could be evaluated. The point is that the more we know about the cause of the person's problem, the easier it is to select a practice model and intervention methods.

The different theories and practice models discussed in Chapters 2 to 4 contain principles for organizing our thinking about the client's problems and how to approach them. We choose a theory on the basis of how well it explains the client's problems and how effectively it helps us solve them. Allen's theory of cognitive disabilities is very useful for evaluating how well a person with chronic schizophrenia can function in an independent living situation and for detailing how to modify the environment so that it better supports the person's functioning. However, this theory helps little in designing a work adjustment program for an intelligent but depressed middle-aged woman whose children have grown up and left home. For this situation, the model of human occupation or the role acquisition model is a better guide for planning. No one theory is adequate to address every problem, and so it is important to choose the best one for the particular situation.

Intangible factors such as self-esteem can and often should be considered in this stage of intervention planning. Several of the theories covered in this text are based at least in part on ideas about the client's feelings and internal psychodynamics. The client's sense of personal causation (model of human occupation) or narcissistic needs (object relations) may provide clues about what principles we might follow. Although these intangibles cannot be directly measured and so should not be written into the goals, they can guide our selection of intervention methods. If we believe, for example, that the person is neglecting hygiene because self-esteem is low as a result of being laid off from work for the second time in 18 months, we will direct our energies toward raising self-esteem and procuring work opportunities, assuming that the hygiene will follow.

## SELECTING INTERVENTION METHODS

Once we have chosen the theory and the principles we believe best explain the client's problems, we can choose methods based on them. The method specifies the activity to be used, the environment in which it will be performed, and the approach the therapist will use to present the activity. Each of these—activity, environment, and therapeutic approach—is examined separately.

### Activity

Activities are chosen on the basis of the stated principles identified in the plan. Activities are selected primarily for their ability to address the intervention goal. We determine this through activity analysis. Analysis and adaptation of activities for psychosocial problems is the subject of Chapter 23. Knowledgeable analysis must be the basis of activity selection if we expect to produce the desired therapeutic effect. For example, if we suspect that the person has trouble making decisions because other people have always decided for him or her, we will look for an activity that involves making choices rather than one that requires absolute adherence to a sequence of rules or directions; ceramics, leathercraft, cooking, gardening, and shopping could be adapted to fit this principle. On the other hand, if the person has been fired from many jobs because he or she did not follow the rules, perhaps an activity with lots of rules and restrictions and serious consequences for ignoring them will help the client explore his or her feelings about following them. Working in wood, a notoriously unforgiving medium, or with slip casting in ceramics might be appropriate for this.

Although occupational therapy practitioners use other therapeutic tools, such as counseling and environmental modification, activity or engagement in occupation should always be a prominent feature of intervention. Activity and occupation have the power to heal and to create change in a way that verbal therapies simply cannot. When a person actually *does* something, he or she explores and experiences his or her own effect on the world; when a person talks, he or she only imagines it (8). By participating in activities, people learn about themselves, about their abilities to use tools and materials, about the pleasure of working directly with their hands and bodies and minds, about the reactions of others to what they have done. They discover, refine, and shape their images of themselves; they discover what they can and cannot do. And they become better at the things they desire to do,

It is essential that the activities chosen for therapy provide the person with experiences that are pleasurable and that reinforce and enhance a sense of competence and mastery (1, 6). This does not mean that the activities should be easy; to engage the person's interest and drive toward competency they must provide a reasonable challenge. Activities, occupational tasks, and occupations themselves will be discussed in detail in Chapters 18 to 22.

## Environment

The conditions under which the activity takes place influence the client's response. An individual's home environment and performance contexts (see Chapter 15) and the treatment setting (see Chapter 7) must be considered. Environments communicate demands but also provide supports for activity performance. An *environmental demand* is an expectation for a certain kind of behavior or action that is evoked by something in the environment. Allen (1) gives the example of the American flag stimulating a person to salute. Another environmental demand might be a family member who expects specific behaviors from the client (e.g., the parent who requires the child to obtain straight As).

An *environmental support* is a feature of the environment that encourages and assists the individual to perform a particular behavior. A machine that dispenses premeasured packets of detergent and fabric softeners is an example of an environmental support in a self-service laundry. Environmental supports may also be social, such as a case manager who regularly calls on clients to make sure they have taken their medication. Occupational therapists and assistants can alter the demands and supports within the environment by adding or removing objects or people, by changing the arrangement of the furniture or the lighting, or by other factors. The purpose of this environmental manipulation is to stimulate clients to perform activities, to engage in occupations, to develop skills, to acquire habits, and to enhance their sense of personal causation by providing opportunities for success. How to modify the environment and choose the proper level of stimulation is discussed within the context of activity analysis and adaptation in Chapter 23.

## Therapeutic Approach

The principles of the therapeutic approach are covered in considerable detail in Chapters 3, 4, 10, 11, and 13. When selecting which approach to use with a particular individual, the therapist must consider the client's values, learning style and preferences, and motivation for change.

## IMPLEMENTING AND MONITORING INTERVENTIONS AND MODIFYING THE PLAN

Once developed, the plan must be carried out; the client engages in activities or exercises using the chosen methods. The OT is responsible but may delegate portions to the OTA (2, 4, 5). Thus the OTA is often responsible for some aspects of this part of the process, known as *treatment implementation* or *intervention implementation.* After explaining to the person what will be happening and why, the assistant engages the person in an activity or series of activities in a rather specific way. Once the intervention has been implemented, the important questions are, How well is it working? and Should it be changed?

Monitoring the treatment/intervention to determine effectiveness is relatively straightforward when clearly stated objectives exist. If the objectives have not been stated in terms of what is observable and what is realistic to achieve during the time provided, measuring success is next to impossible. There are two ways in which effectiveness is monitored: informal observation and formal evaluation.

*Informal observations* are made almost automatically, as the assistant or therapist notes the client's reaction to the intervention. The person's behavior and remarks will provide clues if the task is too easy, too difficult, or just off the mark for the client's needs. On noting that the person can easily accomplish the activity, the OTA should consult with the therapist about how to change the plan; similarly, if the person is observed leaving early, not coming on time, or finding excuses to avoid treatment, the OTA should consult with the therapist, as these behaviors may signify a need to change the plan. And if the person appears to be struggling, confused, or otherwise unable to engage in treatment, this also must be reported. The therapist can then advise whether to continue with the plan or how to modify it. Implementation review and modification are a natural and frequent aspect of the intervention process.

*Formal reevaluation* is the responsibility of the OT. The progress of an individual client is best measured by re-administering the assessments that were used in the original evaluation. Improvements in the person's performance since the time of the initial evaluation may be considered evidence of treatment effectiveness; however, medications, spontaneous remission of symptoms, and many other factors can also account for these changes. Depending on the results of the formal evaluation, the therapist may decide to continue with the plan, to change it in some way, or to discharge the client from therapy.

## OUTCOME ASSESSMENT

Outcomes are the changes that are brought about by occupational therapy intervention. The core of any outcome for occupational therapy should be engagement in occupation. The ideal is for the outcome measure to be selected at the evaluation phase (3, 5). The occupational therapist is responsible for outcome assessment; the OTA must be aware of the client's goals and targeted outcomes and report on outcomes to the OT (2, 4).

## CONTINUITY OF CARE ACROSS SETTINGS

In addition to planning interventions for the client within the current treatment setting, occupational therapy practitioners must also consider the person's future needs and possible future environments of care (treatment settings). It is in making the transition from one setting to another that consumers are likely to fall through the cracks in the mental health system. Continuity of care necessitates that clinicians anticipate how the individual client will respond to the transition. The practitioner should obtain permission from the client to speak directly with the occupational therapist or other service provider in the next setting about the client's needs. The occupational therapy practitioner can then follow up after transition via phone calls to the client and to the service provider to check that the transition has been made and to answer any questions.

## QUALITY ASSURANCE

Measuring the effectiveness of the occupational therapy program or of intervention activities or groups within the program is also the responsibility of the therapist and is usually designed and guided by the manager of the occupational therapy program. Often this is part of a larger *quality assurance* program, which may involve other clinical departments (10). Quality assurance (QA) is a "systematic approach to the evaluation of patient care that enables the identification, assessment, and resolution of problems in order to improve health care benefits for patients" (15). In other words, QA is a way of measuring how well we are doing so that we can improve what we are doing for our clients. Rather than focusing on an individual, QA looks at the entire program, seeking to identify problems in patient care and to resolve them. It is a system review, rather than an individual review.

Therapy practitioners looking to strengthen or expand their practice may employ QA strategies. For example, Smith (22), a therapist at a community mental health agency, used a referral log as a QA tool to determine why the rate of referrals was low. She found that only her immediate co-workers were referring clients. Having this information, she developed a brochure and embarked on an education campaign to reach out to other professionals in the agency. At 6 months, her referral rate had increased by 110%.

One of the obstacles to implementing QA in psychiatric settings has been the vague and highly subjective nature of mental illness and the difficulty of measuring improvements in mental health. Nonetheless, very specific and measurable criteria can be established to assess some aspects of occupational therapy patient care in mental health settings (Table 16-3).

Thien (23) notes three major areas that should be assessed in QA programs for mental health occupational therapy: progress toward goals, patients' satisfaction with care, and behavior rating scores. *Progress toward goals* is most easily measured when the goals are behaviorally observable and measurable. In other words, a criterion that is a five-point improvement on the Scorable Self Care Scale (7) is far easier to measure than "the patient will improve in recognition of common safety hazards." *Consumers' satisfaction with care* can be measured through exit interviews, but the most objective and easily assessed measures are surveys with rating scales. Figure 16-2 gives an example of such a scale. *Behavior rating* can be achieved by using numerical rating scales such as the *Comprehensive Occupational Therapy Evaluation* scale (see Chapter 15).

While not responsible for designing a QA program, the OTA will be expected to contribute in various ways. The first is in collecting data for QA by reviewing medical records. The assistant might be directed to search the charts of all clients who participated in a given program (e.g., independent living skills) and to compile a list of ratings (e.g., on the *Kohlman Evaluation of Living Skills*) for these clients before and after participation in the program. Data collection must be done accurately and completely if it is to have meaning. All of the charts must be reviewed, including those that seem deficient. Another area for the OTA's participation in QA is as a member of the occupational therapy staff selecting measures for QA and developing action plans to respond to areas that need improvement. The assistant often brings a unique practical perspective to the planning process.

**TABLE 16-3 QUALITY ASSURANCE EXAMPLES FOR OCCUPATIONAL THERAPY MENTAL HEALTH PATIENTS**

| OCCUPATIONAL THERAPY MONITORING INDICATOR | MEASURE | APPLIED TO . . . | THRESHOLD AND CRITERIA |
|---|---|---|---|
| Prompt assessment of patient | Time lag between occupational therapy referral and assessment | All psychiatric patients | 90% of patients will be assessed within 24 hrs of referral to occupational therapy |
| Patient's participation in goal-directed activities | Time per day spent in occupational therapy and unit activities with specific treatment goals | All patients in acute-care psychiatric unit | 75% will spend 3 hrs daily in goal-directed activity |
| Increased independent functioning by patients | Mean difference between admission and discharge on *COTE* scale | All psychiatric patients | 80% of patients will decrease score by 10 or more points |
| Improvement in successful placement in independent living | *SSCE* administered before discharge | Psychiatric patients going into independent living | 100% of patients will have overall score of 30 or less before being considered for independent living |

*COTE, Comprehensive Occupational Therapy Evaluation; SSCE, Scorable Self-Care Evaluation.*



Despite its intended purpose as a patient care improvement scheme, the very mention of QA may strike fear in the hearts of staff. One of the reasons is concern about repercussions to themselves or to fellow workers. Staff may suspect that if a program is found lacking, someone will be blamed for it. But QA is not about fault finding and blaming; it is about improving systems of service. Only by looking realistically at what has happened can improvements be made. Most likely, deficiencies will be greeted sympathetically by senior staff, who will recognize their own responsibility for improvement of care. Other reasons for avoiding QA activities include fears of increased documentation and demands on already limited time. It is important to trust and believe that in the long run, QA leads to better time use and decreased documentation. Time spent on learning how to write measurable objectives and criteria pays off in time saved documenting the effectiveness of care.

## CONTINUOUS QUALITY IMPROVEMENT

Continuous quality improvement (CQI) is another quality management process. CQI monitoring is ongoing (constant) rather than retrospective (looking back). It is more interdisciplinary than QA, and it looks at outcomes (results) rather than problems. It is also more client centered than system centered. For example, a CQI program might monitor clients' satisfaction through daily response surveys. If clients' satisfaction is lower than expected, CQI

| | STRONGLY DISAGREE | DISAGREE | UNDECIDED | AGREE | STRONGLY AGREE |
|---|---|---|---|---|---|
| I felt I was treated with courtesy and respect in OT. | 1 | 2 | 3 | 4 | 5 |
| OT treatment helped me work on my problems. | 1 | 2 | 3 | 4 | 5 |
| My occupational therapist involved me in developing my goals. | 1 | 2 | 3 | 4 | 5 |
| I felt my occupational therapist understood my problems. | 1 | 2 | 3 | 4 | 5 |
| The time spent learning relaxation techniques was adequate. | 1 | 2 | 3 | 4 | 5 |
| My participation in living skills group was helpful to me. | 1 | 2 | 3 | 4 | 5 |
| I understood my OT treatment plan. | 1 | 2 | 3 | 4 | 5 |

**Figure 16-2. Examples of questionnaire statements related to patients' satisfaction with the delivery of occupational therapy care.** (Reprinted with permission from Thien M. Assessing occupational therapy care in mental health. In: Joe BE, ed. Quality Assurance in Occupational Therapy. Rockville, MD: American Occupational Therapy Association, 1991. Copyright © 1991 by the American Occupational Therapy Association, Inc.)

would seek to identify the sources and correct them. If, for example, clients said that what they learned in the clinic was not carried over into their lives in the community, the staff might plan more client education or community outreach activities. CQI can give feedback to intervention planning by providing more immediate information about the results of interventions. Interventions that are ineffective can be more quickly identified and adjustments can be made.

## SUMMARY

Intervention planning requires careful thought. The causes of most psychiatric problems are not yet clearly understood; therefore, it is often difficult to figure out exactly how to help persons with psychiatric disorders function better in life and feel better about themselves and what they can do.

Intervention planning involves identifying specific problems and functional goals that the client and staff agree are important. Both problems and goals must be stated in terms that are relevant to the client's needs, understandable, measurable, behavioral, and achievable. Above all, goals should be observable and reachable within the time allotted. There are many ways to approach a given goal; various theories and practice models contain principles for selecting and modifying intervention methods. Methods must take into account the activity used, the environment, and the therapeutic approach that will be most effective for engaging the client. Once intervention has begun, it should be monitored to determine whether it is effective or should be changed. This may be done by informal observation or formal reevaluation. It is helpful to identify measurable outcomes early in the process so that change can be monitored and progress assessed. A QA program may be used to monitor and improve the effectiveness of systems of patient care within a setting or service.

## REVIEW QUESTIONS AND ACTIVITIES

1. Why is planning intervention for persons with mental disorders more difficult than planning for persons with physical disorders?
2. Explain how looking at the causes and contributing factors for the client's problems can help in planning intervention.
3. What is the role of theory and practice models in intervention planning?
4. What should be done when the client appears unmotivated for treatment?
5. At what point in the process are the outcomes first considered? Why at this time?
6. What period of time differentiates a short-term goal from a long-term goal?
7. In what ways are short-term goals related to long-term goals?
8. At what point should the occupational therapy practitioners communicate with the rest of the team about the OT plan?
9. Define *treatment* or *restoration of function.* Give an example.
10. Define *maintenance of function.* Give an example.
11. Define *rehabilitation.* Give an example. By contrast, what is *habilitation*?
12. Define *prevention.* Give an example.
13. Explain and give an example to illustrate each of the following attributes of a good goal: *relevant, understandable, measurable, behavioral, achievable.*
14. Describe goal attainment scaling.
15. Contrast the roles of the OT and the OTA in implementation of intervention.
16. How does activity analysis contribute to planning intervention?
17. Contrast the roles of the OT and the OTA in review and modification of intervention.
18. Give some examples of the kind of situations in which the OTA should notify the OT the that the plan may need to be modified.
19. Contrast the roles of the OT and the OTA in outcome assessment.
20. Define *quality assurance* and state its purpose.
21. What is the difference between quality assurance and continuous quality improvement?
22. *Review activity:* Look at Table 16-1 and read it carefully. Of the listed goals, are there any about which you have questions? Write down your questions to share in class.
23. *Review and practice activity:* Look at Box 16-2 and read it carefully. Practice writing goals that have both a measurement and a time frame. Share any questions in class.
24. *Challenge question:* Create a goal attainment scale using a goal other than those given as examples in this book.
25. *Challenge activity:* Use any of the goals listed in the chapter and show how it can be addressed in two entirely different ways, using different intervention principles and methods.

## REFERENCES


1. Allen CK. Occupational Therapy for Psychiatric Diseases: Measurement and Management of Cognitive Disabilities. Boston: Little, Brown, 1985.
2. American Occupational Therapy Association. Guidelines for supervision, roles, and responsibilities during the delivery of occupational therapy services. Am J Occup Ther 2004;58:663–667.
3. American Occupational Therapy Association. Occupational therapy practice framework: Domain and process. Am J Occup Ther 2002;56:609–639.
4. American Occupational Therapy Association. Roles and responsibilities of the occupational therapist and the occupational therapy assistant during the delivery of occupational therapy services. OT Practice 2002;7(15):9–10.
5. American Occupational Therapy Association. Standards of practice for occupational therapy. Am J Occup Ther 2005;59:663–665.
6. Barris R, Kielhofner G, Watts JH. Psychosocial Occupational Therapy: Practice in a Pluralistic Arena. Laurel, MD: Ramsco, 1983.
7. Clark N, Peters M. The Scorable Self-Care Evaluation (SSCE). Thorofare, NJ: Slack, 1984.
8. Fidler GS, Fidler JW. Doing and becoming: Purposeful action and self-actualization. Am J Occup Ther 1978;32:305–310.
9. Gaines BJ. Goal-oriented treatment plans and behavioral analysis. Am J Occup Ther 1978;32:512–516.
10. Joe BE, ed. Quality Assurance in Occupational Therapy. Rockville, MD: American Occupational Therapy Association, 1991.
11. Kielhofner G, ed. A Model of Human Occupation: Theory and Application. 3rd ed. Baltimore: Lippincott Williams & Wilkins; 2002.
12. Kiresuk TJ, Sherman RE. Goal attainment scaling: A general method for evaluation of comprehensive mental health programs. Community Ment Health J 1968;4:443–453.
13. Lancaster J, Mitchell M. Occupational therapy treatment goals, objectives and activities for improving self-esteem in adolescents with behavioral disorders. Occup Ther Ment Health 1991;11(2–3):3–22.
14. Law M, Baptiste S, Carswell A, et al. Canadian Occupational Performance Measure. 2nd ed. Toronto: Canadian Association of Occupational Therapists, 1994.
15. Lawlor MC. A conceptual framework for quality assurance. In: Joe BE, ed. Quality Assurance in Occupational Therapy. Rockville, MD: American Occupational Therapy Association, 1991.
16. Maloney FP, Mirrett P, Brooks C, Johannes K. Use of the goal attainment scale in the treatment and ongoing evaluation of neurologically handicapped children. Am J Occup Ther 1978;32:505–510.
17. McLeod K, Robnett R. Psychosocial documentation: Are your objectives functional, measurable and reimbursable? Occup Ther Ment Health 1998;14(3):21–31.
18. Payton OD, Ozer MN, Nelson CE. Patient Participation in Program Planning: A Manual for Therapists. Philadelphia: Davis, 1971.
19. Peloquin SM. Sustaining the art of practice in occupational therapy. Am J Occup Ther 1989;43:219–226.
20. Scott AH, Haggerty EJ. Structuring goals via goal attainment scaling in occupational therapy groups in a partial hospitalization setting. Occup Ther Ment Health 1984;4(2):39–58.
21. Spencer JC, Davidson HA. The community adaptive planning assessment: A clinical tool for documenting future planning with clients. Am J Occup Ther 1998;52:19–30.
22. Smith K. States move forward with assisted living regulation. OT Practice Online, Apr 16, 2001. Available at: www.aota.org/featured/area3/links/f-041601.asp Accessed Mar 2007.
23. Thien M. Assessing occupational therapy care in mental health. In: Joe BE, ed. Quality Assurance in Occupational Therapy. Rockville, MD: American Occupational Therapy Association, 1991.
24. Tiffany EG. Psychiatry and mental health. In: Hopkins HL, Smith HD, eds. Willard and Spackman's Occupational Therapy. 6th ed. Philadelphia: Lippincott, 1983.


## SUGGESTED READINGS


Brinson MH. Continuous quality improvement: Developing a therapeutic milieu in an acute psychiatric hospital. Am Occup Ther Assoc Ment Health Special Sect Q Newslett 1993;16(1):6–8.

Lloyd C. The process of goal setting using goal attainment scaling in a therapeutic community. Occup Ther Ment Health 1986;6(3):19–30.

Moorhead P, Kannenberg K. Writing functional goals. In: Acquaviva JD, ed. Effective Communication for Occupational Therapy. 2nd ed. Bethesda, MD: American Occupational Therapy Association, 1998.

Ottenbacher KJ, Cusick A. Goal attainment scaling as a method of clinical service evaluation. Am J Occup Ther 1990;44:519–525.

Peloquin SM. Linking purpose to procedure during interactions with patients. Am J Occup Ther 1988;42:775–781.

CHAPTER 17

# Medical Records and Documentation

***Keep thinking and writing and rewriting. If you force yourself to think clearly you will write clearly. It's as simple as that. The hard part isn't the writing; the hard part is the thinking.***

WILLIAM ZINSSER (16, P. 56)

## CHAPTER OBJECTIVES

After studying this chapter, the reader will be able to:

1. Explain why documentation is important and what purposes it serves.
2. Recognize different types of medical records and different documentation forms.
3. Identify the kinds of information to be included in contact notes and progress reports.
4. Understand how to document in narrative, SOAP, and DAP formats.
5. Identify and discuss the complementary roles of the occupational therapist and occupational therapy assistant in documentation of services.

The medical record is a legal document. It testifies to the appropriateness and effectiveness of treatment and can be subpoenaed by the courts. It justifies reimbursement and communicates essential information to others involved in the person's care. The importance of accurate and timely documentation is impossible to overstate. After direct service to clients, documentation is *the* most important task of the occupational therapy practitioner. Without proper documentation it is impossible to receive reimbursement, to justify the need for additional services, or to defend against a malpractice suit. More fundament, there is no way to be sure that an intervention worked or why, or whether it even occurred, unless it is accurately documented.

Although the occupational therapist (OT) has the overall responsibility for managing and maintaining accurate and complete records on patient services, occupational therapy assistants (OTAs) are responsible for recording the results of services they provide to patients and consumers. This chapter discusses some of the kinds of medical records the OTA might encounter and delineates the roles of the OT and the OTA in documentation of service. Guidelines as to who is to document various aspects of the OT process may vary among jurisdictions and practice settings, depending on laws, federal guidelines, certification requirements, and reimbursement policies and procedures. The OTA is legally and ethically responsible to stay informed of relevant guidelines and to practice within them. Specific guidelines for writing notes and examples of different kinds of notes will be provided later in this chapter.

## PURPOSE AND USES OF MEDICAL RECORDS

The medical record serves multiple purposes and addresses many audiences. Each chart chronicles the story of a person's care in the medical system. The chart tells why treatment was sought, what problems were identified, what treatments or interventions were attempted, and how well these interventions worked. Everyone who provides patient services and records information may be held accountable for the quality of treatment received, *based on what is documented;* this applies equally to the psychiatrist and the OTA. Each is responsible to practice in a manner that reflects current standards in his or her respective field and to document provided services and their effects on the patient.

The purposes of the occupational therapy portion of the psychiatric medical record[1] are as follows:

- To explain why occupational therapy services were needed and how these services contributed to the outcomes for the person
- To show the professional clinical reasoning behind the therapy plan
- To communicate an occupational therapy perspective on the client
- To provide a chronological record of the services provided and the outcomes.

When writing for the medical record, the occupational therapy practitioner might consider some possible audiences and readers (Box 17-1). In economic terms, practitioners may consider third-party payers the most important audience, and much documentation seems reimbursement driven, meaning that it is phrased so that it meets the standards of the person or agency paying for the services (14). In many cases, the standard applied is that of the *Medicare Part B Guidelines for Outpatient Occupational Therapy;* Kannenberg (9) states that these are the most rigorous and specific guidelines; by meeting this standard, the OT practitioner will usually meet the standards of other third-party payers (8).

[1] Summarized and adapted from the American Occupational Therapy Association (3).

**BOX 17-1**

**WHO READS THE CHART?**

- *The treatment team* (e.g., psychiatrists, nurses, social workers, peer counselors) to understand what is happening with the patient and the treatment
- *Documentation reviewers* (OT practitioners and others) to evaluate the quality of OT service provided
- *Third-party payers and reimbursement reviewers* (case managers in HMOs, fiscal intermediaries, hospital-based utilization reviewers) to determine whether services as documented meet the normal and customary standards and hence whether payment will be approved
- *Accrediting agencies* (JCAHO, CARF, and others) to determine whether documentation and service meet the standards of the accrediting body
- *Consumers* (the patient, client)
- *Legal system* (lawyers, judges) in cases related to work injury, disability claims, accidents, and malpractice
- *Researchers* (OT practitioners and other professionals) seeking, for example, to establish which services are effective in which cases

*OT,* occupational therapy; *HMOs,* health maintenance organizations; *JCAHO,* Joint Commission on the Accreditation of Health Care Organizations; *CARF,* Commission on Accreditation of Rehabilitation Facilities.

Adapted with permission from Robertson SC. Why we document. In: Acquaviva JD, ed. Effective Documentation for Occupational Therapy. 2nd ed. Bethesda, MD: American Occupational Therapy Association, 1998.

## TYPES OF RECORDS

Before discussing OT documentation specifically, let us first consider the several ways in which the medical record may be organized: source oriented, integrated, problem oriented, and computerized or electronic.

### Source-Oriented Records and Integrated Records

In source-oriented and integrated records, each source, or clinical discipline such as nursing or OT, documents information in a separate section of the chart. The first part of the chart contains the patient's name, case number, identifying information, and admission records. This section may also include legal documents, such as court orders for involuntary hospitalization. Next there are evaluation reports and treatment plans from each of the different services concerned with the patient's care; these may be psychiatry, nursing, psychology, social work, OT, and recreation therapy. A section for laboratory reports and records of medical and other consultations may follow this or may be placed at the back of the chart. There is also a section for doctors' orders and medication records.

All of these take up only a minor fraction of the chart, however, the bulk of which consists of sequential notes written by all of the different services involved in the patient's care. Each staff member writes notes at assigned intervals, according to the standards that apply to the facility. For example, nurses may be required to write a note on each patient every day; this may apply to all three shifts in an inpatient setting. OT practitioners, on the other hand, may be required to write notes only every 2 weeks. Frequency varies with the setting; some require daily notes or notes every time a service is rendered.

There are two approaches to organizing this material. In the *source-oriented record* the notes are organized into smaller sections, each for a different discipline, so that for example all of the OT notes are in one place, such as between the social work and psychology notes. A variant on this format uses color-coded pages to indicate progress notes of each discipline (e.g., green for nursing, orange for OT).

In the *integrated record,* all of the notes from different disciplines are in one section; the notes are written one after the other, so that a given page in the chart might contain two nursing notes, a medication order from the physician, and an OT progress note.

One of the problems with both source-oriented and integrated records is that locating specific information about a patient's progress is difficult without reading *all* of the sequential notes, most of which probably have none of the desired information. Consider the case of someone who has been hospitalized repeatedly over many years and whose record is correspondingly lengthy. A physician who wanted to know the effects of various medications the patient has received would have to read all of the notes from OT and nursing to see how the patient functioned and whether the staff noticed any side effects. Only a few of those notes would contain information related to medication. As another example, suppose that the OTA wanted to know what kinds of independent daily living skills programs the patient has attempted and what the results were. The OTA would have to start at the beginning of the chart and read every OT note.

It was largely in response to this difficulty that the problem-oriented medical record was developed. Although some psychiatric settings have not changed over to the problem-oriented record, it is important to know how its format differs from that of the traditional record.

## Problem-Oriented Medical Record

The *problem-oriented medical record,* or POMR, was introduced in 1969 by Lawrence Weed as a possible solution to the problems of the source-oriented record. The POMR is organized into three major sections: the database, the problem list, and the reports of plans and progress. The database contains the same sorts of information that might be included in the admission report, the psychiatrist's evaluation, and the social history. The database is developed within the first 48 hours of hospitalization or outpatient treatment and is usually coordinated by the patient's primary therapist.

The problem list is developed from the database. It identifies all of the patient's problems. The primary therapist may write the problem list, usually with recommendations from other disciplines, or the treatment team might develop the list together. The OTA can suggest problems to the primary therapist, to the OT supervisor, or to the treatment team. Some problems that might appear on the list in a psychiatric record are difficulty expressing feelings, suicidal ideation, poor self-care, and lack of employment. Each problem is given a number, and the date the problem was entered in the chart is recorded.

The reports section includes all of the notes from different disciplines. The problem to which each note refers is indicated in a separate column next to the note. For instance, the OTA writing a note about the patient's progress in an activities of daily living group writes the number of the problem (poor self-care) next to the note. If the note refers to more than one problem, the OTA records all the relevant problem numbers. Organizing the chart in this way enables someone who is interested in the treatment of a particular problem to find all of the notes that pertain to that problem without reading those that do not. The notes in the problem-oriented record are generally written in subjective-objective assessment plan (SOAP) format, discussed later in this chapter.

## Computerized Documentation

As this text goes to press, most documentation in mental health settings is still done manually, written with a pen by hand on paper. A grand vision of

**BOX 17-2**

**COMPUTERIZED DOCUMENTATION: THE FUTURE IS ALMOST HERE**

Vinh arrives for work at the day hospital and downloads to his personal digital assistant (PDA) his daily schedule from the OT department computer. For his first assignment, he meets separately with two new admissions and administers the Allen Cognitive Level (ACL) test, using each patient's identifier code to enter the test scores directly into an ACL form in the patient record via a laptop computer plugged into the local area network.

While he's working, his PDA vibrates to alert him to an OT staff meeting just scheduled for noon at the main hospital building. He text messages the art therapist saying he will have to reschedule lunch for another day. Vinh then leads two groups, entering attendance and participation into preformatted grids in the laptop, which sends the information to the network computer and logs it into the billing system and the records of all 17 patients in the two groups.

Wondering whether anyone has responded to his query about a patient with Tourette's syndrome and substance abuse, Vinh checks his e-mail and finds six messages from the American Occupational Therapy Association's Mental Health Listserv. He saves to read later the two that are of interest. Finding that he has a half hour remaining before he has to leave for the noon meeting, he files biweekly progress notes on six patients, using preformatted phrases from the database and notes he has stored on the laptop. (After the meeting, he and his supervisor will co-sign his notes electronically at one of the signature stations in the main hospital.)

Vinh grabs his PDA, so he can take notes, and rushes off to the meeting.

the electronic health record (EHR) in which each individual's lifetime health records are stored in a computerized database is not yet a reality. Nonetheless, today's OT practitioner should expect to be documenting electronically within the decade. Box 17-2 illustrates how the OTA might use computerized documentation.

Computerized documentation promises significant benefits: speed of information recording and retrieval, more universal availability because many people can read the record simultaneously, centralized information, and ease of entering data. The primary concerns are with security of information: how to limit access only to those who have legitimate rights to the information and how to safeguard the integrity of information so that it cannot be altered.

## DOCUMENTATION OF OCCUPATIONAL THERAPY SERVICES

The different kinds of OT documentation in the patient's permanent record are classified as follows (3):

- Evaluation report
- Intervention plan
- Contact, treatment, or visit note
- Progress report
- Reevaluation report
- Transition plan
- Discontinuation report

*Evaluation reports* identify the assessments that were used, the results of these assessments, the therapist's interpretation of the results, and the therapist's treatment plan; the emphasis is on obstacles to the client's engagement in occupation. The *intervention plan* spells out the goals established, the methods to be used, the frequency of treatment, and the time by which the therapist expects the goals to be reached; the emphasis is on the client's goals for engagement in occupation and the ways in which occupational therapy service will address these. A *contact, treatment,* or *visit note* documents individual OT sessions or contacts and the service provided. A *progress report* documents treatment periodically, updating information on progress toward functional goals, changes to the plan, and coordination of care. This includes a record of the patient's attendance and participation, any change that has occurred since the last note and the probable causes of the change, and any modification of the treatment plan. A *reevaluation report* documents the results of the reevaluation, compares these to the initial evaluation, and recommends changes or continuations in the plan. A *transition plan* is written in preparation for a move from one setting to another; it summarizes all of the pertinent information and recommendations. A *discharge or discontinuation report* gives a concise description of the entire course of OT intervention since first contact and includes assessment of outcomes.

Other types of documentation that the OTA may encounter are consultation reports, special reports, and incident reports. A professional who does not have sufficient expertise to understand a patient's problem and recommend treatment will request a consultation with someone who does. Occupational therapists may receive consultation requests from physicians and others, and the *consultation report* records the therapist's assessment of the patient's problems, including recommendations for treatment or other interventions. The entry-level OTA is not qualified to serve as a consultant and, therefore, does not need to know how to write consultation reports; this is a role reserved for OTs and for OTAs with considerable experience and expertise. *Special reports* include various records that the law requires to be in the permanent chart. Examples are referrals to other programs and agencies, summary reports for legal reasons, home programs, and correspondence.

A *critical incident report* or *note* documents the facts of an emergency in which, for example, a patient was injured or eloped while under the supervision of an OT staff member. Specific legal requirements govern the way such reports are written, and the staff member is given precise instructions by a supervisor about how to write up the incident.

The OTA may also contribute to appeal letters and may write letters of advocacy. The purpose of an *appeal letter* is to request review of a denied reimbursement. The purpose of a *letter of advocacy* is to speak on behalf of a client, group, or population to request funding or services or political action.

## Documentation Responsibilities of the OT and OTA

The OT oversees the documentation of patient treatment. The OT is responsible for assessment reports, treatment plans, reevaluation reports, and discharge or discontinuation reports; the OTA may assist in providing information or portions of these reports. The OTA most often will write contact, treatment, or visit notes and progress notes. When required by law or by the facility, the OT must countersign all notes written by OTAs and students (3, 6).

However, the OTA's documentation responsibilities may become more extensive as the he or she gains experience. The OTA may contribute to the treatment plan and even write sections of it, for example, on activities of daily living. The OTA may write a discharge or discontinuation summary, as for example when the patient completes a 10-week money management group led by the OTA.

The OTA also keeps records on each treatment service he or she provides. Sometimes this is referred to as a *therapy log* (3). An attendance record for each group must be completed daily or after each session. In addition, records of assessments, interviews, and other services to each patient must be maintained. These may be combined in a monthly report, which tabulates all patient service sessions for the month and is used for financial reporting and quality control. Each staff member's monthly report is given to an OT supervisor or director, who compiles reports on the entire department.

The most basic documentation responsibility for the entry-level OTA is to write *contact, treatment,* or *visit notes,* which concisely describe either a single service or a course of treatment over time. In this text, they are called *simple summary notes* or *simple observation notes.* The purpose of these notes is to present a clear picture of the service provided, the client's response, and the assistant's plans and recommendations for the future. These notes are classified according to their content, which may be the initial contact with the patient, an evaluation, or a single treatment session. The OTA would also be expected to write a contact note to document telephone calls, communications with other health professionals about the client, and contacts with any family members or others concerned with the patient (13). Two other forms of documentation that will also be discussed and for which examples will be given are the *progress report* and the *discharge or discontinuation report.* Before looking in detail at these forms of documentation, let us first consider some basic rules that apply to all clinical documentation.

## Guidelines for Note Writing

Writing a simple note is not generally a simple task for the beginner. Because it becomes part of the client's permanent record, it must be accurate and complete; future decisions about the patient may be based on the contents of the chart. Besides being accurate and complete, the note should also be concise, brief, and to the point; otherwise, given human nature and the busy schedules of most health professionals, no one (except possibly the supervisor) will read the whole thing. Simple observation notes are intended to convey an accurate picture of what happened so that someone who was not present can understand it almost as well as if he or she were there. The novice note writer may benefit from the following *stylistic* advice:

- *Record observations, not interpretations.* Let the reader draw his or her own conclusions based on the facts you present.
- *Avoid judgmental language.* Judgments are open to varying interpretations. What is a good job to one person may not meet the standards of another, for example. Moorhouse and Doenges (11) cite five types of judgmental statements that should be avoided. These are presented in Box 17-3.
- *Avoid jargon.* Your note will be seen (and, one hopes, read) by many people, most of them not OT practitioners. Other mental health professionals and paraprofessionals cannot be expected to understand OT jargon such as *virtual context, habit dysfunction,* or *Snoezelen room.* Unless these terms are well understood by all staff, they should not be used in material for the chart without a brief explanation of their meaning.
- *Omit extraneous detail.* Many of the things that consumers do they do more than once. By grouping like observations together, the note writer can shorten the note. The reader does not have to know everything that happened in the exact order it happened, but only a general sense. Therefore, rather than writing a *process* note, which records every behavior in sequence, the assistant should write a summary note.
- *Be brief.* This, more than anything else, will ensure that your notes will be read by the doctors, nurses, social workers, and other professionals working with the patient. And *that* is the point of writing the note in the first place.

**BOX 17-3**

## MAKE DOCUMENTATION STRONGER: AVOID WEAK WORDS!

- *Undefined references to time.* Words like *often, frequently,* and *seldom* should be replaced by measurable and defined periods, such as "five times per hour" or "twice during a 6-hour work session."
- *Undefined quantities.* Words like *some, many, and enough* should be replaced by numerical quantities, as, for example, "5," "10," or "1."
- *Qualities.* Adjectives that convey opinions, such as *hostile, spaced out,* or *bored* should be replaced by actual observations. "Patient clenched his fists and said to OTA, 'I'll knock your teeth down your throat'" is an observation. So is "Patient stared out the window for three-quarters of the hour, did not participate in discussion, and responded to her own name only after two calls."
- *Failure to provide an objective basis for judgment.* A statement such as "Patient likes trains" does not give evidence to support it. A more effective statement is, "Patient stated that he likes trains and that he will read anything on the subject."
- *Inappropriate use of clinical terminology.* Only the physician can diagnose the patient. Similarly, the assistant should not use medical terms to describe behavior or symptoms unless he or she is absolutely certain the usage is correct. Even when certain, the assistant must place the description within the context of what he or she observed. For example, it is incorrect to state, "The patient was hallucinating." This should instead be recorded as "The patient may have been hallucinating; she was conversing when no one was there."

Adapted with permission from Moorhouse MF, Doenges ME. Nurse's Clinical Pocket Manual: Nursing Diagnosis, Care Planning, and Documentation. Philadelphia: Davis, 1990.

It is normal and expected to have to write several versions of a note when one is learning this skill. Figure 17-1 gives three versions of a note that documents an observation of a patient making a mosaic ashtray; the third version is similar to what the OTA might write into the chart. Can you see why this is the preferred version?

The first version is written in an informal style. The writer refers to himself as "I," which is not usually done in the chart. The information is poorly organized, but the writer has captured some details that are very descriptive of the patient's behavior. The reader understands immediately how the patient behaved in the group. With rewriting, this has the potential to become a very useful note. But look what happened in version two: the writer introduced medical jargon, added interpretations, and omitted some of the descriptive details that made version one so compelling and convincing. The reader no longer has a clear picture of what happened. The note is shorter but less useful.

Version three, while almost twice as long as version two, is still shorter than version one. More important, it retains many of the details contained in version one. The writer has saved space by grouping like observations (e.g., of gluing tiles to the wrong side) and by choosing descriptive single words instead of phrases (e.g., regarding the patient's conversations with others). And, it is interesting to note, in this version the writer included new details that were omitted from version one.

Although narrative-style notes for the medical chart should be written in the style of version three,

**Three Versions of an Observation Note**

These are three versions of a note on a single observation of a patient making a mosaic ashtray. Version three is the final rewrite and is suitable for entering in the medical chart.

*Version One*

Marilyn came into the room very slowly. She held on to the chair when she sat down. She didn't know where she was. When I asked her name, she knew it, but she didn't know the answers to any of the other questions about her age or address. She was willing to make an ashtray when I showed one to her. She wanted to make a checkerboard pattern, but she couldn't figure out how to do it, so she just did a little bit in one corner, and then she turned the tray over and glued a tile to the wrong side. Then she turned it back to the right side and put white tiles over the rest of the tray. Then she glued another tile to the bottom of the tray. I told her that was wrong and showed her the sample, but she wanted to leave it the way it was. Her tray was a real mess, with glue and gluey fingerprints all over it. She got a lot of glue on the table too, and on her face. She cleaned up, though, when I told her to, but we had to wait for her because she was so slow. She held onto the sink and the table when she moved around. She didn't talk to any of the other patients at the table except once when someone asked her if she liked snow; she said "Yes." She concentrated totally on her tray. Another patient took her glue bottle when his got stuck, and she let him. I had to get it back or she would have just stopped right there. She didn't say anything at all unless someone asked her a question.

*Version Two*

Marilyn participated in an occupational therapy group to make a mosaic tile ashtray. She had psychomotor retardation and disorientation. She used good concentration but poor planning. Her work habits were poor. She put some tiles on the wrong side of the tray. She was bored. She let another patient take one of her supplies and didn't say anything.

*Version Three*

Patient attended OT group 1X since admission. She was neatly dressed, but her hair was uncombed. She moved slowly and held onto furniture, appeared confused, was able to state her name but not her age or address. Working with apparent concentration, she completed only a few tiles in the checkerboard pattern and finished with plain tiles. She did not speak to others except to answer questions in one or two words. She stopped working when another patient took her glue bottle (saying nothing to the patient), but resumed work when the therapist retrieved it. She twice glued tiles to the wrong side of the tray, did not recognize this error, and refused to change it when it was pointed out to her. She used more glue than was needed, dripped some on the table, and smeared some on her face. She helped clean up but continued to move very slowly.

**Figure 17-1. Observation note.**

less formal notes are sometimes written into a communication book kept in the nursing station in inpatient settings or a central office in outpatient settings. The purpose of these notes is to communicate important information to staff coming onto the ward or into the center later in the day or evening. An example is noting that the patient got a paper cut in OT; although this may sound trivial, it may be very important for someone who has diabetes or a circulatory disorder, who is immunocompromised, or whose hygiene habits are poor.

In addition to these stylistic requirements, the following rules and guidelines apply to notes written by the OTA:

- The note should be organized in a logical fashion. Similar ideas should be grouped—for example, all statements about the patient's self-care and physical appearance should appear in the first paragraph. Each paragraph addresses a different area, and the final paragraph should contain a brief summary and statement about the plan for further treatment; the plan should flow logically from the information that precedes it.
- Notes must be written neatly so that they are legible or typewritten or printed if necessary. Correct grammar and spelling are mandatory.
- The note should be as brief as possible without omitting essential information or ideas.
- The note should be precise and factual, providing objective and truthful information about the patient's condition rather than vague generalizations or interpretations.
- Notes should be written within the deadlines that apply in the particular facility. If notes are to be written every 2 weeks, the assistant must make time to complete the notes by the date they are due. If not, the assistant is likely to be cited for noncompliance. If this happens often enough, it can damage the person's performance rating.

For legal purposes, each note must contain the patient's name and case number on each page and the date of the note, including month, day, and year. Without this identifying information notes can be lost or misfiled. Then when the chart is audited, the note may be cited as missing when in fact it was done. The assistant should title the note with the name of the department and the type of note (e.g., "Occupational Therapy Biweekly Progress Note"); in some facilities this information is on the form already. The assistant is required to sign the note with full name and the professional designation of OTA; the signature must come directly after the note, with no space left between the last line of the note and the signature.

Because it is only human to make mistakes, the assistant should expect a few in the writing of notes. If an error has to be corrected, the correct and legally required procedure is to draw a line through it so that it can still be clearly read and then insert the correction and initial it. Finally, the note must be countersigned by a therapist. Box 17-4 provides a checklist of important points for all documentation.

**BOX 17-4**

**DOCUMENTATION CHECKLIST—DID YOU . . . ?**

- Use **black ink?** And have patients use black ink to complete forms? (Other colors do not photocopy well.)
- **Write legibly?**
- **Date** your entry?
- **Sign** your entry with no space between last sentence and signature?
- **Indicate errors** by drawing a single line through, initialing, and dating the entry?
- Include **patient's name and case number** on each page?
- Document every **telephone contact?**
- Document the **outcome** of the contact and the **plan?**
- Document **immediately** or as soon as you could?
- Think about whether the **third-party payer** will understand what you have written?
- Think about **reading the entry in court?**

## ESSENTIAL CONTENT FOR OCCUPATIONAL THERAPY NOTES

While version three in Figure 17-1 is clearer, more objective, and more concise than the earlier version, it does not state *why* the patient needs OT or *what benefit* the patient might expect to receive from OT. These elements are essential to document both the need for OT services and the results to be expected. We must explain clearly so that other disciplines or third-party payers such as insurance companies and the federal and state governments will understand the point of our observations. The observations have to be connected to problems that will affect the patient's ability to function and to a plan for addressing these problems. Figure 17-2 shows version four of the note, including the assessment of deficits in functional performance and the plan (how these deficits will be addressed). The situation in this note is that the patient has not yet been evaluated, nor has the treatment plan been developed. Both of these tasks are the responsibilities of the OT. The OTA, in writing this note, is suggesting particular evaluation instruments and a focus for evaluation, based on experience and observation of the patient. The note would be countersigned by the OT.

### Focus on the Patient's Goals

Wherever possible, the client's views of his or her problems and goals should be included in notes. When asked, patients may give very general goals, "to get out of here" or "to feel better." Skillful questioning based on observation of the client and some knowledge of the person's background can elicit more detail, even from individuals who are not good talkers. Asking a concrete question, focusing on a specific observed or known behavior or interest, is most likely to result in a specific response. In the case of the confused patient described in Figure 17-2, one might ask her tactfully whether she combed her hair today. She might indicate that she did so and that her appearance is important to her. This can be restated as a functional goal: "Patient wants to 'look nice.' By the end of a week patient will independently complete essential grooming tasks (hair care) without reminder."

**Incorporating Performance Deficits and Functional Goals into an Observation Note**

*Version Four*

Patient attended OT group 1X since admission. She was neatly dressed, but her hair was uncombed; moved slowly and held onto furniture, appeared confused; able to state her name but not her age or address. Working with apparent concentration, she completed only a few tiles in the checkerboard pattern, finished with plain tiles. She did not speak except to answer questions in one or two words. She stopped working when another patient took her glue bottle (saying nothing), but resumed work when the therapist retrieved it. She twice glued tiles to the wrong side of the tray, did not recognize this error, and refused to change it. She used more glue than was needed, dripped some on the table, and smeared some on her face. Patient helped clean up but continued to move very slowly. ASSESSMENT: Patient demonstrates possible cognitive disability, indicated by grooming errors, errors in task execution with failure to recognize or correct errors, impaired situational awareness. Mobility deficit suggested by using furniture for support. PLAN: Administer cognitive level test and assess mobility deficit (within 48 hours).

**Figure 17-2. Incorporating deficits and goals into an observation note.**

### Focus on Functional Goals

Functional goals should follow logically from goals the patient or client identifies. The example about hair care is one such functional goal.

### Focus on Deficits and Solutions for Problems in Occupational Performance

The reader wishes to know why the patient has difficulty with such routine tasks and what solutions the practitioner has identified. By identifying these clearly and briefly in the note, the OT practitioner verifies the need for OT services. For example, the sentence "Patient says she forgets to look in the mirror after dressing" suggests that the problem is either with memory or with habit.

### Cognitive Deficits

Persons with psychiatric disorders may display cognitive deficits such as unreliable memory, errors in judgment, impulsivity, and difficulty making decisions. Observing and reflecting on the person's performance of tasks and asking the person about it will often suggest the nature of the problem; documenting the problem clearly is very helpful in finding solutions and communicating to other staff. An example is, "Patient interrupts tasks when distracted, is easily distracted by sounds, other people, etc. Patient performs self-care routines without error *only* in a distraction-free setting."

### Need for Assistance, Supervision, or External Structure

Individuals with cognitive problems and other performance deficits may benefit from the assistance of other people, from notes or signs in the environment or other external structure. An exact description of the nature of the helpful assistance or structure should be documented. For example, "If distracted, patient will resume self-care routine if given simple one-word cues, such as 'teeth!' to indicate she should brush her teeth."

## SPECIFIC TYPES OF DOCUMENTATION

The following sections address in more detail the specific types of notes the entry-level OTA may be asked to write: contact, treatment, *or* visit notes, which may include *initial notes, assessment reports, progress reports,* and the *discontinuation or discharge report.*

### Contact, Treatment, or Visit Notes

Contract, treatment, or visit notes document a single contact or visit, such as a telephone call or a treatment session. Such a note includes the following (3):

- The patient's name and case number and the date, including year
- Person's attendance and participation, including any reason for therapy not occurring as scheduled
- Kinds of interventions used
- Any equipment, assistive devices such as memory aids, given to the person; also the instructions given to a patient or caregiver
- Outcome of session in terms of patient's response
- The OTA's signature and title
- The OT's countersignature

An example of such a note is given in Figure 17-3.

### Initial Note

The purpose of an initial note is to record that the OT practitioner has received and acted on the referral for service. The note includes the following:

- The patient's name and case number and the date, including year
- The source of referral, the reason for referral, and the date referral was received
- The information obtained and behavior noted at the first contact

12/3/07
Case #34711

Patient participated in cooking group, was goal-directed in familiar task of making hamburger patties in familiar environment, but needed frequent check for safety (placement of knife, washing hands). Attention span WFL for task, but needed verbal cuing and c/o feeling sleepy. Cooperates well in group. ASSESSMENT: Patient when returns home will benefit from daily check on environment to remove safety hazards and solve problems when minor changes occur. PLAN: No change to main plan. Will schedule home visit and meeting with spouse by 12/6.

J.B. Black COTA

**Figure 17-3. Contact note.** *WFL,* within functional limits; *c/o,* complained of.

- Plan for further contact
- The OTA's signature and title
- The OT's countersignature

The sort of initial note the OTA might write is shown in Fig. 17-4, which refers to case 1 in Appendix A.

## Assessment Report

The OTA performs various structured assessments and from time to time may be required to document them in a simple summary note. This is not to be confused with the evaluation reports in which the OT compiles and interprets the results of all OT assessments the patient has received (3, 5, 6). An assessment report should contain the following information:

- The patient's name and case number and the date, including year
- Tests and assessments administered and the results
- A summary and analysis of the patient's specific impairments and the areas of function affected (in regard to engagement in occupation)
- Anticipated functional outcome after intervention. Functional outcome should address area of occupation (activities of daily living, work, leisure, social participation) and a specific kind of performance (e.g., "return to work as bookstore cashier for 3 hours per day")
- The OTA's signature and title
- The OT's countersignature

In many settings, particularly those with restrictive reimbursement guidelines, the OT is held responsible for all documentation of assessment and evaluation data. The OTA may be prohibited from any assessment documentation. In other settings,

**Spruce Valley Hospital, Occupational Therapy Department, Initial Note**

5/5/07
Case #186302

Patient referred to OT by Dr. Zamorska (5/4/07) for evaluation of independent living skills.
Pt. seen briefly to schedule and discuss evaluation. Patient expressed "It won't help"
but agreed to eval. at 10 AM Wed., 5/6/07.

Jerry Doe COTA

**Figure 17-4. OT department, initial note.** *Pt,* patient; *eval,* evaluation.

**Spruce Valley Hospital, Occupational Therapy Department, Assessment Report**

5/6/07
Case #186302

Patient cooperative during testing with KELS. Required refocusing to complete test 2° to ↓ attention span. Patient stated "I've got a lot on my mind." KELS results indicate patient independent in all areas except money management. Patient states desire to get job as a physical education teacher.

ASSESSMENT: Patient capable of independent living in community; has been independent in the past. Patient acknowledges difficulty managing money: "My mother won't give me any. I never have enough."
PLAN: Continue evaluation by OT to be completed by 5/11/07.

Jerry Doe COTA

**Figure 17-5. OT department, assessment report.** *KELS, Kohlman Evaluation of Living Skills;* 2°, secondary; ↓, decreased.

such as long-term care or substance-abuse or community treatment, the OTA may expect greater involvement in selecting, recommending, or administering assessments, and documenting the results. Figure 17-5 presents a note documenting the results of an assessment using the *Kohlman Evaluation of Living Skills (KELS)*.

An example of how the OTA might write up a more complex report on the results of a daily living skills evaluation is presented in Figure 17-6. This report is based on case 5 in Appendix A. (The home arts evaluation was performed because the patient and his wife decided that he would take on the homemaker role in their household.) This evaluation report incorporates the intervention plan, focusing primarily on the areas of self-care and homemaking. An entry-level OTA would not be responsible for writing such a plan. This might be expected of the OTA with a year or more of experience and proven competency in the particular area of intervention, depending on the treatment setting.

## Intervention Plan

Less common than the combined assessment report and intervention plan note is the separate intervention plan. The OT is responsible for developing and documenting the overall intervention plan (4–6). A OTA with sufficient experience and service competency may be asked to formulate and document a portion of the plan, applying to a particular area of occupation such as self-care. The basic information to be included in a note that documents the plan consists of the following (3):

- The client's name and case number and the date, including year
- Measurable long-term functional goal or goals, "directly related to the client's ability to engage in occupation" (3, p. 647), as determined by the consumer and the therapist or assistant
- Measurable objectives or short-term goals related to the long-term goals
- Intervention approaches, activities
- The frequency and duration of planned interventions, the person who will provide the interventions, and where
- The anticipated completion date
- The projected outcome, or end result of treatment
- The OTA's signature and title
- The OT's countersignature

An example of how a treatment plan should be recorded is shown in Fig. 17-7, which relates to case 5 in Appendix A.

**Occupational Therapy Department, Home Arts Program Evaluation Report and Intervention Plan**

12/18/07
Page 1 of 1
Case #291083

Patient was evaluated for independent daily living skills in six sessions of 1 hour each (12/7, 12/8, 12/10, 12/14, 12/15, 12/17). Patient arrived on time, neatly dressed in casual clothes and well groomed. The CEBLS checklist was used. A score of 135 of possible 176 points was obtained in the personal care and hygiene section. Patient scored independent level in toileting, brushing teeth, bathing, hair care, dressing. Patient needed assistance with shaving, missing areas on the right side of face (probably because of visual deficit). He did not perform any of the personal housekeeping tasks correctly and could not trim fingernails and toenails using clippers or scissors. Patient sat with a slouched posture and walked with a shuffling gait.

On the practical evaluation, patient scored 90 of possible 240 points. Patient independent in use of telephone but showed poor social behavior on phone. Patient able to use bus with some assistance in interpreting route and schedule. He did not have any idea of how to plan, shop for, or prepare a meal and did not know how to serve a meal. Patient ate appropriately, independently, helped in cleaning up after meal, but needed much assistance (e.g., reminders to wash backs of plates, instruction in how to scrape dishes). Patient occasionally bumped into objects on his right because he failed to notice them.

When patient did not know how to proceed, he appeared very anxious, began pacing and wringing his hands, and asked to stop the evaluation and be taken back to the unit. This occurred when the bus failed to arrive on schedule and was 20 minutes late. Patient stated that he tends to panic under stress.

ASSESSMENT: Patient independent in most areas of self-care; unable to perform most housekeeping and cooking tasks correctly unless directly supervised. He fails to compensate for absent vision in the right eye; this is a serious safety risk. Patient also tends to panic when confronted with a problem he is not immediately able to resolve.

**GOALS**

1. Patient states desire to overcome visual deficit so he can assume home management tasks.
   a. To learn compensatory techniques for navigating in home environment and for placement of tools and other objects (by 2 weeks).
2. Patient stated desire to help his wife around the house.
   a. To learn to maintain kitchen in clean, safe manner (by 2 weeks)
   b. To learn to prepare a simple meal (by 3 weeks)
   c. To learn to plan and shop for weekly groceries (by 6 weeks)
   d. To learn to keep home clean and tidy (by 5 weeks)
   e. To learn to launder and care for clothing (by 8 weeks)
3. Patient verbalized desire to learn to shave face accurately.
   a. To learn compensatory techniques for visual deficit (by 1 week)
4. Patient wants to be able to travel in community and deal with household emergencies without "losing it."
   a. To learn stress management techniques and apply these to situations encountered in daily life (by 10 weeks)

PLAN: Enroll patient in 10-week Home Arts Program, 4 hours per day (9 AM to 1 PM), 4 days per week, 12/28/07 through 3/8/08. Schedule individual half-hour sessions twice weekly to instruct in visual compensatory techniques. Schedule patient for stress management group one evening per week with wife. Encourage wife to help patient practice and reinforce new skills. Reassess progress in 1 month (1/18/08).

B White COTA

**Figure 17-6. Evaluation report and intervention plan.** *CEBLS,* comprehensive evaluation of basic living skills.

**Occupational Therapy Department, Home Arts Program Intervention Plan**

12/18/07
Page 1 of 2
Case #291083

*Long term objectives:*

1. Patient will carry out home management role.
2. Patient will plan, organize, and execute basic household tasks.
3. Patient will use social skills in basic communication, will relate effectively to others in small groups, and will assert self appropriately.
4. Patient will use techniques to compensate for visual deficit.
5. Patient will use stress management techniques.
6. Patient will develop leisure interests and leisure habits.

*Method:*

Patient to attend Home Arts Program (M, T, T, F, 9 AM to 1 PM) beginning 12/28/07 for 10 weeks' instruction in meal preparation, nutrition, housekeeping, self-care skills, play and leisure skills, sewing, social skills, and use of community resources. Patient will receive individual training and reinforcement in visual compensation techniques.

*Short-term objectives:*

1. Patient will plan and prepare a simple meal independently, including the following steps: preparing shopping list, grocery shopping, food storage, kitchen safety, food preparation and cooking, table setting, meal cleanup, and use of kitchen equipment, utensils, and appliances (by 4 weeks).
2. Patient will compensate for visual deficit, independently and without cuing, in performance of meal preparation tasks (by 4 weeks).
3. Patient will identify at least two situations that he finds stressful and will discuss why.

*Plan:*

Patient will receive instruction in basic methods of meal preparation as a member of a small group in the kitchen of the Home Arts Center and in the community (e.g., grocery store). OTA will explain purpose of visual compensation, will teach patient to turn and look to the right before moving any part of the body to the right, and will reinforce use of this technique through praise and verbal encouragement. Through group discussions focusing on recognizing and analyzing stress, patient will learn to identify his own reactions to stressful situations and will develop awareness of which situations he finds stressful. Reevaluate in 1 month (1/18/08).

B White COTA

**Figure 17-7. Arts program intervention plan.**

## Progress Report

Most notes written by OTAs are progress reports, documenting treatment and changes in the patient's condition since the last note. Obviously, the specific content of these notes varies with the setting, the client, and the type of intervention provided by the OTA. It is suggested (3) that all progress notes contain the following information:

- Patient's name and case number and the date, including year
- Record of patient's attendance, including number of sessions and inclusive dates
- Summary of treatment procedures and methods used and goals addressed
- Statement of patient's response to therapy (e.g., participation, behavior, whether change has occurred, what change has occurred)
- Any changes in goals or time to achieve goals and explanation
- Statement and explanation if treatment has not occurred as planned
- A copy of any home program given to patient and of any instructions to a caregiver
- Summary of any conferences or communications (e.g., with family, agencies) related to patient in which OT practitioner has participated
- Plan for continued treatment, including any modifications needed and specific procedures to be used
- OTA's signature and title
- OT's countersignature

Thoughtfulness and planning are the first steps in preparing a progress note. Allen (2) breaks down the separate processes of thinking, doing, and writing as they apply to the clinical reasoning used to document patient progress. Figure 17-8 shows this breakdown. Taking the steps listed one by one and assembling the information in an orderly fashion makes the actual writing of the note quite straightforward. Examples of progress reports are shown as Figures 17-9 to 17-12. These notes refer, respectively, to cases 1, 2, 3, and 5 in Appendix A.

Progress reports should record what actually happened, not what you wish had happened or what you planned but were not able to do. One of the realities of work with severely disabled clients is that they do not always show improvement from session to session. In fact, some individuals, like Mrs. Anderson in the note presented in Figure 17-10, actually function less well despite the best efforts of the staff.

One of the purposes of writing accurate and careful progress notes is to document reasons treatment should be continued or stopped. If the patient is making progress toward goals that have been established in the treatment plan or in previous notes, it is easy to show why treatment should be continued. Figure 17-11 presents a note that documents progress in a measurable way by including the results of a periodic reevaluation. On the other hand, if the note shows that the patient has been consistently uncooperative—missing treatment sessions, for example—the plan should be reviewed and modified or perhaps discontinued.

Increased case loads and demands to document more objectively have led to the development of forms used for charting progress. A common type is the checklist format with several columns and a coding system for indicating level of assistance required (1, p. 369).

## SOAP Note

Progress notes are most often written in the narrative form shown in Figures 17-9 to 17-12, but in problem-oriented medical records and in some integrated records notes may be written in the SOAP format. These letters stand for *subjective-objective assessment plan.*

The *subjective* section of the plan contains what the patient reports he or she feels or believes, based on what he or she tells the therapist. This section usually begins with the words, "The patient states [or similar verb of speech] . . ."

| Where OT Documents | What the Therapist Thinks! | What the Therapist Does! | What the Therapist Documents! |
|---|---|---|---|
| Daily notations on chart<br>Weekly progress note<br>Monthly summary notes | • Constantly reassessing goals:<br>• Are treatment services covered?<br>• Are you duplicating services?<br>• Are you providing maintenance care?<br>• Are you changing plans as necessary?<br>• Also consider:<br>• Should patient be put on hold for a while owing to illness?<br>• Should you design a maintenance program for residual deficits? | Chart review<br>Provide treatment<br>Observe performance in requested activities<br>Modify treatment according to patient's response to STG and LTG<br>As patient's goals change, you modify treatment<br>Verify new short-term and long-term goals with patient/caregivers<br>Discontinue patient temporarily<br>Instruct in-home program | Record briefly: date, type, length of treatment<br>State change in meeting short-term goals and the effect on long-term goals<br>Record changes in goals in weekly or monthly notes<br>Every 30 days summarize changes in patient's ability to perform functional activities and changes in underlying factors<br>State when patient reaches goals. Explanation if patient does not reach goals and how that affects treatment plan<br>Recertification of Medicare<br>Record temporary discontinuation of treatment and reason<br>Record home program and any follow-up recommendations made |

**Figure 17-8. Therapist's short-term goals and changes in goals.** *STG,* short-term goal; *LTG,* long-term goal. (Modified with permission from Allen CK. Clinical reasoning for documentation. In: Acquaviva JD, ed. Effective Documentation for Occupational Therapy. 2nd ed. Bethesda, MD: American Occupational Therapy Association, 1998. Copyright © 1998 by the American Occupational Therapy Association, Inc.)

**Spruce Valley Hospital, Occupational Therapy Department, Weekly Progress Report**

5/22/08

H. Page Case #186302

Ms. Page present at 6 of 8 mtgs. of Money Management Gp. Absent X2 for lab tests. Patient says she is bored; frequently converses with another female patient (T.M.); computation skill and banking knowledge are WFL for independent living; patient acknowledges problem with impulsive spending in past ($2500 credit card bill).

Patient to continue in group until discharge, tentatively scheduled for 5/29. Goal: Patient to identify three ways to stop self from impulse purchases by 5/29. Patient scheduled for visit to Safe Haven (group home) with this writer on 5/25.

Treatment sessions attended: 5/13, 5/14, 5/18, 5/20, 5/21, 5/22.

Jerry Doe COTA

**Figure 17-9. Weekly progress report.** *Mtgs,* meetings; *Gp,* group; *WFL,* within functional limits.

**Green Manor Nursing Home, Occupational Therapy Department, Biweekly Progress Report**

J. Anderson Case #9801
3/12/08 Treatment given: 2/26, 3/1, 3/2, 3/3, 3/4, 3/5, 3/8, 3/9, 3/10, 3/11, 3/12.

Patient seen 1:1, 5X/wk since 2/26 (10 sessions). Condition continues to deteriorate. Patient usually found seated in a gerichair in the dining room. She appears alert and interested in her surroundings, but on approach by OTA is consistently disoriented to time, place, and person. She responds to simple familiar activities like tossing a ball and will imitate motions (exercises) that are demonstrated. *Plan:* Train aide to perform daily visits to provide social and sensory stimulation and basic movement experiences to orient patient to environment, limit extent of contractures, and encourage as much independent function as possible. Aide training to be completed by 3/19/08.

Nelly Cortland COTA

**Figure 17-10. Biweekly progress report.** *Wk,* week.

The *objective* section describes observable or measurable behavior noted by the therapist. This may include evaluation results and observations of the patient's performance. This is the section in which most of the information usually contained in a narrative progress note is written.

The *assessment* section summarizes the therapist's understanding of the patient's problem. (Remember that everything in the problem-oriented record is organized around the problem list.) Here the therapist draws upon the subjective and objective information contained in the first parts of the note and analyzes whether the plan needs to be modified.

The *plan* section describes the action the therapist will take in response to the patient's problem. Here the therapist records the plan for continued treatment, including modifications to the previous plan, and any new objectives and methods.

The note given in Figure 17-11 has been rewritten in SOAP format and presented in Figure 17-13. Because notes in the problem-oriented record are

**County Hospital, Occupational Therapy Department, Weekly Progress Report**

10/7/07
L. Lammamoor Case #082751

Patient has selectively attended general ward activities over the past week (11 of 18 activity group sessions). She states she does not need the socialization group or the community meeting, and efforts to involve her have been unsuccessful. She participates in the daily crafts group, the senior stretch exercise group, and the semiweekly cooking group. Patient continues to rely inappropriately on help from group leaders but fails to seek help when she truly needs it. In cooking, she asked for assistance and approval in measuring and mixing ingredients although she did so correctly and quickly, but then reached for a pot handle without a potholder. Her crafts projects are neat and attractive, but she hoards materials and criticizes other patients. Periodic c/o leg pain (reported to J. Brown, R.N., on 10/2/07). *Plan:* Continue to engage in exercise, craft, and cooking activities and observe for safety. Continue to encourage participation in social and verbal groups with one-on-one escort of OTA student. Reassess 1 week.

M.A. Teun COTA

**Figure 17-11. Weekly progress note.** *C/o,* complaint of.

**Occupational Therapy Department, Home Arts Program, Biweekly Progress Note**

D. Kennedy Case #291083

1/8/08 Sessions attended: 12/21, 12/22, 12/23; 12/28, 12/29, 12/30; 1/4, 1/5, 1/7, 1/8

Patient has attended all scheduled sessions over the past 2½ weeks. At first seemed uncomfortable with other members of the group but has begun to interact spontaneously during the past week. Patient has mastered all of the meal preparation tasks (see plan 12/18/07), obtained a score of 92 of a possible 100 points on sections 4, 5, and 6 of the Practical Evaluation, and appears able to carry out routine cooking safely. Patient still tends to panic in difficult situations; for instance, when he was $1.50 short to pay for groceries, he ran out of the store. He was able to discuss this later with the group and explore other ways he could have handled the problem. Patient says he needs to stop and think before acting; OTA feels this shows insight and growth. OTA contacted patient's wife, who is pleased with his progress and willing to allow him to take over meal preparation responsibilities at home.

*New short-term objectives:*

1. Patient will demonstrate knowledge of nutrition as evidenced by ability to plan balanced meals.
2. Patient will demonstrate ability to organize and perform basic household cleaning tasks, including dusting, vacuuming, sweeping, cleaning, and knowledge of household products.
3. Patient will demonstrate ability to compensate for visual deficit in performance of household cleaning.
4. Patient will report his reactions to stress and his use of alternative responses.

*Method:*

Continue group instruction in basic nutrition and methods of household cleaning in the Home Arts Center and local shops. Continue to teach and reinforce visual compensation techniques. Group discussions on stress and stress management will continue. It is expected that objectives will be reached by 2/1/08, at which point patient will be able to plan balanced meals and perform housekeeping tasks independently.

B White COTA

**Figure 17-12. Home arts program, biweekly progress note.**

written in response to specific problems, other information unrelated to these problems is omitted in the SOAP note and documented separately.

Some versions of the SOAP note allow for the omission of the S, or subjective, component, which is useful when patients are nonverbal. It is also possible to combine the S and the O, or objective, components into one section, as shown in Figure 17-14, which restates information found in Figure 17-2. Here the combined S and O are termed *D*, which stands for "data."

## Discontinuation or Discharge Report

The discontinuation or discharge report reviews the entire course of the person's treatment. It includes the kinds of assessments and treatment the person received, the number of OT sessions, progress toward goals, and the individual's functional level at discharge. The person's condition at the beginning of treatment and at discharge are compared, and recommendations for continued care or referrals to other agencies are included. A discharge or discontinuation report includes the following (3):

**County Hospital, S.O.A.P. Note**

10/7/07
Note #64

Problem #4, Possible cognitive disability

**S:** Patient continues to request assistance from group leaders to perform simple exercises, craft activities, and meal preparation tasks in occupational therapy groups.

**O:** Patient performs well in many tasks, as evidenced by completion of a complicated main dish and detailed braiding of a basket based on a diagram in a book. However, patient also has acted unsafely in kitchen (reaching for pot without potholder to protect hand).

**A:** Patient is working in unfamiliar kitchen with unfamiliar equipment. Patient seems to know task well. Reasons for errors may be related to unfamiliar environment.

**P:** OTA will arrange for evaluation of patient's cooking behaviors in patient's home kitchen.

M.A. Teen COTA

**Figure 17-13. Subjective-objective assessment plan (SOAP) note.**

- The patient's name and case number and the date, including year
- A summary of the OT process, including the number of sessions, goals achieved, and final outcome regarding engagement in occupations
- A comparison of patient's status at admission to the program with that at discharge
- Follow-up plans and recommendations
- The OTA's signature and title
- The OT's countersignature

The OT is responsible for documenting the discontinuation or discharge from occupational therapy (6). The OTA might write a discharge

**Clearview Hospital, D.A.P. Note**

2/1/08
OT Note #1

Problem #1, Possible cognitive disability

**D:** Patient arrived for OT group with uncombed hair. Made errors in simple tile task, gluing tiling to wrong side. Dripped glue and did not recognize that she had smeared glue on face. Moved slowly, holding on to furniture.

**A:** Patient demonstrates behavior consistent with cognitive level 4.

**P:** Administer ACL and further assess cognitive deficit.

C. Sample COTA

**Figure 17-14. Data assessment plan note.** *ACL,* Allen Cognitive Level.

**Occupational Therapy Department, Home Arts Program Discharge Report**

3/31/08
page 1 of 2

D. Kennedy
Case #291083

Mr. Kennedy completed 44 sessions of instruction in the occupational therapy home arts program. Four sessions missed because of illness were made up during the past week. Patient achieved the following goals during the program:

1. Patient has learned to plan, organize, and carry out basic household tasks and states he feels comfortable in role of homemaker.
2. Patient has learned to participate in and initiate simple social conversations and to assert self appropriately in social situations.
3. Patient has learned techniques to compensate for his visual deficit and uses these techniques consistently.
4. Patient has learned progressive relaxation and the use of imagery to control the effects of stress.
5. Patient has identified music as a major leisure interest and has enrolled in a guitar study course at the local YMCA.

Patient is capable of functioning independently in the community in the role of homemaker while his wife continues to work full-time. Wife states that patient has "really turned his life around," that she looks forward to coming home to a clean house and a hot meal every day. Patient expresses satisfaction with his accomplishments and his new role. On final reevaluation Mr. Kennedy obtained a score of 173 of 176 possible points on the personal care and hygiene section and 234 of a possible 240 points on the practical evaluation section of the Comprehensive Evaluation of Basic Living Skills. This compares with scores of 135 and 90, respectively, prior to admission to the program.

3/31/08
page 2 of 2

D. Kennedy Case #291083

*Plan:* Follow-up visits to the patient's home at 1 month intervals for 3 months to ensure that patient continues to carry over learned skills to home environment. Reassess 3 months (6/08).

B White COTA

**Figure 17-15. Home arts program discharge report.**

or discontinuation report when a patient is discontinued from or completes a program the OTA supervises. An example of such a discharge or discontinuation report, relating to case 5 in Appendix A, is presented in Figure 17-15.

## Special Reports

Occasionally the OT department may wish to include additional records or reports in the patient's chart, or these may be required for legal reasons. Some examples follow:

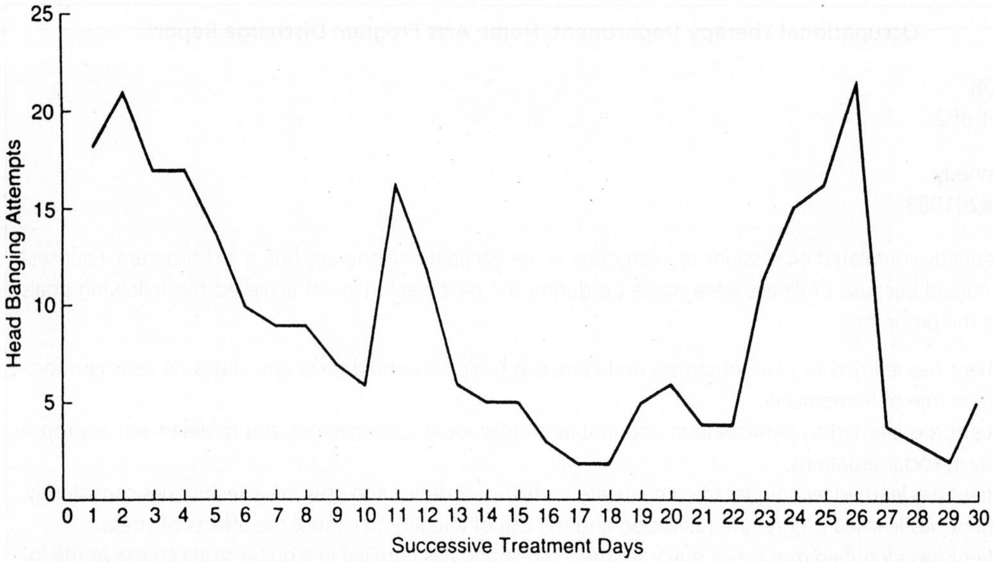


**Figure 17-16. Head banging per half hour.** Behavior chart used to record data related to change in a patient.

- Referrals to other programs or agencies
- Letters about or from the patient that relate to his or her condition and treatment, including appeals and letters of advocacy
- Copies of home programs given to the patient or the family
- Reports to the court
- Behavioral counting scales

Most of these items should be familiar or self-explanatory, with the exception of the *behavioral counting scale.* This is a grid-like chart used to record a specific aspect of a patient's behavior. For instance, the rater might count the number of times an autistic child bangs his or her head during a 1-hour session or how many minutes a consumer in a work group can attend to a task. The rater counts the number of times the behavior occurs during the selected period and records it on the vertical axis of the chart. The horizontal axis is used to show changes over time, as the behavior is counted day after day. This gives a clear visual picture of whether the behavior is increasing or decreasing. An example of this kind of record is shown in Figure 17-16.

The OTA may on occasion become involved in writing letters of appeal or advocacy, to argue for additional services or continuation of services (7, 10). Examples of such letters with good examples are shown in other texts (15), which the reader is encouraged to consult.

The therapist makes the final decision about which documents from OT will be included in the patient's chart. The OTA should, therefore, bring any correspondence or other special reports to the OT's attention.

In addition to the kinds of notes covered in this chapter, there exist many checklist or grid types of documentation formats, in which information for a number of different sessions can be checked off on one sheet. The *Comprehensive Occupational Therapy Evaluation (COTE)* scale (see Chapter 15) is a popular example. Other flow sheets or documentation summaries may be particular to individual facilities.

## DOCUMENTATION REVIEW AND QUALITY ASSURANCE

Quality assurance (see Chapter 16) is the term given to methods and programs designed to ensure accountability in health care. Quality assurance programs investigate whether treatment was provided in a timely fashion and in keeping with the accepted standards of practice in the various professional disciplines involved. Another purpose of quality assurance is to demonstrate which interventions were effective and which were not.

Chart audit is one method of quality assurance. The general procedure for chart audit is first to develop a set of criteria or standards for patient care and then to review charts to see whether patients received the care that is required by the criteria. For example, one of the criteria developed by the OT department is likely to be that every patient must receive an OT evaluation on referral. When the charts are reviewed (audited), it is easy to demonstrate whether this has happened (12, pp. 155–157).

## SUMMARY

Keeping accurate and complete records is an important part of the OTA's job. The patient's chart is a legal document and an important tool for communication among different disciplines involved in the patient's care. Increasingly strict reimbursement guidelines have made it more important than ever before to record measurable objectives and objective signs of progress; written evidence of clear goals (related to engagement in occupation) and reasonable efforts to achieve them are the only way to persuade public and private insurers to continue to pay for OT services.

## REVIEW QUESTIONS AND ACTIVITIES

1. Why is documentation an important activity for the OTA? List several reasons.
2. What are four major purposes of the psychiatric medical record?
3. How does the problem-oriented medical record differ from the source-oriented medical record?
4. Describe each of the following types of occupational therapy documentation: initial note, assessment note or plan, intervention plan, progress report, treatment record, therapy log, discontinuation report, critical incident report, letter of advocacy, letter of appeal.
   - What is the role of the OTA in regard to each type of document?
   - What is the role of the OT?
5. Explain why progress notes do not always indicate that the patient has made progress.
6. Identify and describe the information that should be included in each of the four sections of the SOAP note.
7. What is the difference between SOAP and DAP notes?
8. How does chart review relate to quality assurance?
9. *Challenge activity:* After reading the chapter, identify areas in which you feel you need to develop more skill. Make a plan for improving your skills. Share in class.
10. *Challenge activity:* Using the cases in Appendix A or in Chapters 2 and 3, write examples of initial notes, intervention plans for an area of occupation, progress notes, and discontinuation summaries.

## REFERENCES


1. Acquaviva JD, ed. Effective Documentation for Occupational Therapy. 2nd ed. Bethesda, MD: American Occupational Therapy Association, 1998.
2. Allen C. Clinical reasoning for documentation. In: Acquaviva JD, ed. Effective Documentation for Occupational Therapy. 2nd ed. Bethesda, MD: American Occupational Therapy Association, 1998.
3. American Occupational Therapy Association. Guidelines for documentation of occupational therapy. Am J Occup Ther 2003;57:646–649.
4. American Occupational Therapy Association. Occupational therapy practice framework: Domain and process. Am J Occup Ther 2002;56:609–639.
5. American Occupational Therapy Association. Roles and responsibilities of the occupational therapist and the occupational therapy assistant during the delivery of occupational therapy services. OT Practice 2002;7(15):9–10.
6. American Occupational Therapy Association. Standards of practice for occupational therapy. Am J Occup Ther 2005;59:663–665.
7. Brennan C, Robinson M. Documentation—Getting it right to avoid medicare denials. OT Practice 2006;11(14):10–15.
8. Centers for Medicare and Medicaid Services Therapy Overview. Available at: http://www.cms.hhs.gov/TherapyServices/. Accessed October 9, 2007.
9. Kannenberg K. Special considerations: 3. Mental health. In: Acquaviva JD, ed. Effective Documentation for Occupational Therapy. 2nd ed. Bethesda, MD: American Occupational Therapy Association, 1998.
10. Lloyd LD. Medicare denials—Fight denials with knowledge. OT Practice 2004;9(10):CE1–8.
11. Moorhouse MF, Doenges ME. Nurse's Clinical Pocket Manual: Nursing Diagnosis, Care Planning, and Documentation. Philadelphia: Davis, 1990.
12. Pinson CC. Documentation review. In: Acquaviva JD, ed. Effective Documentation for Occupational Therapy. 2nd ed. Bethesda, MD: American Occupational Therapy Association, 1998.
13. Ranke BEA. Documentation in the age of litigation. OT Practice 1998;3(3):20–24.
14. Robertson SC. Why we document. In: Acquaviva JD, ed. Effective Documentation for Occupational Therapy. 2nd ed. Bethesda, MD: American Occupational Therapy Association, 1998.
15. Sames KM. Documenting Occupational Therapy Practice. Upper Saddle River, NJ: Pearson Prentice Hall, 2005.
16. Zinsser W. Writing to Learn. New York: Harper & Row, 1988.


## SUGGESTED READINGS


Acquaviva JD, ed. Effective Documentation for Occupational Therapy. 2nd ed. Bethesda, MD: American Occupational Therapy Association, 1998.

Allen C. Clinical reasoning for documentation. In: Acquaviva JD, ed. Effective Documentation for Occupational Therapy. 2nd ed. Bethesda, MD: American Occupational Therapy Association, 1998.

Borcherding S. Documentation Manual for Writing SOAP Notes in Occupational Therapy. 2nd ed. Thorofare, NJ: Slack, 2005.

Borcherding S, Morreale MJ. The OTA's Guide to Writing SOAP Notes. 2nd ed. Thorofare, NJ: Slack, 2005.

Kannenberg K. Special considerations: 3. Mental health. In: Acquaviva JD, ed. Effective Documentation for Occupational Therapy. 2nd ed. Bethesda, MD: American Occupational Therapy Association, 1998.

McGuire MJ. Documenting progress in home care. Am J Occup Ther 1997;51:436–445.

McLeod K, Robnett R. Psychosocial documentation: Are your objectives functional, measurable and reimbursable? Occup Ther Ment Health 1998;14(3):21–31.

Moorhead P, Kannenberg K. Writing functional goals. In: Acquaviva JD, ed. Effective Documentation for Occupational Therapy. 2nd ed. Bethesda, MD: American Occupational Therapy Association, 1998.

Pinson CC. Documentation review. In: Acquaviva JD, ed. Effective Documentation for Occupational Therapy. 2nd ed. Bethesda, MD: American Occupational Therapy Association, 1998.

Robertson SC. Why we document. In: Acquaviva JD, ed. Effective Documentation for Occupational Therapy. 2nd ed. Bethesda, MD: American Occupational Therapy Association, 1998.

Sames KM. Documenting Occupational Therapy Practice. Upper Saddle River, NJ: Pearson Prentice Hall, 2005.

SECTION V

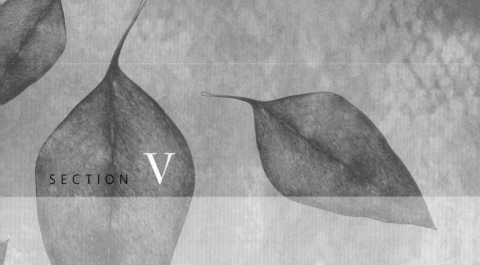

# Occupational Therapy Methods

CHAPTER 18

# Activities of Daily Living

***Caregivers must visit often to ensure that patients take their medication appropriately. Patients frequently need help so that they clean their clothes and their living spaces, and so that they have an opportunity to socialize.***

FREDERICK J. FRESE (6, P. 2)

## CHAPTER OBJECTIVES

After studying this chapter, the reader will be able to:

1. Recognize that knowledge, skills and attitudes are aspects of learning.
2. Identify and analyze the kinds of difficulties that persons with mental disorders may have with daily living skills.
3. Differentiate between personal and instrumental activities of daily living.
4. Select appropriate contexts in which to train and practice daily living skills.
5. Identify cognitive and sensory reasons why clients may perform poorly in some activities of daily living.
6. Discuss the effects of family background, social support, financial means, and culture on performance of daily living skills.
7. Identify training activities and environmental compensations for a range of daily living skills.
8. Discuss the role of practice, repetition, and varying conditions on the development of habits and routines.

The five chapters in Section V present an overview of the areas of occupation (1) most frequently targeted by occupational therapists (OTs) and occupational therapy assistants (OTAs) working in psychiatry. Chapter 23 discusses activity analysis. Performance skills and patterns are also addressed. It is crucial to remember that *doing* is the core experience of occupational therapy. Engagement in valued occupation makes occupational therapy unique among the health professions. It is through participation and involvement in chosen and necessary activities that clients develop and practice skills, learn about themselves and other people, increase their sense of competence, express their feelings and ideas, and develop confidence in their own ability to have an effect on the world.

The occupations and activities in which OTAs support clients, and the methods they use, are presented in five chapters. Many other excellent methods and activities cannot be discussed because of space limitations. Chapter 18 focuses on activities of daily living and instrumental activities of daily living, two of the seven areas of occupation (1). Chapter 19 gives an overview of the areas of education and work. Chapter 20 examines the areas of leisure and play and social interaction. Chapter 21 describes the role of occupational therapy in developing the client's communication and interaction skills. Chapter 22 discusses the development of process skills, presents those skills used to manage and modify actions, and includes information on some client factors related to mental and sensory functions. Considerable overlap exists among the topics in these chapters. Performance skills (to organize, to communicate, to move self and objects) and mental and sensory functions (memory, sensory processing) support one's ability to function in the occupations of daily living skills, work, leisure, social participation, and so on. Occupational therapy practitioners use activities as broad instruments of practice; Although we must analyze activities carefully and always know what we are doing and why, it is rarely useful to classify activities too rigidly.

In each category and when needed for individual activities within the category, the following information is covered: general purposes of the activity, prerequisite skills, environment and context factors, habits and patterns, and precautions and considerations that apply to persons with psychiatric disorders. The reader will find additional detail in the references and other resources listed at the end of each chapter.

## FACTORS IN LEARNING AND USING SKILLS

Before discussing the activities themselves, we will examine why and how specific activities can be used. At first glance, it seems that all that is needed is for the therapist or assistant to teach someone whatever skills are lacking and then gradually withdraw support to encourage the person to function independently. However, although many clients need to learn specific skills, others already possess the necessary skills but fail to use them for various reasons. Even sadder, some people go through the motions of everyday life with a high degree of skill in the activities they attempt but feel miserable and disconnected from any meaning or purpose. To understand why these problems can exist, it is helpful to think about the three basic categories of learning: knowledge, skills, and attitudes.

*Knowledge* is acquired *information* (facts about reality). For instance, individuals preparing to live on their own for the first time may not understand the basic facts and methods of homemaking. They may not know what tasks are involved, what tools and supplies they will need, or how often and how thoroughly various tasks should be done. A person who has spent the past 20 years in hospitals and supervised board-and-care homes may not know, for example, that bed sheets should be changed regularly.

*Skills* are *actions* or behaviors that are learned. For example, some clients may not know how to change a bed, perhaps not even how to make a bed.

They may not know how to wash sheets, wash dishes, wring out a mop, or clean a toilet. Skills are the "doing" part of the activity.

*Attitudes* are learned *feelings,* values, and beliefs. Schwartzberg (23) suggests that clients may have difficulty staying motivated to use skills they already possess because of various intrapsychic (within the mind) and emotional factors. For instance, low self-esteem or a feeling that one is a failure can undermine motivation and sabotage any chance of success. In other words, the person lacks the energy even to get started, and previous failures have convinced the person there is little point in trying. A related problem is that impaired ability to express feelings may lead to anger and frustration. Schwartzberg quotes one patient:

> I have recently, since I got sick, for the first time been able to get angry. I have never been able to get angry before. I know I have a lot of anger in me. When I let go of some of it I usually get an anxiety attack after it. Perhaps, I feel, it is not the way one should act. You should act nice. Anger is something that I feel is evil. I should be a good girl. 'Cause of the neck tightening and the phobias I can't go to the store, I can't buy groceries, I can't do anything to take care of myself. I'm not able to walk anywhere (23, p. 15).

Schwartzberg also notes the positive effect of social contact on healthy occupational behavior and maintenance of habits. She suggests that people who become socially isolated are deprived of an important environmental stimulus and so may find normal activities much less gratifying. In addition, whereas good habits depend on following a routine, too much of the same thing can lead to boredom and diminished motivation. She quotes another patient:

> I'd get up at 8:30 in the morning, make the beds, and I'd do the dishes. This is all after I ate breakfast, of course, and washed up, put on my makeup and put my dentures in. Then I'd dust around, if it needed to be dusted, and then I'd spend most of my time watching TV. I prepared breakfast and lunch for myself and I was always alone. That's how I became very depressed. When my husband came home from work I'd prepare his supper and then he would go and listen to his C.B. while I went into the living room and watched TV. Then around 8:00 or so I'd go in my room, I mean our room, and watch the colored TV in there because I got tired of watching black and white all day. So I'd watch the colored TV until around 10:00 and then shut the light off and go to bed. It became very depressing for me. I was very lonely. I had anxiety attacks. I live in a younger neighborhood and they work. They are in their thirties and I am left alone. There is no neighbor to come in and talk to me or anything. I don't even have anyone to talk to on the phone because my children work too. I'd say, Oh God the same thing tomorrow and the next day and the next day! (23, pp. 16–17).

In addition, roles and patterns and values learned from one's parents can influence one's willingness to attempt and maintain certain skills. For instance, someone reared in a wealthy household would be accustomed to having personal and housekeeping needs taken care of by paid servants and might have some negative feelings about being required to learn and use basic housekeeping skills. Similarly, a woman whose mother was obsessively tidy in her housework may find it hard to break the habit of spending most of her waking hours cleaning; indeed, she may not even recognize this as a habit and a choice. Schwartzberg proposes that people may have difficulty sustaining activities that were not approved of or just not done by their parents. Values and beliefs that arise in one's cultural and ethnic heritage may have a similar effect on motivation for activities.

Similarly, personal learning preferences and habits can affect new learning. For example, some individuals enact a lifelong pattern of helping or advising other people while avoiding having to demonstrate their own ability. A difficulty in asking for and receiving help can seriously interfere with learning new skills from a therapist or peers.

Feeling inadequate or unworthy of help or unwilling to reveal inadequacy are all possible reasons for this kind of behavior. There may be a feeling that having to rely on another person is a big risk, too frightening to attempt. Underlying beliefs and feelings such as these can impair both the ability to function and one's general feeling of well-being and mental health.

Thus a careful analysis of the knowledge, skills, and attitudes of a particular client is necessary. The therapist or assistant must ask these questions:

- How important is it for this person to be involved in this activity?
- What will it do for him or her?
- Does the patient know when, where, why, and with whom to use this activity?
- Does the person know how to do it and has he or she practiced it enough to remember how to do it independently? Has the person made it a habit or part of a routine?
- Does *the person* think it is important to do this activity, and *why* is it important? (What does it mean to him or her?)

As stated previously, Chapter 23 describes further how to analyze and adapt activities to meet the needs of different individuals and groups.

## DAILY LIVING ACTIVITIES (BASIC AND INSTRUMENTAL)

Daily living activities include all of the tasks the average adult needs to perform to manage life on a daily basis. These are divided into two groups. The first is called *activities of daily living* (ADLs) or *personal or basic activities of daily living* (PADLs, BADLs). Occupations classified as activities of daily living in the American Occupational Therapy Association's (AOTA's) *Occupational Therapy Practice Framework* (1) are listed in Box 18-1. The second group, *instrumental activities of daily living* (IADLs), comprises more complex occupations requiring greater cognitive skill and involvement with others in the community. IADLs are listed in Box 18-2. Throughout this chapter we will combine activities from the two areas when appropriate. For example, clothing selection is part of

**BOX 18-1**

### ACTIVITIES OF DAILY LIVING

- Bathing or showering
- Bowel and bladder management
- Dressing
- Feeding and eating
- Functional mobility
- Personal device care (e.g., contact lenses)
- Personal hygiene and grooming
- Sexual activity
- Sleep or rest
- Toilet hygiene

Reprinted with permission from American Occupational Therapy Association. Occupational therapy practice framework: Domain and process. Am J Occup Ther 2002;56:609–639.

**BOX 18-2**

**INSTRUMENTAL ACTIVITIES OF DAILY LIVING**

- Care of others (including selecting and supervising caregivers)
- Care of pets
- Child rearing
- Communication device use
- Community mobility
- Financial management
- Health management or maintenance
- Home establishment and maintenance
- Meal preparation and cleanup
- Safety procedures and emergency response
- Shopping

Reprinted with permission from American Occupational Therapy Association. Occupational therapy practice framework: Domain and process. Am J Occup Ther 2002;56:609–639.

dressing (an ADL) and clothing maintenance and shopping for clothing are classified as IADLs. All three will be discussed together.

Many persons diagnosed with mental disorders have adequate basic ADL skills and do not require occupational therapy intervention for personal ADL occupations. Higher-functioning individuals frequently demonstrate adequate to excellent personal care and daily living skills. However, persons with chronic conditions or severe psychotic disorders may appear indifferent to their personal hygiene; bathing so infrequently and toileting inattentively so that they have a strong body odor; combing and washing their hair rarely, if at all; and dressing bizarrely in clothes that are out of date, ill-matched, or inappropriate for the season or the occasion. Clients who have acceptable skills in grooming and hygiene may have other problems that are less immediately obvious but that present serious impediments to carrying out a normal daily routine. Inadequate knowledge of nutrition, poor eating habits, and excessive use of cigarettes, drugs and alcohol, caffeinated beverages, and over-the-counter medications (antacids, diet pills, laxatives, sleeping pills) contribute to malnutrition and chemically induced anxiety.

Problems become more apparent in instrumental activities of daily living. Persons with cognitive disabilities may be unable manage money successfully and will be caught short before they have paid for basics like food, rent, and utilities. Without knowing how to get around their communities on foot or on public transportation, many clients remain isolated in impoverished environments. These are only a few of the problems encountered by those whose daily living skills are deficient. Increasing skills in these areas can dramatically enhance the quality of the lives of the mentally ill and in many instances prevent future hospitalizations.

Those most likely to need help with daily living skills are persons diagnosed with chronic schizophrenia and organic mental disorders. In a review of the literature, Hayes (10) indicated that living skills taught to such individuals carried over well to community life, provided opportunity was given for transfer to the new situation and for generalization of learning. Transfer and generalization of learning are not reliable when skills are taught in a clinical environment; the person is not likely to use the skills in a home environment, which is different. We will stress throughout this chapter that learning and habit are linked to context—in other words, the skills should be evaluated, taught, and practiced in the real life situation whenever possible.

## Bathing, Showering, Hygiene and Grooming, Toilet Hygiene

Individuals requiring occupational therapy intervention in this area may be further considered in terms of functional level, length of illness and hospitalization, previous knowledge and skills, and social support available. At one extreme, the very regressed chronic patient who has been hospitalized for long periods may need training and reinforcement in basic hygiene habits, such as proper use of the toilet, use of toilet tissue, washing of hands and face, and so on, and may require ongoing assistance or cuing from a caregiver (5, 22). Some individuals whose illnesses are equally severe but who come from middle-class backgrounds may have adequate skills or sufficient social support from their families, so that they always appear presentable (even though they may need reminders or actual physical assistance from family members or paid caregivers). At another extreme, some individuals who have reasonable personal care skills but low self-esteem may benefit from the experience of pampering themselves in a grooming group, experimenting with samples of new self-care products, and receiving praise from their peers.

Personal hygiene and grooming may be taught on a one-on-one basis. This is appropriate for individuals with very poor skills and those who wish or need to learn some aspect that is private or not of general interest. Most commonly, however, hygiene and grooming are taught in groups that may be restricted to clients of one sex or the other, depending upon the specific skill content.

Activities that may be covered include bathing, toilet hygiene, skin care, use of deodorant, hair care (including when to get a haircut), care of the teeth and use of mouthwash, and shaving or use of depilatories. Following the principle that context contributes to developing habits, all of these skills should be taught in the bathroom or an area that simulates it. Ideally, skills should be taught in the consumer's home, using the tools and equipment to which he or she is accustomed. Lower-functioning individuals may have to be reminded to pay attention to parts of the body that are not immediately visible, such as the back of the head or body, the underarms, the soles of the feet. The use of a full-length mirror, a three-part folding mirror, and various

> **POINT-OF-VIEW**
>
> ***We fight about showers. I put a mark on the calendar, and I keep reminding her; then after a couple days I have to insist. I'll take her arm and lead her to the bathroom, and I'm firm about it. After the shower, I take her in my arms. Sometimes she'll actually say "thank you."***
>
> A caregiver of a spouse with dementia, quoted by Hasselkus and Murray (9, p. 14)
>
> - What does this story tell you about the patient and her husband?
> - What does his holding her after the shower communicate?
> - How might you (would you?) share this story with caregivers who are experiencing problems in caring for their loved ones?

handheld mirrors is helpful. Shatter-proof mirrors may be required in some settings and are safer generally, although the image in such mirrors is less clear than an image in a glass mirror.

An important precaution should be mentioned. Because health problems (bacterial, viral, parasitic) can be transmitted via shared personal care products, either each person should have his or her own items or disposable sample sizes should be used.

In addition to these basic personal care skills, occupational therapy practitioners may also teach the use of makeup and nail care. Some female patients use excessive amounts of makeup or apply it in old-fashioned or bizarre ways; skill development may focus on matching make-up color to complexion, choice of flattering shades, and methods of application and removal. The goal is to help these women learn to use makeup in an attractive and socially acceptable way. The use of mirrors, including magnifying mirrors, and feedback from peers can rein- force what is appropriate and what is not. Fashion and beauty magazines can be helpful, but those that picture extreme makeup styles sometimes used in high-fashion modeling should be avoided.

Nail care at its simplest entails cleaning and trimming the nails wherever they need it and pushing back the cuticles. Teaching clients these skills and reinforcing their continued use will contribute greatly to their making a positive impression on other people. The use of cuticle removers and colored nail polish, on the other hand, are optional practices that are sometimes overused as activities in self-care groups. It seems odd to have patients apply nail polish when they have other self-care problems that are more serious and when their nails will be dirty again and the polish chipped within a day's time. However, applying nail polish can be useful for clients who have done this in the past or who may get a needed boost to their self-esteem from doing it. The act of caring for one's body by cleaning and enhancing the appearance of one's nails can stimulate increased attention to other areas of self care.

In working with clients around self care tasks, the OTA should observe carefully for sensory processing problems. Clients with sensory processing problems may react adversely to the scents of deodorants and other toiletries. They may avoid bathing, and may dislike touching their own skin, simply because the sensation is unpleasant to them. Another obstacle for clients who have experienced abuse in bathrooms is that they may avoid bathing or showering because the context reminds them of the abuse. The OTA should refer any concerns to the OT, for further evaluation. If indicated, the OTA may speak with the client to try to find out what is behind the aversion and avoidance.

### Selection and Maintenance of Clothing

A large part of the impression one makes on others depends on being dressed in clean, neat, well-fitting clothes that are appropriate for the season and the occasion. A brief glance at magazine covers on the supermarket checkout stand will testify that people in general have a more than casual interest in how they look. Those with severe mental disorders often lack even the basic skills necessary to present a good personal appearance. Persons who are indigent may be used to wearing clothes selected for them by others or donated to charity; these clothes are rarely in fashion and often appear bizarre because they are out of date and cannot be coordinated with each other. Persons with cognitive disabilities or limited life experience may wear ill-fitting clothes because they do not know what size they wear or because they did not adjust their wardrobes when they gained or lost weight. They may not know how to care for their clothing, with shrinkage, wrinkling, and run colors the result. They may not have the means or skill to repair ripped seams and missing buttons.

Clothing selection and maintenance activities focus on how to select clothes for a given occasion, how to shop for clothing, and how to maintain it. Specific activities may start with learning what clothes are appropriate and flattering. Clients may start by taking their measurements and figuring out sizes. This may be followed by a trip to see what is available locally in a clothing store or thrift shop, as a part of learning to budget and comparison shop. Another approach is for members to bring in garments from their own wardrobes and use a mannequin for the group to assemble and discuss appropriate outfits. Alternatively, the assistant can create visual aids from photographs in magazines to illustrate appropriate clothing for different occasions. Attention should be given to seasonal differences and to the differences among casual, dressy, and work attire.

Dressing neatly and appropriately in a reasonably brief space of time requires skill and practice. Clients may need help setting up combinations of clothes that work together. They may benefit from developing routines of laying out clothing the night before, laundering and ironing on a weekly basis, hanging up or folding clothes or placing them in the hamper when they undress, and so on. Much work may need to go into habit development in this area. Repeated practice with feedback under varying conditions will be necessary, particularly for clients with cognitive disabilities.

Learning to shop for clothing requires that clients know their sizes for all garments, including shoes and underwear. For example, being measured for a brassiere may seem overwhelming to a person with depression or with cognitive or sensory problems. Accompanying clients on shopping trips allows the OTA to provide support so that the client learns what is customary, develops confidence, and obtains the correct size. Instruction in how to recognize whether a garment is well made and easy to care for is especially important because people on disability assistance have limited funds to replace damaged clothing. Clients may need help in planning their purchases to fit in with other clothing they already own and in selecting flattering styles and colors.

In addition to being able to select and shop for clothing, one needs to know how to maintain it, clean it, and repair it. Clothing care requires reading care labels and recognizing when something needs special care such as washing by hand, dry-cleaning, or drip or flat drying as opposed to machine drying. The necessary laundry skills vary, depending upon where the client lives, whether the client or someone else is responsible for the client's laundry, and whether the client has access to a home washing machine or must use a commercial laundry. Knowing how to control water temperature and use various laundry products is necessary. All clients should know the rudiments of mending if they are to live on their own; being able to repair a hem or a ripped seam or sew on a button or a snap can make the difference between looking relatively normal and looking like a patient.

Shoe care includes matching polish color to shoes, knowing when to polish shoes, and knowing when and where to take them for repairs. All of these skills can be taught by a combination of verbal instruction, demonstration, and actual practice; photographs and written guidelines that can later be used as reminders are often helpful. Again, development of habits of shoe care is critical. The OTA may help the client set up an area for shoes, with racks or bags as preferred. Organizing shoes and other garments so that they can be located helps in achieving a neat appearance.

It's important for the OTA to bear in mind that clients may not have had the kinds of experience and support we think of as "normal" for learning these tasks. Providing information, giving demonstrations, allowing time for questions, and creating opportunities to practice will support client achievement of these skills.

Cognitive disabilities compound problems with dressing. Disorganization and clutter magnify the problems a person with a cognitive disability experiences. Environmental compensations such as using see-through organizers, pull-out shelves, color coding items, can help reduce disorder and improve performance. The client may need to obtain additional dressers or other storage; alternately, the client may need support and supervision to discard or store elsewhere clothing items that no longer fit, are no longer in fashion, don't work with the rest of the wardrobe, and so on.

## Nutrition and Weight Control

Basic nutrition and weight control are a concern both for those who have weight problems—anorexia and bulimia (7), obesity—and for those whose eating habits result in an unbalanced diet. Nutrition may be taught either as part of a cooking program or within the general area of self-care. Methods of teaching may include the use of flash cards and worksheets (15) and other commercially available educational aids (companies that supply primary and secondary school teachers are good sources); therapist-created educational aids, such as posters and collages; and group discussion. Another activity is making a file of recipes that are nutritious, inexpensive, and uncomplicated. Most important is actual practice. Clients can practice by planning and preparing a meal or by going out to eat and ordering a balanced meal in a restaurant. Multiple practice sessions, with gradual introduction of variations, will help clients achieve mastery.

A nutrition program provides an opportunity to teach clients about the psychotropic effects of caffeine and cigarette consumption. Both caffeine and nicotine are drugs, classified as such by the American Medical Association. The *Diagnostic and Statistical Manual of Mental Disorders*, fourth edition, text revision *(DSM-IV-TR)* category of substance-related disorders includes both of these drugs. Research evidence conclusively shows that ingestion of large amounts of caffeine in coffee, soft drinks, and chocolate is associated with increased anxiety, irritability, aggression, and psychomotor agitation and that it may counteract the effects of prescribed sedative medication (24). Nicotine has similar stimulating effects, and the other negative health effects of tobacco products are well known.

Weight control activities should inform patients about the relationships among calorie consumption, exercise, and weight. Successful weight control requires strong habits of calorie restriction and moderate exercise. Because high-protein, low-carbohydrate diets are known to increase demands on liver metabolism and to cause increased fatigue, dehydration, and mental depression, clients should be cautioned to avoid fad diets. Instead, they should be encouraged to follow diets that are high in complex carbohydrates but low in fat and calories and to eat reduced portions at regular meals. A good educational activity is planning a weekly calorie-conscious menu within budget limitations. Skills can be reinforced and monitored through weekly weigh-ins and by encouraging members to keep daily records of food consumption and exercise.

Some psychotropic medications (e.g., olanzapine) are associated with significant weight gain. Clients taking such medications may be upset with themselves for gaining weight and may cite this as a reason to discontinue the drug. Other medications such as monoamine oxidase (MAO) inhibitors require changes in diet and avoidance of specific foods. Grapefruit juice may alter the effects of psychotropic medications if taken at the same time. The OTA should encourage clients to learn more about their medications and to consult with the prescribing physician before making any changes.

The issue of weight control is sensitive and difficult for many people to confront. Weight control is related to *body image,* which is one's sense of one's own body and how it looks to other people. Body image includes feelings about physical coordination and sexual attractiveness. It takes a very long time to change body image, which may remain constant despite weight loss or weight gain. A change in the way one looks may mean, for example, that members of the opposite sex suddenly become interested, and this unaccustomed social pressure may feel threatening.

## Medication Management and Health Maintenance

One of the least obvious but potentially most damaging problems faced by a person with a psychiatric disorder who is living in the community is mismanagement of medication. At present, some psychiatric disorders are controllable only with continued use of medication; a person who stops taking pills will become ill as soon as the drugs wear off, and this may result in rehospitalization or worse, including suicide and acts of violence toward others. There are many reasons why a person might not take prescribed medication; the client may forget, lose track of doses, run out of pills, or stop deliberately.

One reason some clients give for stopping deliberately is that the side effects of psychotropic medication can be uncomfortable; these side effects and how to help patients manage them are discussed in Chapter 8. Individuals may give other reasons, such as "getting better, don't need it" or wanting to "see if I could get along without the pills." Clients who are members of Alcoholics Anonymous or other 12-step groups may erroneously believe that they are supposed to avoid all drugs, including those that are prescribed by physicians. The cultural trend toward holistic and alternative medicine may engage some clients in thinking that they can substitute herbal and nutritional therapies for prescription drugs.

Any effort to help a client manage medication independently should begin with a discussion of his or her feelings about it; group discussion with peers can provide feedback based on the direct experience of others. Some individuals need instruction and practice in specific skills, such as where to go or whom to call when they need more medication. Those who cannot remember to take their medication can be taught to use various environmental supports and memory aids such as compartmentalized pillboxes, signs, lists, and timers. Injectable medications that last as long as 2 weeks can sometimes be used for those who are unable to manage their own medication. Clients who cannot remember whether they took their medication might learn to use a diary to record each dosage. In any medication management program the OTA should work closely with the prescribing physician and should *never* give the patient advice that contradicts or countermands the doctor's orders.

Related to medication management is the issue of relapse prevention. Clients feel (and are) empowered when they learn to monitor the signs and symptoms of their own illnesses and recognize and respond effectively to signals of impending relapse. Precin (21), Korb and associates (17), and Linehan (19) provide worksheets to help clients analyze the triggers that may set off a relapse and the measures that they can use to prevent a relapse (Box 18-3). Another source for ideas is Linehan's (19) manual for skills training in borderline personality disorder.

Health maintenance also requires the ability to respond to the minor and major health problems that occur in daily life. It includes the important skills of knowing where to go to obtain medical care and how to respond to emergencies. Clients should be taught how to deal with minor health problems such as splinters, blisters, colds, burns, cuts, fever, indigestion, sprains, bruises, and headaches.

**POINT-OF-VIEW**

***Sometimes they help, sometimes they don't. Sometimes they make me feel like another person, like not normal.***

Paul Williams, quoted by Benedict Carey (4)

- Paul's reaction is similar to that of many clients, who find the effects of medication unpleasant and fluctuating. What would you say to Paul if he said this to you?
- What, if anything, would you document?

**BOX 18-3**

**FOCUS: RELAPSE PREVENTION**

Clients can learn to monitor the course of their mental disorders and prevent relapse that may lead to hospitalization. Help clients see this as a necessary health management activity, just like monitoring blood sugar levels in diabetes.

*Typical triggers* include the following:
- Life changes (e.g., getting a job, going back to school)
- High levels of expressed emotion (e.g., family gatherings)

*Measures to prevent relapse* include the following:
- Telephoning one's physician or case manager
- Seeking support from a peer or family member
- Specific cognitive-behavioral strategies, such as thought stopping

Information should also be available on how over-the-counter (OTC) medications can impair motor ability and judgment (important for driving) and interact with prescribed medication. Also, clients need information about how to read labels and consult with the pharmacist about, for example, the many OTC medicines that should not be combined because they all contain acetaminophen.

## Sexual Activity, Sexual Needs, and Hygiene

Skills related to sexuality include, for women, care of menstruation and breast self-examination. For both sexes, knowledge of the basic mechanisms of sexual reproduction, the use of contraception, methods for avoiding and recognizing sexually transmitted diseases, the use of condoms, the dangers of unprotected sexual relations, and awareness of socially acceptable behaviors are important. Strange as it may seem, women have occasionally gotten pregnant because they did not know that sexual intercourse had anything to do with having a baby; therefore, it is especially important for persons with psychiatric disorders (who may have more difficulty coping with raising a child than does the average person) to learn the basic facts. Instruction is directed at the person's level of understanding, and the use of detailed anatomical vocabulary or elaborate diagrams is not necessary.

Helping clients acquire knowledge about sexually transmitted diseases is critical. Some disorders, such as substance abuse and impulse-control personality disorders, are associated with promiscuous or sexually impulsive behaviors. Some clients may be so passive and submissive that they have sexual relations with anyone who asks. Topics to be covered include what to look for and how to examine a potential sexual partner as well as why, when, and how to use condoms. Male homosexuals may need instruction in which sexual practices to abstain from to avoid transmission of human immunodeficiency virus (HIV), which leads to acquired immunodeficiency syndrome (AIDS). Concerns about gender identification may also be addressed. Histories of sexual abuse may be an issue for persons with cognitive disabilities and those who abuse alcohol or other substances; they may submit to sexual activities unwittingly or may be threatened or abused (20). Therapists and assistants who feel uncomfortable or unknowledgeable in these areas might seek the assistance of a nurse as a co-instructor. In some settings, instruction in issues relating to sexuality is the responsibility of the nurse or the social worker, not the occupational therapy practitioner.

Finally, individuals may need instruction and training in basic social standards such as not exposing oneself or masturbating in public or talking in public about masturbation or soliciting sexual acts from others. This can be very confusing for persons with cognitive disabilities because the broadcast media (television, radio) feature so much sexually explicit content. Ideas and worksheets for activities on relationships can be found in Korb and associates (17) and Korb and Leutenberg (18).

## Exercise

Exercise has many documented health benefits. It reduces the effects of stress and tension; provides outlets for frustration, anxiety, and aggression; speeds up metabolism; burns calories; reduces appetite; improves cardiovascular health; and increases strength, flexibility, and endurance. It improves balance, coordination, and other sensory integrative functions. Finally, it enhances self-satisfaction and creates a feeling of well-being. Persons with psychiatric disorders should be encouraged to learn about the benefits of exercise and to develop the habit of regular exercise at least three to four times weekly.

A variety of approaches can help clients learn to meet their exercise needs. One is to provide instruction in the basic facts of physical health and fitness; understanding the value of exercise motivates some clients to attempt it. Another is to assist clients in working out a schedule for exercise. Other approaches include actually providing instruction in a sport or physical fitness activity, arranging for a volunteer or fitness instructor to teach an exercise activity, and arranging for a visit to a community fitness center. Nonprofit organizations such as the YMCA and YWCA may have inexpensive membership options that can accommodate those who have financial needs.

Exercise and physical fitness activities must be selected carefully. The goal is for clients to enjoy and value exercise sufficiently that they will follow through on it on their own, and make it a habit and part of their routine. The exercise must be inexpensive and convenient enough for them to practice without turning their lives upside down. Running; doing calisthenics or yoga; swimming at a public, YWCA, or YMCA pool; bicycling; and brisk walking are examples of exercises that require little investment of money, equipment, or space. Normal daily activities, if done consciously and deliberately, may provide significant exercise benefits; clients can be encouraged to take the stairs rather than the elevator, to walk rather than use motorized transportation, to consider housecleaning as an opportunity for exercise, and so on. Selection of exercise must also take into account any medical precautions or drug side effects that may impair a person's ability to perform certain exercises safely.

## Communication Device Use

Clients may have some understanding of how to use the telephone system and the postal system. Cell phones and computers may present challenges to older consumers who have not previously been exposed to them.

Answering the telephone and/or placing a phone call can be overwhelming and disturbing to some mentally disabled people. Those who have difficulty conversing with others face to face are even more disconcerted by the prospect of carrying on a conversation with a disembodied voice. Following and responding to recorded instructions and using decision trees (e.g., "for sales press 1, for customer service press 2") require attention and memory and can be confusing and tedious. A person unfamiliar with telephone answering machines and voice mail may begin speaking before hearing the beep and thus fail to have the message recorded.

Receiving nuisance calls, such as telemarketing calls or calls intended to obtain personal information, is annoying to the average person, but may be confusing and alarming to someone with a cognitive disability. Clients need instruction and practice with simulations of these types of call so that they develop ways to protect themselves from being exploited.

Consumers who have been hospitalized for long periods or whose lives have been regulated by family members or professional staff may have little experience in using the telephone. Basic telephone skills needed for independent community living include answering and making telephone calls, taking messages accurately, using the telephone book (White Pages and Yellow Pages), using a pay telephone, and knowing how to make an emergency call. Each of these skills consists of several subskills; recognizing the differences among a dial tone, a busy signal, and a fax tone is just one example. Several exercises that teach telephone communication skills are included in Kartin and Van Schroeder (13). Examples of other exercises include calling the telephone number for time, weather, or other information and reporting the information to the group; calling a store and asking for information; and finding the correct number and phoning for bus information. It is a good idea to create an index card file of such exercises for the patients' use.

Because using the telephone requires a combination of communication skills (3), process skills, and manual skills, actual practice is essential. Although clients can try out their telephone skills on any phone that is available in the treatment setting, this has some problems. First, the occupational therapy practitioner working with the patient can hear only half of the conversation and, therefore, may not be able to give accurate feedback. Second, the person may feel anxious because the situation is a real one. Finally, phones in treatment centers are used and needed by many people and cannot be monopolized by telephone training. An alternative is to use disconnected telephones to practice dialing and conversational skills. Clients may be eligible to receive cell phones for emergency use, and need instruction in their use.

Clients may also need some instruction about various aspects of the postal system. In particular, because they may receive registered or certified mail from various government agencies or from their landlord, they need to know the legal implications. In addition, they may need to purchase stamps and recognize when a letter needs extra postage. If they wish to send packages, they need to know how to wrap them, whether to insure them and for how much, and what options are available for sending them through the post office or other package delivery services. They should be able to locate mailboxes and the post office in their own neighborhoods. Finally, clients need to learn to refuse unsolicited packages and to recognize and avoid solicitations and rip-offs in the mail and over the phone.

At another extreme, some clients have access to e-mail and are highly proficient in using a computer. Some of these individuals need assistance in recognizing and ignoring unsolicited e-mail, in practicing good body posture and ergonomics, and in limiting use of the Internet so as to leave time and energy for other activities, such as face-to-face communication.

## Mobility and Transportation

Being able to get around in one's local community considerably enhances the range of resources and experiences available. Without specific training, some clients may be reluctant to venture beyond a one- or two-block radius of their homes. Depending on the geographical area in which the person lives and the extent of the person's disability, transportation skills (also called *functional mobility* and *community mobility skills*) may focus on either public or private transportation or a combination of the two. Many clients can drive a car but benefit from practice in reading maps and planning routes. Others who are unable to drive or who do not have a car available must use the public bus or transit system or a private car service or taxi. Subskills that may be important are knowing where the bus stop or train station is, how to obtain and read the bus schedule, the correct fare and how to use bus transfers, and how long one must allow to reach the bus stop from one's home or the treatment center. Those with severe cognitive disabilities or memory impairment will need repeated supervised practice to learn how to get from their homes to some other location (e.g., the treatment center) and back. This should be considered situation-specific training; in other words, the person learns only this one destination and route. Those who cannot master this will have to use a private car service or rely on rides from others.

Getting around on foot also merits attention. Some people with long-standing disabilities have no idea of what is available in their immediate neighborhoods; activities that can be used to develop awareness of the immediate environment include walking around and reading or making maps. It is especially important to include safety when walking at night. In rural and suburban areas where there are no sidewalks, this means wearing light-colored clothing and walking facing the traffic; in the city, it means being street smart and wary of unlit areas and possibly dangerous people.

## Money Management

Knowing how to use money to make purchases and provide for one's basic needs is absolutely essential if a person is to function independently in the community for any length of time. Yet it is not unusual for someone with a chronic mental disorder to run out of money long before the next disability check is due to arrive. Without money, the person may become desperate, perhaps so anxious as to become psychotic and need to be rehospitalized. Or the person may resort to panhandling and become a public nuisance.

People with psychiatric disorders, especially those with cognitive disabilities, have many kinds of problems dealing with money. They may lend it or give it away or be swindled out of it in con games. They may have no concept of budgeting money and no awareness that overspending today will mean going without tomorrow. They may make impulsive or extravagant purchases, take taxis instead of public transportation, eat in restaurants too frequently, or gamble their money away. Some people may demonstrate accurate arithmetic and computational skills and be able to give correct answers on a written evaluation but fail to make or recognize the correct change in a store.

Kaseman (14) reports that it may take as long as 3 to 6 months of supervised practice for these clients to learn to budget their money to meet their needs. Individuals with memory impairments or severe cognitive disabilities may never be able to handle their money independently and will have to rely on family members or court-appointed custodians. Earhart (5) provides a highly structured guide to money management skills using Allen's cognitive levels. For clients below level 4 all financial planning must be done by a caregiver.

Kaseman (14) developed a program for training psychiatric outpatients to manage their money. The first step is assessment of the person's cognitive and money management skills. The program consists of a 12-week course of modular instruction (Table 18-1). Additional money management activities can be found in Korb and associates (16).

Some of the issues that have to be addressed in a money management training program are awareness of how much money is available, the priorities for spending it, and how it is being spent.[1] Once these basic facts are established, clients may need help to develop a budget and stick to it; those with schizophrenic and organic

[1] Exercises designed to develop awareness of spending habits and budget priorities can be found in Hughes and Mullins (12).

**TABLE 18-1 LESSON PLAN FOR 12 SESSIONS: MONEY MANAGEMENT**

| SESSION | CONTENT |
|---|---|
| 1 | Give general information and introduction to course<br>Have client fill out assessment of money management form |
| 2 | Have client fill out asset information sheet; discuss assets and liabilities<br>Ask each client, What do you wish to learn in this class? (answers and their ability to learn will set pace of course)<br>Homework for week should be to keep an account of expenditures; give each client a weekly budget record sheet |
| 3 | Discuss budgeting; examine present use of funds, possible changes in expenditures that will better meet needs of each client<br>Homework: Continue budget-keeping records but use revised record; visit a bank and bring to class literature from bank |
| 4 | Discuss banking; share literature brought in |
| 5 | Practice using banking forms |
| 6 | Discuss and practice balancing checkbook<br>Review banking procedures |
| 7 | Review balancing checkbook<br>Homework: Each client brings to class a list of two things he or she would like to do if he or she had enough funds |
| 8 | Discuss savings plans and items clients included on lists they brought to class |
| 9 | Review budget to include some kind of savings plan<br>Homework: Draw up a new budget plan |
| 10 | Discuss and examine new budget plan |
| 11 | Discuss methods of keeping to a budget<br>Provide encouragement<br>Review budgets and banking |
| 12 | Again have clients fill out assessment of money management form question and answer period |

Reprinted with permission from Kaseman BM. Teaching money management skills to psychiatric outpatients. Occup Ther Ment Health 1980;1(3):66. Permission of The Haworth Press.

disorders may not be able to adhere to a budget because they become distracted or forget. Keeping a daily record of expenditures can help some clients become more aware of the need to conserve their funds. There are many levels at which budgeting can be taught. Persons with severe disabilities may need to keep daily records, as discussed earlier; those with good cognitive skills may benefit more from monthly or yearly or long-range planning. Paper and pencil exercises are more concrete and, therefore, more effective for actual budgeting than are group discussions.

Although some persons with mental disorders may say that they would rather not keep their money in a bank, they should be encouraged to do so because it is much safer. Savings accounts have fewer procedures and do not generate transaction fees, so they require less scrupulous bookkeeping than checking accounts and are thus easier to learn. Also, with savings accounts there is no danger of getting in trouble by bouncing checks. Clients will need instruction in how to fill out various deposit, withdrawal, and application forms; banks are usually quite willing to provide blank forms for practice. It helps to role-play situations in which a client might interact with bank personnel, for instance to open an account or withdraw money. Obviously, trips to the bank and supervised practice in a real situation should be included.[2] With electronic transfers of benefit checks becoming more common, the OTA may devise activities to help clients learn about this and become more comfortable with the notion that their money will be there even if they cannot physically hold the check in their hands.

Another aspect of money management is concerned with the ability to judge where and how to spend money; this includes knowledge of comparison shopping and consumer rights and understanding the pros and cons of using credit cards. Information about how and where to shop for bargains and where and how to complain about a defective product should be covered. Group discussions of how to handle difficult situations involving money can help clients focus on why they sometimes have trouble sticking to their budgets. Some of the situations[3] that might be considered are these:

- You receive a circular in the mail that says you have been selected to receive a check for $500 if you purchase a particular sewing machine by mail.
- You have been invited to a dinner dance and have nothing to wear. You are considering buying a dress and shoes, but the ones you have chosen would use up all your spending money for 2 months.
- Your child is constantly begging you for a new bicycle. The old one was stolen.
- A missionary comes to your door asking for a contribution for children starving in Africa. He shows you pictures that make you want to cry.
- You have always had trouble losing weight and are considering investing in a reduction plan advertised in the newspaper. It costs only $39.98 and promises a 10-pound weight loss in a week.

Depending on an individual's judgment and experience, situations like these can present real dilemmas and temptations. Willson (25) emphasizes that we cannot realistically expect to prepare clients for every situation they may encounter but that we can help them develop general skills in identifying the real issues, generating alternatives, and selecting realistic solutions.

## Home Management

Taking care of a home and family is as demanding as most paid employment. In fact, the job of homemaker and caregiver is *more* difficult than many jobs, because the person has to structure and organize the entire process; there is no one to tell the homemaker or caregiver what to do and when. There are so many subtasks within the job and so many possibilities about how to do them that the homemaker or caregiver can easily become overwhelmed or discouraged. Programs that help clients learn, practice, and maintain

[2] Additional banking and budgeting exercises for patients at all levels can be found in Kartin and Van Schroeder (13).

[3] Additional discussion topics can be found in Hughes and Mullins (12).

their homemaking and child care skills are usually vocationally oriented, meaning that they view the job of homemaker as a work role.

Activities covered in a home management training sequence include making and changing beds, emptying of ashtrays and trash, airing of rooms and linens, use of a broom and mop and dust rag and other household cleaning tools, storing dangerous products out of reach of children, and procedures such as how to change a light bulb and how to turn off the water if there is a leak. Clients with cognitive impairments may have to be reminded to clean areas that are out of sight, for example under the toilet and the bed. Not everyone owns a vacuum cleaner, so its use should be taught judiciously. Other topics that should be covered in housekeeping are knowing when to repair something yourself and when and where to get help from the superintendent, plumber, or handyman.

Clients also need to learn which cleaning products, paper products, and other house-keeping products provide the best value for the money. Many popular references are available (see Suggested Readings at the end of the chapter). Such books may be kept in the clinic for clients to consult. Alternatively, the OTA may use these references to develop materials for presenting psychoeducational programs in home management. Finally, videotapes on specific home management or home repair tasks may be borrowed from the public library.

In teaching or reinforcing homemaking skills, the OTA must respect the culture and values of the client. Cuisine, home furnishings, habits, and routines vary enormously from culture to culture. Recent immigrants from Third World countries may wish to continue to keep house in the manner to which they are accustomed. This should be accepted as long as the particular practices do not violate social norms in a manner that would infringe on the rights of neighbors. Alternatively, immigrants from rural or poor areas may fail to understand the purpose of technological aids and, for example (in a true case), attempt unsuccessfully to use a dishwasher to do laundry.

Detailed objectives and goals for home management can be found in Hemphill and associates (11). Barrows (2) gives suggestions for home adaptations for persons with severe mental or cognitive disorders who may also have a sensory or physical disability. The compensations suggested by Barrows, such as using a dark-colored hamper for dark clothing and a light-colored hamper for light clothing, are simple and logical. By observing and listening to clients, the OTA can learn of their particular obstacles, the first step toward finding effective and inexpensive solutions.

## Meal Preparation and Cleanup

A *meal preparation* training program may have an educational or classroom format. Kitchen safety, food storage and handling, nutrition concepts, and meal planning are the first skills taught. Basic cooking skills and use of convenience foods are taught next. Proper mealtime manners and how to set a table and clean up afterward are practiced within the context of actually consuming a meal. Grocery shopping and cost comparison skills and the use of measures (cups, spoons) and weights are often also included. Clients are taught to use a dishwasher and other kitchen appliances (e.g., microwave, food processor) only if they will actually have these appliances at home. Obviously, it makes sense to teach these skills in the appropriate environments (kitchen, dining area, grocery store). Electrical appliances, knives, and other sharp implements should be used only under close supervision.

Cleanup after meals should include instruction about washing, drying, and putting away for storage all of the implements used and safe storage of food leftovers. Hand washing and either air drying or towel drying; use of a dishwasher, if the client will have one in the home; and special techniques for washing glassware, flatware, sharp implements, and pots and pans should be covered. The client should be given the opportunity to practice under supervision. Wiping of counters and surfaces, sweeping and mopping should be included. As with other ADLs, repeated practice with gradual variations will promote the development of effective habits and routines.

Clients with cognitive disabilities will need environmental compensations and, in some cases, the ongoing supervision of another person to make sure that spoiled food is discarded, that food is stored safely, and so on. Forgetting to turn off the stove or walking away and losing track of cooking time are common problems and require safe and permanent solutions. Clients who cannot remember or who do not routinely use safe procedures will need in-home supervision; alternately, the knobs can be removed from the stove.

## Shopping

Shopping presents unique challenges to people with mental disorders. For some, it creates a temptation to buy impulsively and beyond one's means. For others, it overwhelms with information and sensation to the point of being intolerable. Clients with cognitive or sensory issues generally find big-box stores and crowded hours very difficult. Hamera and Brown (8) are in the process of developing a test of grocery shopping skills. They address the problem of the overwhelming environment of the supermarket or grocery store and the difficulties involved in remembering and locating items.

Clients need to learn (and they need support to practice) many aspects of shopping. A short list of subtasks includes working within a budget, listing what you intend to buy, choosing a store than you can tolerate, shopping at a time when the store is less crowded, asking for assistance, reading and following signage, finding what you want, making choices among competing items, paying for items with cash or debit card, and keeping receipts in case of returns.

## Care of Others

Hiring and supervision of caregivers is included in this category. Caregiving and work with caregivers has been covered in Chapter 9. The situation in which a person with a mental disorder is also charged with the caregiving for another person requires special mention. A family member with the psychiatric diagnosis may have more time than others in the family to care for an elderly or disabled relative. If the person also has the interest and the skills, this can be a rewarding role. But it is a stressful role. Consequently, ample social support, respite services, and skills training should be available.

## Care of Pets

Pets and companion animals serve many needs, including comfort and physical touch. Consumers need to know how to perform all routine care for their pet, how to recognize when special care is needed, and where to obtain care. Consumers who have allergies should receive guidance in avoiding the choice of a pet that will aggravate this condition.

## Child Rearing

Supporting the developmental, physical and emotional needs of children may be a challenge for the parent who has a mental disorder. Parents need to know about children's basic needs and how to provide for them. Some parents have had inadequate parenting themselves, having suffered from neglect, violence, or poverty, and need time and support to learn new ways to behave. These parents may say, in effect, "*My* parents did okay by me, and they loved me, so I'm going to do things the way *they* did." Such parents may not recognize that their abusive behavior and failure to provide appropriate nurturing may result in developmental deficits in their children (13).

Others need to learn to talk to their children, how to praise and nurture them, how to discipline them effectively, or how to help them structure their time. They may be unaware of community resources, from which they can receive guidance and ongoing support. Still others may have trouble thinking of things they can do with their children. These skills may be taught through group discussion, paper and pencil exercises, review of videotaped situations, role playing, and actual practice with children. Again, suggested readings on these topics are provided at the end of this chapter.

Some parents with severe psychiatric disabilities have trouble keeping their children properly cleaned, clothed, and fed; these clients need supervision on a daily basis. With enough practice and reinforcement, they may learn enough to function more independently. A social worker usually works closely with the occupational therapist or assistant in such cases, because of the real possibility that the child may be harmed by the parent's neglect.

A more common problem, shared by parents from all social classes and all levels of disability, is how to communicate with children. Parents need to know what children of a given age are capable of understanding, what they are likely to be interested in, and what their emotional needs are. Discussion groups, augmented by printed reminders with developmental issues listed for each age, are often used. This is also a good way to help parents identify appropriate toys for their children and to help them think of activities they and their children might do together.

Another problem many parents share is their concern over children's behavior and appropriate discipline. Discussion with other parents is extremely valuable in helping parents develop a sense of what constitutes a reasonable punishment for a particular misdeed committed by a child of a given age. This is especially important for parents with delinquent adolescent children, many of whom feel frustrated, overwhelmed, and helpless in dealing with their child's behavior.

Unfortunately, relatively few lesson plans and activities for developing child care skills have been described in the OT literature. Those that do exist (12, 15, 16, 18) provide only a few exercises focusing on limited areas of need. Therefore, the occupational therapy practitioner must create materials and activities from the available developmental literature and other sources. The OTA should work under the supervision of, or at the very least in consultation with, a registered occupational therapist with pediatric training and experience.

In working with parents, OTAs will be more successful when they appreciate that parenting values and attitudes vary and that the parent and the OTA may hold different views. Furthermore, practitioners who are themselves parents will be viewed as more credible than those who are not.

## PRACTICE, REPETITION, AND HABIT DEVELOPMENT

Effective performance of the occupations discussed within this chapter requires habit and routine. Habit develops with repeated performance, so that the actions are fixed in memory. We have stressed the importance of providing multiple opportunities to practice and refine skills. When the basic skills are established, variations in conditions will promote mental flexibility and the ability to solve problems. Again, many practice opportunities will ensure better mastery. Always, skills should be practiced and refined in the contexts in which they will be used. The OTA must not rely on paper and pencil activities, or on clinic-based simulations. Actual practice, over and over again, in the client's environment, is essential.

## SUMMARY

This chapter presents activities in the broad categories of personal activities of daily living and instrumental activities of daily living. Many of the topics discussed here overlap with work activities, leisure activities, and activities of social interaction. Each activity has benefits and potentials besides the obvious ones. Exercise, for example, is not only a health maintenance activity but can be a leisure or socialization activity or a rehabilitative activity structured to develop sensory processing skills or even social skills. A simple daily living activity such as sweeping the floor can be structured to promote postural balance or to develop concentration and attention span (or to provide exercise). Thus it is not so much the activity itself that is the therapy but its skillful application by the occupational therapy practitioner. This will be explored further in Chapters 19 through 23.

## REVIEW QUESTIONS AND ACTIVITIES

1. What are three categories of learning? Give an example of each.
2. Discuss the effect of roles and values learned from one's parents on one's occupational functioning.
3. In what way does the ability to ask for and receive help affect the ability to function in daily life occupations?
4. Contrast activities of daily living with instrumental activities of daily living. List activities within the two groups.
5. Describe the personal care problems that are common in persons with severe mental disorders.
6. Discuss the effect of social support on the personal care of someone with mental illness.
7. Describe the environment in which personal care skills are most effectively practiced.
8. Identify some possible reasons for a person with a psychiatric disorder presenting a poor personal appearance.
9. List some activities that could be included in a program to teach clothing selection and maintenance. Place these skills in the order in which you would teach them.
10. List some activities and topics that might be included in a program to teach nutrition.
11. Define *body image.*
12. Discuss the relationship between body image and weight control.
13. List some reasons why a person might not take his or her prescribed psychiatric medication. Explain how the OTA might respond.
14. What is *relapse prevention*? What kinds of topics should be included?
15. List the benefits of exercise. List four approaches to helping clients meet their needs for exercise.
16. How might you teach a client to use the telephone skillfully?
17. List some activities that might be part of a community mobility training program.
18. Analyze the factors that might contribute to poor money management.
19. Identify topics that should be included in a money management program.
20. Explain why group discussions about difficult problems in money management are recommended.
21. List some of the skills and activities that should be included in a program about meal preparation and cleanup.
22. State some topics and activities to help clients acquire shopping skills.
23. What kinds of activities might be included in a child care and parenting skills program?
24. Why is repeated practice recommended in training clients in daily living skills?

## REFERENCES


1. American Occupational Therapy Association. Occupational therapy practice framework: Domain and process. Am J Occup Ther 2002;56:609–639.
2. Barrows C. Home adaptations—Creating safe environments for individuals with psychiatric disabilities. OT Practice 2006;11(18):12–16.
3. Bellack AS, Mueser KT, Gingerich S, Agresta J. Social Skills Training for Schizophrenia. New York, Guilford, 1997.
4. Carey B. What's wrong with a child? Psychiatrists often disagree. New York Times, Nov 11, 2006, A1, A11.
5. Earhart CA. Analysis of activities. In Allen CK, Earhart CA, Blue T, eds. Occupational Therapy Treatment Goals for the Physically and Cognitively Disabled. Rockville, MD: American Occupational Therapy Association, 1992.
6. Frese FJ. Occupational therapy and mental illness: A personal view. Am Occup Ther Assoc Ment Health Special Sect Q Newslett 1998;21(3):1–3.
7. Giles GM. Anorexia nervosa and bulimia: An activity-oriented approach. Am J Occup Ther 1985;39:510–517.
8. Hamera E, Brown CE. Developing a context-based performance measure for persons with schizophrenia: The test of grocery shopping skills. Am J Occup Ther 2000;54:20–25.
9. Hasselkus BR, Murray BJ. Everyday occupation, well-being, and identity: The experience of caregivers in families with dementia. Am J Occup Ther 2007;61:9–20.
10. Hayes R. Occupational therapy in the treatment of schizophrenia. Occup Ther Ment Health 1989;9(3):51–68.
11. Hemphill BJ, Peterson CQ, Werner PC. Rehabilitation in Mental Health: Goals and Objectives for Independent Living. Thorofare, NJ: Slack, 1991.
12. Hughes PL, Mullins L. Acute Psychiatric Care: An Occupational Therapy Guide to Exercises in Daily Living Skills. Thorofare, NJ: Slack, 1981.
13. Kartin NJ, Van Schroeder C. Adult Psychiatric Life Skills Manual. Kailua, HI: Schroeder Publishing, 1982.
14. Kaseman BM. Teaching money management skills to psychiatric outpatients. Occup Ther Ment Health 1980;1(3):59–71.
15. Korb KL, Azok AD, Leutenberg EA. Life Management Skills: Reproducible Activity Handouts Created for Facilitators. Beachwood, OH: Wellness Reproductions, 1989.
16. Korb KL, Azok AD, Leutenberg EA. Life Management Skills: 2. Reproducible Activity Handouts Created for Facilitators. Beachwood, OH: Wellness Reproductions, 1991.
17. Korb KL, Azok AD, Leutenberg EA. Life Management Skills: 3. Reproducible Activity Handouts Created for Facilitators. Beachwood, OH: Wellness Reproductions, 1993.
18. Korb KL, Leutenberg EA. Life Management Skills: 4. Reproducible Activity Handouts Created for Facilitators. Beachwood, OH: Wellness Reproductions, 1997.
19. Linehan MM. Skills Training Manual for Treating Borderline Personality Disorder. New York: Guilford, 1993.
20. Neville-Jan A, Bradley M, Bunn C, Gehri B. The model of human occupation and individuals with co-dependency problems. Occup Ther Ment Health 1991;11(2–3): 73–98.
21 Precin P. Living Skills Recovery Workbook. Boston: Butterworth Heinemann, 1999.
22. Rogers JC, Salta JE. Case report: Documenting functional outcomes. Am J Occup Ther 1994;48:939–945.
23. Schwartzberg SL. Motivation for activities of daily living: A study of selected psychiatric patients' self-reports. Occup Ther Ment Health 1982;2(3):1–26.
24. Wells SJ. Caffeine: Implications of recent research for clinical practice. Am J Orthopsychiatry 1984;54:375–389.
25. Willson M. Occupational Therapy in Long-Term Psychiatry. Edinburgh, UK: Churchill Livingstone, 1983.


## SUGGESTED READINGS

### General


Allen CK, Earhart CA, Blue T. Occupational Therapy Treatment goals for the Physically and Cognitively Disabled. Rockville, MD: American Occupation Therapy Association, 1992.

Barrows C. Home adaptations—Creating safe environments for individuals with psychiatric disabilities. OT Practice 2006;11(18):12–16.

Earhart CA. Occupational therapy groups. In: Allen CA, ed. Occupational Therapy for Psychiatric Diseases: Measurement and Management of Cognitive Disabilities. Boston: Little, Brown, 1985.

Hasselkus BR. The meaning of daily activity in family caregiving for the elderly. Am J Occup Ther 1989;43:649–656.

Hemphill BJ, Peterson CQ, Werner PC. Rehabilitation in Mental Health: Goals and Objectives for Independent Living. Thorofare, NJ: Slack, 1991.

Henry AD. The needs of parents with mental illness and their families. OT Practice 2005;10(20):8–12.

Kasl CD. Women, Sex, and Addiction. New York: Harper Perennial, 1990.

Knis-Matthews L. A parenting program for women who are substance dependent. Am Occup Ther Assoc Ment Health Special Sect Q Newslett 2003;26(1):1–4.

Maslen DM. Rehabilitation training for community living skills: Concepts and techniques. Occup Ther Ment Health 1982;2(1):33–49.

Weissenberg R, Giladi N. Home economics day: A program for disturbed adolescents to promote acquisition of habits and skills. Occup Ther Ment Health 1989;9(2):89–103.

## Home Management, Meal Preparation, Shopping

Graham AL, Wolfe NC. Identifying person-context factors in meal planning for persons with severe and persistent mental illness. Am Occup Ther Assoc Ment Health Special Sect Q Newslett 2000;23(3):1–4.

Hamera E. Grocery shopping habits of persons with schizophrenia. Am Occup Ther Assoc Ment Health Special Sect Q Newslett 2000;23(4):1–4.

Household Hints and Handy Tips. Pleasantville, NY: Reader's Digest, 1997.

Pinkham ME. Mary Ellen's Complete Home Reference Book. New York: Crown, 1994.

Primeau LA. A woman's place: Unpaid work in the home. Am J Occup Ther 1992;46:981–988.

Rogers L. Book of Forms for Everyday Living. 3rd ed. Lincolnwood, IL: National Textbook, 1997.

## Parenting

Bettleheim B. A Good Enough Parent. New York: Vintage, 1987.

Crary E. Pick Up Your Socks . . . And Other Skills Growing Children Need. Seattle: Parenting, 1990.

Crary E. Without Spanking or Spoiling: A Practical Approach to Toddler and Preschool Guidance. 2nd ed. Seattle: Parenting, 1993.

Faber A, Mazlish E. How to Talk so Kids Will Listen and Listen so Kids Will Talk. London: Picadilly Press, 2001.

Gordon T. P.E.T.: Parent Effectiveness Training. New York: Three Rivers Press, 2000.

Krueger CW. 1001 Things to Do with Your Kids. Galahad, 1999.

Loukas KM. Motherhood, occupational therapy, and feminism: Weaving or unraveling the fibers of our lives? [The Issue Is]. Am J Occup Ther 1992;46:1039–1041.

Nelsen J. Positive Discipline. New York: Ballantine, 2006.

Nelsen J. Positive discipline A to Z: 1001 Solutions to Everyday Parenting Problems. New York: Three Rivers Press, 2007.

CHAPTER 19

# Education and Work

***To be successfully employed, one must view oneself as employable.***

CRIST AND STOFFEL (7, P. 435)

## CHAPTER OBJECTIVES

After studying this chapter, the reader will be able to:

1. Appreciate the ability to engage effectively in education and work as a developmental process.
2. Recognize the place of habit and skill development in occupational engagement in school and work.
3. Identify the challenges faced by children, adolescents, and adults with mental disorders as they attempt to engage in the roles of student and worker.
4. Discuss context or environment as a factor in engagement in school and work.
5. Describe three approaches to supported education.
6. Understand the basic provisions, in regard to employment and education, of the Americans with Disabilities Act of 1990.
7. Recognize and differentiate a variety of work-related programs.
8. Describe supported employment, and explain why it is considered best practice.
9. Discuss the value of worker cooperatives and volunteer work as alternatives to competitive employment.
10. Describe appropriate roles for occupational therapy practitioners in assisting clients to succeed in education and work and in the transition to retirement.

This chapter gives an overview of occupational therapy (OT) programming related to education and work for persons with mental disorders. Overlap between the scope of occupational therapy services and those of other education and mental health disciplines is significant. In educational settings, the special educator, the vocational counselor, and the other therapy services may take lead roles. With work and job performance, the disciplines of vocational counseling, drug and alcohol counseling, psychotherapy, social work, and psychiatric rehabilitation will be involved. The challenge of delineating an appropriate focus for the occupational therapy practitioner will be addressed. Typically, the occupational therapy assistant (OTA) provides services under the supervision and guidance of the occupational therapist (OT) and should expect to receive specific direction.

## EDUCATION

The American Occupational Therapy Association (AOTA) in the *Occupational Therapy Practice Framework: Domain and Process (OTPF)* defines the occupational performance area of *education* as "activities needed for being a student and participating in a learning environment" (2). The occupations nested within the category of education are shown in Box 19-1. Before considering how the OTA may contribute to programs to develop or maintain the client's ability to participate in educational activities, we will take a broader look at how children and adolescents acquire the skills that support their participation in education and work. This information was introduced in Chapters 5 and 9.

### Acquiring Skills for Success in School and Work

As was discussed in Chapter 5, skills and habits learned during childhood and adolescence lay a foundation for the roles of student and worker. Consequently, occupational therapy programs for young people with mental health problems generally include activities that provide opportunities to learn and practice these skills. Young children and grade school students can acquire work habits by carrying out household chores and school assignments. In a hospital setting, it is sometimes difficult to create opportunities for every child to perform a task that contributes to the family or the community, but requiring children to clean up after themselves, to put away toys and games and

**BOX 19-1**

**EDUCATION**

- **Formal educational participation** in academic, nonacademic, extracurricular, and vocational programs
- **Educational exploration (personal, interest related),** such as investigation and selection of ways to learn about skills and topics of interest
- **Informal personal education participation** in classes and programs that provide growth or training in areas of interest

Modified with permission from American Occupational Therapy Association. Occupational therapy practice framework: Domain and process. Am J Occup Ther 2002;56:609–639.

materials, and to wipe the tables and sweep the floor after an activity is a start. Children also need opportunities to fantasize about adult roles. These can be provided through unstructured costume play and child-initiated games that involve imitation of adult worker roles. Films, field trips, and visits by adults in different occupations also increase children's awareness of the role of the adult worker.

Adolescents are faced with important decisions about future occupational roles. To choose a career that suits one's interests and abilities, adolescents need to identify and appreciate what these are; this knowledge can be developed through participation in a wide range of activities. It is very important to allow adolescents to explore areas that interest them and to expose them to other activities of which they may not be aware because they will choose their careers on the basis of what they know.

## Students with Mental, Emotional, and Cognitive Disorders

Occupational therapy service supporting the role of student for children, adolescents, and adults with mental health problems is an area for potential growth, but few therapy practitioners actually work within school settings with the emotionally disturbed population (5, 17). What kinds of services are needed? What are the problems these young students face?

Primary and secondary school students (kindergarten through grade 12) should be developing and establishing skills and habits that will support them in college and in the work world. Yet, habit and skill development typically lags behind in young people who have mental and emotional disorders. Staff reports about students enrolled in alternative educational environments showed that the students had multiple problems that interfered with engagement in the role of the student and participation in the school setting (9). The problems included the following (9):

- Deficits in executive cognitive functioning (planning, organization, decision making)
- Difficulties with multitasking and following multistep directions
- Unhealthy habits and lifestyle practices, such as poor nutrition and lack of involvement in fitness or hobbies
- Problems with attention span, memory, and coping
- Inadequate or ineffective nonverbal behaviors and communication generally

A common complaint about students with emotional disorders (EDs) is their "bad" behavior, which disrupts the educational process and makes the teacher's job difficult. Untangling the causes of the misbehavior is an important first step. Some students have sensory processing factors that make it hard for them to concentrate. Many students have strong feelings that they have no words for and that they can't control. Few special education students have much experience of successful self-determination; they have been controlled by others, restricted from certain activities, and so on. The first step in helping the struggling student is to identify which of these many possibilities is the cause of the difficulties.

For the postsecondary student (college level and beyond) the challenges may be different, especially if the person was normally developing until a first episode of a serious mental disorder in his or her late teens or early 20s. Schizophrenia and bipolar disorder typically first manifest in late adolescence. The young person with one of these conditions may be intellectually ready for college, may have a good academic record from high school, and may have established student habits and a strong motivation. However, the ups and downs of mental illness interfere with management of the student role. The student may experience exacerbations with psychotic features, such as hallucinations or preoccupations, that make concentration difficult. Stress may provoke a relapse or an increase in symptoms. The side effects of medications such as sleepiness or motor restlessness will affect the student's ability to be present (both physically and mentally) in the classroom when required. Cognitive processing may be slowed by the illness or by the medications, making it hard for the student to follow lectures or to complete examinations in the typically allotted time.

## Supporting and Developing Readiness for the Student Role

We will consider first the problems of primary and secondary school students, whose need is for skill development and acquisition of habits that support the student role. Occupational therapy task groups (discussed later in the chapter) can reinforce basic task skills and study habits. For example, a middle school student whose attention span is less than 10 minutes cannot succeed in a regular school program; by participating in a basic task skills group, he or she can work on concentrating for longer periods while enjoying an activity that is less stressful than school. At the same time, if hospitalized, he or she would attend classes taught by special education teachers in the hospital; if an outpatient, he or she might attend a regular public school but be in a special class, go to a resource room for extra help during certain class periods each day, or have a reduced schedule.

In the elementary or secondary school, the student will have an individualized education program (IEP), a plan with specific goals developed jointly by the special educator, medical and therapy personnel, and the family. The IEP is required under the Individuals with Disabilities Education Improvement Act of 2004 (IDEA) (40), which covers children aged 3 through 21 who have disabilities. The IEP will identify educational objectives. Psychosocial or emotional needs may not be addressed clearly but are intended to be covered under the law. This is an area in which occupational therapy practitioners can provide needed services.

In the United States, the current practice is to *mainstream* (place in regular classrooms) students with special needs. Two models used in mainstreaming are *pull-out,* in which the student leaves the class to go to the resource room, and *push-in,* in which the resource room teacher or other specialist goes to the classroom to meet with the student. Using the push-in model allows the OT practitioner to observe and suggest interventions for the classroom environment, a place in which peer and authority interactions occur repeatedly and naturally. Because social skills are a frequent concern for students with psychiatric disorders, it makes sense to work on these skills in their natural environment.

Effective occupational therapy services should support the student in the student role and at the same time help the teacher manage the ED student in the classroom (6). For students who behave in a way that disrupts the classroom, the functional behavioral analysis (FBA) approach may be used. The OT analyses the behavior, the events leading up to it, and the consequences that follow, attempting to answer the question: What function is this behavior serving for the student? Next, the OT and the teacher identify other ways to meet the student's needs, using an approach called positive behavioral support (PBS) (6).

Specific recommendations for adjusting the classroom environment to meet the needs of students who have behavioral issues can be found in Haack and Haldy (16). Outside the classroom, the OT practitioner may provide individual help by structuring an environment in which the student can do homework and sometimes by teaching study, note-taking, and test-taking skills. This may include work with the parents to improve understanding of the environmental compensations that best support the student's completion of homework (34, 35). Box 19-2 lists some strategies to help children diagnosed with attention deficit-hyperactivity disorder (ADHD) succeed with homework; many of these strategies are appropriate, with minor adjustments, for children with EDs (35), and may also be helpful to older students.

**BOX 19-2**

**STRUCTURES FOR HOMEWORK SUCCESS**

- *Match environment to student.* Student may need to eliminate all distractions; parents can provide quiet area, visual shields, sound-proof headphones; alternately, student may require specific auditory experience such as music in order to focus.
- *Break homework tasks into manageable units.* Plan ahead; divide long assignments into sections or into tasks to be done in sequence with a time frame; work in smaller units of time but increase time as student is able.
- *Get help with nonessential tasks.* For students with poor handwriting or poor keyboarding, consider having someone else type the work (that person should take care *not* to correct the student's work)
- *Provide a model.* When the student can't figure out how to do a problem, the parent or tutor can show this once, or even twice; then the student must be helped to do the task by himself or herself
- *Supervise and refocus.* Parents must learn to redirect student to the task, which may require repeating instructions several times.
- *Use meaningful and relevant consequences.* The naturally occurring negative consequence is failing in school; because this consequence is long term and harmful to the student, more immediate and less punitive consequences should be chosen (e.g., not being able to do or have something that is desired, such as watching a favorite TV show, unless the homework is completed; a positive consequence is being able to do what one wants because the homework is done); consequences should be adjusted to the attention span and impulse control of the child.

Data from Segal R, Hinojosa J, Addonizio C, et al. Homework strategies for children with attention deficit hyperactivity disorder. OT Practice 2005;10(17):9–12.

Supporting students in the student role requires individual programming and careful attention to the child's or adolescent's capacities, needs, and goals. Segal et al. (35) give the following example, involving the use of meaningful consequences (Box 19-2). For an older student who has the concept of time and who can appreciate the value of finishing 20 algebra problems before watching TV, the promise of being able to watch a show makes sense. For a younger child, the promise of being able to play with a toy may seem too far away. To make this more real, the parent can place the toy on top of the refrigerator as a reminder of the promised reward (35).

Students who have difficulties with sensory regulation require interventions that address these problems. In other words, they must learn how to identify what they are experiencing, how it is affecting them, and how to change the way they respond. The Alert Program for Self-Regulation (also called How Does Your Engine Run?) helps students learn about their level of arousal and alertness and change it using sensory strategies (44).

## Communication Skills for Educational Success

Some children and adolescents labeled as having an ED do fairly well at academic tasks and get good grades. But they experience great difficulty getting along with their peers and communicating with adults. Students with Asperger's syndrome and related autism-spectrum disorders typically misread social cues and do not understand nonverbal language or social customs. These individuals require intensive instruction and remediation to learn and practice effective communication. Students who have problems with impulse control will get into trouble when they ignore boundaries and rules. A variety of approaches have been used and recommended for helping students with these and other social and communication problems.

Salls and Bucey (31) reported on the Lifelong Communication Skills Lab designed for middle school students. This psychoeducation program taught in a regular class period focused on topics such as observing, listening, reading body language, and other communication related skills. Again, the needs of the individual student should guide what is taught and how it is demonstrated and practiced.

Schultz (33) points out that students labeled as having an ED or emotional behavioral disorder (EBD) may receive negative messages from the school environment—for example, that the student will cause trouble, will not succeed, will break rules, or will be unreliable. The student's work is not hung on display; he or she is barred from certain activities; classmates grimace and sigh and teachers frown when the student enters the room. The student may develop a repertoire of behaviors that contribute to a vicious circle of mutual negativity. When encountering a difficulty or entering a new situation, the student might get angry or create a disruption or start telling jokes and acting silly. To help the student succeed in the student role requires, Schultz believes, a change in the environment. By providing students with tasks in which they can be successful, by responding realistically and constructively, and by helping students explore the consequences of their actions, the therapist can provide the conditions in which change is possible. This is a slow process involving a great deal of patience.

## Supported Education

For the college level student, practitioners should be aware that the Americans with Disabilities Act of 1990 (ADA), discussed later in this chapter, applies to educational settings as well as to work and community. Students younger than 22 years of age are covered under the IDEA of 2004. Three types of approaches to assist the young adult to succeed as a student have been attempted under the general rubric of supported education (SEd). The first type is the *self-contained classroom* (38). Gutman and colleagues (14, 15) provided such a program, with occupational therapy students serving as instructors and mentors. The program consisted of a 12-week curriculum, 3 hours per day, with a psychoeducational orientation to prepare the participants to assume the role of college student. Modules of instruction included time management, stress management, study skills, reading skills, use of the Internet, computer skills, library skills, communication and public speaking, writing skills, and college exploration. The self-contained classroom is an appropriate model for people who are not yet in school, and who need to acquire skills, habits and confidence before entering the college environment.

The second type of supported education program is the *on-site support model* (38). In this model, professionals on the college campus help the student use services already available at the college and help the student interface with faculty and administration to obtain necessary supports. For example, under the ADA, the college student with a psychiatric disability may approach a professor to request reasonable accommodations. The student should be prepared to provide medical documentation. In the on-site support model, an office for students with disabilities provides an interface between the student and the professors by documenting the disability and providing support services. Examples of reasonable accommodations for a college student with mental health problems include the following:

- A quiet environment in which to take examinations
- Extra time on examinations
- Extended time to complete assignments

The third type of approach, the *mobile support model,* is associated with the clubhouse model described in Chapter 7. Here, peer counselors provide support on and off campus, tailored to the needs of the individual student.

## WORK

Work is a major life role for the average nondisabled adult; it consumes at least half of most people's waking hours and provides a sense of self-worth, identity, and a place in the social structure. By using time in ways that are valuable to others, workers affirm their contributions to the world and their place within it. Spencer and associates (36) determined that work provides benefits to self and to others. Benefits may be short term (e.g., enjoyment, income) or long-term (identity, social contribution). These benefits are shown in Table 19-1. People who are unable to work for whatever reason are, therefore, deprived of a major life role and potential source of personal satisfaction and social identity. AOTA identifies services to facilitate work performance in its official documents (3). For persons with cognitive disabilities and mental disorders, the services may include supported employment strategies, discussed later in the chapter. The categories of occupation classified in the area of work are presented in Box 19-3.

Many individuals with psychiatric disorders have problems with work. Those who have been ill for a long time may have little or no experience of working and thus no real understanding of the behaviors expected in a work setting. Nonetheless, even among the chronically mentally ill, the desire to work and to have an identity as a worker is quite strong. Others may have cognitive disabilities that prevent their making sense of a typical work environment or of tasks that require even minimal decision making. Still others (this is true particularly of those with personality disorders) fail over and over again because they act without thinking, relate hostilely or negatively to others, fail to organize their tasks, or do not take responsibility for their own behavior.

Work evaluation and interventions in occupational therapy are designed to assess the client's work potential, assist the client in developing basic task skills and work behaviors, and help the client make the transition to a productive worker role or to further training for a vocation. Such programs target the needs of clients who have a history of failure at work or no work history at all or who need a different kind of work that is more suited to their interests and functional level.

**TABLE 19-1 POTENTIAL ADAPTIVE BENEFITS OF ENGAGEMENT IN WORK**

| SOURCE OF BENEFIT | SHORT-TERM BENEFIT | LONG-TERM BENEFIT |
|---|---|---|
| Self | Intrinsic enjoyment for its own sake | Identity (accomplishment, independence), valued lifestyle |
| Others | Immediate extrinsic rewards (social recognition, income) | Contribution to purposes larger than oneself |

Reprinted with permission from Spencer J, Daybell PJ, Eschenfelder V, et al. Contrasting perspectives on work: An exploratory qualitative study based on the concept of adaptation. Am J Occup Ther 1998;52:474–484.

**BOX 19-3**

**WORK**

- Employment interests and pursuits
- Employment seeking and acquisition
- Job performance
- Retirement preparation and adjustment
- Volunteer exploration
- Volunteer participation

Modified with permission from American Occupational Therapy Association. Occupational therapy practice framework: Domain and process. Am J Occup Ther 2002;56:609–639.

Work-related programming typically involves other professionals and paraprofessionals. Vocational counselors, rehabilitation counselors, job coaches, work adjustment specialists, work evaluators, and job placement specialists all provide services that overlap those provided by OT. The role of OT and of the OTA will be affected by the availability of these specialized personnel, the needs of the client population, and the relevant local and federal regulations affecting the service delivery agency. As in any other professional situation, it is important to work cooperatively with other staff, offering services in a manner that is noncompetitive and in the best interests of those to be served.

## Americans with Disabilities Act of 1990

Title I of the ADA (39) protects persons with physical and mental impairments from discrimination in employment due to disability. Employers are required to provide *reasonable accommodations* to disabled employees. A reasonable accommodation is a change in the workplace environment or in the job itself that enables a person to work despite a disability that would otherwise make the job difficult or impossible. Under the law, the accommodation must be *reasonable.* The employee's needs and the requested accommodation must enable adequate functioning in the job. However, the person must be able to perform the *essential functions* of the job, given the accommodation. Furthermore, the accommodation should not result in *undue expense or hardship* to the employer. Also, there should be no *direct threat* of substantial harm to the person or to others from performing the job with the accommodations (43).

It is up to the employee to disclose the disability and make the request for accommodation. The employer typically will ask for medical documentation, which the employee must provide to claim protection under the ADA. In the case of mental health problems, clients may be reluctant to disclose a disability or to seek accommodations (32). Nonetheless, in 1997 claims related to mental disability constituted the largest category (15.3%) under the ADA (30). In addition to claims against employers for failing to provide accommodations, the number of disability-related bias cases has risen (1, 45). Co-workers and managers may resent the special provisions given the client or may stigmatize the disability.

What are some reasonable accommodations? An example of a reasonable accommodation is a ramp for a person in a wheelchair. Table 19-2 provides examples of reasonable accommodations for some of the problems associated with psychiatric disorders.

For the ADA to be effective, OTs and OTAs may be called upon to assist the individual to fit

**TABLE 19-2 EXAMPLES OF ACCOMMODATIONS THAT HAVE BEEN CONSIDERED REASONABLE**

| PROBLEM | SOLUTION(S) |
|---|---|
| Distractibility | Isolated cubicle; schedule to work off-peak hours |
| Anxiety | More frequent breaks to calm down; option to use vacation days as needed |
| Depression | Reduced work load; flexible scheduling |
| Dry mouth | Permission to sip on drink at work station |
| Limited work tolerance | Reduced workload; flexible scheduling; option to do work from home |
| Learning disability | Provision to read work out loud to self or to make audio recordings of meetings and other information; extended time to perform task; option to use color coding or other device in lieu of alphanumeric organization |

the work environment or vice versa (13). Crist and Stoffel (7) described three tasks for occupational therapy in assisting persons with mental disabilities to enter and remain in the workforce. The first is to provide *advocacy training* for clients as well as for employers and co-workers. Advocacy training promotes the acceptance of persons with disabilities, encourages alliance with the value that work is a right for all, and teaches strategies that assist the nondisabled to work effectively with persons with mental impairments. The second is to increase, through training, the mentally disabled worker's *self-efficacy,* or belief about one's own skills and competence. The third is to help employers with *job analysis,* to identify essential functions of a particular job and work out accommodations so that it can be performed by a disabled individual.

**POINT-OF-VIEW**

***Recovered mentally ill persons often contact me about whether to reveal their condition to others, especially employers. I usually encourage them to show their boss an article about me or another recovered person as a way to gauge that person's receptivity—and then to be guided by the reaction they elicit.***

—Fred Frese (10)

- Why would it be useful to test an employer's reaction before revealing a history of mental health problems?
- How might different people react to this news?

Lysaght (26) points out that job analysis as performed by OT practitioners has not been consistent. A job may be analyzed according to its physical demands or some other parameter. No structure has been developed for classifying or describing jobs in which the demands vary significantly from day to day or within the same day. Furthermore, forms for documenting or for ensuring reliability and validity of an analysis have yet to be developed.

We will now consider how OT practitioners assist individuals to enter the world of work.

## Employment Interests and Pursuits

The AOTA, in *OTPF,* defines *employment interests and pursuits* as "identifying and selecting work opportunities based on personal assets, limitations, likes, and dislikes relative to work" (2). The client is aided in exploring and choosing work-related opportunities that match his or her capacities, or that prepare for future employment within expected future capacities. Commonly, vocational and rehabilitation counselors also perform this function for clients. It is not unique to occupational therapy. However, occupational therapy practitioners are skilled in activity analysis and for this reason can assess the match between the client's abilities and the demands of the work.

## Work Potential Evaluation

The *work potential evaluation* is designed to assess the individual's present work skills and to estimate potential for work. The areas evaluated include such basic task skills as these:

- *Attendance, punctuality, and productivity* (rate of production)
- *Work attitudes and social and interpersonal behaviors,* such as accepting responsibility for oneself, accepting direction from a supervisor, and relating to peers
- *Cognitive factors,* such as memory, organization, and sequencing of a task
- *Physical factors,* such as tolerance for standing, stamina, and eye–hand coordination (which may be impaired by disuse, drug side effects, or the disease process)

Work potential evaluation is different from *vocational evaluation,* which assesses the individual's interests, talents, and skills for a particular kind of work.

Evaluation methods include the use of *aptitude tests,* which assess the client's talent or capacity for different kinds of work. Job samples (also known as work samples) and work simulation experiences may also be used. A *job sample* is a selected piece of the kind of work that is done in a particular job—for example, a job sample for an electrician might include cutting, stripping, twisting, and taping wire connections. This work would be timed and compared with the average time a working electrician would take. Several systems of prepared job samples are commercially available. Such systems (Valpar is one example) are expensive, but because they are standardized, they can provide a normed result. Job samples prepared ad hoc by a therapist may give useful measures of a client's work potential for an immediate local situation (e.g., a sheltered workshop with specific jobs), but these may not help in comparing the client's work abilities with those of the nondisabled population. *Work simulation* is a method of assessment that involves placing clients in a worklike setting (work group) on the hospital grounds, in a sheltered workshop, or in the community to see how they adapt to it; thus the OT is able to predict whether the clients could succeed in a job.

Work potential evaluation should be performed by an OT with specific training or experience in selection and design of job samples and other evaluation methods. The OTA may be designated to carry out parts of the evaluation. The purpose of the evaluation is to arrive at a *realistic* assessment of the individual's potential for work; it is important for any evaluator to be objective and to follow standardized procedures exactly for the results to be useful.

Owing to years of disability and relative inexperience, some clients have limited understanding of possible vocational choices. For such individuals, intervention should focus on vocational exploration and vocational decision making. Diamond (8) describes the format for such a group.

Several important issues should be considered in any work potential evaluation or work-related program. One is whether it is realistic or feasible for a particular client to work in competitive employment now or in the future. The determination of what is reasonable or feasible should respect the client's wishes while considering the clients strengths and supports as well as his or her disabilities and the general employment climate. When unemployment is high, one must consider whether persons with mental disabilities will be able to compete for jobs. Similarly, the prospect of guaranteed disability income may dampen a client's motivation to work. Certainly if the likelihood of a client's obtaining and keeping a job seems insecure, it is unethical for the therapist or assistant to recommend that the client seek employment and thereby jeopardize rights to disability income. Depending on the answers to these questions and the results of the evaluation, the client is referred to a service that meets the client's particular needs. If the person is eligible for assistance, services may be funded and arranged by the state office of vocational rehabilitation.

## Vocational Evaluation and Training

Clients may be referred for evaluation of their potential for different kinds of work. Clients whose basic task skills and work behaviors are adequate but who have no marketable or usable job skills may also enter vocational evaluation directly after prevocational evaluation. Vocational evaluation may be performed by a certified rehabilitation counselor or vocational evaluation specialist, by a occupational therapist, or sometimes by all three.

The client is given paper and pencil tests that measure interests, such as the *Career Assessment Inventory;* other evaluations that measure specific job-related skills, such as the *Minnesota Paper-Form Board Test,* which measures visual-spatial abilities; or tests that measure overall achievement, such as the *Wide Range Achievement Test.* The purpose is to assess the client's potential for and interest in various kinds of work, to explore these through discussion, and to select an area for further training. Helping the client substitute more realistic choices for interests that are unrealistic (e.g., astronaut, judge, neurologist) occurs at this step. Assessment of what is realistic for a particular client must also consider the possible work environment. For example, an environment that is noisy or full of distractions may be an impediment.

The next step is to arrange for the client to enter a training program—for example in a trade school or community college. Financial, administrative, and advisory support from the state office of vocational rehabilitation should be available.

## Employment Seeking and Acquisition

*OTPF* defines *employment seeking and acquisition* as "identifying job opportunities, completing and submitting appropriate application materials, preparing for interviews and following up afterward, discussing job benefits, and finalizing negotiations" (2). Given the cognitive disabilities and impaired social behaviors associated with psychiatric disorders, this is a daunting list of tasks. Occupational therapy practitioners may assist clients to identify job opportunities that are a suitable match for the individual and may coach clients on how to fill out job applications and what to expect on a job interview. They may assist them in completing applications, advise them on ADA-related concerns, help them understanding health benefits, and so on.

Those who already have adequate and marketable job skills but who do not have a job may be referred to a job search skills group in which they work toward obtaining a job. Clients with good job skills sometimes have trouble getting work because their social skills are poor and they behave oddly during telephone inquiries or job interviews. Still others do not know how to find job leads or write résumés or complete job application forms. Another problem is the difficulty many have in explaining why they have not worked for long periods during hospitalization. (A client who does not wish to disclose a psychiatric disability might be counseled to say that he or she was caring for a sick relative, for example.) All of these problems are compounded by feelings of insecurity and anxiety.

There are several ways to approach the task of teaching clients job search skills. Worksheets and activities are available (22, 23). Discussion groups by themselves have limited value unless they include expectations and opportunities to practice skills both within and outside of the group meeting. Groups that use an educational (classroom) format seem more effective. Kramer and Beidel (25) developed a series of 10 classroom lessons designed to teach interviewing, finding and following up on job leads, résumé writing, and other skills; interviews of group members by hospital staff who were simulating the roles of employers were videotaped and reviewed to improve performance. Homework was assigned in each session, to be completed before the next lesson; exercises included filling out job application forms and coming up with answers to difficult questions an interviewer might ask.[1]

A similar classroom or seminar format was used in the Altrusa Work Readiness Seminar (27). This program, designed for female clients with chronic psychiatric disorders, consisted of five seminars on work readiness and community living. Community leaders and business people provided the instruction, which focused not so much on job search skills as on self-awareness, consumerism, and money management.

Even with a highly structured format that requires member involvement and participation, some clients will not follow through with the skills they learn and actually obtain a job. Some may need more practice, and others may not be motivated to work.

## Job Performance

*OTPF* describes *job performance* as "including work habits, for example, attendance, punctuality, appropriate relationships with coworkers and supervisors, completion of assigned work, and compliance with the norms of the work setting" (2). The OT practitioner may first assist the person to acquire basic work behaviors and then help the person transition to some sort of meaningful productive employment.

### Task Groups

Groups in which participants work on simple tasks (*task groups*) have been used as a setting for development of work behaviors and for work adjustment. The underlying assumption is that basic task skills such as attention span, neatness, speed, and attention to detail are needed for all kinds of jobs; in other words, these skills affect the quality of the work whether the person is sewing a pincushion, keyboarding a letter, taking orders over the telephone, or transplanting seedlings. Therefore, any task that is structured and that has recognizable standards can be used to evaluate and teach these basic task skills. These simple, humble activities may be less threatening initially for someone who would be overwhelmed by the idea of having a real job or by being assessed for one.

Traditionally, task groups and work groups were different terms for the same kind of group; today, however, it appears that therapists generally use the term *task group* to mean a highly structured group in which very low-functioning clients learn basic task skills. Among the basic task skills taught or reinforced in task groups are the abilities to do the following:

- Attend to a task long enough to complete it
- Use tools and materials safely and without waste
- Work at a consistent and productive rate
- Recognize errors and problems
- Work neatly and with attention to detail

Such task skills are basic to functional success across many life roles—student, worker, homemaker, hobbyist, and so on. In such a group, each client works independently on his or her own

[1] The exercises and corresponding homework sheets can be found in Kramer (24).

project and receives individual attention from the therapist or assistant leading the group. Clients may all do similar projects or different ones; projects are designed to be completed in a relatively short period.

Although clients in such groups are encouraged to work on neatness, attention span, and other basic skills, they are not expected to perform complex tasks, work for long periods, or interact much with others. The task skills that they develop or relearn in these groups are a foundation for more complex work behavior, just as the work habits acquired by the preschool child are the skills needed later to succeed in school and ultimately on the job.

Helping a client develop task skills requires intense concentration from the OTA. It is important first of all to analyze exactly what the client needs to do to improve performance and to communicate this clearly. For example, someone who fails to notice errors must be taught how to check for them and to understand what an error looks like and how to correct it. Some clients become distracted, confused, or overwhelmed if asked to work on more than one problem at a time, so the OTA should design the learning experiences in steps or stages. Close supervision and immediate feedback are essential. Positive feedback and praise encourage learning and help to support development of task skills.

## Work Groups

*Work groups* are designed to simulate a work environment; such groups actually produce a product or provide a service. Clients who have at least parallel-level group interaction skills and some basic task skills are generally eligible (28). Participants are assigned specific tasks and various levels of responsibility. Behavior appropriate in a work setting is expected, and acting out is discouraged. The group leader designs and analyzes the tasks the group will perform and divides and assigns them to members. Clients are expected to do the jobs they are assigned and to work during the entire period, just as they would in paid employment. These groups generally meet at least three times a week and for relatively long periods, 2 hours or more. Activities that are suitable for a work group are those that can be structured into clear tasks and work roles. Among the many possible tasks are refinishing furniture, cleaning the treatment center, preparing food for others, and doing office work.

### Production Line

One popular format is the *production line*, in which a product is manufactured by dividing the task into steps that are performed by different members. Each person does only a part of the process and then passes the item along to the person who does the next step. For example, in a jewelry production line, one member might design the beading sequence for two or three styles of necklaces. Another client might be assigned to attach the jump rings to the cords; others would actually string the beads, following the designed samples; and one or two others would finish the necklaces by knotting the cords and attaching the catches. Other jobs in this group might include acting as foreman or work supervisor, counting supplies and finished necklaces, and boxing or packaging them. It is also possible to structure a production line to teach the team, or group, a work style that is becoming more common in the workplace. In group work, the group is responsible jointly to achieve a task; responsibilities are fluid and are determined by the group. A problem that sometimes arises in work groups is that many of the members want the glamorous jobs, designer or foreman; discussion of this issue after the group's work is finished for the day gives members a chance to work through their feelings about this and about equivalent situations in the work world.

Production lines may employ many media, including woodwork, ceramics, leathercraft, horticulture, and printed matter as well as assembly, sorting, or packaging of items produced elsewhere. Some production lines sell their products through hospital gift shops or concessions or bazaars; other provide services through contracts with departments in the treatment setting or with outside companies. Many are paid for their work. For a production line to work well, the jobs within it must be designed so that each worker has enough work; it may be necessary to assign several jobs to one person or to give several individuals the same job. Producing a salable product or one that is useful to others (e.g., assembling a mailing for the hospital) is also important. The staff member in charge of the group is responsible for ordering and obtaining supplies, for maintaining the environment and equipment used by the group, and for monitoring the quality of the product. At times, a higher-functioning client may take over these duties, which are similar to those of an administrator, supervisor, foreman, or manager.

Safety is a concern in production lines that employ power tools, heat, or toxic substances. Safety equipment that complies with Occupational Safety and Health Administration (OSHA) regulations should be used, and clients must be instructed in safety guidelines and emergency procedures. Clients who have visual disturbances, seizures, or motor incoordination should be watched closely and not assigned to work in which they may injure themselves. Similar precautions should be taken for clients who have poor judgment or other cognitive deficits or who may be violent or suicidal.

### Clerical Groups

*Clerical groups* focus on office skills. They may be designed around a division of labor similar to a production line; in fact, they are sometimes called office production lines. The activity is the production of printed matter; tasks might include typing forms or word processing, taking dictation or transcribing from a machine, using a computer for numerical entry or data base work, using duplicating equipment, collating, stuffing envelopes, or sorting outgoing mail by ZIP code. It is necessary to have computers and other electronic devices if clients are actually to be trained to provide office services in the business world. Clients who already have word processing skills also need opportunities to practice, maintain, and upgrade them. In competitive employment, a job in word processing can be scheduled for off hours and thus is suitable for the client who cannot tolerate the interpersonal stresses of the nine-to-five shift.

A *newspaper* or *journal group* is a variation on the clerical group, but it requires more initiative, creativity, and decision making from its members. The group's major activity is to write, edit, type, print, and distribute a newsletter or similar publication. Although many job functions and levels of responsibility can be designated within the group, it is often left up to the members to decide who does what on a day-to-day basis. In some senses this type of group may be more effective for teaching interpersonal skills than work behaviors. Nonetheless, negotiations among members about what to report, what to print, and what to censor provide opportunities to practice group interaction skills. This sort of group is feasible only in long-term or community settings, where membership can remain constant for some time.

### Service Concessions

Service concessions for the treatment center or for the community are yet another type of work group. A *food service* or *coffee shop* work group provides food and beverages, usually for only a few hours a day. The staff member in charge is responsible for making sure that proper health and sanitary precautions are followed in regard to food storage and handling and maintenance of the equipment and the food preparation area. Accounting and managing of the proceeds from sales is finally the group leader's responsibility, although clients may be assigned these tasks under supervision. Other service concessions that are sometimes used as work groups in psychiatric settings are a *library* and a *child care service;* the latter is possible only where legal requirements permit. Other work groups may be based on the sale in a *boutique* or *thrift shop* of goods made in production lines or items received through donations. These groups provide an opportunity for members to practice interpersonal skills needed to relate to the public.

In summary, all of these different kinds of work groups provide a milieu in which clients can practice behaviors appropriate for the work world. Although the same basic work behaviors are reinforced in all of these groups, there are also opportunities for different kinds of learning in different groups. Placement of clients in groups and assignment of clients to particular jobs within groups should be based not on the client's preference for the particular medium or activity used in that group but on the group's ability to provide experience that will help contribute to the individual's ability to perform productive work. Detailed examples of goals and objectives for work behavior can be found in Hemphill and associates (18).

## Work Adjustment Programs

A work adjustment program (sometimes called *personal adjustment training*) helps clients acquire basic work habits, work attitudes, and social skills. Such programs are directed toward the functionally impaired client who needs to reach a socially acceptable level of performance before competitive employment can be a realistic option. Both inpatient and outpatient programs exist, some permitting or requiring attendance for 30 to 40 hours weekly. Such programs may include training in activities of daily living (especially grooming and hygiene), social skills training, communication skills development, and work behaviors. Work groups, including assembly lines and service groups (e.g., to provide meals to the homebound or to clean the park), are used to simulate a real work environment and to allow participants to practice work behaviors. Clients are assigned tasks and job responsibilities and are expected to behave and perform as they would be expected to on the job. Behavioral methods such as feedback and reinforcement are widely used in these programs. Videotape is very popular as a feedback medium; clients can critique themselves and their peers at the end of the work day.

The OTA in a work adjustment program may lead discussion groups or work groups or provide counseling and feedback on an individual case management basis. For example, the assistant may help a very impulsive client learn to stop to think before acting; it may take many conversations for this message to get across. Or the assistant might help someone with limited work tolerance explore why he or she is so easily bored by the work and avoids work by leaving early. There are many, many issues involved in successful work adjustment that require sensitivity on the part of the assistant. A client's problems with work may be based on expectations learned from parents or cultural background, on personal beliefs, or simply on lack of positive prior experience and lack of knowledge of what is expected. Successful intervention must be based on accurate assessment of the problem.

## Sheltered Work Programs

Sheltered work programs provide a work-like experience for persons whose disabilities are so limiting that they will never be able to enter competitive employment. Such programs help clients achieve a sense of direction, purpose, and productivity by performing simple tasks in a relatively stress-free environment. Long-term placement gives participants a feeling of being productive and making a contribution to the extent they are capable; this is very important for a person's sense of self-worth. Pay is generally based on the amount of work or number of pieces completed, as a fraction of what a nondisabled worker might complete in the same time. Sheltered workshops are not a preferred type of programming for persons with serious mental illness because they are stigmatizing and do not connect the client with the desired goal of paid employment in the community (19).

Sheltered work programs are sometimes found within hospital settings, especially in large public institutions, and also in the community; many are operated by charitable organizations such as Goodwill Industries, the Lighthouse, and others. The work itself is usually highly structured and divided into measurable units; assembly and packaging of small items are typical activities. The rates at which workers are paid for their work vary across the country; court decisions have interpreted the Fair Labor Standards Act of 1966 to mean that working patients must be paid when their work benefits the hospital or agency. Generally, payment is below minimum wage and usually based on some measurable criterion such as the number of pieces produced (as compared with workers in competitive employment) or hours worked. Because the needs of clients in these programs remain relatively constant, OTAs can administer sheltered work programs with only modest amounts of supervision from an OT.

Some sheltered work programs are designed so that participants who qualify may graduate into placement in community jobs. Howe and associates (21) created a program in which the sheltered work component involved a choice of either house and grounds maintenance work or food services. Classes in daily living skills and various work skills were also included. Clients who consistently demonstrated strong basic task skills and cooperative work attitudes were encouraged to join a transitional employment program, in which they could work first on a volunteer basis and then as a paid employee in an entry-level job, for example at McDonald's.

## Trial Employment and Transitional Employment

One approach that has been used with some success is placing the client temporarily in a job within the treatment setting or in a volunteer job in the community. Some community employers have been willing to fill a part-time position with a series of clients, each of whom rotates through it for a short period; once the client becomes comfortable with the idea of working, he or she is encouraged to move on to a regular job.

*Transitional employment programs* (TEPs) provide time-limited job placements with the goal of enabling the client to hold a regular job. The client can try out several TEPs in succession. For example, for 6 months the client may work in a janitorial service and for the next 6 months, in a retail store as a stock clerk. Urbaniak (41) points out that clients may have to try several placements before they feel ready to consider competitive employment.

Negotiating with an employer to establish a TEP requires the OTA to learn and understand the employer's business and to teach the employer about the special concessions needed for the client to succeed. Serving as a placement manager, the OTA would be responsible for learning the position, training the client, and providing support and job coaching as needed (41).

## Job Sharing

Another model that is sometimes used is *job sharing*, in which several clients share the same job, possibly a TEP. As a group they may work more total hours than a nondisabled worker, but as a group they are paid at the same rate. Their wages are divided according to the relative contributions of each person sharing the job. Typically, a staff member serves as *job coach* and learns the job, teaches it to the clients, and even fills in when the client is absent and there is no one else to do the job.

## Supported Employment

Many of the approaches previously discussed have been criticized by consumers and psychiatric rehabilitation professionals. The criticisms

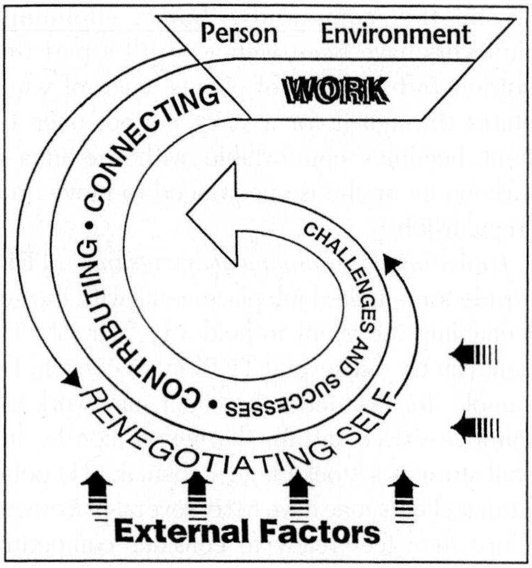


**Figure 19-1. Work and the change process.** (Reprinted with permission from Strong S. Meaningful work in supportive environments: Experiences with the recovery process. Am J Occup Ther 1998;52:31–38.)

focus on the prolonged period of time that participants stay in make-work and prevocational settings and the delay in getting to competitive employment. The current best practice acknowledged by professionals, including occupational therapy practitioners, is *supported employment* (SE), which has strong research evidence of effectiveness with persons with serious mental illness (12, 19). A model of SE called Individual Placement and Support (IPS) is commonly used in psychiatric rehabilitation. The client is placed directly into competitive employment and the services and accommodations are built around the client and the job. Clients do not have to be "well" to participate. The SE program provides supports similar to those of TEP (i.e., job coaching, clinical services) over the long term. Occupational therapy practitioners are trained to analyze the transactions among the person, the work environment, and the job task; this analysis of how to modify the environment to suit the client is extremely helpful. Furthermore, OTs and OTAs can provide specific suggestions and concrete recommendations to help employers support the worker who has a psychiatric disability (4).

Strong (37) points out that supported employment and other work experiences enable the client to "negotiate a new sense of self." Figure 19-1 demonstrates the spiraling feedback loop that arises from transactions among the worker, the work, and the environment.

**POINT-OF-VIEW**

***It is a pleasure to be and to feel needed. We get no personal financial profit. We have social goals, like a Christmas buffet, a crayfish party, and then a trip once a year, and when it is someone's birthday, we'll always have a cake.***

—Unnamed worker cooperative member, quoted by Gahnstrom-Strandqvist et al. (11)

- How do you reconcile this statement with the argument that supported employment is the best model for persons with disabilities?
- What needs are met by the worker cooperative model?
- What needs might be better met in a supported employment situation?

## Worker Cooperatives

Worker cooperatives are owned by workers, who share in the profits and decide jointly how to spend or invest what they have earned. A study in Sweden (11) of three working cooperatives, each with 20 to 30 mentally ill participants, showed that the cooperative model met the participants needs for meaningful occupation, productivity, social support, belongingness, self-determination. The tasks performed by the cooperatives included catering, making and selling craft products, and packing and other subcontracted jobs. Most of the supervisors were occupational therapists.

### Volunteer Positions

Serving as a volunteer worker provides many of the benefits of competitive employment while permitting significantly greater flexibility for someone with a psychiatric disorder. House (20) cites the following specific advantages:

- Volunteers can set their own schedules.
- Volunteers are always appreciated.
- Volunteers have more flexibility to respond to the changing symptoms of their psychiatric disability.

Volunteer positions within mental health advocacy programs are particularly supportive for the client because the nature of one's condition can be freely discussed and accepted. Furthermore, a volunteer job provides a way to begin exploring the possibility of competitive employment while retaining medical and disability benefits that would be discontinued if the client entered paid employment full-time.

### Role Maintenance

Clients who are employed may find extended hospitalization (whether as inpatient or outpatient) very disruptive to their work habits and skills; they can be helped to maintain their role responsibilities and skills by participating in a role maintenance group (42). The purpose of such a group is to help the client identify which responsibilities can be continued during hospitalization and to assist the client in communicating and negotiating with the employer and family (important for homemakers). The therapist and the group discuss ways in which the worker's tasks can be redesigned or if necessary delegated to others.

Later, the client and the therapist arrange for a gradual transition back to the worker role by gradually increasing the amount of time the client spends out in the community working. For example, a secretary might go back to work first on a part-time basis.

Richert (29) described a vocational transition group whose co-leaders were an occupational therapist and a vocational counselor. The purpose of this group was to assist psychiatric inpatients to make the transition back to work after discharge. Activities and focuses of this group included identifying personal goals, discussing and problem solving job stressors, and exploring fears of stigma and prejudice from coworkers.

### Transition to Retirement

Retirement may lead to mental health problems in persons who previously functioned well. The loss of the social structure of work and of the benefits listed in Table 19-1 is significant. However, the retiree may not think of retirement as a loss and thus may fail to anticipate the psychosocial stresses. Depression is a common result. The OT practitioner may assist the retiree in the following ways:

- Facilitating expression of the meaning of work and of the feelings of loss
- Bringing closure to the work experience
- Providing links to enable part-time, consultative, or volunteer work to continue the experience of productivity

## SUMMARY

This chapter focuses on education and work. The ability to engage effectively in these activities depends on a foundation of task skills and work habits that typically are acquired in a developmental progression. School provides knowledge and additional skills to enable work, through which a person can contribute to the human community. The adult's self-esteem is deeply rooted in a sense of productivity and a belief about one's own contributions and achievements. Occupational therapists and assistants can enhance and maintain their clients' self-concept and ability to function by supporting them as they engage in the work of a student, and in productive roles in supported or competitive employment.

## REVIEW QUESTIONS AND ACTIVITIES

1. Describe how children learn the skills to succeed in school and work.
2. List some challenges faced by children and adolescents with mental disorders in their attempts to engage in the role of student.
3. In what ways do the problems of the student who develops mental illness in late adolescence differ from those of students whose mental illness dates from childhood?
4. What is an IEP?
5. What ages are covered under the IDEA?
6. Describe how occupational therapy services to children with mental disorders might be provided in a school setting.
7. Environmental management may be the key to success with school and with homework. Discuss this statement, giving examples to illustrate your points.
8. What is supported education? What three models are used?
9. For which clients is the self-contained classroom recommended?
10. Discuss how the ADA may apply to college students with mental disorders.
11. Name some functions of work.
12. What are some challenges encountered by persons with mental disorders in the world of work?
13. What are the provisions of the ADA in regard to workers with mental disorders?
14. Define the following in regard to the ADA: *reasonable accommodation, essential function,* and *direct threat.*
15. Describe how occupational therapy practitioners can assist persons who have a mental disorder in obtaining accommodations under the ADA.
16. Differentiate the following programs: work potential evaluation, vocational evaluation, vocational training, employment seeking/acquisition, task group, work group, work adjustment program, sheltered work, transitional employment, job sharing, supported employment, and worker cooperatives. Identify the roles of the OT or OTA in each.
17. Why do consumers and psychiatric rehabilitation professionals embrace the supported employment approach?
18. A role maintenance program is recommended for what clients and situations?
19. What are the challenges of retirement and how can the occupational therapy practitioner assist clients in making this transition?
20. *Challenge activity:* Observe a classmate during class and study time and write a summary of that person's task skills. With the person, develop a plan for improving skills. Share your experience with the class.
21. *Challenge activity:* Imagine that you are working in a community mental health center that serves a group of young adults who have serious mental disorders. You have been asked to help transition the clients to jobs in the community. How would you achieve this goal? Describe the specific steps you would take.

## REFERENCES


1. Abelson R. Employers increasingly face disability-based bias cases. New York Times, Nov 20, 2001. Available at: query.nytimes.com/gst/fullpage.html?sec=health &res=9A05E6D7113BF933A15752C1A9679C8B63. Accessed Apr 2007.
2. American Occupational Therapy Association. Occupational therapy practice framework: Domain and process. Am J Occup Ther 2002;56:609–639.
3. American Occupational Therapy Association. Occupational therapy services in facilitating work performance. Am J Occup Ther 2005;59:676–679.
4. Basler RM, Harvey BM, Hornby H. Building employer support for hiring persons with psychiatric disabilities. Am Occup Ther Assoc Ment Health Special Sect Q Newslett 1998;21(4):2–4.
5. Beck AJ, Barnes KJ, Vogel KA, Grice KO. The dilemma of psychosocial occupational therapy in public schools: The therapist's perceptions. Occup Ther Ment Health 2006;22(1):1–17.
6. Chandler BE. Hidden in plain sight—Working with students with emotional disturbance in the schools. OT Practice 2007;12(1):CE1–8.
7. Crist PAH, Stoffel VC. The Americans with Disabilities Act of 1990 and employees with mental impairments: Personal efficacy and the environment. Am J Occup Ther 1992;46:434–443.
8. Diamond H. Vocational decision making in a psychiatric outpatient program. Occup Ther Ment Health 1998;14(3): 67–80.
9. Dirette D, Kolak L. Occupational performance needs of adolescents in alternative education programs. Am J Occup Ther 2004;58:357–341.
10. Frese F. Coping with schizophrenia requires effort. Available at: fredfrese.com/?q=node/view/2&PHPSESSID=6e4a85f28fd6311d15bde3d1433ffbca. Accessed July 2007.
11. Gahnstrom-Strandqvist K, Liukko A, Tham K. The meaning of the working cooperative for persons with long-term mental illness. Am J Occup Ther 2003;57: 262–272.
12. Gray K. Evidence-based employment services for persons with serious mental illness. Am Occup Ther Assoc Ment Health Special Sect Q Newslett 2005;28(3):1–2.
13. Gupta J. Workplace accommodations—Challenges and opportunities. OT Practice 2006;11(11):9–14.
14. Gutman SA. Schindler VP. The effectiveness of a supported education for adults with psychiatric disabilities: The Bridge Program. Occup Ther Ment Health 2007:23(1):21–38.
15. Gutman SA. Schindler VP. Supported education for adults and adolescents with psychiatric disabilities: Occupational therapy's role. OT Practice 2007;12(5):CE1–8.
16. Haack L, Haldy M. Making it easy: Adapting home and school environments. OT Practice 1996:1(11):22–28.
17. Hahn C. Building mental health roles into school system practice. OT Practice 2000;5(21):14–16.
18. Hemphill BJ, Peterson CQ, Werner PC. Rehabilitation in Mental Health: Goals and Objectives for Independent Living. Thorofare, NJ: Slack, 1991.
19. Henry AD. Employment for people with serious mental illness—Barriers and contemporary approaches to service. OT Practice 2005;10(5):CE1–8.
20. House G. A consumer speaks out: The beneficial realities of volunteer employment. NAMI Advocate 1998–1999; 20(3):11.
21. Howe MC, Weaver CT, Dulay J. The development of a work-oriented day center program. Am J Occup Ther 1981;35:711–718.
22. Korb-Khalsa KL, Azok SD, Leutenberg EA. Life Management Skills: 3. Reproducible Activity Handouts Created for Facilitators. Beachwood, OH: Wellness Reproductions, 1994.
23. Korb-Khalsa KL, Leutenberg EA. Life Management Skills: 4. Reproducible Activity Handouts Created for Facilitators. Beachwood, OH: Wellness Reproductions, 1996.
24. Kramer LW. SCORE: Solving community obstacles and restoring employment. Occup Ther Ment Health 1984;4(1):1–135.
25. Kramer LW, Beidel DC. Job seeking skills groups: A review and application to a chronic population. Occup Ther Ment Health 1982;2(2):37–44.
26. Lysaght R. Job analysis in occupational therapy: Stepping into the complex world of business and industry. Am J Occup Ther 1997;51:569–575.
27. Mauras-Corsino E, Daniewicz CV, Swan LC. The use of community networks for chronic psychiatric patients. Am J Occup Ther 1985;39:374–378.
28. Mosey AC. Activities Therapy. New York: Raven, 1973.
29. Richert GZ. Vocational transition in acute care psychiatry. Occup Ther Ment Health 1990;10(4):43–61.
30. Rosenberg G. When the mind is the matter: Mental disability cases pose painful workplace issues. New York Times, Nov 7, 1998, C1–2.
31. Salls J, Bucey JC. Self-regulation strategies for middle school students. OT Practice 2003;8(5):11–16.
32. Schneider D. When do I disclose? ADA protection and your job. Occup Ther Ment Health 1998;14(1–2): 77–87.
33. Schultz S. Psychosocial occupational therapy in schools. OT Practice 2003;8(17):CE1–8.

34. Segal R, Hinojosa J. The activity setting of homework: An analysis of three cases and implications for occupational therapy. Am J Occup Ther 2006;60:50–59.
35. Segal R, Hinojosa J, Addonizio C, et al. Homework strategies for children with attention deficit hyperactivity disorder. OT Practice 2005;10(17):9–12.
36. Spencer J, Daybell PJ, Eschenfelder V, et al. Contrasting perspectives on work: An exploratory qualitative study based on the concept of adaptation. Am J Occup Ther 1998;52:474–484.
37. Strong S. Meaningful work in supportive environments: Experiences with the recovery process. Am J Occup Ther 1998;52:31–38.
38. Unger KV. Supported postsecondary education for people with mental illness. Am Rehabil 1990;16(2):10–15.
39. U.S. Congress. Americans with Disabilities Act of 1990 [Public Law 101-336]. Available at: www.usdoj.gov/crt/ada/adahom1.htm. Accessed Apr 2007.
40. U.S. Congress. Individuals with Disabilities Education Improvement Act of 2004 [Public Law 108-446]. Available at: frwebgate.access.gpo.gov/cgi-bin/getdoc.cgi? dbname=108_cong_public_laws&docid=f:publ446.108. Accessed Apr 2007.
41. Urbaniak M. Yahara House: A community-based program using the Fountain-House model. Am Occup Ther Assoc Ment Health Special Sect Q Newslett 1995; 18(1):1–3.
42. Versluys HP. The remediation of role disorders through focused group work. Am J Occup Ther 1980;34:609–614.
43. Wells SA. The Americans with Disabilities Act of 1990: Equalizing opportunities. OT Practice 2000;5(6):CE1–8.
44. Williams MS, Shellenberger S. How Does Your Engine Run? A Leader's Guide to the Alert Program for Sensory Regulation. Albuquerque NM: Therapy Works, 1996.
45. Zimmerman E. On the job, learning disabilities can often hide in plain sight. New York Times, Dec 17, 2006. Available at: select.nytimes.com/search/ restricted/article?res=F50C14FC38550C748DDDAB0994DE404482. Accessed Apr 2007.

## SUGGESTED READINGS

### General

Allen CK, Earhart CA, Blue T. Occupational therapy treatment goals for the physically and cognitively disabled. Rockville, MD: American Occupational Therapy Association, 1992.

Earhart CA. Occupational therapy groups. In: Allen CA, ed. Occupational Therapy for Psychiatric Diseases: Measurement and Management of Cognitive Disabilities. Boston: Little, Brown, 1985.

Fidler G. The task-oriented group as a context for treatment. Am J Occup Ther 1969;23:43–48.

Kartin NJ, Van Schroeder C. Adult Psychiatric Life Skills Manual. Kailua, HI: Schroeder Publishing, 1982.

### Education

Haack L, Haldy M. Making it easy: Adapting home and school environments. OT Pract 1996:1(11):22–28.

Soyden AS. Frequently Asked Questions by Educators about Students with Psychiatric Disabilities. Boston: Center for Psychiatric Rehabilitation, Boston University, 1997.

### Work

Alexander CK. Work programs practice—Aiming for successful context management. OT Practice 2004;9(7):CE1–8.

Burson KA. Work as purposeful activity: The vocational program at Rock Creek Center. Am Occup Ther Assoc Ment Health Special Sect Q Newslett 1992;15(4):2–4.

Gray K. Evidence-based employment services for persons with serious mental illness. Am Occup Ther Assoc Ment Health Special Sect Q Newslett 2005;28(3):1–2.

Henry A. Employment services reference list. Am Occup Ther Assoc Ment Health Special Sect Q Newslett 2005;28(3):3.

Joe BE. Psychiatric disabilities and the workplace. OT Week, July 31, 1997, 11:14–15.

Johansson C. New opportunities in mental health. OT Week, Oct 22, 1998, 12:14–15.

Johansson U, Tham K. The meaning of work after acquired brain injury. Am J Occup Ther 2006;60:60–69.

Kakutani K. New life expresso: Report on a business run by people with psychiatric disabilities. Psychiatric Rehab J 1998;22(2):111–115.

Lucca AM, Henry AD. Barriers to employment and recommendations for change: What do consumers and providers say? Am Occup Ther Assoc Ment Health Special Sect Q Newslett 2004;27(1):1–3.

Man Hong Siu A. Predicting employment outcomes for people with chronic psychiatric illness. Occup Ther Ment Health 1997;13(4):45–58.

Tryssenar J. Vocational exploration and employment and psychosocial disabilities. In: Stein F, Cutler SK, eds. Psychosocial Occupational Therapy: A Holistic Approach. 2nd ed. Albany, NY: Thomson Delmar, 2002.

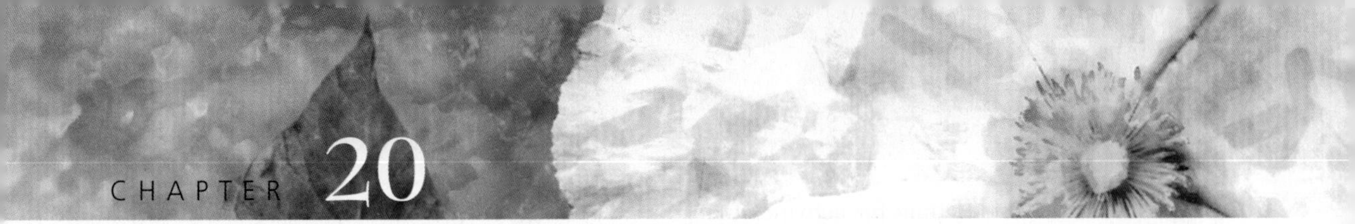

CHAPTER 20

# Leisure and Social Participation

***The popular assumption is that no skills are involved in enjoying free time, and that anybody can do it. Yet the evidence suggests the opposite: free time is more difficult to enjoy than work. Having leisure at one's disposal does not improve the quality of life unless one knows how to use it effectively, and it is by no means something one learns automatically.***

MIHALY CSIKSZENTIMIHALYI (6, P. 65)

## CHAPTER OBJECTIVES

After studying this chapter, the reader will be able to:

1. Examine obstacles to effective participation in leisure and social interaction for persons with mental disorders.
2. Recognize general principles that guide interventions to assist clients with leisure and social participation.
3. Guide clients in exploring and participating in leisure and social activities.
4. Analyze the benefits and disadvantages of a variety of leisure activities.

Leisure is the use of time for activities that are personally satisfying and for most people, not related to work. Social participation is the activity of interacting with others in various social situations, including peer and family relationships and community relations. These areas of occupation are recognized as distinct from each other, according to the *Occupational Therapy Practice Framework (OTPF)* (1). Most people use some of their leisure time for pleasurable association with other people, and so these two areas of occupation sometimes overlap.

Leisure or recreation actually re-creates the capacity to work by restoring lost energy and refreshing the spirit. Leisure activities reflect the personal preferences, values, and interests of the individual. Unless these activities are chosen by the client, there is no reason to believe that he or she will find them satisfying or refreshing. Therapy staff may be surprised that some clients enjoy activities that other people consider boring, childish, or unpleasant. You need only think about your own family, friends, and acquaintances to realize that not everyone likes listening to rock music or opera and that some people prefer playing bingo, collecting stamps, or riding mountain bikes. It should be obvious that to improve clients' use of leisure time you have to help them do the activities that *they* want to do.

The American Occupational Therapy Association (AOTA) in the *OTPF* defines *leisure* as "a nonobligatory activity that is intrinsically motivated and engaged in during discretionary time, that is, time not committed to obligatory occupations such as work, self-care, or sleep" (1). The AOTA recognizes that two interrelated processes are involved in leisure activities. The first is *exploration,* defined as "identifying interests, skills, opportunities, and appropriate leisure activities" (1). In other words, to identify preferences in leisure activities, one must have some experience of the different options. The second is *performance,* which includes the following three aspects:

Planning and participating in play or leisure activities
Maintaining a balance of play or leisure activities with work and productive activities, and activities of daily living
Obtaining, utilizing, and maintaining equipment and supplies" (1)

We will consider *exploration* first.

## LEISURE EXPLORATION

Leisure can be a source of personal identity and can provide a continuous thread of meaning over a lifetime (4, 11). Exploration of leisure requires energy and initiative; it is difficult to learn about (or to remember and restart) different activities while sitting staring into space or at the television. Leisure is a particular challenge for persons who have psychiatric disorders, many of whom are unemployed or underemployed and have large amounts of time on their hands. People who do not have major mental disorders value leisure much more than do those who have mental disorders (5). Clients with mental health problems may undervalue leisure and fail to recognize its importance (5) or may describe it as not relevant to their lives (13). Some clients may not know or cannot remember what they enjoy doing in their spare time.

A study of adolescents with criminal records showed that they spent significantly more time in passive leisure (watching television, listening to music) than they did before becoming involved with drugs and crime (7). These adolescents mourned the loss of activity and engagement but felt unconnected to their prior leisure selves and unable to structure their own time to include formerly valued leisure activities. Another challenge occurs for older persons who have recently retired and whose patterns of time use have changed dramatically. Homemakers whose children are grown may have difficulty filling the hours formerly spent in parenting and may have little idea of their own interests.

The occupational therapy practitioner may take a two-step approach to assisting clients with leisure exploration. The first step is a leisure evaluation, which may include one or more assessments. The occupational therapist (OT) or the occupational therapy assistant (OTA) may ask the client to complete an *interest inventory*, described in Chapter 15. Through interviewing, the OT or OTA may review the person's history, perhaps even back to childhood, or speak with family members to identify activities that the person used to engage in.

The second step is to involve the client in one or more leisure activities or in a group designed to present leisure opportunities. Discussion can focus on which activities were enjoyed and why. This is perhaps the best approach when clients are not familiar with many activities and have no clear sense of their own preferences and competencies. Alternatively, worksheets and exercises can provide a beginning point for planning and selecting leisure activities (15, 17, 24).

Because different people have different needs for leisure, the preferred context and style of activity should be explored extensively. For example, does this person want to be alone or with others? Would it bring more pleasure to do the activity in one's home, in a special environment, or in a combination? Exercises and worksheets to develop these and other aspects can be found in various sources (10, 12, 15, 16, 24).

## LEISURE PERFORMANCE

Leisure exploration does not automatically result in sustained leisure performance. Consumers experience many obstacles, both internally generated and external (from the environment), that may interfere with successful use of leisure. The OTA must understand the skills and abilities that support leisure performance, analyze the source of any difficulty, and identify and provide appropriate interventions. The following discussion examines some of these points.

### Planning and Participating

Leisure planning and leisure counseling activities must take into account clients' ability to make decisions and follow through on them, their financial and time resources, and the recreation and leisure opportunities available locally. Clients who find it difficult to make decisions and to follow through on choices will benefit from increased structure. A buddy system or group approach may help; the person may be more committed to the activity if someone else is going along (9).

Clients may also have trouble initiating a search for leisure opportunities. One approach is to make a list of possible activities, including classes at the YWCA or YMCA or the local community college, sports, crafts, games, expressive activities, and domestic activities (cooking, gardening). This helps structure leisure choices for people who have difficulty coming up with ideas; the list can be abbreviated or expanded to suit the client's age and ability to make decisions. Because limited income may be an issue, the list should include some free or low-cost activities. When possible, clients should learn to generate their own lists.

For clients who need or wish to develop new leisure pursuits or to explore scheduling more time for leisure, intervention might focus on helping them identify pleasurable activities, discover reasons why pleasurable activities are avoided, and locate community recreation resources. Even though it is possible and sometimes necessary to counsel clients individually, group counseling is probably more effective because members can get ideas and support from each other.

### Maintaining Balance in Life Activities

A related problem is that some people do not manage their time well and, therefore, appear to have no leisure time even though in fact they have too much. On the other hand, workaholics may actually not have any time for leisure because they spend so much time working. Although there is no magic formula or minimum weekly requirement that we can apply equally to all individuals, it appears that each person should spend enough time relaxing to feel restored and refreshed and able to work again. This is an area in which the OTA must be careful to follow the lead of the client. Classifications of activity as work or leisure are culturally bound and highly individual (25). Furthermore, women may be especially reluctant to make time for leisure until they have met the needs of others and so need particular support and encouragement to examine and meet their own needs (20).

Activity configurations such as the *Barth Time Construction* (see Chapter 14) and the Balance Your Life exercise in Korb and associates (16) are useful in promoting self-awareness of leisure habits in that they give a vivid picture of exactly how time is being used.

Passive activities present a special problem. Some depressed persons say they watch television and read in their leisure time. It may be helpful to supplement these activities with others that provide social contact and the opportunity to express one's own competence through active doing. Active leisure (doing) provides more experience of "flow" than does passive leisure (e.g., reading popular magazines, watching television). Csikszentimihalyi (6) defines *flow* as a "sense of effortless action" and states that the flow experience has three characteristics:

- A clear set of goals that require appropriate responses
- Provision of immediate feedback
- Use of skills to meet a challenge that is just about manageable (pp. 29–30)

The experience of flow is not restricted to leisure activities, and many people find their greatest experience of flow in work (6). Nonetheless, clients can learn to increase their experience of flow by changing the balance of leisure to include more *active* leisure experiences that provide these three characteristics.

### Obtaining and Maintaining Supplies and Equipment

Many leisure activities require some equipment or supplies. For the client on a limited income, obtaining the necessary items may be a problem. Sometimes vendors are willing to make donations if the situation is explained to them; and last season's unsold merchandise is often steeply discounted. Supplies and equipment last longer if properly maintained; clients may benefit from specific instructions and demonstrations (e.g., how to clean and store a paintbrush) as well as written reminders.

## LEISURE ACTIVITIES

We will now consider some activities that may provide a leisure experience. Trends in leisure are constantly evolving. Traditional activities that have been ignored for decades may suddenly be revived, and new activities appear frequently. For example, knitting and other needlecrafts were popular through the 1960s and then fell out of favor but came back into fashion after 2001. Scrapbooking as it has been practiced in the past 10 years is quite different from the ways scrapbooks were used previously. The new scrapbooking is much more artistic and craft-like and highly demanding of manual skills and organizational judgment. Thus the OTA must stay alert to popular culture and fads and fashions in leisure. Although we will discuss the teaching of leisure activities, it is more common for the occupational therapy practitioner to connect the client with a leisure opportunity than actually to instruct it.

### Crafts

Crafts have been used in occupational therapy since the beginning of the profession. However, some people actively dislike crafts; other leisure opportunities must be available to meet their needs. Discussion here will focus on the use of crafts for leisure; the use of crafts to develop task skills and work habits has been discussed separately.

Some factors that should be considered before using any craft as a leisure activity with a client are the requirements in time and money, the traditional sexual orientation of the craft, the level of expertise required in manual and cognitive skills, the length of time needed to complete the activity, and the likelihood of successful completion. Some crafts, such as needlework, have a strong feminine identification, and some men may be offended by any suggestion that they might do them. Leathercraft, woodwork, electronics, and metal crafts are more likely to be accepted by men.

Some activities require a greater degree of manual dexterity than is immediately obvious—for example, threading a needle, knotting the thread, and making the first stitch are more difficult than continuing a stitch that has already been started. The OTA should analyze activities carefully before recommending them. If instructing a craft, the OTA should practice each step, including completing a sample, before teaching it to clients; in this way problems can be identified in advance and adaptations made (e.g., prethreading needles). Other activities require cognitive skills that the client may lack; using a ruler to measure is one example. Again, modifications can be made once the problem is recognized; the OTA might teach ruler and measurement skills or provide premeasured project pieces.

To enable clients to carry on with leisure activities in their expected or future environments, the OTA should help them choose activities that are practical there as well as in the clinic or hospital. Impractical choices include crafts that require a special environment or expensive tools or materials or that are successful only if the client uses therapist-prepared materials.

Students and new graduates may wonder how best to respond in a leisure-focused program to clients whose projects have errors. The suggested approach is first to say something complimentary about the project or the effort that went into it and then offer a single suggestion for improvement. Some people may reject this advice; if so, that's fine. They may be more receptive tomorrow or next week. Others may seek further help. The important thing is that the experience should be pleasurable and successful in the client's view; too much criticism or advice from staff can sabotage the use of crafts as a leisure activity.

## Hobbies

In addition to crafts, hobbies that entail collecting or creating appeal to many. Model railroading, stamp and coin collecting, baseball card collecting, antiquing, doll collecting, scrapbooking, miniatures, bird watching, and other pastimes are not only entertaining but also intellectually challenging. Some of these hobbies provide opportunities to relate to others with similar interests through clubs, exhibitions, competitions, and special events. Specialized magazines addressing these interests may be found in local libraries and used to generate contacts and activities.

## The Arts

Painting, music, and literature are major sources of personal pleasure for many. Whether the involvement is receptive (viewing, listening, reading) or creative (making art by painting, dramatizing, playing an instrument, singing, or writing), these pastimes are valued for their capacity to create an alternative reality in which the day-to-day world recedes as the created world of the artist becomes the focal point of perception. In working with clients for whom these activities have been a source of pleasure in the past, the OTA should first assess why these pastimes have been abandoned. Clients who are or have been depressed may feel undeserving of the experience of beauty or may lack the energy to take the first step. The process of making art may invoke fear and hesitation for a variety of reasons (2, 21). The assistant may have to cajole, persuade, or otherwise entice the client to open a door. Interest and willingness can sometimes be facilitated by a trip to a museum, library, or musical performance. Clients with multiple roles and time management problems may need assistance to structure time for pleasure and will need support to make a personal commitment to the pursuit of such activities.

During the 1990s, reading groups became popular with the general public. Reading groups for clients with psychiatric disorders may serve several purposes in addition to the pleasure of reading:

- Improved literacy skills
- Increased concentration skills
- Opportunity to explore first-person accounts of mental illness
- Improved self-expression and group skills

## Gardening and Horticulture

Working with plants and the earth is deeply fulfilling to many people. It is interesting that gardening may be a more powerful aid to mental health than previously suspected; recent scientific research suggests that exposure to harmless soil microbes may alleviate depression (27). In inpatient settings and in cities the assistant must use ingenuity to provide gardening experiences. A successful program requires that plants be chosen carefully, based on the available light and the size of the pot or container. Gardening is an infinitely diverse activity with tremendous therapeutic potential. It can provide physical exercise (spading, planting seedlings, weeding) as well as intellectual stimulation (learning the names of plants, their needs for light and water and fertilizer, control of pests, methods of propagation, and so on). Horticulture can be structured as a prevocational experience, with assigned tasks such as transplanting seedlings, cleaning pots, watering, and the like. Helping plants grow can also fulfill an emotional and psychological need to nurture and create. It may also have a positive effect on life satisfaction and general well being (22).

## Other Connections to the Natural World

For clients who are not interested in gardening but who would like an experience of nature, there are many possibilities, such as hiking, trips to the beach or zoo, activities in the park, and trips to the mountains.

## Games

Like crafts, games have been used in occupational therapy since the beginning. They are seen as a way to learn about the world and how to function in it. Games can provide relaxation and socialization and promote the development of physical and cognitive skills. Which particular game should be used for a particular client and a particular purpose requires an analysis of the characteristics of the game and of the client's attitudes about play. It may be helpful to use Moore and Anderson's (19) three categories: games of chance, games of strategy, and puzzles. Moore and Anderson developed these categories to classify play experiences that help the child acquire knowledge and competency for real-life situations.

*Games of chance* provide experiences whose outcome is based mostly on luck. Bingo, which has long been very popular with some client groups, is an example. Games of chance give everyone an equal shot at winning, and those who lose know that it was not their fault they lost; varying educational and functional levels among clients cannot influence the outcome. Games of chance simulate real-life events that are random, unpredictable, and beyond the control of the individual. Some games of chance involve an element of skill or strategy—for example, the contestant can improve his or her chances to succeed at the popular game show *Wheel of Fortune* by his or her knowledge of words and spelling and by choosing the most common letters first.

*Games of strategy* give participants the opportunity to use skill and planning to influence the outcome. Such games have definite goals and rules, and the players each have a role. The outcome is determined by how the players interact. In this way games of strategy simulate real-life situations that involve interactions with other people. These games can be used to teach such basic social skills as following the rules, staying in one's role, being aware of the roles of others, negotiation, cooperation, and so on.

Two types of games of strategy appropriate for use in psychiatric settings are team sports, such as volleyball, softball, and relay races, and simulation games. Simulation games provide imaginary roles or situations to which the players try to respond. Commercially available simulation games include The Ungame, which encourages sharing of opinions, goals, and ideas; Roll-A-Role, in which players' roles are determined by the roll of large dice that have different roles on each side; and Scruples, in which players must respond to situations requiring tough ethical choices. Many computer games involve simulation. Generally these games are for single play and, therefore, are socially isolatingl but some allow two or more players to play together. For example, playing interactive fiction games can be a team effort. The goal of these games is to solve a puzzle, find treasure, or unravel a mystery. Some of them are so difficult that the help of many people is a necessity.

Several role simulation games that teach expressive and interpersonal skills and that require little or no equipment have been published in the social science literature (23, 26). A game like Balloon Debate (26), for example, can help develop self-expression; in this game each player chooses to be a famous person and then must prove to the others why he or she (rather than they) should be allowed to stay in the basket of a hot air balloon that will crash unless everyone but one person jumps overboard.

*Puzzles* provide an experience of discovery, exploration, and problem solving. Unlike games of strategy, puzzles have a definite outcome or solution that can be reached only by following a correct procedure. Puzzles thus simulate real-life situations in which the individual or group must analyze and deal with a problem such as changing a lock or putting a child's toy or piece of furniture or barbecue grill together.

Regardless of which type of game is used, it is up to the group leader to structure a therapeutic experience. This may mean, for example, minimizing the importance of winning and losing by emphasizing sportsmanship or team interaction or fun. In some games it is appropriate to discuss the concept of handicapping the more skilled players so as to give everyone an equal chance. Games can teach skills that are needed for the real-life situations they imitate. They can also increase a client's sense of mastery and competence; winning a game cannot make up for other losses, but it does provide a successful experience that can balance minor disappointments and frustrations.

### Sports and Exercise

In addition to team sports, discussed earlier, other physical activities may provide a leisure experience. These activities—which include individual sports, yoga, tai chi, qi gong, Pilates, calisthenics, and aerobics—often have other purposes, such as developing body awareness or sensory integrative skills or maintaining good physical and mental health or achieving integration of body and mind. Activities may have to be adapted when there are not sufficient numbers for a group (e.g., one-on-one basketball). For those who need to explore exercise options or understand how to make a commitment to exercise, the worksheets in Korb and associates (15) are useful. In some treatment facilities, many physical activities are provided by recreation therapists. The use of physical and sports activities to develop sensorimotor skills is discussed in Chapter 22.

For many, watching sporting events (normally a passive activity) provides opportunities for release of tension and for socialization with others. The experience of rooting for one's team and sharing an event with friends gives vent to emotions, promotes social identification, and provides material for discussion after the event.

## SOCIAL PARTICIPATION

Many people with mental health problems feel lonely yet are uncomfortable when they are with other people; in some cases they just do not know how to act or what is required of them or how to express what they want. Besides games and the social skills groups described in Chapter 3, many other activities can provide a social experience. Kuenstler (18) developed a format for a planning group for psychiatric clients that helped participants acquire social skills needed to plan and follow through on leisure activities. Behaviors such as asking for help from others and learning what to say and what not to say to other people were discussed, rehearsed, and reinforced in weekly meetings.

Other socialization experiences include parties, topical discussions, and community excursions. Planning a party requires the accomplishment of many small tasks that give everyone a chance to participate. Skills in leadership, negotiation, and compromise can also be exercised; this becomes educational and therapeutic when staff involve the group members in a discussion of the interactions that have occurred. Relating to others during a party at the treatment setting or clubhouse can serve as a rehearsal for life outside; it is important for staff to pay attention to clients' behaviors so they can follow up or give feedback later.

Discussion groups that focus on a general topic are a good way for clients to learn how to converse with other people. Generally, such groups are organized around a theme such as sports, current events, or music appreciation. The leader selects topics for each meeting or arranges for members to bring in topics; appropriate conversational behavior is taught by modeling and reinforcement during the discussion.

**POINT-OF-VIEW**

***People with schizophrenia tend not to look at the [other] person. . . . We're more easily distracted, and the other person's facial expressions can make it difficult to focus on what we are trying to say. Because we're slower to process information our recognition of what the other person says is often delayed.***

—Fred Frese (8)

- Dr. Frese recommends that consumers explain this and other cognitive and sensory problems of schizophrenia to new acquaintances so they will understand the peculiar behaviors that may occur. What do you think of this suggestion? Is it helpful, neutral, or potentially problematic?

Some clients require a more structured and individualized approach. Basic skills for social interaction and conversation can be taught by a four-step method: coaching (motivation), behavior modeling (demonstration), behavior rehearsal (practice), and feedback. This approach was discussed in Chapter 3. Instruction should focus on the basic skills of starting and ending conversations, asking for or giving help, listening, and responding (14). Clients may need instruction and feedback about the nuances of nonverbal behavior, such as eye contact, minimal response, body language, and maintaining appropriate body distance. Excellent resources are available for sequencing instruction in social and conversational skills (3, 14, 28) and for developing nonverbal communication skills (3, 23, 26). In any program that aims to develop clients' social and self-expressive skills, the OTA works under the supervision and guidance of the OT.

## SUMMARY

Being able to choose and enjoy leisure activities is essential to health. People with mental health problems sometimes have difficulty using their spare time to meet their leisure needs. Occupational therapists and assistants can help them select meaningful leisure activities, schedule time for leisure, and explore new leisure experiences. These therapeutic services may also be provided by recreation therapists.

## REVIEW QUESTIONS AND ACTIVITIES

1. Define *leisure* and describe its purpose.
2. Define *social participation.*
3. In what ways do leisure and social interaction overlap? In what ways are they distinct from each other?
4. Identify three aspects of leisure.
5. Explain why it is important for the client to select his or her leisure activities rather than allowing someone else to do this.
6. How can the OTA facilitate the client to identify possible leisure interests to explore?
7. Why might leisure be a problem area for someone with a mental disorder?
8. Give examples of active and passive activities and explain the effects of each type.
9. Identify three factors that should be considered when counseling clients about leisure.
10. Discuss the advantages and disadvantages of crafts as leisure activities.
11. Explain what you would do if a client doing a craft for leisure enjoyment made an error. What is the reasoning behind your action?
12. Discuss the advantages and disadvantages of games as leisure activities.
13. What factors would you consider in recommending or selecting a game for a client?
14. Discuss the advantages and disadvantages of gardening and horticulture as leisure activities.
15. Discuss the advantages and disadvantages of social activities as leisure.
16. Write a short essay detailing how you would help someone in the area of social participation.
17. Discuss the advantages and disadvantages of sports and exercise as leisure activities.
18. *Challenge question:* Imagine that your supervisor has asked you to develop a leisure activity program for each of the following cases: Hilary Page (Appendix A, Case 1), Mrs. Anderson (Appendix A, Case 2), Mr. Velasquez (Appendix A, Case 4), Howard (Chapter 3). Describe how you would go about designing such a program for each client and what it might include.

## REFERENCES


1. American Occupational Therapy Association. Occupational therapy practice framework: Domain and process. Am J Occup Ther 2002;56:609–639.
2. Bayles D, Orland T. Art & Fear—Observations on the Perils (and Rewards) of Artmaking. Santa Barbara, CA: Capra Press, 1993.
3. Bellack AS, Mueser KT, Gingerich S, Agresta J. Social Skills Training for Schizophrenia. New York: Guilford, 1997.
4. Charmaz K. The self as habit: The reconstruction of self in chronic illness. Occup Ther J Res 2000;2:31S–41S.
5. Crist P, Davis CG, Coffin PS. The effects of employment and mental health status on the balance of work, play/leisure, self-care, and rest. Occup Ther Ment Health 2000;15(2):27–42.
6. Csikszentimihalyi M. Finding Flow: The Psychology of Engagement with Everyday Life. New York: Basic Books, 1997.
7. Farnworth L. Time use and leisure occupations of young offenders. Am J Occup Ther 2000;54:315–325.
8. Frese F. Coping with Schizophrenia Requires Effort. Available at: fredfrese.com/?q=node/view/2&PHPSESSID=6e4a85f28fd6311d15bde3d1433ffbca. Accessed July 2007.
9. Haertl K, Minato M. Daily occupations of persons with mental illness: Themes from Japan and America. Occ Ther Ment Health 2006;22(1):19–32.
10. Hemphill BJ, Peterson CQ, Werner PC. Rehabilitation in Mental Health: Goals and Objectives for Independent Living. Thorofare, NJ: Slack, 1991.
11. Howie L, Coulter M, Feldman S. Crafting the self: Older persons' narratives of occupational identity. Am J Occup Ther 2004;58:446–454.
12. Hughes PL, Mullins L. Acute Psychiatric Care: An Occupational Therapy Guide to Exercises in Daily Living Skills. Thorofare, NJ: Slack, 1981.
13. Ivarsson AB, Carlsson M, Sidenvall B. Performance of occupations in daily life among individuals with severe mental disorders. Occup Ther Ment Health 2004;20(2):33–50.
14. Kartin NJ, Van Schroeder C. Adult Psychiatric Life Skills Manual. Kailua, HI: Schroeder Publishing, 1982.
15. Korb KL, Azok AD, Leutenberg EA. Life Management Skills: Reproducible Activity Handouts Created for Facilitators. Beachwood, OH: Wellness Reproductions, 1989.
16. Korb KL, Azok AD, Leutenberg EA. Life Management Skills: 2. Reproducible Activity Handouts Created for Facilitators. Beachwood, OH: Wellness Reproductions, 1991.
17. Korb-Khalsa KL, Leutenberg EA. Life Management Skills: 4. Reproducible Activity Handouts Created for Facilitators. Beachwood, OH: Wellness Reproductions, 1996.
18. Kuenstler G. A planning group for psychiatric outpatients. Am J Occup Ther 1976;30:634–639.
19. Moore OK, Anderson AR. Some principles for the design of clarifying educational environments. In: Goslin DA, ed. Handbook of Socialization Theory and Research. Chicago: Rand McNally, 1969.
20. Nahmias R, Froelich J. Women's mental health: Implications for occupational therapy. Am J Occup Ther 1993; 47:35–41.
21. Orland T. The View from the Studio Door—How Artists Find Their Way in an Uncertain World. Santa Cruz, CA: Image Continuum, 2006.
22. Perrins-Margalis NM, Rugletic J, Schepis NM, et al. The immediate effects of a group-based horticulture experience on the quality of life of persons with chronic mental illness. Occup Ther Ment Health 2000;16:15–32.
23. Pfeiffer JW, Jones JE, eds. A Handbook of Structured Experiences for Human Relations Training. Vols 1-10. La Jolla, CA: University Associates, 1977–1985.
24. Precin P. Living Skills Recovery Workbook. Boston MA: Butterworth Heinemann, 1999.
25. Primeau LA. Work and leisure: Transcending the dichotomy. Am J Occup Ther 1996;50:569–577.
26. Remocker AJ, Storch ET. Action Speaks Louder: A Handbook of Nonverbal Group Techniques. 3rd ed. Edinburgh, UK: Churchill Livingstone, 1982.
27. Than K. Depressed? Go Play in the Dirt. Available at: www.livescience.com/humanbiology/070411_happy_bacteria.html. Accessed May 2007.
28. Weaver RL. Understanding Interpersonal Conversation. Glenview, IL: Scott, Foresman, 1981.


## SUGGESTED READINGS


Carlson J. Complementary Therapies and Wellness—Practice Essentials for Holistic Health Care. Upper Saddle River, NJ: Prentice Hall, 2003.

Erikson JM. Activity, Recovery, Growth: The Communal Role of Planned Activities. New York: Norton, 1976.

CHAPTER 21

# Management of Emotional Needs: Self-Awareness Skills and Coping Strategies

***There is an art to facing difficulties in ways that lead to effective solutions and to inner peace and harmony.***

JON KABAT-ZINN (19)

## CHAPTER OBJECTIVES

After studying this chapter, the reader will be able to:

1. Discuss the relationship between management of emotional needs and engagement in occupation.
2. Identify a unique role for occupational therapy in interventions related to management of emotional needs.
3. Identify and define aspects of self-awareness.
4. Identify and describe a variety of approaches to management of emotional needs, including self expression, stress management, time management, assertiveness training, anger management, and mindfulness practices.

Occupational performance extends beyond the mechanical aspects of carrying out tasks. The social interactions and the feelings with which activities are done also require attention. This chapter provides an overview of *management of emotional needs* to support successful engagement in occupation. Two main aspects are addressed: self-awareness and coping skills. Although not expressly included in the *Occupational Therapy Practice Framework (OTPF)* (2), these concepts have long been a part of occupational therapy practice in mental health. Within the *OTPF*, the reader may find related information within the client factors, classified within the subcategory of mental functions as *emotional functions*. Some related information is also classified within performance. And some is classified within contexts (cultural, personal, spiritual).

## NEEDS

All creatures have needs. Successful functioning depends on recognizing and gratifying needs without unduly compromising the needs of others. Many persons with psychiatric disorders have difficulty identifying and expressing their needs. Those unable to identify, express, or gratify needs may resort to impulsive acting out of unrecognized feelings. Or they may feel deadness or dullness in their attachment to reality, as if living out a sentence on earth rather than making a life for oneself. A useful approach to understanding needs was developed by Abraham Maslow (32). Maslow's hierarchy of needs consists of five levels, built upon each other, so that the lower levels must be satisfied before the higher levels (although in some individuals the higher-level needs at times take precedence). The lowest level, *physiological*, refers to needs for food, shelter, sleep, sex, exercise, light, and air. *Safety* needs are at the second level; these include psychological as well as physical safety. At the third level are *love and belongingness* needs; these are the needs to be accepted and loved as a unique human being, unconditionally for what one is. The fourth level is for *esteem* needs, or the need to be recognized by others. *Self-actualization*, or the need to accomplish personal goals, is at the fifth level (Fig. 21-1).

White (40) identified a need for *mastery* or *competence*, which includes the desire to explore and make sense of the world, to control one's environment, and to make a difference. This may be seen as an aspect of esteem and self-actualization needs or as separate.

Intimately connected with needs are feelings and emotions. Frustration of needs results in frustrated emotions (anger, depression, fear, boredom, withdrawal, irritability). Need gratification may result in positive emotions (happiness, elation, contentment, pride, relief) but may generate mixed feelings (guilt, indecision, regret, confusion) when needs are in conflict. The failure to monitor, recognize, accept, and examine one's feelings and needs impoverishes life and often contributes to a negative cycle of acting out without understanding the reasons for one's actions.

While the development of awareness of one's own needs and emotions is primarily the province of trained psychotherapists, it is also an important aspect of occupational functioning and thus is a concern of occupational therapy practitioners.

## OCCUPATIONAL THERAPY'S DOMAIN OF CONCERN

Throughout this chapter we will examine areas of treatment that overlap with those of other professions. To avoid confusion in presenting our skills and expertise both to clients and to other mental health practitioners, it is useful to review some of the differences between occupational therapy and the other health professions. First, occupational therapy practitioners are concerned primarily with how people function in their daily life activities and occupations. Interventions we make related to psychological and psychosocial skills aim to

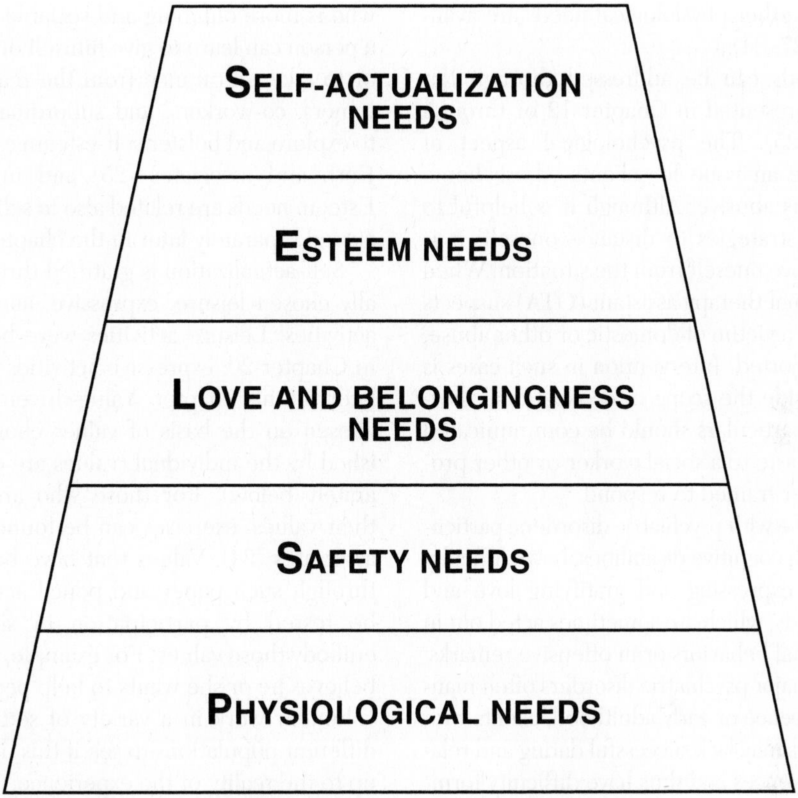


**Figure 21-1. Maslow's hierarchy of needs.** (Reprinted with permission from Maslow A. Toward a Psychology of Being. Princeton, NJ: Van Nostrand, 1962.)

improve clients' ability to function in work, home life, school, leisure, and other occupational areas. Second, ours is a "doing" therapy more than a "talking" therapy. While we *do* discuss with clients the problems in their lives, and while we do present much information verbally, the main vehicle for therapeutic intervention in occupational therapy is activities. Third, because of both historical and reimbursement-driven factors, we tend to provide treatment for mental health problems in groups rather than individually. Thus some techniques may be limited to those that can be presented in a group format. Often, for specific skills such as time management or stress management, we use a psychoeducational approach (see Chapter 3), in which we employ a classroom style for delivering information and engaging clients in classwork and homework to apply it to themselves. We generally do not, therefore, use techniques that require long-term one-on-one verbal interaction. This is not to say that we do not take the individual into account; we individualize therapy by fine-tuning our general approach to the person's presenting problems and occupational performance issues.

Earlier chapters present much information on activities that gratify physiological needs (see Chapters 18, 19, 20). In addition, for clients having difficulty in specific areas, worksheets and exercises to examine sleep, exercise, healthy lifestyles, and other physiological needs are available (24, 26, 27, 34).

Safety needs can be addressed through the information presented in Chapter 12 or through worksheets (25). The psychological aspect of safety may be an issue for clients whose home environment is abusive. Although it is helpful to learn coping strategies to distance oneself, it is better to remove oneself from the situation. When the occupational therapy assistant (OTA) suspects that a client is a victim of domestic or other abuse, it must be reported. Intervention in such cases is generally outside the scope of occupational therapy, and the particulars should be communicated with utmost haste to a social worker or other professional better trained to respond.

Some people with psychiatric disorders, particularly those with cognitive disabilities, have difficulty appropriately expressing and gratifying love and belonging needs, which are sometimes acted out in impulsive sexual behaviors or in offensive remarks. Because the major psychiatric disorders often manifest in adolescence or early adulthood, clients with these disorders may lack successful dating and relationship experiences and thus have difficulty forming intimate relationships. Social skills training (see Chapter 3) and role plays can help illustrate the difference between behavior that is appropriate and likely to succeed and that which is not.

Esteem needs are generally met through work and related activities (see Chapter 19). However, other problems in gratifying esteem needs have to do with a mismatch between the esteem desired and the source from which it is sought. For example, a woman may desire respect from her family for her work as an artist. But if the family places low value on artistic work, preferring scientific or academic or business careers, the desired esteem may not be forthcoming. Thus sometimes people have to learn to look elsewhere for esteem. This might involve, for someone who desires praise from a gruff and business-like boss, recognizing the need to find a new job working for someone who is more outgoing and sociable. Alternatively, a person can learn to give himself or herself praise or to take nurturance from the reactions of customers, co-workers, and subordinates. Exercises to explore and bolster self-esteem can be found in Korb and associates (25) and in Precin (34). Esteem needs are related also to self-concept, discussed separately later in the chapter.

Self-actualization is gratified through individually chosen leisure, expressive, and value-driven activities. Leisure activities were been discussed in Chapter 20; expressive activities are presented later in this chapter. Value-driven activities are chosen on the basis of values chosen and cherished by the individual (values are discussed separately below). For those who are unaware of their values, exercises can be found in Korb and associates (24). Values that have been identified through such paper and pencil activities should be tested by participation in situations that embody those values. For example, someone who believes he or she wants to help people might try volunteer work in a variety of settings and with different populations to see if this desire will hold up to the reality of the experience.

Mastery needs are best met through experiences that permit practice, repetition, and experimentation. To learn to do something well requires time and opportunity. Once the preferred activity has been identified, the client can be helped to achieve a feeling of competence by scheduling repeated and prolonged experiences, assisted by someone who can provide feedback and suggestions. It is important for the staff member to tailor the activity to maintain the experience of challenge without going beyond the client's limits and endurance to the point of failure. For those who catastrophize or evaluate experiences in black-and-white, either-or terms, group discussion may be valuable to help the person to put failure in perspective and to accept occasional setbacks as an inevitable and educational aspect of the journey toward competence.

## SELF-AWARENESS

Three aspects of self-awareness will be discussed (values, interests, and self-concept). Values and interests are addressed to some extent in Chapters 4, 19, and 20.

### Values

Kielhofner (21) defines values as "what one finds important and meaningful" (p. 15). While some people have clear understanding of their own values, this is not always the case. *Values clarification* is an approach to helping individuals and groups understand their values. Worksheet exercises (24, 27) can be completed individually but are perhaps more effective in a group format, as members can give and receive feedback and refine their thinking in response. Another approach to helping someone identify or clarify values might be a discussion of a theme or a videotape or reading. Clients can be encouraged to enact their values by scheduling and participating in an activity or event that represents those values. For example, a client who feels that helping other people is important might arrange to volunteer in a library or a homeless shelter.

### Interests

Interests are "what one finds enjoyable or satisfying to do" (21, p. 53). Like values, interests are developed from experience. The OTA can help clients to identify interests by using interest checklists, such as the one given in Figure 15-5, but clients must recognize and have some sense of the activities listed for this to be useful. Alternately, the OTA can encourage and assist the client to identify and participate in activities in the community and to acquire experience and preferences in this way. Clients should be encouraged to express whether they liked or disliked a given experience and to talk about the activities at length so that they increase their understanding of their choices.

### Self-Concept

*Self-concept* is "the composite of ideas, feelings, and attitudes that a person has about his or her own identity, worth, capabilities, and limitations" (1). This includes ideas, beliefs, feelings and attitudes about the physical, emotional, and sexual self. Self-concept is acquired through interactions with others and the environment. Childhood experiences and the responses and opinions of family and peers contribute to the development of self-concept. Thus self-concept is deeply held and not easily changed.

Paradoxically, people are not always aware of their ideas and attitudes about themselves. Furthermore, the self-concept may include both positive and negative valuations. Negative valuations tend to undermine effective engagement in occupation because they set up an expectation of failure and this can become a self-fulfilling prophecy. The person internally believes, "I can't do this; I've never been any good at this," and sure enough, the person fails.

Occupational therapy practitioners seek to enable successful engagement in occupation. To do this we sometimes must help the client recognize a negative aspect of the self-concept that is undermining the ability to function. Once it is recognized, the client may have a revelatory experience and be able to change behavior simply because he or she recognizes how limiting and false the negative valuation has been. However, the client may not appreciate that the negative valuation is incorrect, and then it is necessary to help the client challenge the negativity. Cognitive-behavioral approaches (see Chapter 2) are particularly effective.

As should be clear, interventions related to self-concept must address both *self-awareness* (understanding the self) and *self-esteem* (valuing the self). Workbook exercises (24–27, 34) can be used one-on-one or in groups. However, there is some danger that clients will respond only superficially to a workbook exercise. Deeper and more lasting benefit can be achieved if the OTA consciously and deliberately attends to the client's performance of an activity and to what the client says about that performance and then guides the client by gentle questioning to consider whether the client's statements are accurate.

## ISSUES RELATED TO ENGAGEMENT IN OCCUPATION

The ability to participate effectively in the occupations of ones choice is affected by habits and roles, communication skills, and in particular by the ability to assert and express oneself.

### Patterns: Role Performance

Roles are defined in the *OTPF* as "a set of behaviors that have some socially agreed upon function and for which there is an accepted code of norms" (2, p. 623). Many ordinary people complain of *role stress* (a feeling that one cannot meet the expectations of one's roles) and *role conflict* (a feeling that one's roles are in conflict). Worksheets related to roles, role stress, and role conflict are available (24, 26). A psychoeducational approach is effective, as is a group format. It is particularly helpful for clients to see that others experience the same demands and feelings of inadequacy and that steps can be taken to change or to accept the situation.

### Social Conduct: Communication and Interaction Skills

The *OTPF* (2) gives considerable detail that will assist the OTA in analyzing the social behaviors that together make up communication and interaction. The concepts of physicality (the body language of communication), information exchange (the delivery of communication), and relations may seem abstract until you apply them to a client who is having difficulty in this area. Social success requires complex interrelated semiautomatic skills such as gesturing, use of physical space, listening and responding, and applying the manners and social customs that match the situation. The social skills training section of Chapter 3 and the socialization and communication section of Chapter 20 consider several aspects of social conduct. Gentle and specific feedback given immediately following a social interaction is most effective. Workbook exercises can also be used (25–27, 34).

It is important to analyze very carefully the performance of clients who demonstrate deficiencies in social conduct. Frequently, the client "knows" the desired behavior but misreads environmental cues and thus fails to choose the effective behavior for achieving the desired result. The OTA must engage the client in a discussion of what was happening and what the client perceived. Only by repeated experience, with the OTA providing friendly observation and feedback, will the client be able to differentiate the signs and contexts of different environments and choose the effective behavioral response.

There are many ways to communicate—verbally and nonverbally, clearly and confusedly, directly and obliquely, effectively and ineffectively. Clients with mental health problems may need assistance to learn to communicate effectively so others will help them meet their needs. Again, it is important to recognize that occupational therapy should be concerned with these skills only where they directly affect the person's occupational functioning. More general treatment of need expression falls under the scope of psychotherapy rather than occupational therapy.

A variety of media and approaches have been used. Role plays and small group discussions are the most common. Hemphill and associates (16) provide a list of step-by-step goals for this area. Videotape is a popular medium for facilitating self-expression and personal awareness (15, 17). Clients can create and record their own dramas; if done as a group activity, this can develop communication and group interaction skills as well as personal expression. Video can also be used to teach social functioning. Clients can watch videotaped models of effective social skills and discuss what is effective about them. More important, they can review and analyze their own recorded behaviors to identify their strengths and weaknesses and select areas for change. Alternatively, Korb and associates (24) and Precin (34) provide worksheets for understanding and communicating verbally and nonverbally. Regardless of the medium used, it is most important to help clients analyze their own behavior, to understand what worked and what didn't, and to formulate a plan for the next social encounter.

## Assertiveness

Assertiveness is the ability to state one's needs, thoughts, and feelings in an appropriate, direct, and honest way (11). When one reflects on the life experience of persons with psychiatric disorders, one quickly appreciates how repeated hospitalization and involvement with the mental health system may thwart personal assertiveness. Thus clients may need to learn or relearn these skills. Assertiveness is often taught through a structured set of exercises in assertiveness training (18, 24, 25, 34). The usual format is to begin by defining assertiveness, usually by illustration, in a variety of social encounters. The next step is to help clients identify their own assertiveness patterns. This may be done through a questionnaire or a diary or log. Next, obstacles to assertiveness (fear, shyness, self-doubt) are identified and tackled. Specific assertive strategies and behaviors are taught and practiced in hypothetical role plays. Then participants are asked to put these strategies to use in their own lives and to keep records in a diary. Experiences are reported to the group, which engages the members in problem-solving and feedback.

## Self-Expression

*Self-expression* is showing, demonstrating, or revealing ones thoughts, feelings, and needs. Self-expression assumes some awareness of self. For a variety of reasons, many clients need help in this area. Some have experienced extreme emotional deprivation as children and, therefore, habitually turn off or ignore their feelings. Others, because of the symptoms of their disease, tend to extremes of emotion (euphoria and despair) and lack appreciation of the subtle distinctions of emotions in the middle range (e.g., contentment, serenity, satisfaction, confusion, mischievousness, shyness, boredom). Korb and associates (24) give some paper and pencil exercises to develop and expand the ability to identify emotions.

In addition, occupational therapy has always included creative activities that help clients express their inner thoughts, feelings, beliefs, anxieties, and perceptions. Depending on their purpose and the needs of the client, these activities may be used to teach basic communication skills or leisure and social skills. More typically, however, they are used to develop the clients' self-concept and self-identity, their awareness of themselves and of their own feelings and needs (3). Activities from the arts are most often used, although communication games and exercises can be used effectively also. Settings that have large numbers of staff may employ creative arts therapists to run these expressive activities. Creative art therapists have special training in one or more of the arts, such as dance, music, art, or poetry, and in how to use the arts as therapy.

Graphic and fine arts media, such as drawing, painting, collage, and clay, are familiar to most people from experiences in school and during childhood. These media are unstructured and can feel overwhelming and complex unless the OTA imposes some structure. The client may be totally paralyzed if presented with numerous choices, unfamiliar tools and materials, and a blank canvas or lump of clay. Adults may feel insecure or anxious about engaging in art because they feel their work will be seen as childish or unsophisticated or because they fear it will be analyzed for unconscious content.

One approach is to provide structured paired or group activities with a specific procedure, purpose, or theme. For example, in Pass-A-Drawing (36) each participant draws something to represent himself or herself; the drawings are passed around the room so that everyone has an opportunity to add to everyone else's drawing. Discussion focuses on why people sometimes see each other differently from the way they see themselves. As another possible activity, each person can trace his or her hands on a piece of paper, labeling one of them "present" and the other "future"; the clients then draw in the hands the things that they believe they have now and the things they would like to have in the future. Clients in turn discuss their drawings with the group.

Creative writing and the study and appreciation of the written word can also be used expressively in occupational therapy groups. Clients can perform plays or write and act out their own, thus learning not only to express ideas but also to identify with the emotions of a particular role. Those who are too self-conscious to act out a role themselves may enjoy using puppets to express their feelings and ideas (37). Groups that work with poetry may include both appreciation and writing; writing a poem can be an individual or group project.[1] Keeping a daily journal can give clients a structure to record and explore what happens in their lives and how they react to situations and experiences; when clients later review what they have written, they may see patterns that they otherwise might not have recognized. For example, clients may learn that they get depressed around family holidays or that episodes of tension and outbursts at home tend to follow disappointments at work.

Another valuable writing exercise is life review (22, 35). Most often used with older adults, life review consists of the recording of a personal biography. Going over the events of one's past and thinking about the things one has done can help the depressed older adult resolve the developmental crisis of ego integrity versus despair (see Chapter 2) by revealing that his or her life did indeed have meaning, purpose, and direction. Volunteers can assist those who are unable to write. Alternatively, tape recorders can be used.

Playing musical instruments or moving to music through dance or exercise can help those who are unable to express themselves verbally. Keeping the beat or creating one's own beat with a rhythm instrument is an example. It is not a good idea, however, to make a practice of having music on continuously in the background during all different kinds of occupational therapy groups. Although music can serve as a kind of acoustical wallpaper to create a mood, not everyone enjoys it, and some find it distracting. Music and dance are often used in sensorimotor activity groups, discussed in Chapter 22.

## SELF-MANAGEMENT SKILLS

Coping skills, time management, and self-control help one balance one's own needs and feelings with the demands of life and time.

### Coping Skills

*Coping* is "a process by which a person deals with stress, solves problems, and makes decisions" (1). Many practitioners use a cognitive-behavioral approach (see Chapter 2) to teach or enhance coping skills. In this approach what matters is what the client *believes* and *thinks* about the situation and how capable the client feels. In other words, whether one can cope or not depends very much on how one evaluates or *appraises* the problem and one's own resources (12, 13).

It is not enough to try to persuade clients that they are capable of dealing with situations that challenge them. Direct experience in performing challenging activities or dealing effectively with troubling situations is much more effective (13). Thus the client who steadfastly maintains that he or she is not ready to return to work is unlikely to be convinced by the OTA's repeated reassurances that the client has sufficient concentration and skills to

[1] Ideas on how to structure exercises for a poetry writing group can be adapted from those in Koch (23).

do so. It would be best for the OTA to help the client set up a trial experience (e.g., for the client to go to work for half a day or a day only) so that the client can appraise his or her own readiness.

## Stress Management

Most readers recognize the experience of stress, yet the condition is hard to define. Stress occurs when a threat is perceived. The threat, or stressor, may be a life event (marriage, birth of a child, death of a parent), an environmental factor (hurricane, economic recession), a hassle or series of hassles (having to run out to buy milk, a child staying home from school, a parking ticket, a challenging examination or school assignment), or the individual personality style in reaction to normal events (e.g., a tendency to catastrophize or to be hypervigilant). Stress that is not effectively managed in time leads to a variety of problems—physical illnesses (such as cardiovascular disease and asthma and intestinal disorders) and mental symptoms (such as irritability, depression, mood swings, and impulsivity) (4).

Cotton (9) provides a thorough analysis and description of stress and techniques for stress management. She divides these into techniques that are *problem focused,* that aim to change the stressful situation, and those that are *emotion focused,* that aim to change the stress response to the situation. For each of these two areas, she further delineates techniques based on whether the focus of intervention is primarily physiological (aimed at the body's stress response), cognitive (aimed at the negative thoughts), or behavioral (aimed at the actions taken by the patient). The attentive reader will immediately recognize that occupational therapy, with its activity orientation, will most likely employ techniques that are behavioral in their focus. Because activities are rarely simple or one-dimensional, we will see that these techniques also affect the physiological and cognitive processes.

Some of these techniques have already been mentioned in this and earlier chapters. Exercise, particularly aerobic exercise, seems to yield improved responses to stress. Breathing and progressive muscle relaxation, yoga, meditation, and stretching exercises also reduce stress (4). All of these techniques affect the physiological response and provide an activity focus that diverts attention from cognitive ruminations over stressful events. Assertiveness training and anger management training can also mediate stress by increasing skills in recognizing and dealing with feelings and needs.

A format that seems popular in the occupational therapy literature is the *psychoeducational stress management group,* in which patients are instructed in the effects of stress and in personal stress analysis and stress management. This approach creates step-by-step change by first helping individuals identify what they find stressful and how their own stress response manifests itself. Then techniques for changing one's response to stress in terms of how one thinks, feels, and acts can be presented one by one and can be applied in homework assignments and reported in a diary or log. An outline for such a group can be found in Cotton (9, p. 16), and a more detailed description is given in Courtney and Escobedo (10). Exercises in Korb and associates (23, 24) Korb-Khalsa and associates (26), and Korb-Khalsa and Leutenberg (27) provide structure for teaching and reinforcing specific aspects of stress management, such as the use of diversional activity, problem solving, and putting things in perspective. Stein (38) provides a short and practical guide. The popular press also offers many books on this topic (6, 19, 20).

Perhaps the most widely available and effective stress management technique is the use of *social supports,* people and institutions that may help by providing feedback, socialization, information, and material support. A single parent may, for example, benefit from meeting with other parents, either formally in a group or self-help format or informally at the playground or in the neighborhood. Interaction with other parents provides the opportunity to confirm and validate feelings, to learn others' parenting strategies, and to work out play dates and child care swaps. An isolated elderly person may blossom if given the opportunity to meet with peers in a social situation or to work as a volunteer. In addition, people in all sorts of situations may obtain relief from stressful situations by investigating and using resources in their own communities, such as YMCA, YWCA, and other organizations.

Brief descriptions of other stress management techniques are found in Table 21-1. The reader is cautioned as follows in regard to some of these stress management techniques:

- Clients must have medical clearance to engage in aerobic exercise.
- Any exercise done with closed eyes may increase psychosis; do not use these techniques with clients who are actively psychotic or who have a history of psychosis.
- Yoga and tai chi require study; practitioners who wish to use these with clients should first obtain certification as a practitioner and teacher of the discipline.
- Some yoga asanas (poses) are contraindicated for specific medical problems. Clients should be advised to find a certified teacher and to share pertinent health information.
- Biofeedback requires knowledge of electrical machines and their operation; it is not an entry-level technique. Use of biofeedback requires established service competency and occupational therapist (OT) supervision.

**TABLE 21-1 STRESS MANAGEMENT TECHNIQUES**

| TECHNIQUE | DESCRIPTION |
|---|---|
| Verbalization | Talking out one's problems, preferably with a neutral or supportive listener |
| Humor | Laughter and facial expressions associated with humor; believed to promote release of endorphins (neurotransmitters that produce pleasurable feelings) |
| Regular and sufficient sleep | Sleep on a regular schedule to prepare the body to cope with stress |
| Proper nutrition | Conscious consumption of foods that are nutritious and not harmful (e.g., eat a balanced diet, avoid stimulants like caffeine) |
| Aerobic activity | Exercise or sports activity that requires an aerobic level of exertion, releasing physical tension and increasing levels of endorphins |
| Meditation | Mental exercise that entails quiet sitting for a period to empty the mind or just quietly observe the mind's activity |
| Progressive relaxation | Method of systematically tensing and releasing muscles in successive body parts to promote relaxation; generally done with eyes closed |
| Visualization or guided imagery | Sitting or lying with closed eyes and imagining a pleasant scene or cherished goal; audiotapes often used |
| Yoga | Physical and spiritual discipline that promotes relaxation through stretching, physical postures, awareness and control of the breath |
| Tai chi | Physical and spiritual discipline that promotes relaxation through guided movements and quiet breathing |
| Biofeedback | Use of a machine to feed back to the person information about some measure of physiological stress (e.g., galvanic skin response) |

## Managing Grief and Loss

Sometimes life deals a blow in the form of loss of something that we never expected to be taken from us. Whether the loss is of a family member or friend, a pet, a job, the possibility of future pregnancies, or a normal life span, the response is the same. Grief and loss derail normal activities with turbulent and distracting emotions that demand attention and that interfere with business as usual. The typical dysfunctional pattern of responding to grief is to deny it, or stuff it. This does not remove the pain. Grief settles in the body and spirit and may manifest as physical symptoms, cognitive deficits, and other impairments. Constructive, honest, and self-respecting techniques for responding to loss must often be learned. Korb and associates (25) give some exercises that can be useful. The life review activities suggested earlier in this chapter can also be used to express and release feelings of loss.

## Mindfulness Practices

Mindfulness practices provide another route to self-awareness and self-control. Mindfulness practices teach acceptance and self-restraint. Jon Kabat-Zinn (20) defines mindfulness as "paying attention in a particular way: on purpose, in the present moment and non-judgmentally" (p. 4). Mindfulness brings one back to the present and keeps one focused on the here and now. Practicing mindfulness reveals that daydreaming and dwelling on the past are empty of meaning because they are not real. Through mindfulness practice, one can appreciate that the way things are is the way that they are, and that this is okay. The practice of mindfulness helps reduce the compulsion to change things, improves tolerance of discomfort, and cultivates a sense of contentment.

Linehan (30, 31) employs mindfulness skills as a core element of dialectical behavior therapy (DBT), used primarily for treatment of persons with borderline personality disorder (BPD). Like the other impulse control disorders, BPD is characterized by acting on uncomfortable feelings without exploring or understanding what the feelings are (the opposite of self-awareness). Persons with BPD cut and otherwise mutilate themselves and have a high risk of suicide. When a person with BPD learns mindfulness, she is more equipped to identify her feelings and to "sit with the feeling" than to act out in self-destructive behavior.

Mindfulness has applications with psychiatric disorders and with adjusting to physical pain, to loss, and to death. It helps reduce the urge to change things, helps contain the impulses to act out feelings, and aids in acceptance. A simple and concise explanation of mindfulness practice by Braza (5) is a good place for the interested reader to start. Books by the American Buddhist nun, Pema Chodron, provide additional practice ideas (7, 8).

How can the occupational therapy practitioner apply mindfulness practices for persons with psychiatric disabilities? The most basic and important way is to help the client to become and remain present in the performance of a task. Being present leads to noticing, observing, reflecting, being contented,

**POINT-OF-VIEW**

***So, now I know that when I'm really depressed I just tell myself, "I know that this is just my mood right now," and I know that I will get out of it. . . . [W]hen it starts to feel endless I have to remind myself that it's only going to last for a while.***

—Belinda, quoted by Fran Babiss (3, p. 81)

- The consumer is describing a coping strategy she learned as part of DBT. What would you call this strategy?
- How could you help a client learn such a strategy?
- What other kinds of problems could this strategy be helpful for?

and appreciating that doing is being. It takes the client away from thoughts such as comparing self to others, comparing present self to past self, worrying about future outcomes, and the like. Helping the client to be present requires that the OTA attend to the client's experience of the task and to listen to what the client is saying both in words and in body language. The OTA might ask, "What are you thinking about now? Are you paying attention to what you are doing, or are you getting ahead of yourself or thinking about something else?" The OTA may also redirect the client: "Focus all of your mind on what you are doing. Try not to think about other things." Preparing a peanut butter sandwich while practicing mindfulness lets one truly see the bread, the jelly, the peanut butter, the knife, the motions involved, and so on. One becomes receptive to the quality of the air, the light, the cool smooth hardness of the knife, the softness of the bread, the fluid spreading of the peanut butter, and all aspects of things as they really are. Mindfulness opens a path to complete engagement in occupation.

## Time Management

It was Benjamin Franklin who coined the phrase Time is money." Although time may not translate into money for patients who are not gainfully employed, nonetheless time is like money in that there is a fixed amount of it in each day and in each person's life. However we spend it, once spent, it is gone forever; understanding the value of time and knowing how to make the best use of it are important aspects of mental health.

Time management requires that one recognize one's values and priorities, structure a daily routine, schedule one's time, and organize tasks efficiently. Both skills and habits are necessary. Clients may need help with time management for a variety of reasons. The first is that the sense of time itself is sometimes distorted by psychiatric illness, especially organic illness. Patients may perceive time as long and stretched out, seemingly endless. The future may seem bleak, empty, or incomprehensible. The second reason is that having one's daily habits disrupted by a long illness or hospitalization or retirement or the death of a spouse may make previously familiar routines feel odd and awkward. Third, some clients have developed ineffective time habits; they may be chronically late for things, never have time for leisure, or spend long hours in unproductive activity (taking drugs, drinking, gambling, watching television).

When working with clients' use of time, it is critically important to remember that time use must reflect personal values and that the values of the client may be different from those of the therapist. Another consideration is that some individuals with severe cognitive disabilities cannot be expected to manage their own time. Any time management program should begin with an assessment of how the person uses time; the *Barth Time Construction* (see Chapter 14) is probably the best assessment because the contrasting colors give clients direct feedback about how they allocate their time among various activities. Other areas that should be assessed include clients' values and goals and how these are (or more frequently are not) reflected in their use of time.[2] Clients who have trouble identifying values and goals might be asked to write a future biography, in which they describe what they will be doing at some point in the future.

A frequent complaint heard from persons who are stressed is that they don't have enough time. This complaint should be taken seriously because the subjective experiences is legitimate. Since occupational therapy assistants, like everyone else, have to manage time, some strategies are given in Chapter 25. These strategies can effectively be taught to clients as well.

[2]Exercises for this can be modified from those in Lakein (28).

One of the most common approaches to teaching time management is the psychoeducational approach described in Chapter 3 and in the stress management section earlier in this chapter. A multisession time management group might begin by defining time management and analyzing each person's time use patterns. Later sessions would focus on developing specific skills such as setting priorities, using lists, and organizing one's day. A protocol for a psychoeducational type of time management group can be found in Gibson (14).

Clients can be helped to structure their time by using daily schedules, monthly calendars, and flowcharts. Lower-functioning individuals may need to post their daily schedules prominently in their homes; many ordinary people find this is a relatively stress-free way of keeping family members informed of their schedules. Monthly calendars should be chosen according to need; large wall calendars can serve as general remainders in the treatment setting or in the client's home; those whose daily activities require traveling to various locations may find a pocket calendar or a personal digital assistant (PDA) more helpful.

Flowcharts are plans that show the steps that have to be taken to reach a goal and the time frame for each step. For example, if one of your goals is to travel to South Africa, you could make a flowchart showing the dates by which you expect to have saved enough money, secured your passport and received your inoculations, made your plane and hotel reservations, and so on. For a client with the goal of getting a job, the charted activities might include writing a résumé, responding to advertisements, practicing interviewing, planning what to wear to an interview, and so forth. Using a flowchart organizes time around a desired goal while clarifying what has to be done to reach it. It is important to remember that time management aids by themselves will not change a person's time behaviors; clients need to learn to use organizational tools and to get in the habit of referring to them and updating them.

Worksheets and exercises on time management activities can be found in Korb and associates (24, 25) and Hughes and Mullins (18) and Precin (34).

## Self-Control

*Self-control* means that one can "shape or contain emotions and thought and exercise control over one's actions" (21, p. 48). There are many levels at which one might consider self-control. For example, to eat only until full or to consume only a reasonable amount of food given the number of people present. Self-control is also required when one has a strong emotional reaction but the time and place do not permit its expression. In both of these examples, the ability to recognize the demands of the situation is critical. Thus one of the first questions one must ask when considering a client's self-control or lack thereof is whether the client *recognizes* the need for self-control. If not, intervention should begin with a dialogue with the client about various features of the environment and how these may send messages about appropriate behavior.

### Anger Management

Of all self-control issues, anger has received the most attention, perhaps because it can be so disturbing to others. Furthermore, clients may feel ashamed or embarrassed after expressing anger in an inappropriate way.

Anger is a feeling that most people recognize. The problem for many is that the feeling is recognized only when it is expressed. Recognizing that one is angry *before* the urge to express it is acted out is essential to success in work and social situations. Difficulties in identifying, managing, and appropriately expressing anger may arise for persons who had poor role models in their own families or who were never expected to express it appropriately because of their illness.

Anger management can be taught in a step-by-step format similar to that of assertiveness training (25). The first step is to define anger and help the client to identify typical patterns of dealing with it (e.g., stuffing, escalating). Next, strategies for managing anger through techniques such as visualization, empathizing, relaxation, and conflict resolution are taught. Then clients are asked to put the strategies to use in their own lives and to report on the results, which are discussed.

Taylor (39) described the application of an anger intervention model in occupational therapy. This model, initially developed by Novaco (33), begins with a very thorough individual assessment of anger as felt by the client. Elements such as physiological reactions, specific thoughts, environmental factors that provoke the client, and the client's behaviors when angry must all be documented. The treatment phase focuses on developing in the client an awareness of the relationship between stress and anger and on increasing the client's stress management skills and actual use of those skills. Taylor advocates the use of activities to divert attention from negative, anger-producing thoughts. Two elements are essential here. First, clients must recognize that anger is being aroused and that they must shift attention to something else. Second, the activities chosen for this purpose must be pleasurable, not ones that will lead to other negative thoughts. Taylor specifically mentions that some activities that occupational therapists have traditionally expected to provide outlets for anger (e.g., woodworking, metal hammering) may actually increase anger. Gardening, socializing, watching television, and other more passive or less forceful activities may provide more relief, at least in some individuals. A study by Larson (29), however, suggests that such passive occupations, particularly if solitary and if used excessively, may bring on depression.

## SUMMARY

Occupations are not just actions. They are actions driven by needs, feelings, and desires, and they generate feelings as well. Being able to identify, express, and act on one's feelings, needs, and values contributes to a sense of personal identity and improves the quality of one's life. The abilities to assert oneself, manage one's feelings with self-control and dignity, and channel stress into successful outcomes are all useful skills. While many mental health professionals teach these skills to clients, occupational therapists and assistants have a unique perspective in their emphasis on functional outcomes in daily life activities. It is important, when addressing these areas, to remain within the scope of occupational therapy practice. Even more important, one should provide a good role model to clients by demonstrating the qualities of self-control and self-expression, satisfaction of needs, and management of stress. Personal experiences, especially those that are immediate and germane to the situation, can be shared with clients to help them understand that we are people too and that these techniques really do work.

## REVIEW QUESTIONS AND ACTIVITIES

1. Name and describe, in order, the needs in Maslow's hierarchy.
2. How is the need for mastery related to expressive and coping skills?
3. List activities and interventions that address each of the five needs in Maslow's hierarchy.
4. Contrast the role of occupational therapy with that of other professions in interventions related to management of emotional needs.
5. Explain how values, interests, and self-concept are related to self-awareness.
6. What is values clarification?
7. How does self-concept develop?
8. What is the relationship between role performance and management of emotional needs?
9. What is the relationship between self-awareness and social interaction skills?
10. Describe assertiveness and assertiveness training.
11. What is self-expression?
12. What sorts of activities promote self-expression?
13. What is a creative arts therapist?
14. Discuss the advantages and disadvantages of unstructured graphic and fine arts media as expressive activities.
15. Describe some ways to increase structure in these activities.
16. Describe several ways in which writing can be used as a structured expressive activity.
17. What is a life review?
18. Discuss the advantages and disadvantages of music and dance as expressive activities.
19. What is the relationship between expressive skills and mental well-being?
20. What are coping skills and how can the OTA assist the client to develop them?
21. Define these terms: *stress* and *stress management.*
22. Relate social support to stress management and name some strategies to help client increase social support.
23. Contrast the problem-focused with the emotion-focused method of stress management.
24. Identify and contrast several stress management techniques.
25. What are precautions for the various stress management approaches?
26. Define *mindfulness.* Relate mindfulness to occupational engagement.
27. List some ways the OTA can promote mindfulness in clients engaging in occupation.
28. Discuss the relationship between time management and stress management.
29. State some time management strategies that can be shared with clients.
30. Relate self-control and anger management to the ability to engage in occupation.

## REFERENCES


1. Anderson RN, ed. Mosby's Medical, Nursing, and Allied Health Dictionary. 4th ed. St. Louis: Mosby, 1994.
2. American Occupational Therapy Association. Occupational therapy practice framework: Domain and process. Am J Occup Ther 2002;56:609–639.
3. Babiss F. An ethnographic study of mental health treatment and outcomes: Doing what works. Occup Ther Ment Health 2002;18(3–4):1–146.
4. Benson H. (ed) Stress Management—Techniques for Preventing and Managing Stress. Boston: Harvard Health Publications, 2006.
5. Braza J. Moment by Moment—The Art and Practice of Mindfulness. Boston: Tuttle, 1997.
6. Carlson RC. The Don't Sweat the Small Stuff Workbook. New York: Hyperion, 1998.
7. Chodron P. The Places That Scare You—A Guide to Fearlessness in Difficult Times. Boston: Shambhala, 2005.
8. Chodron P. When Things Fall Apart—Heart Advice for Difficult Times. Boston: Shambhala, 2005.
9. Cotton DHG. Stress Management: An Integrated Approach to Therapy. New York: Brunner/Mazel, 1990.
10. Courtney C, Escobedo B. A stress management program: Inpatient to outpatient continuity. Am J Occup Ther 1990;44: 306–310.
11. Edgerton JE, ed. American Psychiatric Glossary. 7th ed. Washington: American Psychiatric Association, 1994.
12. Gage M. The appraisal model of coping: An assessment and intervention model for occupational therapy. Am J Occup Ther 1992;46:353–362.
13. Gage M, Polatajko H. Enhancing occupational performance through an understanding of perceived self-efficacy. Am J Occup Ther 1994;48:453–461.
14. Gibson D, ed. Group Protocols: A Psychosocial Compendium. Binghamton, NY: Haworth, 1989.
15. Goldstein N, Collins T. Making videotapes: An activity for hospitalized adolescents. Am J Occup Ther 1982;36: 530–533.
16. Hemphill BJ, Peterson CQ, Werner PC. Rehabilitation in Mental Health: Goals and Objectives for Independent Living. Thorofare, NJ: Slack, 1991.
17. Holm M. Video as a medium in occupational therapy. Am J Occup Ther 1983;37:531–534.
18. Hughes PL, Mullins L. Acute Psychiatric Care: An Occupational Therapy Guide to Exercises in Daily Living Skills. Thorofare, NJ: Slack, 1981.
19. Kabat-Zinn J. Full Catastrophe Living. New York: Dell (Delta), 1990.
20. Kabat-Zinn J. Wherever You Go, There You Are. New York: Hyperion, 1994.
21. Kielhofner G, ed. A Model of Human Occupation: Theory and Application. 3rd ed. Baltimore: Williams & Wilkins, 2002.
22. Kiernat JM. The use of life review activity with confused nursing home residents. Am J Occup Ther 1979;33:306–310.
23. Koch K. Wishes, Lies and Dreams: Teaching Children to Write Poetry. New York: Random House, 1970.
24. Korb KL, Azok AD, Leutenberg EA. Life Management Skills: Reproducible Activity Handouts Created for Facilitators. Beachwood, OH: Wellness Reproductions, 1989.
25. Korb KL, Azok AD, Leutenberg EA. Life Management Skills: 2. Reproducible Activity Handouts Created for Facilitators. Beachwood, OH: Wellness Reproductions, 1991.
26. Korb-Khalsa KL, Leutenberg EA. Life Management Skills: 3. Reproducible Activity Handouts Created for Facilitators. Beachwood, OH: Wellness Reproductions, 1994.
27. Korb-Khalsa KL, Leutenberg EA. Life Management Skills: 4. Reproducible Activity Handouts Created for Facilitators. Beachwood, OH: Wellness Reproductions, 1996.
28. Lakein A. How to Get Control of Your Time and Your Life. New York: Wyden, 1973.
29. Larson KB. Activity patterns and life changes in people with depression. Am J Occup Ther 1990;44:902–906.
30. Linehan M. The Cognitive-Behavioral Treatment of Borderline Personality Disorder. New York: Guilford Press, 1993.
31. Linehan M. Skills Training Manual for Treating Borderline Personality Disorder. New York: Guilford Press, 1993.
32. Maslow A. Toward a Psychology of Being. Princeton, NJ: Van Nostrand, 1962.
33. Novaco R. The cognitive regulation of anger and stress. In: Kendall P, Hollen S, eds. Cognitive-Behavioral Interventions: Theory, Research, and Procedures. New York: Academic, 1979.
34. Precin P. Living Skills Recovery Workbook. Boston: Butterworth Heinemann, 1999.
35. Quigley P. Those Were the Days: Life Review Therapy for Elderly Residents in Long Term Care Facilities. Buffalo, NY: Potentials Development for Health and Human Services, 1981.
36. Ryder B, Gramblin J. Activity Card File. Brookfield, IL: Sammons, 1981.
37. Schumann SH, Marcus D, Nesse D. Puppetry and the mentally ill. Am J Occup Ther 1973;27:484–486.
38. Stein F. Stress management. In: Carlson J, ed. Complementary Therapies and Wellness—Practice Essentials for Holistic Health Care. Upper Saddle River, NJ: Prentice Hall, 2003.
39. Taylor E. Anger intervention. Am J Occup Ther 1988;42:147–155.

40. White RW. Motivation reconsidered: The concept of competence. In: Rabkin L, Carr J, eds. Sourcebook in Abnormal Psychology. Boston: Houghton Mifflin, 1967.

## SUGGESTED READINGS

Benson H, ed. Stress Management—Techniques for Preventing and Managing Stress. Boston: Harvard Health Publications, 2006.

Braza J. Moment by Moment—The Art and Practice of Mindfulness. Boston: Tuttle, 1997.

Precin P. Living Skills Recovery Workbook. Boston: Butterworth Heinemann, 1999.

Vergeer G, MacRae A. Therapeutic use of humor in occupational therapy. Am J Occup Ther 1993;47:678–683.

Wade JC. Socialization groups: Using the Book of Questions as a catalyst for interaction. Am J Occup Ther 1992;46: 541–545.

CHAPTER 22

# Cognitive, Sensory, and Motor Factors: Performance Skills and Activities

*Walking onto a ward of chronic, neurologically and psychiatrically impaired male patients who had seen me often during the past six months, I started a ball throwing activity. Not only did I introduce a large ball, but I requested that the patients stand to participate. Their usual behavior was to sit throughout the group. What a lot I was asking!*

MILDRED ROSS (21, P. 1)

## CHAPTER OBJECTIVES

After studying this chapter, the reader will be able to:

1. Appreciate the effects of cognitive, motor, and sensory factors in performance of skills needed for engagement in occupation.
2. Identify cognitive, sensory, and motor impairments that might be present in persons with mental disorders.
3. Differentiate between remedial and compensatory approaches.
4. Identify compensatory strategies for specific cognitive impairments.
5. Understand the role of sensorimotor activities in treatment of persons with psychiatric disabilities.
6. Identify sensorimotor activities and approaches appropriate for specific sensory and motor deficits.
7. State precautions for sensorimotor activities.
8. Recognize the uses of computers, electronic aids, and multisensory environments for the psychiatric population.

Almost every activity requires cognitive, sensory and motor functions of which we are usually quite unaware. Taking notes in class depends on being able to hold the pen with just the right amount of pressure (managed by our proprioceptive feedback mechanisms), to maintain our balance without having to think about it, to understand the lecturer's words and emotional expression, and to concentrate despite distractions. And these are just a *few* of the countless internal mechanisms that support our ability to perform everyday activities successfully.

These internal functions are impaired in many individuals who have psychiatric disorders. Impairment is most severe in disorders with a known organic basis or neurological symptoms.[1] Psychotropic medications may create additional sensory, motor or cognitive problems.

Impairments of client factors in the cognitive, sensory, and motor areas undermine the development of performance skills. Remember that in the *Occupational Therapy Practice Framework (OTPF)* (2) the performance skills are categorized in three groups: motor, process, and communication/interaction. Deficits or impairments in cognitive, sensory, or motor factors may affect any or all of the performance skills. Take, for example, a motor skill such as calibrating (applying the correct amount of grip pressure to hold on to an object in the hand so that the object is neither dropped nor crushed). The client may demonstrate errors in calibration because grip strength is weak, because proprioceptive feedback is inadequate, because the sensation in the hand is poor, or because the client isn't thinking clearly about the task. As another example, consider the communication skill of gesturing (using body movements to indicate, demonstrate or otherwise give information). To gesture one must have adequate motor function, adequate sensory and proprioceptive functions, the ability to think through how to show something, and some awareness of ones effect on others. These examples illustrate the intricate and interrelated effects of client factors on observable performance skills. This chapter explores some of the approaches and activities occupational therapists (OTs) and occupational therapy assistants (OTAs) employ in their work with clients who have deficits in cognitive, sensory, and motor factors. We are interested here in reducing the effect of these deficits on performance skills and the ability to engage in occupation.

[1]For some interesting case examples, see Sacks (23).

## COGNITIVE FACTORS

Cognitive functions were listed and described in some detail in Chapter 4. The reader is encouraged to review that material before proceeding.

### Roles of the OT and the OTA

In regard to occupational therapy services for deficits in cognitive factors, the OT performs the evaluation and coordinates all interventions. The OT may assign the OTA to conduct specific structured assessments. The OT may also direct the OTA to carry out planned interventions to maintain, compensate for, or improve cognitive functioning. These interventions may be conducted in groups or individually.

### Etiology of Cognitive Impairments

Cognitive impairments have many sources, among them substance abuse, trauma, brain injury or disease, developmental disorders, and psychiatric brain disorders, such as schizophrenia. Many different cognitive deficits are recognized. When providing occupational therapy services to persons with cognitive impairments, the practitioner is most concerned with the effects of the impairment on ability to function in daily life. Table 22-1 lists examples of functional deficits that may result from specific impairments.

**TABLE 22-1 EXAMPLES OF COGNITIVE IMPAIRMENTS**

| IMPAIRMENT | FUNCTIONAL EXAMPLE |
|---|---|
| Confusion | Person responds to a simple question with an unrelated remark |
| Disorientation | Person says the year is 1983 |
| Inability to recognize objects or persons | Man cannot recognize his wife |
| Reduced attention or inattention | Grade school student attends to task for only 5 minutes during math test |
| Difficulty initiating an activity | Homemaker does not start dinner in time for evening meal |
| Difficulty ending an activity | Person with brain injury brushes teeth for 15 minutes |
| Deficits in STM or LTM | Client cannot remember where wallet is (STM); cannot remember wedding date (LTM) |
| Inability to sequence logically | Client dons shoes before socks |
| Difficulty recognizing categories or placing objects in categories | When putting away groceries, client puts items into cabinets and refrigerator, not differentiating those that need refrigeration |
| Difficulty organizing information or recognizing its significance | Client puts all mail in a drawer, mixing advertisements with official notices, bills, and important correspondence |
| Problems understanding how objects relate in space | When asked to make a sandwich, client puts two pieces of bread on top of the piece of cheese |
| Difficulty solving problems | Client tries to move folding shopping cart through narrow doorway but fails to fold it and turn it sideways and so gives up |
| Difficulty learning new information or skills | Client needs cuing and supervision to travel to local pharmacy |
| Difficulty generalizing or transferring skill or knowledge from one situation to another similar one | Client can use a specific bus and route but does not generalize this to other buses and routes |

*STM*, short-term memory; *LTM*, long-term memory.

## Types of Interventions

Interventions for cognitive deficits are classified as either remedial or compensatory. Most therapists attempt to compensate for deficits, to help the client learn strategies to enable better function. For clients with lower cognitive level, the strategies are taught to the caregiver(s). *Compensatory strategies* aim to substitute personal assets and environmental aids when cognitive skills are impaired. The purpose is to provide enough structure and support to enable the person to perform a specific task. For instance, a caregiver may leave a prepared cold lunch on a shelf in the refrigerator for a person with dementia who lives at home; this compensates for the person's inability to prepare food safely and enables the person to eat lunch independently when the caregiver is not home. For more examples, see the recommended strategies given in Chapter 11 for helping clients cope with specific cognitive deficits. Allen and associates (1) provide a highly detailed catalog of compensatory strategies for persons with cognitive disabilities. Medalia and Revheim

(16) give additional strategies in a handbook available on the Web.

Toglia (24) further breaks down compensatory strategies into those in which the *client* learns to use a particular strategy (such as a memory notebook to compensate for memory loss) and those in which the *task* or *environment* is altered to enable performance. The example given in the previous paragraph (the caregiver prepares a lunch in advance) demonstrates the latter type, which Toglia refers to as *adaptation*.

As an example in which the client must learn the strategy, research is under way to determine if electronic aids such as the Planning and Execution Assistant and Trainer (PEAT) can enable clients to be more independent. The PEAT device is similar in size and shape to a cell phone or Blackberry personal digital assistant (PDA). It cues the client to stop and start activities and can store a schedule as well as scripts (directions) to inform the client how to do a task (3). It can be customized for individual needs.

*Remedial training* seeks to enhance underlying abilities and support the reintegration of cognitive functions. This approach is used less frequently than the compensatory approach, because it is time-consuming and not necessarily effective. The Neuropsychological Educational Approach to Rehabilitation (NEAR) for cognitive remediation, which uses computer drills and exercises, shows some (limited) promise; clients attended sessions twice a week. The best results were obtained with clients who already had good work habits and a high level of motivation (18).

Other attempts to remediate cognitive deficits include computer games to improve sequencing. Group and individual activities may be used to improve clients' memory, orientation, concentration, and attention span. A particular difficulty with remediation is that some clients have difficulty carrying skills over from one situation to another (15, 20). For this reason, each skill must be taught separately, and interventions must target one task at a time. Considerable resources in time, money, and personnel may be needed, and they are not always available.

## Some Specific Interventions

Among the approaches that have been in use in recent years are reality orientation, remotivation, and computer software applications.

### Reality Orientation

*Reality orientation* is an educational technique designed to reinforce confused and disoriented individuals' sense of personal identity and help them stay aware of time and place, who they are with, and what they are doing. In a reality orientation program, staff members interact with clients, asking them questions and encouraging them to think about such things as what place this is, what time of year it is, what the next meal will be, and so on. Reality orientation can be done one on one or in groups. It can also be used to organize an entire therapeutic milieu; in this case the environment would be saturated with memory and orientation aids, such as calendars, clocks, and signs, and every activity from bathing to eating would include reality orientation. Personal mementos; items from home; and videotapes, audiotapes, and photographs of family members all can enhance reality orientation (24). Protocols for reality orientation groups can be found in Fidler (13) and Brown and associates (8).

### Remotivation

*Remotivation* is a group discussion technique for helping depressed and confused persons organize and verbalize their thoughts and feelings. Topic selection is based on clients' interests, age, cultural backgrounds, and personal histories. For example, topics that might interest people in their 70s or 80s include music from past decades, what they remember of their first automobile ride, the first time they saw a television, and what it was like to go swimming when they were young. The leader generally opens the group by showing and then passing around an object that is related to the topic for the day's discussion. The object should be immediately recognizable and interesting. For a discussion of ocean swimming, suitable objects might be an old photograph from a seaside resort or a seashell. For a discussion of music, a photograph of a singer (e.g., Billie Holiday, the Andrews Sisters) or a musical instrument (harmonica or tambourine) might be used. The leader then asks a series of simple, prepared questions about the topic, calling on each member by name and involving everyone in the discussion. Wherever possible, the leader encourages individual contributions—for example, a participant who shows the slightest interest in doing so may be asked to demonstrate a dance step, sing a song, or imitate a famous person. Remotivation topics usually draw on long-term memory, which may remain intact and quite sharp despite deterioration of short-term memory and orientation to the present.

## Computer Software

*Computer software* has been used for cognitive rehabilitation of persons with psychiatric disabilities (17). This is an attractive activity for many clients for several reasons. First, the computer is a modern device that is easily mastered. Second, computer games (if properly matched to the task abilities of the client) provide a success experience. Third, computer activities give feedback about performance. And, fourth, computer activities have the look and feel of something that is educational or diversional rather than medical or therapeutic.

Medalia and Revheim (17) suggest the following four *C*s as a guide to selecting software to be used for cognitive rehabilitation.[2]

- *Cognitive.* Which target impairments are addressed?
- *Client.* What are the client's task abilities and interests?
- *Computer.* Will this software play on the computer that is available (e.g., speed, memory, and version of computer)?
- *Creativity.* How versatile is the software? Are there options for adaptation, printing out, changing level of difficulty, and so on?

Availability of computer-based cognitive training and retraining programs is increasing. The Captain's Log system, produced by Brain Train, first released in 1985, is one example. The program has been expanded and revised over the years and claims to provided exercises to improve more than 20 separate cognitive skills. The Captain's Log is designed for persons recovering from traumatic brain injury, but the company asserts that it may help improve cognitive functioning for persons with schizophrenia and attention deficit-hyperactivity disorder (ADHD) as well (6).

Another approach to improving brain functions such as memory, attention, and concentration is *educational kinesiology,* specifically the Brain Gym system (4). The underlying concept is that complex and demanding body movements that cross the midline can reprogram brain centers to be more functional. In this approach, the learner is led through a series of body movements intended to activate specific brain centers and functions. Designed for and used primarily with learning-disabled persons, the system has some supportive research (5). The reader is advised, however, that many other kinesiological activities also very likely will have the effect of improving and maintaining cognitive functions. Tai chi, qi kong, the other martial arts, yoga, and dance are just a few examples.

Although reality orientation and remotivation discussion groups and computer applications are the approaches the OTA is most likely to encounter on the job, many other cognitive activities are used by occupational therapists working in psychiatry. These include puzzles, block designs, problem-solving discussions, and visual and auditory training exercises. The OT may instruct the OTA in how to use such activities to help individuals or members

[2] The wording has been adapted from Medalia and Revheim (17) to match more closely the terminology of this text.

of small groups improve their cognitive functioning. Alternatively, the therapist may evaluate the client and identify a specific cognitive deficit, then work jointly with the OTA and the client to select an appropriate activity to build skills.

### Cognitive Factors and Performance Contexts

When working to compensate for or to remediate cognitive impairments, the occupational therapy practitioner must consider the performance context. Because the aim is to improve functioning in daily life activities, the interventions should occur within this context wherever possible. To take an example, sequencing may be the targeted skill. Computer games that reward the player for putting a series of pictures into a sequence may seem to be an easy and measurable way to teach the skill. But this does not necessarily translate into the ability to sequence another activity. If the goal is for the client to be able to sequence getting dressed or making a meal, the training should involve doing those activities within the environment in which the client will be expected to perform them.

## SENSORY AND MOTOR FACTORS

Sensory and motor factors were described to some extent in Chapter 4, to which the reader is referred for an introduction. More detail is contained in the *OTPF* (2). We assume that these factors are covered in more detail elsewhere in the OTA's training and thus focus here only on those that are commonly addressed in the psychiatric and mental health populations.

### Sensory and Motor Impairments and Psychiatric Disorders

The ability to perceive and respond to sensory stimulation underlies almost all daily life activity. As discussed in Chapter 3, this ability may be impaired in persons who suffer from mental disorders. Very depressed individuals tend to move and respond slowly; those in manic episodes often move quickly and respond rapidly and impulsively. Clients with organic disorders and/or schizophrenia sometimes have very specific sensory and motor problems, which may include stereotyped movements, S-shaped posture, or shuffling gait. Other observable deficits in motor functions are also associated with severe and persistent mental illness; these deficits include reduced grip and pinch strength, impaired coordination and fine motor control, and generally diminished hand function (12). Occupational therapy practitioners use *sensorimotor activities* (activities that provide sensory stimulation and a movement experience) to improve clients' perception of and response to sensory stimuli and to stimulate movement.

### Roles of the OT and the OTA

The sensorimotor interventions must be designed and supervised by an OT. The OTA can carry out selected aspects of the program and can assist in other areas. Activities that an entry-level OTA might be expected to perform independently are addressed here. The specific sensorimotor skills that these activities are designed to develop are as follows:

- Tactile awareness and processing
- Olfactory and gustatory awareness and processing
- Postural control
- Gross and fine coordination
- Range of motion, endurance, and strength

#### Tactile Awareness and Processing

*Tactile awareness and processing* is the perception and interpretation of sensation through the skin. Activities that are used to promote tactile awareness entail applying to the skin objects with various textures and temperatures. Examples include rubbing or being rubbed with textured cloths or lotions, receiving or giving a message, shampooing, manicuring, putting on makeup, finger painting, and matching paired objects by texture while blindfolded.[3] Certain individuals find some of these activities threatening and unpleasant, and the group leader should *never* force tactile stimulation on someone who does not want it. Tactile stimulation has a disorganizing effect on some people, causing them to have trouble sleeping or paying attention. Clients who are unwilling to have the OTA touch them may be more willing to apply the stimulation to themselves.

## Olfactory and Gustatory Awareness and Processing

*Olfactory* (smell) *and gustatory* (taste) *awareness* exercises can also be included. These may involve passing around tidbits of food (e.g., olives, raisins) and things to smell (lemon slices, cotton balls perfumed with peppermint or scented oils). The purpose of all of these activities is to alert and arouse clients to take notice of their environment and participate in activity. These alerting activities are generally used at the beginning of a sensorimotor treatment session and should be done with the group seated or standing together in a circle. This allows for physical contact and promotes a feeling of cohesiveness without putting anyone on the spot.

Olfactory stimulation may also be used to calm agitated clients. Scents such as lavender, chamomile, and vanilla are considered calming.

## Postural Control

*Postural control* is the ability to maintain balance and control of the body while moving. Without adequate postural control, a person will feel insecure in almost any activity. Dance, movement, and exercise are the modalities most often used to promote postural balance. Clients generally enjoy these activities but may have difficulty getting started. Music affects the nervous system at a level below conscious awareness and is, therefore, a good way to stimulate movement or to change a person's level of physical activity. If clients are reluctant to move, start with simple seated movements such as swaying from side to side, swaying back and forth, rolling the neck, raising and lowering the arms.

Because of its central nervous system effects, music should be used cautiously. Karen Miller (19), an occupational therapist with a degree in music therapy, developed guidelines, summarized as follows:

- Match the *tempo* to the client's ability to move. Start with a slow or moderate tempo and adjust the speed up or down as needed. When clients are able to perform a movement easily, gradually increase the tempo.
- Use music with a clear, steady *beat,* and keep the movements in time with the rhythm.
- Adjust the *volume* so that everyone can hear both the music and the group leader's voice.
- Use *instrumental* music rather than vocal music, as clients are sometimes distracted by the words. Use *vocal* music to set a theme or to establish a mood.
- Use good *equipment* and good *recordings* because poor sound quality interferes with comprehension of the tempo, beat, and rhythm.
- Choose music that is *appropriate* for the age, cultural background, and tastes of the group members.
- *Plan* your music—for example, make several audiocassette recordings, using different tapes for music of different tempos. Continue to use the same music in successive sessions, in keeping with the principle that practice and repetition are necessary for learning.
- *Observe* how clients respond to the music. Watch for signs of depression such as indifferent

[3] Other activities can be found in the gray section of Vander Roest and Clements (25).

posture and retarded movement, which may indicate that the music is too slow. Likewise, agitation and uncontrolled movement may be signs that the music is too fast.

Movements and dance routines must be selected carefully so that they are within the clients' range of ability. With regressed or vegetative individuals it may be necessary to start by copying the way one person is moving—for example, the group leader might say, "Let's all rock back and forth in our chairs, like Nelisha is doing." The next step would be to extend the range of the movement (by rocking to a standing position) or to change the speed or direction of the movement. Gradually, other simple movements can be added, always retaining the original pattern. Unfamiliar movements may confuse some people or make them anxious and should be avoided. Movements in which both sides of the body move the same way are the easiest to imitate.

## Coordination, Range of Motion, Endurance, and Strength

*Gross and fine coordination, range of motion, endurance, and strength* can all be developed through physical activities, which are described in detail in the literature (14, 22, 25). Other activities can be designed around specialized equipment like the parachute, the balance beam, and T-stools.

To obtain the greatest benefit from sensorimotor activities, the group leader should create an atmosphere of fun, pleasure, and joy in movement. If the participants pay too much attention to what they are doing, their movements will lose spontaneity. The leader should obtain everyone's attention before demonstrating a new movement and should repeat movements several times, even using the same activities over and over in different treatment sessions. It is a good idea to end an activity by bringing the participants together in a circle to say good-bye.

Sensorimotor treatment activities can overstimulate some clients, and the OTA is cautioned to be alert to clients' condition and response. Signs such as nausea, dizziness, sweating, flushing or blanching, fatigue, and cessation of activity indicate that the person has had too much stimulation and that the activity should be stopped. People who are ill or who are taking medication may fatigue quickly, and the pace of the activity should be adjusted so that they can participate for longer periods. Clients who are uncoordinated or clumsy in their movements are liable to fall or injure themselves, and because of this it is important to pay attention to the condition of the equipment, the floor, the lighting, and the general environment. The OTA must obtain the physician's approval and advice on special precautions before initiating sensorimotor activities with individuals who have medical conditions that might impair their ability to participate safely (e.g., asthma, seizures, or cardiovascular problems).

**POINT-OF-VIEW**

***[I]n a busy restaurant . . . my senses would be overwhelmed and shut down. I had three choices. I could sit in a corner of the restaurant with my back to the room, leave the restaurant and go to another restaurant or leave and come back at a less busy time.***

—Richard Weingarten (26)

- What would you think of someone sitting alone at a restaurant facing a corner?
- In what ways do Mr. Weingarten's solutions make sense? Can you think of other solutions? (Catana Brown's sensory processing model (see Chapters 1 and 6) and Lorna Jean King's sensory integrative model (see Chapter 3) both address this type of sensory sensitivity experienced by some people who have mental disorders.)

## Sensory Processing

Brown and associates (7) have development assessment tools and intervention recommendations for clients who have sensory processing disturbances. These are described elsewhere in the text.

## Multisensory Environments

*Sensory-based treatments* (described earlier in this chapter) and the use of *multisensory environments* have become more common in psychiatric settings since the beginning of the 21st century. Sensory-based treatments use light, sound, smell, and tactile stimuli to arouse, alert, calm, and redirect the attention of clients who are in distress. The multisensory environment provides stimulation of many senses (Fig. 22-1). One example is the Snoezelen (from the Dutch words for "sniff" and "snooze") system. A Snoezelen room might include fiberoptic light tubes and light strings with various color filters, bubble tubes, aromatherapy, mats and comfortable beanbag chairs, patterned fabric ceiling, and music. Occupational therapists have used multisensory environments to help clients who are sensory

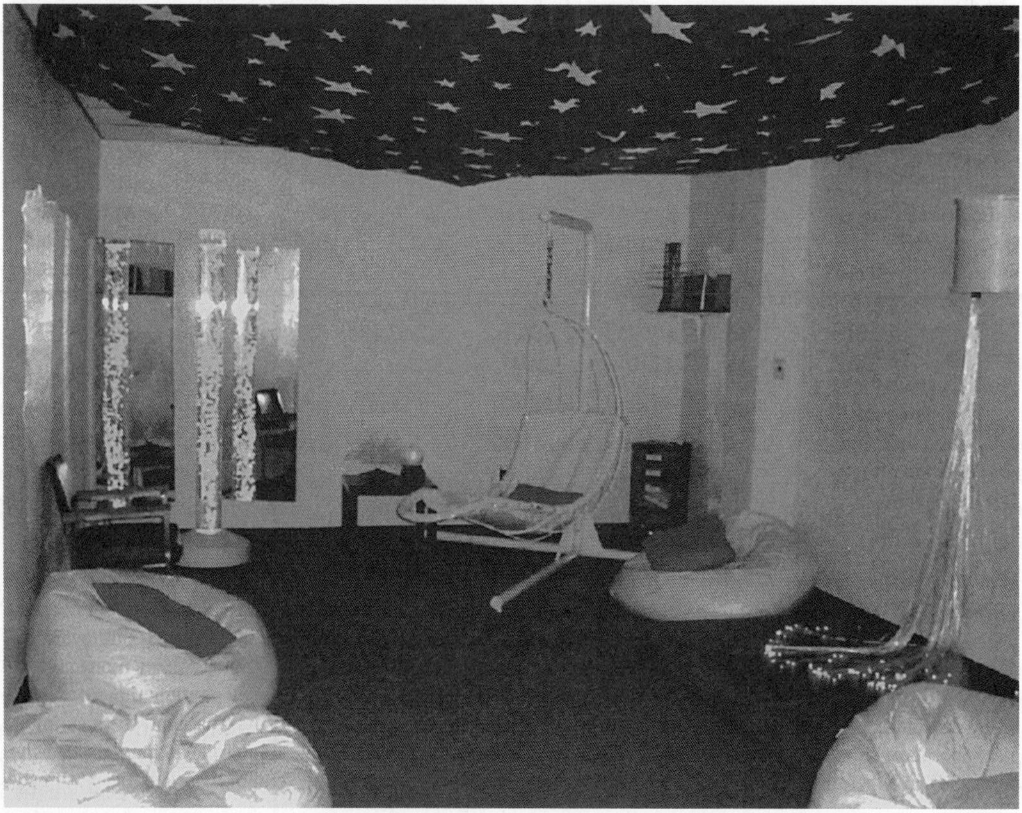

**Figure 22-1. Multisensory room.** Equipment includes a bubble tube with triple mirrors, beanbag chairs, leaf swing, fiberoptic light, music system, fiberoptic light spray, floor mat, and illuminated parachute ceiling cover. (Reprinted with permission of the Central Nassau Guidance & Counseling Services, Inc. and Donna Costa. Original source: Costa DM, Morra J, Solomon D, Sabino M, Call K. Snoezelen and sensory-based treatment for adults with psychiatric disorders. OT Practice 2006; 11(4):19-23, p. 19.)

**TABLE 22-2 SENSORY ROOM EQUIPMENT CONSIDERATIONS**

| GENERAL CATEGORIZATION[a] | EQUIPMENT EXAMPLES |
|---|---|
| Tactile | Stress balls; Koosh balls; Wikki Stix; books and magazines; arts-and-crafts supplies; putty; clay; rubbing stones; T-foam cubes; therapy brushes; beanbags; musical instruments; chalkboard and chalk; massage tools; vibrating gadgets; weighted lap pads, blankets, and vests; seasonal nature items (pumpkins, gourds, pine cones, flowers); beads; puzzles |
| Visual | TV, DVD/VCR player, wall or ceiling projectors, lighted ceiling effects, wall tapestry, books and magazines, laminated scenic pictures, posters, wall mural, colors and textures of wall paints and coverings, mobiles, wind chimes, rock waterfall, fish tank, bubble lamp, water toys, bubbles, glitter wands, colored scarves, target games, Simon game, light box |
| Auditory | Headphones, portable music player, stereo, assorted music selections, musical instruments, singing bowl, karaoke machine, videos, sound machine, rain stick |
| Olfactory | Scented candles, scented lotions and powders, linen sprays, aromatic beads, aromatherapy diffuser, cut flowers, cinnamon sticks, eucalyptus leaves, lavender buds, potpourri |
| Gustatory | Individually wrapped hot balls, sour candies, crunchy and chewy foods, sugar-free gum, strong mints |
| Body awareness, movement, and balance | Weighted blankets, blanket wraps, weighted lap pad, weighted stuffed animals, ankle weights, therapeutic brushing, vibration, self-massage, assorted seat cushions, rocking chair and glider rocker, beanbag chair, yoga videos and mats, therapy balls, medicine balls, a rock climbing wall, vibrating seating equipment |
| Other | Air purifier, locked cabinet, window treatments (blinds, shades, curtains), natural lighting, full-spectrum lighting, book shelf, texturized wall coverings, chalkboard paint, electrical outlets and covers for when not in use |

[a]All experiences are multisensory, and there is much overlap in the categorizations and equipment examples listed. This list is for introductory purposes and is not all inclusive

Reprinted with permission from Champagne T. Creating sensory rooms: Environmental enhancements for acute inpatient mental health settings. Am Occup Ther Assoc Ment Health Special Sect Q Newslett 2006;29(4):1–4.

defensive become aware of their reactions to different sensations and learn to regulate their reactivity by changing the stimulation to which they are exposed (9–11). The OTA would be able to use multisensory approaches under the direction and supervision of the OT and might become responsible for equipping and maintaining the sensory environment. Table 22-2 shows some of the equipment considerations for a sensory room.

## SUMMARY

Occupational therapy practitioners provide interventions to improve or maintain functioning of the cognitive, sensory, and motor aspects for clients who have problems in thinking or moving or being aware of their surroundings. The role of the OTA in such programs is to conduct treatments and programs designed and directed by the OT.

Chapters 18 to 22 describe a range of interventions used by the OTA when providing treatment for persons with psychiatric problems. Almost any activity can be applied therapeutically, but the value of the activity as an occupational therapy intervention is determined by the skilled occupational therapy practitioner's analysis of precisely why and how it is being used. The OTA should be able to explain the purpose of activities to the clients who participate in them and to state the benefits quite clearly. This can happen only when the OTA knows the activity well, has practiced it, has analyzed its effects and demands, and has structured it to meet the needs of clients. Without such careful analysis. It would still be activity, but not occupational therapy. The analysis and structuring of activities are the subjects of the next chapter.

## REVIEW QUESTIONS AND ACTIVITIES

1. Explain how cognitive, motor, and sensory deficits might affect a client's ability to function in desired occupations and activities.
2. List some cognitive impairments that might be found in persons with psychiatric disorders.
3. Contrast the remedial and the compensatory approach for cognitive deficits.
4. Give some examples of compensatory strategies.
5. Why is the compensatory approach more often used than is the remedial approach?
6. Discuss the use of computers and electronic devices in both the compensatory and the remedial approach.
7. Define and describe *reality orientation* and *remotivation*.
8. In addition to computer applications, what other activities can be used to address cognitive deficits?
9. Why is it recommended that cognitive interventions occur in the context in which the skill will be used?
10. Define *sensorimotor activities*.
11. Give examples of interventions to improve the following: tactile awareness and processing, olfactory and gustatory awareness, postural control.
12. List some considerations for selecting music for sensorimotor activities.
13. List some considerations for selecting movement patterns for sensorimotor activities.
14. Why is a "fun atmosphere" important in sensorimotor activities? Why not focus instead on precise and correct movements?
15. State some precautions for sensorimotor activities.
16. What is a multisensory environment? How might it be used?

## REFERENCES


1. Allen CK, Blue T, Earhart CA. Understanding cognitive performance modes. Ormond Beach, FL: Allen Conferences, 1995.
2. American Occupational Therapy Association. Occupational therapy practice framework: Domain and process. Am J Occup Ther 2002;56:609–639.
3. Attention Control Systems. PEAT—Planning and Execution Assistant and Trainer. Information available at: www.brainaid.com. Accessed May 2007.
4. Brain Gym. About Brain Gym. Available at: www. braingym.org/about.html. Accessed May 2007.
5. Brain Gym. Research. Available at: www.braingym. org/BG_Research.pdf. Accessed May 2007.
6. Brain Train. Changing the Way People Think. Available at: www.braintrain.com. Accessed May 2007.
7. Brown C. What is the best environment for me? A sensory processing perspective. Occ Ther Ment Health 2001;17(3–4):115–125.
8. Brown T, Harwood K, Heckman J, Short J, eds. Mental Health Protocols for Occupational Therapy. Baltimore: Chess, 1989.
9. Champagne T. Creating sensory rooms: Environmental enhancements for acute inpatient mental health settings. Am Occup Ther Assoc Ment Health Special Sect Q Newslett 2006;29(4):1–4.
10. Champagne T. Expanding the role of sensory approaches in acute psychiatric settings. Am Occup Ther Assoc Ment Health Special Sect Q Newslett 2005;28(1):1–4.
11. Costa DM, Morra J, Solomon D, et al. Snoezelen and sensory-based treatment for adults with psychiatric disorders. OT Practice 2006;11(4):19–23.
12. Falk-Kessler J, Bear-Lehman J. Hand function in persons with chronic mental illness: A practice concern. Occup Ther Ment Health 2003;19(1):61–67
13. Fidler GS. Design of Rehabilitation Services in Psychiatric Hospital Settings. Rockville, MD: American Occupational Therapy Association, 1991.
14. French R, Horvat M. Parachute Movement Activities: A Complete Parachute Movement Program for Elementary Grades and Beyond. Bryon, CA: Front Row Experience, 1983.
15. Jao HI, Lu S. The acquisition of problem-solving skills through the instruction in Siegel and Spivack's problem-solving therapy for the chronic schizophrenic. Occup Ther Ment Health 1999;14(4):47–63.
16. Medalia A, Revheim N. Dealing with Cognitive Dysfunction Associated with Psychiatric Disabilities. Albany NY: New York State Office of Mental Health, 2002. Available at: www.omh.state.ny.us/omhweb/cogdys_manual/CogDysHndbk.pdf. Accessed May 2007.
17. Medalia A, Revheim N. Using computers in cognitive rehabilitation. Paper presented at Institute 08, the American Occupational Therapy Association annual conference, Baltimore, Apr 3, 1998.
18. Medalia A, Richardson R. What predicts a good response to cognitive remediation interventions? Schizophrenia Bull 2005;31(4):942–953.
19. Miller KJ. Music for movement. Am Occup Ther Assoc Ment Health Special Sect Q Newslett 1983;6(1):1–2.
20. Nakano M. Treatment approaches for attention deficits in schizophrenia. Occup Ther Ment Health 2000;17(2): 35–47.
21. Ross M. Group Process: Using Therapeutic Activities in Chronic Care. Thorofare, NJ: Slack, 1987.
22. Ross M. Integrative group Therapy Mobilizing Coping Abilities with the Five Stage Group. Bethesda, MD: American Occupational Therapy Association, 1997.
23. Sacks O. The Man Who Mistook His Wife for a Hat. New York: Summit, 1986.
24. Toglia JP. Cognitive-perceptual retraining and rehabilitation. In: Crepeau EB, Cohn ED, Schell BAB, eds. Willard and Spackman's Occupational Therapy. 10th ed. Philadelphia: Lippincott-Raven, 2003.
25. Vander Roest LL, Clements ST. Sensory Integration: Rationale and Treatment Activities for Groups. Grand Rapids, MI: South Kent Mental Health Services, 1983.
26. Weingarten R. Calculated risk taking and other recovery processes for my psychiatric disability. Psychiatric Rehabil J 2005;29(1):77–80.


## SUGGESTED READINGS


Allen CK, Blue T, Earhart CA. Understanding Cognitive Performance Modes. Ormond Beach, FL: Allen Conferences, 1995.

Earhart CA. Occupational therapy groups. In: Allen CA, ed. Occupational Therapy for Psychiatric Diseases: Measurement and Management of Cognitive Disabilities. Boston: Little, Brown, 1985.

Fowler RH, King LJ, Snow BA. The use of dance in therapy. Am Occup Ther Assoc Ment Health Special Sect Q Newslett 1984;7(2)2–3.

Kielhofner G, Ankersjo MM, Oakley F, et al. Applying MOHO to clients who are cognitively impaired. In: Kielhofner G, ed. A Model of Human Occupation: Theory and Application. 3rd ed. Baltimore: Lippincott Williams & Wilkins; 2002.

Toglia JP. Cognitive-perceptual retraining and rehabilitation. In: Neistadt ME, Crepeau EB, eds. Willard and Spackman's Occupational Therapy. 9th ed. Philadelphia: Lippincott-Raven, 1998.

CHAPTER 23

# Analyzing, Adapting, and Grading Activities

*[S]eemingly small changes in the . . . materials or instructions can cause large changes in performance.*

DAVID L. NELSON (19)

## CHAPTER OBJECTIVES

After studying this chapter, the reader will be able to:

1. Characterize activity analysis as a skill unique to occupational therapy.
2. Understand the purpose of activity analysis and identify a variety of formats for analyzing activities.
3. Relate activity analysis to theory and practice models.
4. Employ the concepts of adaptation and gradation in analyzing and modifying activities to address intervention goals.
5. Identify and define terms used in Allen's model of task analysis.
6. Understand how to apply dynamic performance analysis while a client is engaged in performing an activity.

To the casual and uninformed observer, psychiatric occupational therapy may appear deceptively natural and easy. What could be more elementary than doing everyday activities[1] or arts and crafts with clients? Despite appearances, these seemingly natural activities are possible only because the occupational therapist (OT) or occupational therapy assistant (OTA) has spent many hours in mental and physical preparation. That clients are willing and able to do an activity cannot be taken for granted. Only by selecting activities carefully, analyzing them thoroughly, and adapting and preparing them to match the needs and interests of the clients can OT practitioners create a task environment that motivates clients and enables them to succeed.

This chapter discusses how to select, analyze, adapt, and grade activities to meet treatment goals for clients with mental health problems. Several methods of activity analysis are described, along with the rationale for choosing one over the others in a particular situation. General principles for adapting activities are outlined, and examples are given. Finally, the chapter discusses the concept of gradation and considers some traditional methods for grading activities to promote a variety of skills and behaviors.

## SELECTION OF ACTIVITIES

Whose job is it to select activities, the OT or the OTA? The answer is both, in collaboration with the client. Although OTs may reserve this responsibility to themselves in some practice models (e.g., sensory integration), more often the therapist calls upon the OTA to propose activities or to work together in discussing which activities could and should be used for a particular client or group.

There are two major factors to consider when selecting an activity. The first is how well it suits its purpose in the OT intervention process. In some cases, the activity must be modified or structured by the practitioner to suit the situation. Unless the activity is going to help provide assessment data or help the client reach treatment goals, there is no reason to consider it further.

The second factor is the match or fit between the activity and the client. Is this client interested in this activity? Is it consistent with the client's values and personal goals? How does the client feel about doing the activity? Is it compatible with the person's age, sex, and sociocultural background? How does it help the client develop or maintain chosen or predicted occupational roles? Can the client do the activity at his or her current functional level?

Only activities that are well matched to the client should be considered. Although it is often possible to alter the way an activity is performed or the materials that are used to do it, these changes cannot be expected to compensate for the client finding the activity irrelevant or uninteresting. There is one clear exception: Treatment related to work and productive activities sometimes includes tasks that the client finds boring or tedious; nonetheless, even these activities must be acceptable within the client's culture.

## ANALYSIS OF ACTIVITIES

To judge whether an activity will meet goals and be acceptable to the client one must first analyze the activity. To do this, the OT practitioner must tear the activity apart, examining each piece against a vast number of concepts and theories drawn from professional and technical education and clinical experience. Every step of the activity, every tool and material used, every social interaction it entails—all of these and many other aspects must be examined to determine whether the activity can do what it is meant to do for the client. (Obviously,

[1] Leaders in our profession periodically urge that we use the word *occupation* instead of *activity* (20, 29). We acknowledge that *occupational analysis* is perhaps more accurate in conveying the occupational nature of ordinary and familiar everyday activities as studied and used by our profession. However, we analyze not just occupations (work, leisure, self-care) but also the purposeful activities that we employ as therapeutic agents; thus, for the purposes of this text, *activity analysis* is the more accurate term.

the client must also be evaluated in the same scrupulous fashion.) An activity analysis, therefore, is the systematic breakdown of something complex (the activity) into its smaller, simpler parts.

Many formats and procedures have been used by occupational therapists to analyze activities for mental health practice. Some of these are based on particular theories or practice models; these activity analysis formats emphasize specific aspects of the activity that are relevant to a particular theory. For example, an activity analysis based on object relations theory would examine the unconscious meanings associated with the motions and materials used in the activity.[2] An activity analysis based on sensory integration theory would stress tactile and kinesthetic stimulation and neuromuscular involvement. Thus wedging clay can be analyzed in relation to anal conflicts (object relations) or in terms of its tactile properties and its motions of shoulder retraction, abduction, rotation, and forward flexion (sensory integration). When a particular theory or practice model is used to plan treatment, the activity must be analyzed from the same perspective.

If an activity is to be used for assessment rather than treatment, the analysis will determine how well it can measure whatever is to be assessed. For instance, if the activity will be used to assess decision-making skills, not only must it provide choices and decision points but the OT practitioner must know precisely what outcomes and responses are possible and what these different outcomes suggest about the client's ability to make decisions. The analysis of activities to be used as assessment is always the responsibility of the OT.

Another type of activity analysis explores all of the possibilities and potentials of an activity without reference to a particular treatment goal or client. Although this exercise can help students appreciate the multiple facets of activity and strengthen awareness of how the activity might be used, it is too broad and vague to be very useful in a real clinical situation (17).

## ADAPTATION OF ACTIVITY

The OTA will most often have to analyze activities so as to adapt them to help a particular client reach an identified treatment goal. Adaptation is *a change that facilitates performance.* Adaptation may entail a change in the task or the environment. To analyze the possibilities for adaptation of an activity, the OTA must start by identifying and describing the activity as exactly as possible. To illustrate, making a leather belt might mean weaving a precut link belt, stamping designs on a precut belt strip, or cutting a strip from a side of cowhide and carving and tooling it. These are three *different* activities. Thus the first step in analysis is a complete description of the materials, tools, and procedures used in the activity. Any equipment needed and the kind of environment where the activity will be performed must also be identified.

The second step is to clarify the relationship between the activity and the intervention goals for the client. Why is this a good activity for this client? What purposes does it serve? What functional outcomes does it address?

The third step is to analyze further all aspects of the activity that might affect the client's performance and to consider how one could modify or design them to better meet the client's needs. For example, repairing ripped hems and seams might be selected for a client who is learning to live on his or her own in the community. How should this activity be taught and over how many sessions? Should samples or photographs be used to demonstrate what has to be done? Is it better for the OT practitioner to teach the activity to the client individually or in a small group? These are only a few of the questions to be answered.

Table 23-1 gives a general structure for analyzing and designing an activity to address specific goals of a particular client. This is a situation the

[2] For examples of an outline based on concepts of object relations and psychodynamic theories, see Fidler and Fidler (9) and Fidler and Velde (10).

## TABLE 23-1 ACTIVITY ANALYSIS OUTLINE

I. General information
   A. Name of activity
   B. Context where this activity *will* occur (specific setting)
      1. Special features of environment (e.g., equipment, safety requirements)
      2. Space per person to do this activity
   C. Breakdown of activity
      1. List of material and supplies
      2. List of tools and equipment
      3. Cost of materials and supplies for one project
      4. Steps and key points of each step

II. Fit or match among client, activity, and intervention goals
   A. Relationship of activity to goals
   B. Relationship of activity to client's interests, values, cultural background, age, sex, activity history, occupational roles, current skills and functional level, previous learning, present and future environment
   C. Motivating reasons for this person to engage in this activity

III. Time and space factors
   A. Time needed for entire activity (estimate for average person and for this client); if more than one session is needed, estimate number of sessions to complete activity
   B. Number of steps in the activity, and time needed for each step
      1. Minimum attention span needed to engage in each step
      2. Opportunity or need to repeat steps
      3. Possibilities for skipping, condensing, or rearranging order of steps
   C. Necessary delays (waiting time)
   D. Demands for rate of performance
   E. Therapist's modifications of environment to facilitate client's performance of activity
      1. Arrangement of furniture to increase or minimize interaction
      2. Provision for task and general lighting
      3. Control of distracting elements (e.g., posters, sample projects, noise)
      4. Control of potential dangers in environment
      5. Positioning of client in relation to activity
         a. Placement of activity, tools, and materials
         b. Opportunity or need for client to move about, get up from chair, etc.

IV. Materials and tools
   A. Potential hazards and precautions
   B. Sensory stimulation available (visual, auditory, tactile, olfactory, gustatory, kinesthetic)
   C. Physical properties (assess in relation to client's abilities and preferences)
      1. Resistance (strength required)
      2. Pliability and maneuverability of materials
      3. Controllability (ease with which material is controlled)
      4. Messiness
      5. Noisiness
      6. Effects on others present in environment (dust, smells, noise)

*(continued)*

## TABLE 23-1 ACTIVITY ANALYSIS OUTLINE *(Continued)*

V. Processes involved
- A. Degree of difficulty of each step or process
- B. Technical knowledge required
- C. Presence of "magical" transformations or other phenomena that may be difficult for those with cognitive deficits to understand (e.g., color change of glaze during firing)
- D. Sensory discrimination required (e.g., of colors, textures)
- E. Perceptual demands (e.g., for matching, spatial relationships)
- F. Physical factors and demands
  1. Coordination, both fine and gross
     a. Muscular control
     b. Dexterity and manipulative skill
  2. Strength
  3. Endurance
  4. Postural balance and control
  5. Range of motion
- G. Cognitive factors and demands
  1. Attention span and concentration
  2. Orientation to time, place, person, and activity
  3. Memory (need to retain or transfer learning from one situation to another)
  4. New learning required
  5. Prerequisite cognitive skills (e.g., literacy, measurement)
  6. Opportunities for reality testing and consensual validation
- H. Social factors and demands
  1. Individual or group activity
  2. Number of people present (staff, clients, family members, others)
  3. Interactions (both possible and necessary)
     a. Level of group interaction skill needed (parallel, project, egocentric-cooperative, cooperative, mature)
     b. Type of interpersonal transactions needed or possible (e.g., giving and receiving help, depending on others, sharing tools or materials, cooperating, competing, providing leadership)
  4. Communication needed (how much, whether verbal or nonverbal)
- I. Opportunities and demands for expression
  1. Expression of feeling, verbally or symbolically
  2. Exploration and discussion of feelings

VI. Design of instruction
- A. Type of directions (demonstration, oral direction, written direction, or diagrams)
- B. Unit of learning (number of steps taught at one time)
- C. Provisions for particular learning experiences (e.g., modeling, feedback, trial and error experiences, practice and repetition, reality testing)
- D. External instructional aids provided (e.g., stimulation, audiovisual aids, activity sample)
- E. Advance preparation of materials by someone other than client

**BOX 23-1**

## ACTIVITY ANALYSIS FOLLOWING THE MODEL OF HUMAN OCCUPATION

- *Environment.* How does the environment affect the person performing the activity? What are the social and cultural meanings of the activity? What objects are used? What tasks are involved and what is their meaning?
- Volitional subsystems
  - *Personal causation.* What is the relationship between the activity and the person's sense of personal causation? Does the activity increase or support feelings of personal competence?
  - *Values.* What values are implied in the performance of the activity? How do these values reflect those of the person doing the activity?
  - *Interests.* In what way does the activity reflect or expand the interests of the individual?
- Habituation subsystem
  - *Internalized roles.* With what important life roles is the activity associated? What is the relationship between these roles and the performer of the activity? What role scripts does the person follow?
  - *Habits.* In what way do habits organize performance of this activity? What habit maps trigger and sustain performance?
- Mind–brain–body performance subsystem
  - *Musculoskeletal.* Which bones, joints, and muscles are typically used in the activity? What possibilities exist for alternate motions?
  - *Neurological.* What sensory and perceptual skills are needed?
  - *Cardiopulmonary.* What are the energy demands of the activity? In which stages?
  - *Communication and interaction skills.* Are communication skills required? What kinds of skills? And with whom?

Adapted with permission from Kielhofner G. A Model of Human Occupation: Theory and Application. Baltimore: Williams & Wilkins, 1st ed., 1985; 2nd ed., 1995; 3rd ed. 2002.

OTA will frequently encounter in clinical practice. The outline in Table 23-1 can be used as a foundation, and other analyses can be added when needed (e.g., if a specific practice model is used). For those using the model of human occupation, the activity must be analyzed for its environmental and personal factors, as shown in Box 23-1.

To use any activity analysis format effectively, the assistant must understand and know how to apply the principles of adaptation and gradation. *Adaptation* has many meanings. As discussed previously, for our purposes it means "the modification of the activity to facilitate performance," generally by modifying the task or the environment. Modifications to the task may include changing the tools, materials, directions, procedures, or rules. For instance, basket weaving is traditionally done with reed, but other materials, such as plastic tubing, which is easier to manipulate, can be substituted. Projects may be made smaller or larger. Adaptation of the environment may focus on physical aspects (the room, the lighting, the furniture) or social demands and social support (number of people involved, their demands on the client, the type and degree of assistance they provide). A game that is usually played by two people might be played by two teams instead. Or a person with cognitive disabilities might participate in meal preparation by peeling and cutting carrots as a part of a group rather than cooking independently.

The OTA may adapt an activity to enable a client to perform it. The client who cannot do the activity in the usual way may be able to do it with modifications. For example, a client with an organic mental disorder and poor postural balance might not be able to execute traditional calisthenics but could do less rigorous exercise while seated in a chair. Or someone with hand tremors, a side effect of some medications, would not be able to paint glaze with a brush on a ceramic project but would be able to dip the project in glaze. Another very common example is that some clients with cognitive deficits find it difficult or impossible to start a stitch in leather lacing or knitting or sewing; however, if the OTA or a volunteer starts the stitch for them, they can continue it.

Another reason the OTA might adapt an activity is to change its demands on the client to make it more effective as an intervention. For instance, if the goal is for the client to assert himself or herself, the OTA might provide fewer supplies and tools so that people have to share. In this task environment, the client must ask for what he or she needs.

Of course, activities are not infinitely adaptable. It is hard to change a crossword puzzle into something that can be done by a large group. One might argue that you could project the puzzle onto a screen so that everyone can see it or give each person a copy of the same puzzle, but these adaptations are extreme. Adaptations should appear reasonable to the client and should support personal dignity and competence. If a group activity is required, an activity designed to be shared should be selected.

OT practitioners must possess both flexibility and good judgment to use the principle of adaptation effectively. They have to envision the versatility of the activity and imagine all of the different ways it could be changed. At the same time, however, they need enough common sense to recognize when the adaptation is excessive, impractical, or unacceptable to the client.

## GRADATION OF ACTIVITY

*Gradation* is defined in the *Oxford English Dictionary* as "the process of advancing step by step; the course of gradual progress." In other words, a goal that is out of reach today can be attained by steady, stepwise movement, as shown in Figure 23-1. Gradation has been employed by occupational therapists since the beginnings of the profession (8). The OTA or OT designs a graded activity program so that clients begin where they are capable and make progress as rapidly as possible. Over the course of the sessions, the assistant gradually adds new challenges so that clients can develop new abilities by building on what they have already done. Figure 23-1 demonstrates some of the ways that activities might be structured to provide increasing opportunities to make decisions; although 5 steps are shown, as many as 20 or 30 might actually be needed. In addition, choices other than those shown could be used to stimulate decisions.

It requires imagination and logic to design a graded program of activities for many of the treatment goals common to psychiatric OT. Range of motion or strength or other typical treatment goals of physical rehabilitation are concrete, visible, and easy to measure; they can be graded by performing simple physical procedures such as changing the position of the activity in relation to the client, or adding weights. Not so with some goals of psychiatric rehabilitation; as discussed several times throughout this text, many important psychiatric goals are intangible and difficult to measure. This imposes a certain vagueness and uncertainty about how to approach them and how to grade activities to make them easier to reach.

The following sections address some of the ways in which activities can be graded to help

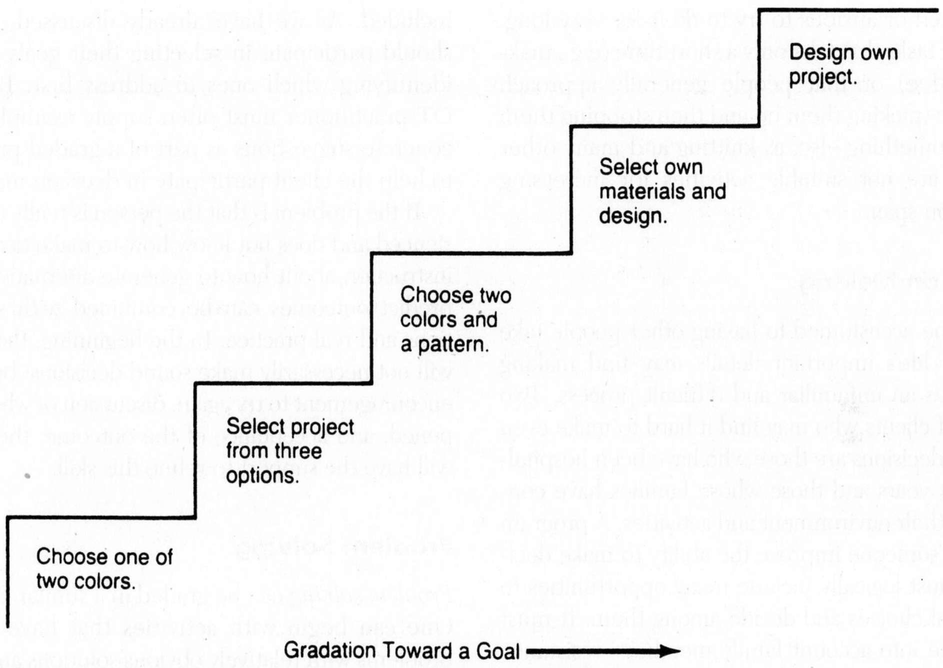


**Figure 23-1. Gradation of decision making.** An example of gradation toward a goal.

clients work toward goals typical of psychiatric OT programs. These include increased ability and performance in the following areas: attention span, decision making, problem solving, self-awareness, awareness of others, interaction with others, and independence and self-responsibility.

## Attention Span

A person can be required to work for increasingly long periods. For example, if the client can work for only 15 minutes without being distracted, the program should begin with 15-minute work periods. Gradually, the client would be asked to work for longer times without taking a break: 20 minutes, 30 minutes, 45 minutes, and so on. The amount by which the period increases and the rate at which the program progresses are based on the client's ability to tolerate increased demands. As a general rule, the clients should be expected to do as much as they can as quickly as they can. One has to assume that clients are eager to reach a goal of increased attention span and that they will work toward it diligently. However, the program should also be designed to accommodate day-to-day variations in ability and motivation that may occur because of medication, stress, or other factors.

If a program is designed to help a client increase attention span, other factors that may interfere with this goal should be eliminated. The task should be one that is meaningful, one that the client is capable of doing, and one that really *does* require constant attention over time. If the client thinks the task is meaningless, it is not reasonable to expect him or her to pay much attention to it. If the task is too difficult, the client is likely to be too frustrated or anxious to try to do it for very long. Finally, tasks that take only a short time (e.g., making coffee) or that people generally approach casually (picking them up and then stopping them to do something else, as knitting and many other crafts) are not suitable activities for increasing attention span.

## Decision Making

Someone accustomed to having other people take care of life's important details may find making decisions an unfamiliar and difficult process. Two kinds of clients who may find it hard to make even simple decisions are those who have been hospitalized for years and those whose families have controlled their environment and activities. A program to help someone improve the ability to make decisions must logically include many opportunities to face real choices and decide among them. It must also take into account family members' resistance to change and must provide ways to deal with it.

It is easy to structure the number and kinds of choices presented to a client in a craft activity. Most crafts can be approached on a very simple level and then made increasingly complex. The assistant can limit or expand choices and possibilities in regard to color, design, tools, size, and amount of detail. For example, clients can be given no choice ("Make a coaster exactly like this one") or can make a mosaic tile coaster in which they choose *only* the color of the tile (the OTA would provide squares of tiles prespaced and mounted on mesh and cut to the exact size of the tray). At the other extreme, by providing a choice of different kinds of tile and mounting surfaces, grout colors, tile nippers, and reproductions of elaborate mosaic work from Italy and Greece, the assistant can make the same activity very complex, requiring many choices and decisions.

Although a craft activity may be a safe place to begin helping a client learn to make decisions, other real-life decisions that are important to the client and functionally relevant should also be included. As we have already discussed, clients should participate in selecting their goals and in identifying which ones to address first. But the OT practitioner must often supply examples and concrete suggestions as part of a graded program to help the client participate in decision making.

If the problem is that the person is really inexperienced and does not know how to make decisions, instruction about how to generate alternatives and predict outcomes can be combined with simulations and real practice. In the beginning, the client will not necessarily make sound decisions; but with encouragement to try again, discussion of what happened, and acceptance of the outcome, the client will have the support to refine this skill.

## Problem Solving

*Problem solving* can be graded in a similar fashion. One can begin with activities that have minor problems with relatively obvious solutions and little chance of failure (e.g., leather stamping, with its need to vary the force of the mallet for stamps of different sizes). Gradually, more problematic activities and situations (e.g., attaching buckles, rivets, and snaps) can be introduced. As with decision making, it is important to work with problems that clients face in their lives (e.g., what to do when a family member asks for money or how to get into one's apartment when the keys are locked inside). Again, specific instruction about how to analyze a problem and generate solutions should be interwoven with opportunities to practice these skills both in simulations and in real life.

## Self-Concept and Self-Awareness

*Self-awareness* is a skill that has many developmental layers. At its most basic, it is the awareness of the body and its effects on the environment. Clients who have severe deficits may need to begin with sensorimotor activities. Usually, however, when we say that someone needs to develop greater self-awareness, we mean that the person is not in touch with personal interests, talents, attributes, and reactions to life events.

A graded program to develop a person's self-awareness and self-concept must include both experiences that allow an exploration of one's effect on the world and opportunities to discuss these experiences with other people. The choice of activities should be based on the interests and experience of the client. Almost any activity can be used, although most people agree that you can learn more about yourself through an art activity or a game played with other people than you can from doing a crossword puzzle or typing a manuscript. This suggests that suitable activities must provide either an expressive medium or interaction with others (or if possible, both). The essential ingredient, however, is the opportunity to verbalize one's ideas and feelings and to receive feedback from others in a safe setting. Thus it is not the activities that are graded but the way the OT practitioner structures the activities to encourage self-reflection and feedback.

### Social Conduct and Interpersonal Skills

When we say that someone needs to develop skills in *social conduct and interpersonal skills,* we usually mean that the person disregards the needs or rights of other people. For the client to develop in this area, the therapist provides activities that require interaction with other people and that include opportunities to discuss and analyze what happens between them. Thus, as with awareness of self, a program to develop social conduct and interpersonal skills is graded in its demands for reflection, discussion, and analysis.

Clients who are socially isolated or who rely on a few rigid patterns of relating to other people can improve their social skills and comfort through a graded program to increase their level of social interaction. Activities are graded on the basis of how much involvement with other people is required and on the nature of the involvement. Box 13-1 lists ways to grade activities to increase interactions with others. As discussed in Chapter 13, the OTA must be careful in grading demands for clients to become involved with other people. Interaction skills take a long time to develop and can improve only when the person is reasonably comfortable. Among the many factors the OT practitioner can vary to accommodate the client's needs are the frequency, length, and intensity of involvement with others.

### Independence and Self-Direction

Programs to help clients develop a greater sense of *independence and self-direction* require activities that can be graded in terms of how much the client must rely on the OT practitioner or other people for help. In other words, the program begins with an activity in which the client requires instruction from the therapist. Gradually, as clients acquire more skills and knowledge, they will need the therapist less. This does not automatically mean that the client will ask for less help than at the beginning; often the therapist must initiate a discussion of what the client is able to do without assistance. Clients who are not accustomed to doing things on their own may not recognize that they are able to do so or that they have done so. In this case, the therapist encourages clients to reflect on what they have done and to think about how little assistance they received. Activities that can be graded to increase independence and self-direction must be ones that require some instruction in the beginning, allow for increased mastery with practice over time, and are complex enough that they include opportunities to develop new skills and to make multiple decisions. Woodworking, leathercraft, and cooking meet these criteria.

## ACTIVITY ANALYSIS BASED ON THEORY: COGNITIVE DISABILITIES

We have discussed in a broad and general way how the principles of adaptation and gradation can be used to tailor an activity to meet the needs

**TABLE 23-2 TASK ANALYSIS FOR ALLEN'S COGNITIVE LEVELS**

| FACTOR | LEVEL 1: AUTOMATIC ACTIONS | LEVEL 2: POSTURAL ACTIONS | LEVEL 3: MANUAL ACTIONS | LEVEL 4: GOAL-DIRECTED ACTIONS | LEVEL 5: EXPLORATORY ACTIONS | LEVEL 6: PLANNED ACTIONS |
|---|---|---|---|---|---|---|
| **Directions** | | | | | | |
| Verbal | Verbs ("Eat"; "Chew") and/or interpolations ("Wait") Directions may have to be shouted | Pronouns (you, I) and names of body parts ("Move your arms") | Add names of concrete objects ("Peel these carrots with this tool like this") | Add adjectives, adverbs ("Cut them in smaller pieces"; "Sand the wood until it is smooth") | Add prepositions and explanations ("This piece goes under, then over"; "The glaze will melt and turn blue") | Add conjunctions and conjectures ("What if you did this and then that; what do you suppose would happen?") |
| Demonstrated | Physical contact, guiding hands, touching, pushing | Gross motor movements, guided movement | Action of hands on an object (stringing beads; peeling carrots) | Several actions on an object if demonstrated one at a time | Up to three steps demonstrated together, including precautions and options (not to strike leather stamps too hard, how to combine them for new designs) | Not required; may follow written directions or diagrams |
| Physical properties of material objects | Subliminal properties, (of food or drink; presence of others) | Patient's own body and your body, confining properties of furniture and clothing | Exterior surfaces of objects (what is visible and touchable) | Color and shape (preferred projects are two-dimensional with contrasting colors) | Space and depth (spacing tiles, rotating leather stamps to produce different patterns) | Intangible and abstract qualities (an engineer designs a wall fastener based on type of wall, weight of object, angle of forces) |

*(continued)*

**TABLE 23-2 TASK ANALYSIS FOR ALLEN'S COGNITIVE LEVELS *(Continued)***

| FACTOR | LEVEL 1: AUTOMATIC ACTIONS | LEVEL 2: POSTURAL ACTIONS | LEVEL 3: MANUAL ACTIONS | LEVEL 4: GOAL-DIRECTED ACTIONS | LEVEL 5: EXPLORATORY ACTIONS | LEVEL 6: PLANNED ACTIONS |
|---|---|---|---|---|---|---|
| **Motor actions** | | | | | | |
| Number | One action (may need prompting to repeat it) | One action (may spontaneously repeat it or do variation) | One action, repetition of same action | One step at a time (add next when first is finished) | Several steps at a time (not more than three if one is new) | Unlimited (can sustain action toward goal for extended time) |
| Tool use | None; may use body parts when stimulated (puts food in mouth) | Uses body parts and may use familiar objects spontaneously (tosses ball) | Uses familiar tools but often poorly (brushes hair, incompletely messily) | Uses tools to make projects or produce an effect but may have trouble with tools that cover up objects (stapler or hole puncher) | Use of tools to produce different effects by varying how they are used (changes angle of blade, force of hammer blow, grade of sandpaper) | Makes own tools, alters existing tools, operates power tools |
| Stimulus for motor action | Alerting stimuli (touching) | Demonstrated action (hand clapping) | Manual action used during task (sanding wood) | Desire to produce exact match of sample project provided | Desire to experiment with or explore how to use materials (may produce several different leather belts) | Independent thoughts and interests Spontaneous |

Adapted with permission from Allen CK. Occupational Therapy for Psychiatric Diseases: Measurement and Management of Cognitive Disabilities. Boston: Little, Brown, 1985.

of clients of varying skill levels. Within a given practice model, OT practitioners employ theory-based activity analysis. Claudia Allen's theory of cognitive disabilities is one example. Table 23-2 delineates the factors that are assessed to determine whether an activity is one that the client can perform successfully at a given level of functioning. Using the same method of analysis, the therapist can make an activity less demanding or more demanding. To use this method of task analysis, it is essential to understand what the various terms in Table 23-2 mean and what they imply about the activity.

Directions are instructions given by another person, most often the therapist or assistant. Verbal directions use words; demonstrated directions instead use physical movements to show what is to be done. The therapist may need to use hand-over-hand guidance or otherwise touch the client to teach what is to be done.

Physical properties of material objects, which Allen calls "perceptibility," are the kind of sensory information that the client must respond to in order to perform the activity. The client can act only upon what is known and perceived, so it is important to present the activity in a way that allows the client to understand it and act on it. The therapist may need to draw attention to the qualities of objects and tools.

Motor actions are behaviors exhibited by clients. The number of actions, both different actions and repetitions of the same action, is considered. Tool use means whether or not tools are used and what kind of tools are used to do the activity. Stimulus for motor action refers to the kind of stimulation that will catch the client's attention and interest and motivate engagement in the activity. Because what we want is for the client to do something (the activity), we need to know what kind of stimulation will get the client started.

Allen (2) explains how to present each of these aspects of the task for each of the six cognitive levels. We can use this information to design activities so that clients will be able to understand and enjoy them.

### Level 1

The person functioning at level 1 is aware only of what penetrates the threshold of conscious awareness. Therefore, shouted one- or two-word directions and physical contact are needed to start the action. The person can do only one action at a time and may not repeat it unless prompted. For example, the OTA might get the person to stand up by tugging on his or her hand and saying "Stand up!" in a loud voice. By contrast, the person probably would not stand up just because everyone else did or because the assistant said "Please stand up" in a normal tone of voice.

### Level 2

Persons at level 2 are aware of their own movements and those of others and are able to perform simple gross motor actions that have been demonstrated by the OTA. Calisthenics and sensorimotor activities can be used. The person will not understand how to use tools but will show interest in simple familiar objects, such as balls and jump ropes. The verbal directions can include names of body parts, but the assistant must also demonstrate the desired action. Each demonstration is limited to one action at a time; repetitions or variations on the same action can be introduced.

### Level 3

The person at level 3 is more aware of surroundings, particularly objects that can be seen and touched. The person enjoys hand movements that are repeated and will participate in activities that have a repetitive manual action. The person enjoys performing the action of the activity but fails to comprehend the end product or goal. For example, the client will string beads but not understand that a necklace or bracelet might be made this way. The directions can include the names of objects used in the action, but the action must also be demonstrated. The same action is repeated over and over.

### Level 4

The person at level 4 is motivated by a desire to make the project rather than by an interest in the motions involved. The person is interested in the color and shape of objects and materials and prefers contrasting colors and clear shapes. The activity can have several steps, but each must be demonstrated separately and then performed by the person before the next step is demonstrated. The spoken directions can include adjectives and adverbs that clarify the standards of performance. The person can use simple tools, such as scissors and hammers, but may be flustered by tools that hide part of the project, as when a stapler covers the pages.

### Level 5

Individuals at level 5 can perform most activities that can be demonstrated, and the demonstrations can include up to three steps at a time. Because the person at this level is aware of space and depth and the relations between objects, the verbal directions can include prepositions and terms about spatial relationships. Activities that require understanding of a spatial pattern (e.g., mosaics) can be introduced. The person can use all hand tools and will spontaneously experiment with different ways to use them to obtain varying results. New learning may be self-initiated.

### Level 6

At level 6, the individual can understand abstract ideas. Written directions and diagrams can be used and demonstrations may not be required. The possible range of activities is unlimited.

Allen's task analysis methods can be used to select, adapt, and grade activities to make it easier for the person to succeed. For example, it is obvious that arranging and spacing mosaic tiles is a poor choice of activity for someone at level 4 but is perfectly suitable for someone at level 5. A level 4 person who says he or she is interested in making a mosaic tile trivet is probably responding to how the project looks rather than the process used to make it. Therefore, the OTA can substitute something that gives a similar appearance but requires less complex thought (e.g., making a trivet but eliminating spacing and grouting from the process). Allen's work (3, 4) addresses the range of abilities (modes) in each of the six levels and provides details on adapting and grading activities to meet individual task abilities.

## DYNAMIC PERFORMANCE ANALYSIS

Analyzing an activity without the client present can introduce errors. The therapy practitioner may assume the client possesses skills that he or she in fact does not have. A mismatch between the analysis and the client's actual capacity to perform will result in frustration for the client. Our goal is always to facilitate accurate and engaged performance; this means we must endeavor to reduce errors and prevent the client practicing things in an ineffective or dangerous way.

*Dynamic performance analysis* (DPA) is a method for analyzing the activity during client performance of the activity (23). Rather than estimating the client's ability to engage in the occupation or activity, the therapy practitioner observes and intervenes while the client is doing the activity. Observation and therapist reflection provide opportunities to re-teach and otherwise adapt the activity to enable more effective performance. Figure 23-2 shows the DPA decision-making process of the therapist observing the client perform an activity.

## ANALYSIS: AN ONGOING PROCESS

Additional tantalizing information about the surprisingly large effects of small adjustments in how activities are presented has come from the research of Nelson and others (1, 5–7, 11, 12, 16,

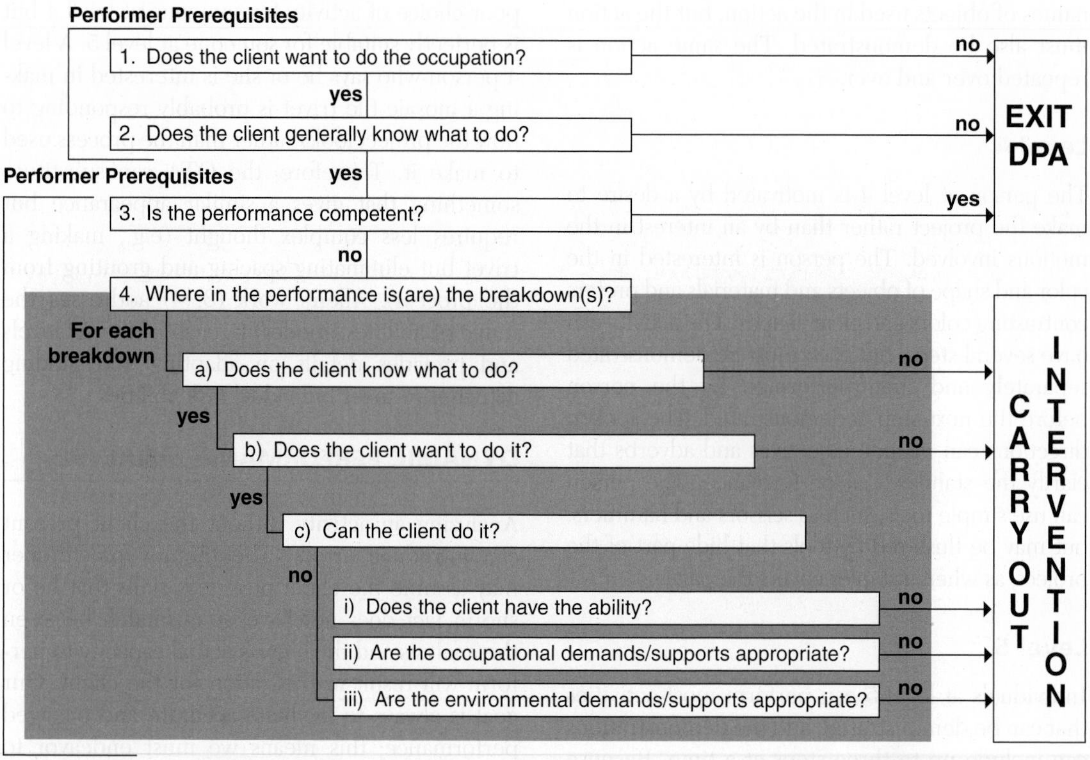


**Figure 23-2. Dynamic performance analysis decision tree.** (Reprinted with permission from Polatajko HJ, Mandich A, Martini R. Dynamic performance analysis: A framework for understanding occupational performance. Am J Occup Ther 2000;54:65–72.)

18, 19, 21, 24–28, 30). Although the studies were performed with small groups (often very different from psychiatric clients), the results indicate, for example, that having a real purpose or outcome enhances enjoyment (27), participation (12), number of exercise repetitions (28), length of performance (26), and positive perceptions of the experience (16). Being allowed to keep what one has made increases positive feelings toward an activity (24) and increases performance (18). Another study (21) demonstrated that for the well elderly, socialization and enjoyment were greater in a project group format than in a parallel group format. Yet another study (25) showed that tool scarcity appeared to increase engagement in the activity compared with the same activity with sufficient tools for each member. A study (5) of college students demonstrated that humorous and silly activities may increase cohesiveness. Having a choice of activities increased efforts by adolescents (22). Middle-school children preferred activities that were creative, related to media production, and involving teamwork (11). Adult males in recovery from substance abuse experienced less boredom, less anxiety, and an increased sense of flow when activity challenges were matched to their capacities (7). These findings should suggest to the OTA that much thoughtful planning and some experimentation with how an activity is presented are necessary to create the best possible outcome.

## SUMMARY

The format used in Table 23-1, the questions asked in Box 23-1, the task analysis presented in Table 23-2, and the decision tree shown in Figure 23-2 at first glance seem highly detailed and complex. But this is the nature of activities, which are themselves very complicated, even though we may feel that we do them almost as second nature. OT practitioners analyze an activity in detail by considering the individual parts and steps. In clinical practice, we generally begin with the client and the client's goals and then analyze how the activity might address these goals. OT practitioners use techniques of adaptation, changing the task itself or the environment, to enable performance by the client. To assist clients to reach goals that are more demanding than their current level of abilities, OTs and OTAs also apply the principle of gradation, or gradual movement toward a goal by successive steps. Adaptation and gradation, based on skillful and thorough activity analysis, permit a range of possibilities for meeting treatment goals.

## REVIEW QUESTIONS AND ACTIVITIES

1. What is the purpose of performing an activity analysis?
2. What are the two most important factors in selecting an activity?
3. Define *activity analysis.*
4. What is the relationship of activity analysis to theories and practice models?
5. What are some considerations in analyzing an activity to be used in assessment?
6. Why should one describe the activity in detail before beginning to analyze it?
7. List the three main steps in analyzing an activity.
8. Define *adaptation* as the term is used in activity analysis.
9. State two different reasons the OTA might adapt an activity, and give an example that illustrates each.
10. Define *gradation* as the term is used in activity analysis.
11. Give an example of gradation that is *not* presented in this chapter.
12. Explain how the OTA would grade an activity to help someone increase attention span.
13. If the person fails to increase his or her attention span, what aspects of the activity should the OTA consider?
14. Explain how the OTA might grade an activity to help someone increase his or her ability to make decisions.
15. State how to grade an activity to increase problem solving.
16. Explain how to grade an activity to provide opportunities to increase self-awareness.
17. Explain how to grade an activity to increase awareness of others.
18. Explain how to grade an activity to increase independence and self-responsibility.
19. In relation to Allen's method of task analysis, define the following terms: *directions, physical properties of material objects, motor action, tool use,* and *stimulus for motor action.*
20. What is dynamic performance analysis?
21. *Challenge question:* Using any of the case examples in the text, select an activity that would address the intervention goals for that person. Analyze the activity using any of the following: activity analysis (Table 23-1), model of human occupation activity analysis (Box 23-1), or Allen's task analysis (Table 23-2).

## REFERENCES


1. Adelstein LA, Nelson DL. Effects of sharing versus non-sharing on affective meaning in collage activities. Occup Ther Ment Health 1985;5(2):29–45.
2. Allen CK. Occupational Therapy for Psychiatric Diseases: Measurement and Management of Cognitive Disabilities. Boston: Little, Brown, 1985.
3. Allen CK, Blue T, Earhart CA. Understanding Cognitive Performance Modes. Ormond Beach, FL: Allen Conferences, 1995.
4. Allen CK, Earhart CA, Blue T. Occupational Therapy Treatment Goals for the Physically and Cognitively Disabled. Rockville, MD: American Occupational Therapy Association, 1992.
5. Banning MR, Nelson DL. The effects of activity-elicited humor and group structure on group cohesion and affective responses. Am J Occup Ther 1987;41:510–514.
6. Boyer J, Colman W, Levy L, Manoly B. Affective response to activities: A comparative study. Am J Occup Ther 1989; 43:81–88.
7. Corvinelli A. Alleviating boredom in adult males recovering from substance use disorder. Occup Ther Ment Health 2005;21(2):1–11.
8. Creighton C. Graded activity: Legacy of the sanitorium. Am J Occup Ther 1993;47:745–748.
9. Fidler G, Fidler J. Occupational Therapy: A Communication Process in Psychiatry. New York: Macmillan, 1963.
10. Fidler G, Velde B. Activities: Reality and Symbol. Thorofare, NJ: Slack, 1999.
11. Frank G, Fishman M, Crowley C, et al. The new stories/new cultures after-school enrichment program: A direct cultural intervention. Am J Occup Ther 2001;55:501–508.
12. Hatter JK. Altruism and task participation in the elderly. Am J Occup Ther 1987;41:379–381.
13. Kielhofner G. A Model of Human Occupation: Theory and Application. Baltimore: Williams & Wilkins, 1985.
14. Kielhofner G, ed. A Model of Human Occupation: Theory and Application. 2nd ed. Baltimore: Williams & Wilkins, 1995.
15. Kielhofner G, ed. A Model of Human Occupation: Theory and Application. 3rd ed. Baltimore: Williams & Wilkins, 2002.
16. Miller L, Nelson DL. Dual-purpose activity versus single-purpose activity in terms of duration on task, exertion level and affect. Occup Ther Ment Health 1987;7(1):55–67.
17. Mosey AC. Occupational Therapy: Configuration of a Profession. New York: Raven, 1981.
18. Murphy S, Trombly C, Tickle-Degnen L, Jacobs K. The effect of keeping an end-product on intrinsic motivation. Am J Occup Ther 1999;53:153–158.
19. Nelson DL. Occupation: Form and performance. Am J Occup Ther 1988;42:633–641.
20. Nelson DL. Why the profession of occupational therapy will flourish in the 21st century [Eleanor Clarke Slagle Lecture]. Am J Occup Ther 1997;51:11–24.
21. Nelson DL, Peterson C, Smith DA, et al. Effects of project versus parallel groups on social interaction and affective responses in senior citizens. Am J Occup Ther 1988; 42:23–29.
22. Oxer SS, Miller BK. Effects of choice in an art occupation with adolescents living in residential treatment facilities. Occup Ther Ment Health 2001;17(1):39–49.
23. Polatajko HJ. Mandich A, Martini R. Dynamic performance analysis: A framework for understanding occupational performance. Am J Occup Ther 2000;54:65–72.
24. Rocker JD, Nelson DL. Affective responses to keeping and not keeping an activity product. Am J Occup Ther 1987; 41:152–157.
25. Steffan JA, Nelson DL. The effects of tool scarcity on group climate and affective meaning within the context of a stenciling activity. Am J Occup Ther 1987;41:449–453.
26. Steinbeck TM. Purposeful activity and performance. Am J Occup Ther 1986;40:529–534.
27. Thibodeaux CS, Ludwig FM. Intrinsic motivation in product-oriented and non-product-oriented activities. Am J Occup Ther 1988;42:169–175.
28. Thomas JJ. Materials-based, imagery-based, and rote exercise occupational forms: Effect on repetitions, heart rate, duration of performance, and self-perceived rest in well elderly women. Am J Occup Ther 1996;50:783–789.
29. West WL, A reaffirmed philosophy and practice of occupational therapy for the 1980s. Am J Occup Ther 1984; 38:15–23.
30. Zimmerer-Branum S, Nelson DL. Occupationally embedded exercise versus rote exercise: A choice between occupational forms by elderly nursing home residents. Am J Occup Ther 1995;49:397–402.


## SUGGESTED READINGS


Allen CK. Activity: Occupational therapy's treatment method. Am J Occup Ther 1987;41:563–575.

Allen CK. Occupational Therapy for Psychiatric Diseases: Measurement and Management of Cognitive Disabilities. Boston: Little, Brown, 1985.

Crepeau EB. Analyzing occupation and activity: A way of thinking about occupational performance. In: Crepeau EB, Cohn ED, Schell BAB, eds. Willard and Spackman's Occupational Therapy. 10th ed. Philadelphia: Lippincott-Raven, 2003.

Friedland J. Diversional activity: Does it deserve its bad name? [The Issue Is]. Am J Occup Ther 1988;42:603–608.

Levy LL. Activity, social role retention, and the multiply disabled aged: Strategies for intervention. Occup Ther Ment Health 1990;10(3):2–30.

Spackman CS. Methods of instruction. In: Hopkins HL, Smith HD, eds. Willard and Spackman's Occupational Therapy. 4th ed. Philadelphia: Lippincott, 1971.

SECTION VI

# Professional Development

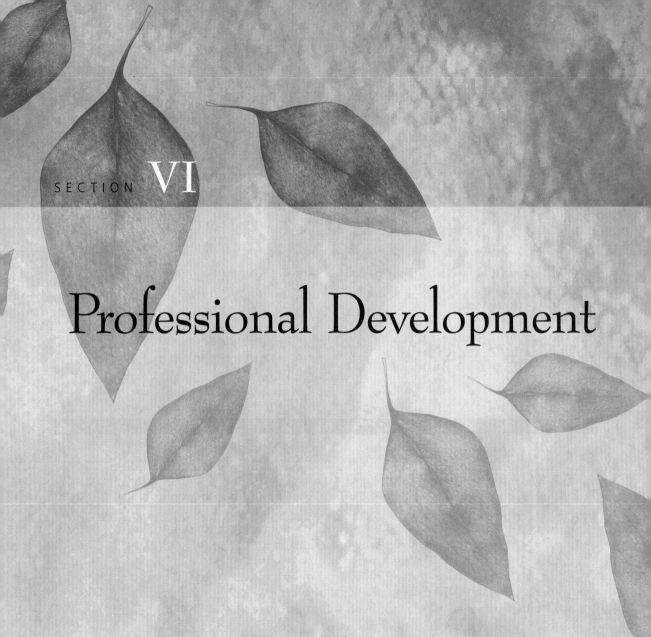

CHAPTER 24

# Supervision

***This system is the most difficult, the least common, and the most thorough way to teach. It is most difficult because it demands constant alertness, invariable good humor, complete earnestness, and utter self-surrender to the cause of truth, on the part of both teacher and pupil. It is least common because it is expensive in time, money, and effort.***

GILBERT HIGHET (12, P. 108)

## CHAPTER OBJECTIVES

After studying this chapter, the reader will be able to:

1. Define supervision and identify its functions and goals.
2. Recognize the complementary responsibilities of supervisor and supervisee.
3. Recognize the purpose of a supervisory contract.
4. Recognize factors that may affect communication in supervisory situations.
5. State ways to analyze and resolve conflicts in supervision.
6. Contrast emerging models of supervision with the traditional model.
7. Recognize the differing supervisory needs of occupational therapist (OT) and occupational therapy assistant (OTA) students, aides, and volunteers.
8. Identify resources for developing supervisory knowledge and skills.

Most students and new occupational therapy assistants (OTAs) enter mental health practice with a desire to help patients and clients and to apply what they have learned in school. But reading about something and actually doing it are different experiences. New practitioners find that clinical practice is more complex than they expected and that it is difficult to apply what they learned in school. It soon becomes clear that new skills are required and that existing skills need more development. One of the best ways to enhance one's skills as a fieldwork student, a new practitioner, or at any time in one's career is through the *active* use of supervision. Chances are that your supervisor will be an experienced clinician, someone with advanced knowledge and skills or at least someone who knows more about mental health practice than you do. A seasoned clinician is an invaluable guide who can increase your understanding of the role of occupational therapy and help you develop your own abilities, skills, and clinical style.

The main purposes of this chapter are to acquaint students and entry-level OTAs with the goals and limits of supervision and to help them learn to use the supervisory relationship effectively to further their own growth and development as mental health practitioners. The following topics will be addressed: the definition and goals of supervision, the responsibilities of the supervisor and the supervisee, factors affecting communication in the supervisory relationship, and the supervisory contract. The chapter also describes how to prepare yourself for the experience of being supervised and how to get the most from supervision.[1]

Because OTAs may become supervisors themselves after a year of practice, an additional purpose of this chapter is to identify some of the issues that concern a beginning supervisor. And because some OTAs work outside of occupational therapy services, we give suggestions for appropriate supervision in that circumstance. Readings and other resources that the novice supervisor might consult are indicated.

[1] Much of the material in this section is derived from Early (9).

## FUNCTIONS AND DEFINITION OF SUPERVISION

Supervision has three functions. You may have thought of a supervisor as someone who tells you what to do and then checks to see whether you have done it and how well. This *is* one aspect of supervision, the *administrative* function. One of the supervisor's responsibilities is to make sure that the work is done well and on time.

The supervisor's second responsibility is to evaluate how well the student or employee is performing on the job. In the case of students, the supervisor must decide whether the student has met the criteria of the fieldwork placement and is ready to go on to the next level. The supervisor must make decisions about whether new employees should be continued on probation or promoted to permanent status and may determine whether or not a staff member should be promoted or given different responsibilities. We will return to this *evaluative* function of supervision later in this chapter.

A third function of supervision is guiding the *learning process*. In occupational therapy and other health professions, a very important goal of supervision is to help the supervisee (person being supervised) grow and develop in a helping role. Supervisor and supervisee must work together toward this goal; it is a responsibility that they share. Combining these three functions—administration, evaluation, and facilitation of learning—Fine (11) defined supervision as "a mutual undertaking to promote the growth and development of the supervisee while evaluating performance and maintaining standards."

## GOALS OF SUPERVISION

What can you hope to get out of supervision? In what ways can you grow and develop? What will supervision help you learn? Some specific goals

**BOX 24-1**

**GOALS OF SUPERVISION**

1. To develop role awareness and self-identity as a OTA and as a member of the occupational therapy profession
2. To independently identify questions, problems, issues, and concerns about your work
3. To accept responsibility for your own behavior and your personal needs as they affect your work
4. To solve problems and make decisions with increased confidence and independence
5. To expand your skills and knowledge about occupational therapy and psychiatry
6. To develop and maintain good working relationships with members of other disciplines
7. To become more aware of yourself and your own behavior, feelings, and needs

you might wish to work toward in supervision are given in Box 24-1. The following sections explore each of these goals in more detail.

## Role Awareness and Professional Identity

*Goal 1: To develop role awareness and self-identity as an OTA and member of the occupational therapy profession.* This goal focuses on your growth and development as a OTA. A OTA is a trained technician who assists and collaborates with the occupational therapist (OT) in the planning and implementation of interventions. The OTA also assists the OT in making the occupational therapy department run smoothly. On your internship or in your first job, you may find yourself in a setting in which no other OTAs are employed or in which OTAs have a role different from what you would want or expect for yourself. The OT who is supervising you may have extensive knowledge of the OTA's role and considerable experience working with OTAs or may have little knowledge or experience of OTAs and what they can do. Together with your supervisor you can explore what your role should be. You can identify possibilities for changes in your role in the future. You can discuss the role and contributions of the OTA to the profession generally, both locally and nationally.

## Identifying Issues and Concerns

*Goal 2: To independently identify questions, problems, issues, and concerns about your work.* The ability to identify your problems and concerns is necessary if you are to make use of the many learning opportunities available to you on the job. It is important to have the confidence to admit that you do not know something, that you do not have all the answers. Sometimes new graduates and students who have finished their coursework feel that they *should* know everything. If analyze this, you may recognize it as a cognitive distortion (cognitive behavioral approach; see Chapter 2). How could *anyone* learn *everything* about occupational therapy in a 2-year program? Even clinicians with advanced degrees and years of experience still have questions. This is one of the things that makes our profession exciting. The questions you raise will help you develop your skills and knowledge and enable you to identify and discuss the central concerns and issues of our profession. The questions we *all* raise help us identify areas for research and new directions for practice. Another aspect of this goal is developing the skill to think through and to verbalize (speak about) the issues and problems you encounter. Supervisors cannot read your mind. You will have to let your supervisor know what you are thinking so that the supervisor can help you work on the problem. If you hold back because you are afraid of sounding ignorant, you miss out on a valuable opportunity to learn.

## Personal Responsibility

*Goal 3: To accept responsibility for your own behavior and your personal needs as they affect your work.* There are times when each of us finds it easier to make excuses for our behavior than to admit that we are in some way responsible. "The bus was late," "I left it at home," and "You didn't give me enough time" are all excuses we have heard others use. Perhaps we have even used such excuses ourselves. Taking responsibility for yourself is an important aspect of mature behavior. It is an essential attribute of a professional. Sometimes the excuses we make are rather subtle. For example, a OTA might be faced with a situation in which only two of the eight patients scheduled for a new group show up on the first day. This is anxiety provoking and could be handled in several ways:

- The OTA could dismiss the patients and not hold the group.
- The OTA could refuse to admit the missing six patients to the next session of the group because they missed the first one.
- The OTA could give the two patients something to do while telephoning around to find out why the others were missing.
- The OTA might just run the group as planned and inquire later about the whereabouts of the missing patients.

Which do you think is the most responsible way to handle this situation? The first solution deprives two patients of a scheduled group. The second deprives six patients for reasons that are not clear. Does either of these solutions seem responsible? Can you think of situations in which they might be justified? The third and fourth solutions seem to be more responsible ones, but deciding which one was better would depend on the type of setting and the kind of patients and group. The key point made by this example is that professionals accept responsibility for their behavior and base their actions on ethical principles. Blaming others or making excuses for not providing services does not solve the problem.

## Problem Solving and Decision Making

*Goal 4: To solve problems and make decisions with increased confidence and independence.* This goal emerges from the previous ones. To solve problems one must first be able to admit that problems exist. One must also accept the responsibility for solving problems and making decisions. There are systematic methods for solving problems and making decisions. You may have learned some of them in school. Your supervisor will be able to help you find ways to develop these skills further.

## Expanding Skills and Knowledge

*Goal 5: To expand your skills and knowledge about occupational therapy and psychiatry.* You will first have to identify more precisely what you wish to learn about occupational therapy and psychiatry. Once you have done this, your supervisor will be able to point out the resources you can use. These may include books and other printed information, websites, distance learning, audiovisual programs, discussions with knowledgeable professionals, and field trips and other activities. Being honest about how you prefer to learn and how you learn best will help your supervisor work effectively with you in selecting resources. (If you don't understand the articles you were given to read, say so immediately—don't wait until you are asked.)

Your supervisor may identify specific learning goals as for a particular patient group or program. Your receptiveness to such direction will have a strong influence on your relationship with your supervisor and on the quality and scope of the services you are able to provide.

## Positive Working Relationships

*Goal 6: To develop and maintain good working relationships with members of other disciplines.* Typically, persons with mental health problems are treated by a team of professionals and paraprofessionals, which may include physicians, nurses, psychologists, social workers, OTs and OTAs, recreation therapists, other activity therapists, counselors, and aides. In community settings there may be fewer medical personnel but more paraprofessionals, such as aides and counselors, and perhaps teachers. Working effectively with these other people ensures that clients receive the best care. Yet it can be difficult to sort out the roles of these different workers and develop good working relationships. Your supervisor can help you analyze or identify specific problems you may be having in this area, specific goals that you can work on, and ways to achieve these goals.

One of the things that frequently happens in mental health practice that does not happen to the same extent in other areas of occupational therapy practice is role blurring. This occurs when members of different disciplines provide very similar kinds of services. For example, the nurse may work with the clients on their activities of daily living, or the social worker or occupational therapy practitioner may take this role. In education settings, teachers and special educators take on this function. Thus students or new occupational therapy graduates are confronted with the uncomfortable idea that the job they went to school for is being done, and done well or not so well, by someone in another discipline. Unless this feeling is identified and discussed, it can fester and perhaps will be acted out in resentment, withdrawal, or defensiveness. Role blurring *is* a frequent concern of students and new graduates. An experienced supervisor can really help you understand the value of shared roles in mental health.

### Self-Awareness

*Goal 7: To become more aware of yourself and your own behavior, feelings, and needs.* As a member of a profession that serves the needs of other people, you will need to observe your own behavior and feelings. Many scary feelings can arise as you encounter clients who are your own age and whose problems do not seem all that different from your own. You will need to know how these and other feelings affect your relationships with other people. You will want to learn how others perceive you. This sort of learning can be difficult and threatening at first. It is hard to open yourself to criticism. It can be hard to face the fact that others see you differently from the way you see yourself. However, by actively working on this goal, you will gain increased confidence and control over your own behavior and your relationships with others.

These seven goals relate to supervision in its function as a learning process. As stated in our definition of supervision, it is a mutual process requiring the attention and energy of both the person doing the supervising and the person being supervised. Let us turn our attention now to the responsibilities of the supervisor.

## RESPONSIBILITIES OF THE SUPERVISOR

The supervisor, as the more experienced person, takes the initiative in setting up the supervisory relationship. This involves the following responsibilities:

- To assign a time for supervision meetings and to be available to the supervisee at the scheduled time
- To identify the specific responsibilities of the supervisee for patient care and indirect services
- To set reasonable expectations for the supervisee's performance of these duties
- To respond to the supervisee as an individual and to encourage the supervisee to begin to identify personal learning goals
- To explain how, when, and by what criteria the supervisee will be evaluated
- To clarify for co-workers and patients the roles and responsibilities of the supervisee
- To orient the supervisee or arrange for someone else to orient the supervisee to the larger institution, its rules and resources

Once the supervisory relationship has been established, which may take a week or two, and the supervisee is more comfortable and oriented to what is expected, the supervisor guides the supervisee in making the best use of supervision as an opportunity for personal and professional growth. This involves additional responsibilities for the supervisor:

- To facilitate the supervisee to identify and focus on specific learning goals
- To provide timely behaviorally focused feedback about the supervisee's progress and any problems that are noted in the supervisee's job performance
- To perform periodic evaluations of the supervisee's performance and to discuss these with the supervisee
- To arrange for appropriate learning opportunities suited to the goals and learning style of the supervisee
- To provide an atmosphere of security, acceptance, recognition, and enthusiasm
- To respect the confidences of the supervisee

Although one of the supervisor's functions is to help the supervisee grow and develop, it is important to remember that clients always come first and that the growth and development of the supervisee is secondary to the provision of clinical services. What this means in practical terms is that the supervisor must make sure that clients are being served *before* turning to the needs of the supervisee. In addition, any evaluation of the supervisee's performance is based on how well the supervisee is providing for clients' needs. Because we have already stated that supervision is a *mutual* undertaking, let us now look at the supervisee's role and responsibilities.

## RESPONSIBILITIES OF THE SUPERVISEE

If you are a student or new graduate, you should be supervised by an OT or an experienced OTA. Because one of the major purposes of supervision is to help you develop and grow as an occupational therapy practitioner in mental health, it is important for you to recognize that *you* have responsibilities in supervision (Box 24-2).

**BOX 24-2**

### RESPONSIBILITIES OF THE SUPERVISEE

- To meet with your supervisor as scheduled
- To follow through with assigned responsibilities to the best of your ability
- To ask for clarification of any responsibilities you do not understand
- To let your supervisor know when you are not capable of doing something you have been asked to do and to make a reasonable effort to learn how to perform tasks that are assigned
- To identify problems in your work
- To respond to your supervisor as a person who is trying to help you learn and to be as honest and open as you can
- To take an active role in setting your own learning goals
- To follow through on learning opportunities suggested by your supervisor
- To ask for assistance when you need it
- To accept performance evaluation as an opportunity for learning more about your own strengths and weaknesses
- To respect the confidences and authority of your supervisor
- To abide by the administrative chain of command
- To abide by the rules of the institution

It should not be surprising that you, as the supervisee, have as many responsibilities as your supervisor does to make the supervisory relationship a good one. Let us look at the supervisee's responsibilities in more detail:

- *To meet regularly with your supervisor at the assigned times.* This responsibility is fairly clear. If for any reason you are not able to attend a scheduled supervision meeting, you should let your supervisor know as soon as possible in advance of the meeting time. You may feel that you need or would like more supervision than is being provided. The reality is that a supervisor probably has no further time to spare.
- *To follow through with assigned responsibilities to the best of your ability.* This requires little explanation. Your supervisor knows that you are just starting out and will not intentionally assign you any responsibilities that are beyond your abilities.
- *To ask for clarification of any responsibilities you do not understand.* If you are not sure exactly what your supervisor wants you to do, ask for an explanation. Trying to interpret what your supervisor means without getting any further clarification can cause serious problems.
- *To let your supervisor know when you are not capable of doing something you have been asked to do.* Occasionally, your supervisor may ask you to do something you have not been trained to do. It is your responsibility to know what you can and cannot do so that your supervisor can decide how to handle it. A supervisor might give you a few days to learn a specific task or might substitute another with which you *are* familiar. If you cannot perform a task for religious reasons, for reasons of a disabling condition, or for any other personal reason, share this with your supervisor promptly so that he or she can make accommodations for your situation.
- *To identify problems in your work.* These may include difficult clients, staff members with whom you disagree, or problems applying techniques and knowledge you have learned. Your goal would be to learn how to improve your ability to handle these problems.
- *To respond to your supervisor as a person who is trying to help you learn and be as honest and open as you can.* If you have worked in the past under supervisors whose main relationship to you was as overseer, boss, and critic, you may feel reluctant to confide in any supervisor. Try to realize that a supervisor *wants* to share knowledge and expertise with a less experienced person.
- *To take an active role in setting your learning goals.* As has already been stated, your supervisor cannot read your mind. It may seem easier to let your supervisor set your goals for you and tell you what you should be learning. But you know a lot about your own learning needs. Share this information with your supervisor so that you can work together to set meaningful and realistic goals.
- *To follow through on learning opportunities suggested by your supervisor.* Once you and your supervisor have identified your learning objectives, your supervisor will help you select methods and resources. It is up to you to follow through on them. If the methods do not suit you or if you would rather approach your learning goals through another method, you should discuss it with your supervisor immediately so that the two of you can develop another plan. Recognize, however, that often you will be required to take direction given by the supervisor and that sometimes there is no room for negotiation.
- *To ask for assistance when you need it.* It is natural to want to function independently, without any help from anyone. This is not realistic, however; we all need help occasionally. Be sure to ask for it. Asking for help does not mean that you are incompetent; it means that you are aware of your own limitations and willing to use the resources that are available. Be aware that help is given with the aim of helping you

become more independent. Therefore, supervisors may be concerned about a second request for help or clarification with the same task.

- *To accept performance evaluation as an opportunity for learning more about your own strengths and weaknesses.* This may sound idealistic. There *are* aspects of evaluation that are unpleasant. It is often hard to listen to criticism. But evaluation is an opportunity for you to hear what others think of your performance. Through evaluation you will become aware of your areas of strength and success and will be able to identify areas that you need to work on further.
- *To respect the confidences and authority of your supervisor.* From time to time your supervisor may share important facts, ideas, or feelings with you and may ask you to keep them confidential. Respect such confidences as you would wish yours respected. Your supervisor may even ask or order you to do something without explaining why. Remember, your supervisor is responsible not just for you but for the smooth operation of the occupational therapy program. A supervisor may not be able to share reasons for decisions with you. If you think about it, you will see why this is sometimes necessary.
- *To abide by the administrative chain of command.* You are responsible to your supervisor, and your supervisor is responsible to someone else in a higher position of authority. And so it goes, up the chain of command to the chief administrator of the hospital or agency (who, by the way, is responsible to the board of trustees, to consumers, to government authorities, and to taxpayers). To abide by the chain of command means *to refrain from* going over your supervisor's head to a higher authority, to *not* take actions that will affect your supervisor or your supervisor's superiors without consulting your supervisor first, and to *not* accept orders and responsibilities from others without consulting your supervisor.

  The only situation in which you may legitimately seek the advice and intervention of a higher authority on your own is when you are having serious problems communicating with your supervisor. Before doing this, though, you should let your supervisor know that you think there is a problem.
- *To abide by the rules of the institution.* Rules are the boundaries that define the rights and responsibilities of people within a social system. The rules of the institution cover routine issues, such as attendance and sick leave policies, and nonroutine ethical questions, such as the rights of patients. You are expected to follow the rules and to question any that you do not understand. Blind obedience is not required; informed compliance is.

These responsibilities of the supervisee and the responsibilities of the supervisor described previously together provide the rules for a relationship that will help the supervisee grow and develop in clinical skills and knowledge. This can happen only if both parties communicate effectively with each other, and so next we consider some of the factors that affect communication in clinical supervision.

## FACTORS AFFECTING COMMUNICATION IN SUPERVISION

Any relationship between two people is affected by the individuals' personal qualities. We will highlight four major factors that often affect interactions in supervision. These are emotional needs, ideas about social and professional roles, personal values and beliefs, and communication style.[2]

### Emotional Needs

The first factor is the *emotional needs* of both people, the supervisor and the supervisee. As a student or new graduate, you may want to

[2] This discussion summarizes ideas expressed by Fidler (10).

depend on the guidance and leadership of your supervisor. If your supervisor needs you to be more independent or autonomous, conflicts will arise. On the other hand, keeping you somewhat dependent may make the supervisor feel more important. If you act very independently, the supervisor may feel threatened or disappointed, or you may think this is so. Conflicts are bound to arise if a supervisee's desire for independence and autonomy is strong and the supervisor perceives the supervisee's skills and abilities as weak. What you do about such situations depends upon how you analyze them. You may decide that it is better to try to change your own behavior without involving your supervisor. However, it is best to work with your supervisor to achieve a balanced and mutual perspective by discussing what each of you thinks is going on.

Related to dependency and autonomy is the issue of self-esteem. Some people take criticism more easily than others. Some appear to take criticism well but inwardly feel devastated. Still others welcome criticism as an opportunity for learning and discussion. These variations apply to supervisors as well as to supervisees. If you discuss with your supervisor how *you* feel about criticism and what kind of criticism is most likely to be acceptable to *you,* this can help set a tone for future evaluations. Be aware that your supervisor has feelings too.

## Social and Professional Roles

Another factor affecting communication in supervision is each individual's *ideas about social and professional roles.* Both you and your supervisor have definite notions, conscious and unconscious, about how an occupational therapist or assistant should act and how a supervisor and supervisee should act. For example, your supervisor may think that dark nail enamel and unusual hair styles are out of place in a psychiatric clinic. You may feel the supervisor is just another nosy parental figure and should stick to business. Or you may want to have a social relationship with your supervisor but your supervisor thinks it would interfere with the supervisory relationship. Or you may think your supervisor should read and correct the first drafts of all of your written work but your supervisor thinks *you* should develop a final draft before submitting it.

Your ideas about social and professional roles frame your beliefs about how a person should act and what a person should do in a given role. If a person's behavior is inconsistent with your opinions about what a role demands, you may feel uncomfortable. Discussing your feelings can help, and it gives you a chance to understand each other better.

## Personal Values and Beliefs

A third factor affecting communication in supervision is the area of *personal values and beliefs.* Even when these are unrelated to the supervisory relationship, they can affect it. For example, if the supervisor is younger than the supervisee, and both come from cultures in which age is a sign of authority, they may interact as though the older person is the one with the greater authority. Or the supervisee, being older, may expect to be treated more deferentially.

Values and beliefs about the nature of occupational therapy and mental health can also affect what occurs in supervision. For example, one person may believe that it does not matter what a client's project looks like in the end as long as the client gets something out of the experience of doing the activity. If the other person believes that the beauty of the final product is a reflection of the person's self-esteem and that everyone should work toward a final product of high quality, there is bound to be some conflict. Clear identification of such conflicts helps limit their influence. You may need to recognize and adjust to the other person's values and beliefs to preserve the relationship.

### Communication Style

*Communication style* has a profound effect on relationships. We each have our own ways of communicating, our own favorite words and ways of saying things. However, a listener who does not know us well may take a very different meaning from our words than what we intended. This can be a special problem for people who have learned English as a second language; they may have problems both in understanding and in being understood, problems that *both* parties in the supervisory relationship need to monitor carefully. Unless we are alert to possible errors in communication, misunderstandings will result. One method for handling this is to ask the other person what he or she understood of your meaning or for you to say what you thought the other person meant. In this way the received meaning can be checked against the intended meaning.

Obviously, supervision is affected by factors other than those we have discussed, but by attending to the four factors—emotional needs, ideas about social and professional roles, personal values and beliefs, and communication style—the supervisee can begin to analyze and understand the major influences on the relationship.

## THE SUPERVISORY CONTRACT

You may wonder what contracts can possibly have to do with supervision. Perhaps you have seen formal contracts, such as leases and bills of sale. A contract is an agreement between two people or among several that lets each person know what to expect from the other and what each is responsible for doing. In supervision, both supervisor and supervisee need to agree upon what they expect to happen in the supervisory process. This is why contracts are sometimes used. The contract may be written, or it may be an oral agreement based on discussion. During your initial meetings, your supervisor may mention the idea of a supervisory contract. You may wish to introduce the idea yourself. Setting up a contract with clear expectations helps prevent misunderstandings.

Written contracts have an important advantage over oral ones: They provide concrete evidence of what was agreed. Therefore, disputes about who said who would do what and by when can be avoided. One way to set up a written contract is to divide a sheet of paper into two columns. One column is headed "supervisor" and the other "supervisee." The expectations for each person are listed in the appropriate column. A sample of part of a supervisory contract is shown in Figure 24-1. Such a contract need not cover every right and responsibility of supervisor and supervisee. The contract can focus on just one aspect of your work and can be updated or rewritten to reflect changes in your interests and learning needs. Supervisors who use supervisory contracts routinely may provide clear and detailed lists of responsibilities (16).

Whether or not you have a formal supervisory contract depends mainly on your supervisor's style of supervision. If you think there may be misunderstandings without a contract or if you have had supervisory problems in the past, it may be a good idea to ask for a written contract.

## GETTING THE MOST FROM SUPERVISION

As a place to learn the clinic is very different from the classroom. In the classroom, your learning was the most important goal; in the clinic, the health and welfare of patients and clients is the primary goal and your learning is secondary. On the other hand, in some settings, learning from a supervisor rather than a classroom instructor can be more individualized and focused on you as a person rather than on a group of people more or less like you. If you are fortunate enough to find yourself with this opportunity, you can learn as rapidly as you wish by practicing the same kinds of skills you used to learn in the classroom: asking questions,

The parties named below agree that they will meet the following responsibilities during the student's three-month internship, which runs from ____________, 20__ to ____________, 20__.

| Supervisee (Student) | Supervisor |
|---|---|
| I will meet every __________(day) with my supervisor at _______(time) to discuss issues that concern both of us. | I will meet with the student at the agreed-upon time. |
| I will follow through with assigned responsibilities, which will include (at a minimum); individual treatment plans on four patients, a group protocol, assisting in four weekly activity groups, running a group three times a week by myself, a written case study that I will present orally to the occupational therapy staff, attendance at OT staff meetings every Tuesday and Thursday from 12 noon to 1 P.M., attendance at team meetings, ordering and maintaining supplies and equipment for my groups. | I will make available to the student all resources needed to carry out assigned responsibilities.<br><br>I will notify the student in advance (when possible) of any additional duties. |
| In addition, I will identify specific areas in which I wish to increase my knowledge and skill, and I will make a separate contract with my supervisor to work on those goals. | I will help the student identify specific learning goals and will provide direction and resources to help the student reach these goals. |
| I will abide by the rules of this hospital, will respect the rights of patients and staff, and will model my actions on the Principles of Occupational Therapy Ethics, as prescribed by the American Occupational Therapy Association. | I will provide ongoing informal feedback on the student's performance, and will discuss my formal evaluation with the student on __________, 20__ (midterm evaluation) and __________, 20__ (final evaluation). |

Signed on ____________________, 20__.

| | |
|---|---|
| ____________________<br>Supervisee (Student) | ____________________<br>Supervisor |
| ____________________<br>School | ____________________<br>Facility |

Figure 24-1. Sample supervisory contract.

reading independently, and following through with available resources. The quality of your learning will depend on the quality of the questions you ask and your motivation, initiative, and resourcefulness in seeking answers.

More commonly, the supervisor will not have the time to answer every question and customize your learning. Effective use of supervision requires that you recognize that your supervisor has other responsibilities. Your willingness and flexibility to respect your supervisor's changes in schedule or inability to meet your needs at a particular time will go a long way toward building an effective relationship. Supervision is a two-way undertaking, and you as supervisee must understand that *you* contribute to the process. As a supervisee, you are *responsible for your own learning.* Your supervisor's role is to facilitate your learning, not to teach you step by step. Thus the supervisee is expected to identify and attempt to solve problems resourcefully and to make independent use of opportunities afforded by the library, the Internet, professional organizations and events, and clinical opportunities such as inservices.

## RESOLVING CONFLICTS IN SUPERVISION

In the ideal supervisory experience, supervisee and supervisor are an exact match. The supervisor provides the precise support needed by the supervisee, who grows by leaps and bounds under this nurturance. The real world of supervision frequently does not match the ideal. Supervisors and supervisees do not always agree, but these disagreements need not become major conflicts. Assignment of responsibilities, differences in treatment preferences and professional values, and disagreements about ratings on evaluations are some possible sources of conflict, and there are many others. Resolving conflicts is not only the supervisor's burden, but yours as well. Orr (13) suggests the following approach:

1. Leave your anger behind you. Don't let hurt and anger and other negative emotions contaminate the situation.
2. Assume that your supervisor is as willing as you are to resolve the problem. Expect a positive outcome.
3. Prepare in advance exactly what you are going to say. Be specific and focus on observable facts.
4. Listen actively, try to understand your supervisor's point of view, and be willing to compromise. A small positive step now can be the first of many to come; you can reach your goal in increments.

## EMERGING MODELS OF SUPERVISION

Traditional one-on-one supervision (one supervisor, one supervisee) requires time and resources and is becoming a rare luxury rather than common practice. With the rapid pace of modern clinical environments and the increased numbers of students and new graduates, this one-on-one supervision is seen as unnecessarily costly. Distance supervision, collaborative supervision, and group supervision are three models that have been employed to reduce costs and use valuable supervisory time more effectively.

### Distance Supervision

Distance supervision relies on technology to provide communication links when supervisors physically cannot be present in the same locations as their supervisees. Distance supervision may use the Internet, videoconferencing, and conference calls to create platforms for dialogue between supervisor and supervisees (4). Given that the American Occupational Therapy Association (AOTA) recommends close supervision (daily on-site direct contact) for OTA students on level II fieldwork, it is unlikely that students will encounter this type of supervision. However, as the OTA practitioner acquires more skill and experience, personal contact with the supervisor can be less frequent and may be supplemented to some extent with distance supervision. Replacing direct supervision with distance supervision is possible only where state practice laws and other regulations permit.

### Group Supervision

In the past, the dominant model of fieldwork was one student per supervisor per fieldwork site, but this model is inefficient given the large numbers of students and the increasing demands on supervisors' time (6). Group supervision is a model in which several students (up to six or eight) are jointly supervised by one or more supervisors. The supervisors may represent several disciplines besides occupational therapy. Supervision occurs in group meetings rather than individually or one on one but may be supplemented by one-on-one sessions. Students learn from each other and learn to facilitate each others' learning—an important skill for the teamwork needed on the job. Clinical issues can be shared; this provides students with opportunities to consider scenarios and cases that they themselves might not otherwise encounter in the few weeks of fieldwork. The group supervision model requires more initiative and greater interpersonal skills from the student than does the one-on-one model. However, the group supervision model also promotes more independent inquiry and greater self-reliance, which build the foundation for an autonomous professional self.

### Collaborative Supervision

Collaborative supervision combines self-directed learning and collaborative group work and is a model that is used in developing programs in the community (16). When no occupational therapy practitioner is available on-site to act as supervisor, the academic fieldwork coordinator from the college may collaborate with non-OT professionals to provide supervision to fieldwork students. Students must be independent in identifying their learning needs and locating resources. Students may work with other students or with agency personnel to give and receive the kinds of feedback and guidance associated with traditional supervision. This model of supervision is appropriate for independent learners, but should not be used in level II fieldwork, in which supervision must be provided by an experienced occupational therapy practitioner (1).

## BECOMING A SUPERVISOR

Helping less experienced people learn how to work with clients can be one of the most satisfying challenges available to the seasoned clinician. Even as a new practitioner, you may be asked to help supervise aides, volunteers, and level I fieldwork students (1, 2). After a year of practice as an OTA, you will be eligible, under the standards of the Accreditation Council for Occupational Therapy Education (1) to supervise level II OTA students.

Wanting to supervise is one thing; knowing how to do it is another. A study by Christie and others (7) revealed that most occupational therapy supervisors learn by experience how to be supervisors and that beginning supervisors feel unprepared and uncertain of their own performance. This section will provide you with some resources and direction, should you wish to undertake the supervision of occupational therapy students and personnel.

### Required Experience

AOTA has identified the level of experience and expertise needed to supervise other occupational therapy personnel at various levels. These are given in Table 24-1. As shown in the table, OTAs even at entry level may be involved in the supervision of level I students, aides, and volunteers. With 1 year or more of experience, the OTA may supervise OTA students on level II fieldwork. Serving as a supervisor requires the ability to understand the roles of others and an ability to assess what skills they need to perform those roles.

**TABLE 24-1 GUIDE FOR SUPERVISION OF OT PERSONNEL**

| OCCUPATIONAL THERAPY PERSONNEL | SUPERVISION | SUPERVISES |
|---|---|---|
| Occupational therapist[a] | Not required<br>Encouraged to seek supervision to grow professionally and develop best practice | OTAs, OT aides, technicians, care extenders, all levels of OTAs, volunteers<br>Level I fieldwork students (from OTA, MOT, OTD programs) if meets role competencies for fieldwork educator<br>With 1 year of experience, may supervise level II fieldwork students from OTA, MOT, OTD programs if meets competencies for fieldwork educator[b,c] |
| Occupational therapy assistant[a] | Must be supervised by an OT to deliver occupational therapy services<br>May be supervised by other professionals when not providing occupational therapy services, depending on state practice acts, regulatory agencies, and other guidelines[a] | OT aides, technicians, care extenders, volunteers<br>Level I fieldwork students (from OTA, MOT, OTD programs) if meets role competencies for fieldwork educator<br>With 1 year of experience, may supervise level II fieldwork students from OTA programs if meets competencies for fieldwork educator[b,c] |
| Aides, who provide support to OT and OTA in some client-related tasks but do not provide skilled services restricted to OT practitioners[a] | Overall supervision plan is developed, documented, implemented by OT<br>OTA may provide direct supervision to the aide[a] | No supervisory capacity |

[a]For further information, refer to American Occupational Therapy Association. Guidelines for supervision, roles, and responsibilities during the delivery of occupational therapy services. Am J Occup Ther 2004;58:663–667.

[b]For details about requirements for supervision of fieldwork students, see Accreditation Council for Occupational Therapy Education (ACOTE). Standards and Interpretive Guidelines. Available at: www.aota.org/nu/docs/acotestandards107.pdf. Accessed Apr 2007.

[c]For details about role of fieldwork educator and required competencies, see American Occupational Therapy Association. Role competencies for a fieldwork education. Am J Occup Ther 60;650–651.

*OTA,* occupational therapy assistant; *OT,* occupational therapy/therapist; *MOT,* masters in occupational therapy; *OTD,* occupational therapy doctorate.

You should be well aware that an *entry-level* OTA is one who has been out of school and in clinical practice for less than a year. The new OTA is usually most interested in learning how to apply and develop clinical skills and in acquiring a professional identity as a competent practitioner. Supervision, therefore, focuses on shaping the supervisee's awareness of what it means to be an OTA and on refining and expanding techniques for working with clients.

## Supervising Aides, Mental Health Workers, and Volunteers

An *occupational therapy aide* (OT aide) is an employee (not a volunteer) who has been taught through on-the-job training how to perform routine maintenance tasks in the occupational therapy department and to perform selected elements of patient-related activities under "intense close supervision" (daily in-person contact) (2). Some of the functions performed by OT aides include transporting patients, preparing supplies and setting up equipment for the therapist or assistant, clerical tasks such as scheduling, assisting in specific simple tasks of intervention, and providing recreational (nontreatment) general activities. In addition, OT aides may be asked to help patients with their personal needs, such as toileting or getting a drink of water. Supervision of OT aides should focus on these specific job tasks and the attitudes and knowledge needed to perform them successfully. The OTA should anticipate that some administrators will exert pressure to have aides assume duties beyond what is appropriate. In a 1998 report, 19% of occupational therapy practitioners responding to a survey indicated that they had had ethical dilemmas relating to the use of aides (14). The OTA and OT must exercise professional judgment in assigning duties to aides and may seek counsel and support from local regulatory bodies (e.g., state licensure boards) and the AOTA.

*Mental health therapy aides* (MHTAs) are technical-level personnel assigned to assist nurses and other staff in general patient care, generally in inpatient settings. They are sometimes assigned to the occupational therapy department to assist in escorting patients and to provide security and additional support if a client becomes disruptive. Frequently MHTAs acquire enough on-the-job experience to function as OT aides in other areas. The focus of supervision for MHTAs is, therefore, similar to that for OT aides. Because OT aides and MHTAs have no formal training, certification, or licensure, they are not qualified to provide skilled OT services. They should not be permitted to perform assessments or treatments, to record client information in the medical chart, or to report to the treatment team (2).

*Volunteers* choose to work in occupational therapy because they enjoy it and want to help or because they want to learn about the field. Volunteers are usually unpaid, but they may receive a small stipend for lunch or carfare. The knowledge and skills of volunteers are varied; some are college graduates; others, high school students. Some are retired people with years of life experience; others are young people whose lives have not exposed them to the variety of experiences persons with psychiatric disorders have encountered. Supervision of a volunteer should focus first of all on that person's motivation for volunteering; when the supervisor knows *why* the volunteer wants to work, the supervisor will be able to make best use of the volunteer's time and energy. A high school student who is volunteering to get work-study credit has different needs and expectations from those of a retiree who is volunteering to help others and to share skills. Supervision of a volunteer should include a thorough orientation to the facility, to occupational therapy, and to the volunteer's responsibilities. With instruction and direction, volunteers can perform many of the functions of an OT aide.

## Supervising Students

Supervising students in education to become occupational therapy practitioners requires a additional knowledge and competencies (3). *Occupational therapy assistant students* (OTA students) are in training to become OTAs. Errors in supervision of students usually lie in one of two areas: expecting too much or expecting too little. Students on level I fieldwork know little or of psychiatric occupational therapy practice and need to observe. The student on level II fieldwork is not yet a trained and skilled assistant but is in the process of becoming one. It is unreasonable to expect a student to perform at the same level as a staff member. On the other hand, the student is more than a volunteer or aide and should be challenged to perform closer to the level demanded in entry-level positions.

*Occupational therapy students* at the masters (MOT) and doctorate (OTD) levels are in training to become OTs at those respective levels of education. The guidelines of Accreditation Council for Occupational Therapy Education (ACOTE) (1) permit the OTA who has supervisory competency to provide supervision to these students on level I fieldwork. As with OTA students, these OT students at Level I need to observe and learn from what they see. Supervising these students is an opportunity for the OTA to educate OT students to the role and responsibilities of the OTA (17).

### Resources and Strategies for Success

Many resources are available to guide the beginning supervisor. These include the Costa's *Essential Guide to Occupational Therapy Fieldwork Education* (5) and an article by Schwartz (15), which gives directions on how to identify and meet the needs of students at various cognitive levels. Workshops and courses on supervision are another possible resource. Your own supervisor should be able and available to give you guidance as well.

In addition, Christie and associates (7) have identified some of the factors that students consider positive in a fieldwork supervisor. The first is an individual approach at the level of the student's needs. The crucial ingredient seems to be the supervisor's ability to present experiences that the student is ready for and finds challenging. Another factor cited by students as positive is the supervisor's ability to organize the fieldwork and to make the student's responsibilities and the objectives of the fieldwork clear. Students also praised supervisors who made themselves available and who provided constructive, timely, and honest feedback. Supervisors who were enthusiastic and sure of themselves were seen as positive role models whom students wanted to emulate.

Farber (9) suggests some strategies supervisors have found helpful in solving problems related to supervision of students:

- Clarifying communications
- Increasing structure
- Using specific interventions to meet specific students' needs
- Seeking support from the academic faculty
- Seeking support from clinical colleagues

The lists of references and selected readings at the end of this chapter contain resources that would be helpful to the beginning or intermediate-level supervisor.

## SUMMARY

Supervision is "a mutual undertaking to promote the growth and development of the supervisee while evaluating performance and maintaining standards" (11). It functions in three ways: as an administrative process for making sure the work gets done, as an evaluative process for ensuring that the work is performed at an acceptable standard, and as a learning process for developing the skills and competencies of those being supervised. Effective supervision requires the active and involved participation of both the supervisor and the supervisee. This chapter explores the goals of supervision and the responsibilities of supervisor and supervisee and addresses some of the factors affecting students and new OTAs in the role of supervisee. The process of becoming a supervisor, as many experienced OTAs finally do, is discussed briefly.

## REVIEW QUESTIONS AND ACTIVITIES

1. State three functions of supervision.
2. Define *supervision*.
3. List seven goals of supervision. Explain each.
4. List the responsibilities of the supervisor and of the supervisee.
5. Explain how the responsibilities of supervisor and supervisee complement each other.
6. List and describe four factors that may affect communication in supervision.
7. What is the purpose of a supervisory contract?
8. List some possible sources of conflict in supervision.
9. Discuss ways to resolve conflicts in supervision.
10. Name and describe three emerging models of supervision. Contrast these models with traditional one-on-one supervision. What are the benefits and drawbacks of each model.
11. What clinic tasks can an OT aide perform?
12. What is the focus of supervision when supervising an OT aide or a MHTA?
13. What tasks can a volunteer perform?
14. If assigned to supervise a volunteer, how would you structure supervision? What would you want to know? What would you be sure to include?
15. List four features identified by Christie et al. as positive qualities in a supervisor.
16. *Challenge activity:* List three specific goals you would like to pursue in supervision while on your next fieldwork (or current fieldwork). For each goal, state the resources and methods you feel would be helpful.
17. *Challenge activity:* Write a description of your own emotional needs as they may affect supervision; your ideas about the social and professional roles of students, OTAs, and OTs; your personal values and beliefs as they may affect your work; and your communication style.
18. *Challenge activity:* After studying the responsibilities of the supervisee, identify an area in which you feel you may have difficulty. Explain. Set a goal for yourself in this area. Share in class.

## REFERENCES


1. Accreditation Council for Occupational Therapy Education (ACOTE) Standards and Interpretive Guidelines. Available at: www.aota.org/nu/docs/acotestandards107.pdf. Accessed Apr 2007.
2. American Occupational Therapy Association. Guidelines for supervision, roles, and responsibilities during the delivery of occupational therapy services. Am J Occup Ther 2004;58:663–667.
3. American Occupational Therapy Association. Role competencies for a fieldwork educator. Am J Occup Ther 60;650–651.
4. Boerkoel D. 21st century clinical management: Strategies for successful leadership and management across distance. Am Occup Ther Assoc Admin Manage Special Sect Q Newslett 1997;13(2):1–4.
5. Costa DM. The Essential Guide to Occupational Therapy Fieldwork Education. Bethesda MD: American Occupational Therapy Association Press, 2004.
6. Crist PA. Nontraditional and group fieldwork models: Their time has come. Am Occup Ther Assoc Educ Special Sect Q Newslett 1993;3(1):3–4.
7. Christie BA, Joyce PC, Moeller PL. Fieldwork experience. 2: The supervisor's dilemma. Am J Occup Ther 1985;39: 675–681.
8. Early MB. T.A.R. Introductory Course Workbook: Occupational Therapy: Psychosocial Dysfunction. Long Island City, NY: LaGuardia Community College, 1981.
9. Farber RS. Supervisory relationships: Snags, stress, and solutions. Am Occup Ther Assoc Educ Sect Q Newslett 1998;8(2):2–3.
10. Fidler G. Five dimensions of the dyad. Paper presented at The Supervisory Dialogue [Forum]. New York, Nov 16, 1979.
11. Fine SB. Using supervision to meet clinical and professional needs. Paper presented at Focus on Mental Health: 2. A Plan for Action [Workshop], New York, Mar 21, 1986.
12. Highet G. The Art of Teaching. New York: Vintage, 1950.
13. Orr M. COTA share. Occup Ther Newspaper 1983; 37(8):13.
14. Russell KV, Kanny EM. Use of aides in occupational therapy practice. Am J Occup Ther 1998;52:118–124.
15. Schwartz KB. An approach to supervision of students on fieldwork. Am J Occup Ther 1984;38:393–397.
16. Walens D, Helfrich CA, Aviles A, Horita L. Assessing needs and developing interventions with new populations: A community process of collaboration. Occ Ther Ment Health 2001;16(3–4):71–95.
17. Walski T. Commission on Education response [Letter to the Editor]. Am J Occup Ther 2001;55:350–352.


## SUGGESTED READINGS


American Occupational Therapy Association. Guidelines for supervision, roles, and responsibilities during the delivery of occupational therapy services. Am J Occup Ther 2004; 58:663–667.

American Occupational Therapy Association. Role competencies for a fieldwork educator. Am J Occup Ther 60;650–651.

Benson KE, Higgins TE. Issues regarding practice and education for certified occupational therapy assistants. Am Occup Ther Assoc Educ Special Sect Q Newslett 1992;2(2):3–4.

Blechert TF, Christiansen MF, Kari N. Intraprofessional team building. Am J Occup Ther 1987;41:576–589.

Costa DM. The Essential Guide to Occupational Therapy Fieldwork Education. Bethesda MD: American Occupational Therapy Association Press, 2004.

Hawkins TR. Supervising the occupational therapy assistant student. Am Occup Ther Assoc Educ Special Sect Q Newslett 1993;3(1):7–8.

Mitchell MM, Kampfe CM. Coping strategies used by occupational therapy students during fieldwork: An exploratory study. Am J Occup Ther 1990;44:543–550.

Yuen HK. Fieldwork students under stress. Am J Occup Ther 1990;44:80–81.

CHAPTER 25

# Organizing Yourself

***Order and simplification are the first steps toward the mastery of a subject—the actual enemy is the unknown.***

THOMAS MANN (7)

## CHAPTER OBJECTIVES

After studying this chapter, the reader will be able to:

1. Explain how being organized improves efficiency and comfort.
2. State a number of simple ideas to improve organization of time, paperwork, and activity areas.
3. Discuss the use of electronic devices and systems as organizational aids and as potential time wasters.
4. Recognize the principles of ergonomic positioning for computer use.

The occupational therapy assistant (OTA) will find only a limited amount of time to meet a diverse range of responsibilities. It is difficult to perform well at such a complex job without being organized. Being organized makes it easier to fulfill obligations, keep up with paperwork, do things on schedule, and carry out long-range projects. When Allen and Cruickshank (1) surveyed 613 newly occupational therapists (OTs) in 1976, they found that of 96 items on a checklist, those rated among the 5 most bothersome were the following:

- Finding ways to treat more patients with limited staff and time
- Finding time to meet all of my work-related responsibilities
- Maintaining an uninterrupted treatment schedule
- Getting systems (such as patient scheduling, transportation, discharge, and transfer) to be more efficient

Furthermore, they rated the following item 11th on the same list:

- Budgeting time for nontreatment tasks such as paperwork, clinic cleanup, fabricating equipment, and so on.

Allen and Cruickshank concluded that therapists need to improve their ability to develop realistic schedules and manage their time. Although this survey was restricted to OTs and is more than 30 years old, we continue to hear the same concerns today from both OTs and OTAs. Pressures for productivity, increased frequency of documentation, and changing reimbursement and regulatory guidelines create a work environment in which efficiency and organization are necessary. This chapter provides information and hints on how to manage your time and environment, with the expectation that being organized will make you feel more competent, energetic, and confident in your work.

The following topics are discussed: priorities, scheduling, paperwork, management of supplies and equipment, organization of space, and delegating. For each, typical problems and suggested solutions are described. Which suggestions to adopt and to what extent are individual choices. The goal of this chapter is not to fit you into a prescribed mold but rather to help you become organized in a way that suits you and your style.

## PRIORITIES

For OTAs who are working in clinical situations, the first priority is care of patients and clients. This means providing treatment and performing interviews and assessments as directed. These tasks come before all others but cannot be an excuse for ignoring documentation, supervision and meetings, and activity preparation and clinic maintenance. In other words, OTAs need to manage their time so that they can take care of clinical responsibilities, paperwork, and meetings with other staff and still leave enough time to get materials ready for treatment activities and make the clinic a clean, orderly, and inviting place.

How can you find the time for all of these major responsibilities? The first step is to assess your habits and how you are using your time. Do you have any nonproductive or dominating habits (2)? Are you spending valuable time doing unimportant tasks? Some relatively unimportant activities are the following:

- Filing and cataloging things that may never be used again
- Chatting with clients and staff outside of scheduled times
- Sharpening pencils and arranging desk supplies
- Listening to and responding to nonessential voice mail messages
- Surfing the Web, diverting from the original purpose, and losing track of time
- Reading and replying to nonessential e-mail

For some people, striving for perfection is a real time trap. Perfection is hardly ever necessary. Here are some examples:

- Rewriting paperwork to make it look nicer
- Deliberating indecisively about how to approach a problem
- Trying to save money by reusing supplies that could be discarded
- Using detailed but cumbersome filing and record-keeping systems

Developing the habit of using time efficiently takes only a little effort, but it has to be consistent effort. An important first step is to *stop* doing the activities that are your particular time traps. Try to get in the habit of monitoring what you are doing. This goes straight to the question of occupational patterns: habits and routines (2). Several times a day, ask yourself, "What am I doing now? Is this the best use of my time? What's really important?"

It is sometimes useful to make a daily to-do list (6). For such a list to work, it should include only things that you really plan to do today; you can make another list tomorrow. You can save time by omitting routine tasks that will get done anyway, noting only those that might be forgotten without a special reminder. You can prioritize the list, giving the must-do items a rating of A, the less important ones a rating of B, and the ones that do not matter much a rating of C (6). Make time to do the A items and try not to be distracted by less important tasks during the day. People who use daily to-do lists report that they feel satisfied by what they accomplish and have a clear and realistic sense of their goals.

To-do lists are not universally helpful, and several variations are possible. You can, for example, list only the A, or must-do items, perhaps listing only those that are critically important or that you are having trouble remembering. Lists on self-stick notes in various sizes can be stuck onto calendars, computers, telephones, mirrors, dashboards, and other places as reminders. Reinforce your feeling of accomplishment by crossing out items when

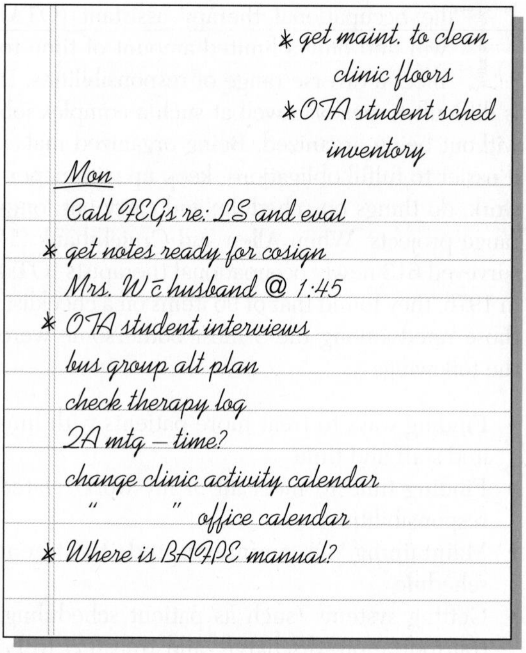


**Figure 25-1. Example of a to-do list.**

they are completed. Figure 25-1 provides an example of a to-do list. The column on the right, though not labeled, is for important tasks that won't be done today but need to be remembered. The asterisks indicate tasks the list maker sees as urgent.

## SCHEDULING

Every OTA needs a schedule, whether or not it is written. Using a schedule is the first step in time management. The OTA's schedule is based on the master schedule for the setting and for the occupational therapy department. In other words, certain hours in the schedule are fixed time slots, set aside for meetings and groups that occur at times determined by others. These include regular treatment groups, supervision meetings, and other staff meetings. Time slots not reserved for these fixed events are flexible time slots. These slots are used to meet the other responsibilities of individual assessments, individual treatment sessions, paperwork, preparation, and clinic maintenance.

It is tempting to assume that these tasks will automatically get done during these times and that there is no need to schedule them for any particular hour. However, doesn't it often happen that you are interrupted by other people or telephone calls or distracted by unexpected things that come up? These interruptions expand to fill the empty time. The only way to avoid this is to schedule time for specific tasks and *actually do them at your scheduled time.* The first step is to make a list of the things you have to do every week or every month. These might include the following:

- Writing progress notes
- Administering interviews or assessments to new clients
- Reading medical records
- Making phone calls or writing letters to arrange or confirm details about supply orders, community activities, or equipment repairs
- Preparing materials for patients to use
- Setting up an area for an activity
- Transporting patients
- Writing up notes on a group
- Taking inventory of supplies
- Unpacking orders and stocking and arranging the supply room and closets
- Cleaning up after activities and general clinic housekeeping
- Writing up monthly statistics

Just one look at the items on this list, which is by no means exhaustive, should prove that the OTA can accomplish them only by organizing time to do so. All of these tasks take time. For example, an empty hour-long time slot quickly dwindles to 20 minutes or less if the OTA must escort patients back to the ward after a group that just ended and then has to get to a meeting in another building. A single phone call can easily consume the remaining time.

## Making a Schedule

A schedule must be accurate and realistic if it is to be of any use to you. Creating a realistic schedule involves the following steps:

1. Get or make a schedule form that you can duplicate so that you can revise it.
2. Fill in the activities that occur at fixed time slots.
3. Around these fixed activities, fill in the time *you* need to perform any tasks that necessarily occur with them. Examples include setting up the activity, escorting patients, and jotting down notes on what happened in the activity.
4. List all of your other routine responsibilities.
5. Leaving at least 2 hours a week for unexpected activities, fill in the rest of your schedule.
6. Live with the schedule for a while to see if it works. Update it as needed.
7. Give a copy of your schedule to your supervisor. Keep another with you and *use* it. Revise it as needed.

When you make up your schedule, give some consideration to how much of what kind of activity you can accomplish in a given time slot. For example, a half-hour slot might not be sufficient for writing progress reports, especially if you have to gather your records first. But this *is* plenty of time to make a few phone calls or begin to write out a supply order.

In addition to the schedule, the OTA should consider using an appointment book. Some prefer one that shows an entire month on a single page, although there are many other formats available. A large stationery or office supply store should have several models to compare. The appointment book is the place to record planned meetings with individual clients and staff, special events, and nonroutine tasks. Personal digital assistants (PDAs), small computers and other handheld electronic organizers are another possibility; these include calendars, alarm clocks, scheduling plans, address book, and other aids.

### Grouping Related Tasks

Gleeson (4) suggests that grouping related tasks can save time. When technology is needed for a given task, consider scheduling the task for a time slotted with other tasks using the same technology. For the OTA, some chunks might be making several phone calls at one sitting, doing several Internet-related tasks in a given time slot, setting up boxes or bins with prepared materials for a few group sessions at one time.

### Scheduling and Planning Nonroutine Events

Some of the OTA's responsibilities may involve events that occur only once a month or once a year. Examples include craft fairs, bazaars, bake sales, holiday parties, student fieldwork, inventory of supplies, and sharpening of saws and knives. Each of these requires some preparation in advance, and time must be allotted for it. Listing these tasks and entering them in an appointment book ensures that you will remember to do them at the appropriate time and that you will not schedule other things that might conflict. You can use last year's appointment book as a guide to setting up reminders in a new book for the coming year. A departmental calendar would be even more efficient; this calendar could be kept or posted in a central location so that all staff, students, and volunteers could be informed of pending events.

Complex nonroutine events (holiday festivals, for example) may feel overwhelming, but are manageable if approached systematically:

1. Break the event down into steps.
2. Consider how much time is needed for each step.
3. Working *backward* from the date of the planned event, schedule each of the steps, leaving a little extra time in each step in case of errors or delay.
4. Use lists and self-stick notes to further detail each step, including the people, supplies, and telephone calls.

## PAPERWORK

As much as you might dislike it (and you are not alone in this), paperwork is an inescapable aspect of clinical work. Timely writing of progress reports and other documentation of clinical services is required. Budgets, purchase orders, requisition requests, maintenance requests, inventories, and statistics are also unavoidable. In addition, occupational therapy staff will be inundated by catalogs, continuing education fliers, memos, and copies of printed matter used in patient activities. The electronic revolution has brought us a flood of e-mail and faxes that also clamor for attention. The four keys to transforming this chaos into an order you can live with are these:

- Have a filing system.
- Make sure you are prepared with whatever supplies you need.
- Set aside blocks of time for paperwork.
- Use the wastebasket.

### Filing System

A filing system can be as simple or as complex as you wish. Avoid making the system too complicated because it will take more time to use. If you keep copies of client records, you will need a locked file drawer; each person should have a separate file folder. Catalogs should be kept together in another location, which could be a shelf, a wall rack, or a file drawer; vertical cardboard magazine file boxes are good organizers for catalogs. Important memos and statements about standard operating procedures belong together; a three-ring or spring-clip binder allows obsolete material to be removed and new material added easily.

Printed matter used in occupational therapy groups, individual assessments, interventions, and home programs rapidly becomes a disorderly mess unless it is organized. The recommended method is to create a series of folders for these handouts and sheets of directions. Another approach is to use heavy accordion files with internal dividers to sort out materials according to how they are used. For example, you might have an accordion file for your money management group and another for your laundry skills group. Materials can be divided into sequential sessions or any other way that makes sense to you. Label everything, though, so that you can find it when you need it.

It is difficult to remember all of the details you want to include in progress reports unless you create a system for managing and retrieving this information. One approach is to keep a daily log with a new page for each day, in which you jot down brief records of the day's events, including a few words on each patient you have seen. Another approach is to use a minicassette recorder or an electronic organizer. Informal notes must be guarded with the same care as any other confidential information about patients. Avoid including any identifiers that can be recognized by someone else; use a private code instead.

Ideally, the OTA writes a contact note immediately after each session or other event (e.g., phone call) that is to be documented. Immediate documentation is less likely to be challenged in court (8). Lengthier progress reports that are supported by frequent contact notes provide evidence of conscientious documentation.

### Preparation

It is amazing how much time is wasted looking for paper clips or running to borrow the hole puncher. Considering how little these things cost, every staff member should have the following: scissors, letter opener or envelope slitter, tape, ruler, paper clips, stapler and staples, staple remover, pencils and sharpener, black and red pens, permanent marking pens, highlighter pen, correction fluid or tape, scratch pad, stationery and forms, envelopes, self-stick notes, rubber bands, dictionary, paper recycling basket, and wastebasket. You should also have immediate access, preferably in the room where you do your paperwork, to a three-hole punch, telephone, shredder, and file folders.

### Making Time for Paperwork

Unless you are an accomplished writer and already a very well-organized person, you will probably find it possible to get your paperwork done only if you allocate large (at least 1-hour) blocks of time for it. This must be time free of interruptions, and if you find the telephone or your co-workers in the office a distraction, you may have to isolate yourself elsewhere.

### The Wastebasket

Lakein (6) writes that one of his best rules is to "handle each piece of paper only once." This is very difficult for some people. Many pieces of paper should go directly into the recycling bin. Not everything is important or should be saved or even read. Discard into the recycling everything you are sure you will not need later. Evaluate each piece of mail or printed matter the first time you see it. Before you save something to read later, consider whether you will actually do so. The benefits of tossing the irrelevant are delightful—psychological freedom and a less cluttered environment.

## THE ELECTRONIC REVOLUTION: MYTHS AND REALITY

We have available many electronic devices that speed storage and exchange of information: desktop and laptop computers, cell phones, beepers, fax machines, PDAs, dictation equipment, and so on. All of these tools can save time and energy if employed deliberately. But they can also consume time and energy (and money) in repairs, upgrading, and misuse. Despite their popularity in the consumer market, the adoption of these devices in clinical mental health settings has been slow. Funding is often insufficient to permit such luxuries; community settings in particular tend to rely on paper-based information systems. However, as electronics become smaller and pricing becomes more competitive, we expect devices will be used more universally. Here are some suggestions to make them serve you best:

- Choose brands and models with proven track records. Read the reports of nonprofit organizations such as *Consumer Reports* to obtain unbiased, comprehensive information.
- Buy computer software that is established and highly rated and that offers consumer support services such as upgrades and toll-free hotlines.
- Integrated packages of software may offer word processing, database management, financial management, and graphics design all in one program.
- In cell phones, PDAs, beepers, and fax machines, look for ringers that can be turned off while the visual display remains active. Cell phones and beepers that signal by vibration may be less disturbing to others. Fax machines can be set not to ring at all.

## The Paperless Office

For many reasons—ecological, organizational, and so on—the paperless office is an attractive ideal. Wouldn't it be wonderful to find everything on the computer? To get rid of all those professional journals, bulky catalogs, and other papers that fill our desks and shelves and cabinets? In truth, many paper catalogs can be discarded, and it's a good idea to request in writing that the vendor stop sending them, as long as the company's website provides sufficient range of items and ease of use. Two reasons for continuing to keep paper catalogs are *(a)* for clients and consumers to consult and *(b)* to provide documentation if the business office will not accept a Web-page document.

We can also stop collecting some professional journals because many are now available online by subscription or through libraries of medical centers and educational institutions. A few journals and newsletters, particularly those that originate in less developed countries and areas, may be accessible only in paper form. So checking as to the availability of an electronic version is important.

## E-Mail Traps

Electronic mail is a reality of the modern business environment, though smaller community settings may not have their own e-mail systems. Reading, writing, and being distracted by nonproductive e-mail are modern workplace dangers. Work efficiency can be speeded by the following strategies related to e-mail:

- Set a timer and plan to spend no more than 10 or 15 minutes on e-mail, first thing in the morning or late in the afternoon.
- Discriminate; look and delete. That's right! Delete spam and other distracting e-mail not related to essential work tasks.
- Read and respond immediately whenever possible.
- If an e-mail requires a response but you need time to think it over, mark the message to be kept as new.
- When the timer sounds, log off of your mail box and walk away.

The occupational therapy assistant who has experienced e-mail previously as a form of social communication should be aware that business and professional e-mail follows a formal protocol. For example, the screen name the OTA chooses for a business e-mail should represent the professional self. In other words, an e-mail address of KathySmith@hcpao.com looks businesslike whereas SweetieLove214@ssmail.com does not. Also, the abbreviations used in instant messaging and casual e-mails are inappropriate in professional communications. The OTA who has questions about how to approach the task of business e-mail should consult with a supervisor.

### Internet Distractions

So you log onto the Internet to locate a resource for a client, a journal article for evidence-based practice, a phone number for an agency, and then . . . ? Many of us find staying focused while on the Internet an ongoing challenge. Having observed students and employees logging onto myspace.com during working hours, playing online games, shopping, and so on, I agree that abuse of computer access in the workplace is a continuing and significant problem. While writing this chapter I have myself checked the weather and my e-mail and the news several times, reviewed my NetFlix queue, and wandered off-task to request a review copy of an unrelated book. With increased computer speed and capacity, the list of temptations grows longer.

I use several strategies that may be of use to the reader. The first is to employ a digital timer (Fig. 25-2). Setting the timer with the number of minutes (perhaps 45) one has to work before indulging in other distractions is helpful. Similarly, when starting down an avenue that will distract, one can set the timer for a short break (15 minutes).

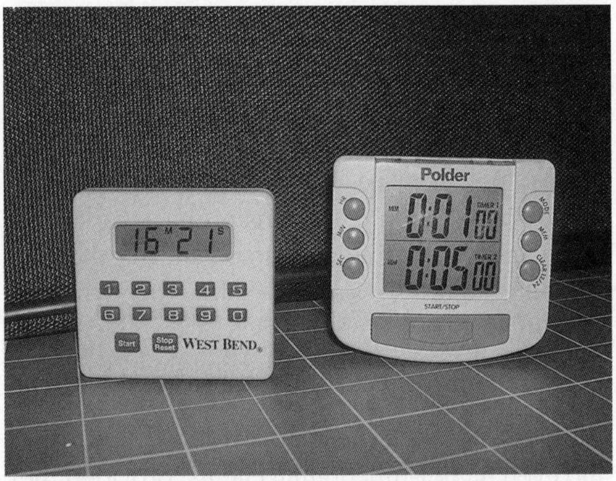


**Figure 25-2. Examples of digital timers.** The one on the right has two programmable memory timers as well as an elapsed time clock and a regular clock.

Another is to turn off or otherwise disable bouncing icons or chimes that signal incoming e-mail.

Hafner (5) reports that several technology companies are exploring development of smart systems that work together with the user to improve attention by (for example) smoothing text that is read by scrolling. But distractions are not all bad. Hafner quotes Dr. Csikszentmihalyi, the flow expert: "'I shouldn't knock distraction completely, because it can be useful,' he said. 'It can clear the mind and give you a needed break from a very linear kind of thinking' " (5, p. 2).

## MANAGEMENT OF SUPPLIES AND EQUIPMENT

Much of the pleasure of doing any task depends on having the necessary supplies and equipment available, prepared, and in working order. In some departments, OTAs are responsible for managing supplies and equipment not only for their own activities but for those of other staff as well.

### Ordering Supplies

The OTA may consider ordering supplies in bulk. Those used frequently and repeatedly should be ordered in quantity. Ordering supplies only a few times a year saves a lot of time. Of course, some items should be ordered only as needed (food and to some extent leather and wood). Copies of previous orders (electronic or paper) are useful reminders of what has to be reordered and from where.

Because many days, weeks, and even months can elapse between the placement of an order and its arrival, the OTA must anticipate this and keep other staff informed of when they can realistically expect to receive orders. Bureaucratic procedures such as paperwork and bidding requirements and policies of vendors (e.g., orders must be prepaid) and of institutions (must see three bids) can create delays.

## Storing Supplies

Storage is an area in which the individual must create a system to meet the needs of the situation. For example, if supplies are ordered only once or twice a year in bulk, a separate supply room must contain those that will not be used immediately. Also, the activities done in occupational therapy require a maddening array of tools and supplies of various shapes, sizes, perishability, and potential for danger. Storage systems have to be designed to accommodate this variety. Small portable electronic devices and other valuables require security locks. Locked storage must be provided for sharp and other dangerous objects and separate vented metal cabinets for flammables. These specialized items are described in more detail in Chapter 12. For storage of other materials, many types of organizers and kinds of storage equipment are available from office suppliers, art supply stores, hardware stores, closet shops, and furniture stores. The following are items that some occupational therapy practitioners have found useful:

- *Stacking bins* are made of plastic, stack on top of each other, and have open fronts so that their contents are easily seen. They can be arranged on open shelves.
- *Sliding wire or plastic baskets* on frames with wheels are good for storing lightweight loose materials such as yarn.
- *Sets of tiny transparent plastic drawers* can store beads, hardware, leather and jewelry findings, and other small items. It helps to label them.
- *Large flat sets of drawers* for large sheets of art paper are available from art and architecture supply stores.
- *Tool racks* can be purchased from hardware stores or be custom-made by an aide, volunteer, or the maintenance staff.
- *Pegboard* with Contac paper tracings of tools can be used to create a shadow board to show which tools belong where. When multiples are hung on the same hook the number of items should be written in large marker.
- *Cubbyholes* can be assigned to each client for storing projects in process.
- *Flat drawers*, easily accessible, can have Contac paper tool shadows for storing sharp objects. These, obviously, must be locked.
- *Bright, eye-catching pressure-sensitive labels* can be used to identify occupational therapy property or give instruction to clients or staff.

Even the best storage system can be defeated by hoarding. Occupational therapy practitioners enjoy a reputation for resourcefulness, for being able to create terrific activities from donations and leftovers. Without discipline, this delightful creativity expands into squirrel-like behavior, compelling its victims to rescue scrap lumber from the trash and save odds and ends of fabric and yarn and supplies left over from kits. Getting rid of this accumulated debris is a liberating experience; not letting it accumulate in the first place is even more energizing. The question that should be asked is whether the material is ever going to be used and, if so, when. Anything that does not have a definite purpose or use within a year should be thrown out, or (if this makes you feel too guilty) given to a local school, after-school program, or scout troop.

## Preparing Supplies

The French have the phrase *mise en place,* which means "put in place." Applying *mise en place* to activity preparation means organizing a work space in advance, gathering and preorganizing the supplies and tools so as to facilitate performance. Certain supplies cannot be used by cognitively disabled clients without some preparation by someone else. This does not necessarily have to be the OTA; these tasks can be handled by aides, volunteers, and even higher-functioning clients, provided they are given sufficient direction. Such tasks include cutting lengths of fabric and leather, attaching hardware, threading needles, unplugging or refilling glue bottles, sorting ceramic tiles, and laying out supplies for an activity. Disposable paper and plastic containers from the cafeteria (e.g., paper bowls, plastic cups) are handy for setting up individual amounts of loose materials such as tiles.

### Making Supplies Portable

OTAs who must carry out activities in a location other than the occupational therapy area need a system for getting the supplies from one place to the other. There are several options. One is to use a small rolling cart with shelves; the shelves should have raised lips to prevent things from sliding off. Another is to use a toolbox with internal trays and compartments. Yet another is to use a special enclosed rolling cart with locked drawers and doors; various models are available from office furniture suppliers, school furniture suppliers, and automotive supply stores.

### Maintaining Equipment

Only people who are skilled at repairing equipment should be charged with doing it; inadequate or slipshod repairs cause accidents. Unless the OTA or the maintenance staff of the facility has expertise with the equipment, it should be repaired by an outside expert. Service contracts should be purchased at the same time as new equipment. For older equipment, it may be possible to arrange a blanket service contract with a company that repairs different kinds of machines.

The OTA may be responsible for coordinating equipment repair for the occupational therapy department. This task can be made easier by providing a place (special notebook or message box) for staff to record a problem with equipment or by creating a special form. Once you are notified of a problem, you should arrange for the repair and let the staff know when they can expect it to be done.

## ORGANIZING SPACE

Entire books have been written on organization of space. This section does not duplicate the contents of these texts, which can be found in any large library, but indicates some of the basic issues involved in the organization and use of space in occupational therapy areas in psychiatric settings.[1]

OTAs do not necessarily make the final decisions about how space will be used and organized, but they should be able to participate in the planning, especially regarding activities they will be conducting. In some situations, as when a OTA is in charge of a skills program such as homemaking or a prevocational work group, the OTA may have complete responsibility for organizing the environment. Because storage areas and office areas have already been touched on, the discussion here focuses on activity areas. Several types of spaces are generally needed, and each has separate requirements.

### Areas for Large Groups

Space is needed for parties, athletic activities, community meetings, other large verbal groups, and perhaps movies and other theater presentations. Making space available may mean doubling up by using a room designed for another purpose, for example the dining room or lounge, and may require removing the usual furniture and bringing in folding chairs and tables. If space is used for more than one purpose, time must be allotted to transform it for its next use.

### Areas for Small Groups

*Small* is a relative concept. The size of the group and the kind of activity determine the kind of space needed. The area should be large enough and sufficiently free of clutter to permit people to move easily within it. On the other hand, it should

[1] This discussion is summarized in part from Bachner and Cornelius (3).

not be so large that a small group seems lost. An area of a larger room can be sectioned off with folding screens.

### Private Areas

A place is needed for interviews and confidential discussions. This can be an office or an activity room that is not otherwise scheduled. In an inpatient setting it may be possible to use patients' rooms for this purpose. The important factors are privacy and freedom from interruptions.

### Computer Areas

Computers are increasingly employed for activities with clients. As an occupational therapy practitioner, the OTA must attend to the ergonomics of the computer environment. Because the online environment is so attractive, a person may lose track of time and stay on the computer for longer than is healthy. Setting a timer for 45 minutes and requiring stretch breaks is a good idea.

The positions of chairs, work surfaces, monitors and keyboards should be compatible with proper body positioning. Specific suggestions are the following:

- Foot rests (even if only stacked telephone books) can help clients with shorter legs.
- Monitors should be positioned so as to minimize glare on the screen from windows and other light sources. Right-angle to windows or other light source is best.
- A open file folder can be taped across the top of the monitor to shade the screen from the glare of overheard lights.
- Keyboards must be placed at least 5 inches lower than the desktop height. Positioning the keyboard on ones knees is an acceptable compromise and far better for the wrists than having it on a tabletop.
- The mouse should be positioned so that the person does not have to reach for it. It should also be at a height lower than desk or tabletop.
- Users who need eyeglasses should consider having an extra pair specifically for computer distance.

### Areas for Messy Activities

Some activities (e.g., ceramics, artwork, woodworking) create so much clutter and mess that they need their own areas. If possible, separate locations should be permanently set aside for *each* of these major activities. Because this is not generally possible, the occupational therapy department should carefully evaluate whether conducting such a varied range of messy activities is worth the time and effort needed to clean up the area each time an activity is done.

### Inviting Functional Performance

The appearance of a room profoundly (if subliminally) affects the way people feel when they first approach it and while they are in it. If you want clients to want to *be* in your activity area and to *work* in it, it is up to you to make it inviting, comfortable, and appropriate for the particular activity. This is not difficult. You need only close your eyes and ask yourself, "Would *I* feel like working in a place like this?" When you open your eyes you will know what you have to do to make the place better. Here are some specific suggestions:

- Reduce clutter. Projects on display should be recent and attractive.
- Send unused equipment to deep storage or see if it can be auctioned off.
- Provide coat racks or wall pegs for clients' outerwear and for aprons and smocks.
- If the place looks drab, give it a paint job. If the maintenance staff cannot do it, see if the clients can.
- Repaint the furniture too, if it needs it. This can be a project for a work group.
- Cover old desktops and tabletops with contact paper or painted Masonite.

- Use display cases and corkboard to show off clients' projects and samples of crafts that are frequently used. Because these can be distracting to those with limited attention span, place them so that they can be screened off when necessary.
- Instead of displaying a sample of every craft available, keep a photo album of Polaroid shots of projects that clients can browse through.
- Keep wall displays simple, cheerful, and attractive. A felt banner or wall hanging or a large framed poster can set the mood for the room.

Maintaining an inviting therapeutic environment requires constant vigilance. Finished and half-finished projects and scraps of various materials tend to pile up. Dust and dirt inevitably accumulate. If the housekeeping staff cannot be relied upon to clean the room properly, you can do it yourself or organize a work group of clients to do routine cleaning chores such as wiping tables, dusting, sweeping, and mopping. Seasonal redecorating parties provide a structure for changing or updating the look of the environment on a regular basis.

## DELEGATING

The OTA does not have to do it all. Volunteers, aides, clients, family members, and other staff can be asked to contribute. Interdependence and community are fostered by shared responsibilities. Depending on the situation, the OTA might delegate these tasks:

- Making phone calls to get information
- Collating, filing, organizing nonconfidential papers
- Sorting and organizing supplies and materials
- Following up on details of tasks that have already been laid out
- Researching and gathering information
- Locating community resources

## SUMMARY

In our work with clients we try to energize and motivate them so that they are able to accomplish what they want and need to do in the time available. Clients find this thrilling and a boost to their confidence and feelings of competence. If this is true of our clients, it is only fair to admit that it applies equally to ourselves. Chaos in the environment can detract from the skill with which an activity is performed. Therefore: Avoid chaos! Embrace order! Use the suggestions here to take charge of your time and space and create a daily environment that makes sense for you.

## REVIEW QUESTIONS AND ACTIVITIES

1. Briefly explain in your own words the value of being organized.
2. Would you or do you use a to-do list? Explain.
3. Do you use a personal digital assistant or other electronic organizer? A paper datebook or organizer? Both? Neither? Discuss.
4. Discuss some of the factors that should be considered in the timing of orders for supplies.
5. How should one decide which items to save and which to discard?
6. Give some examples of supplies that may need to be prepared in advance for clients to use them.
7. What do you think of the paperless office? Do you find the concept attractive? Or scary? Explain.
8. What e-mail address do you use for occupational therapy correspondence? Does it fit your image of yourself as a professional?
9. What do you think about Internet distractions? Do they represent a personal challenge for you? Discuss.
10. Compare the setup of the computer(s) that you commonly use with the positioning recommendations in this chapter. Is there anything you think you should change? Explain.
11. State one alternative to keeping samples of every available project.
12. *Challenge question:* What is your most significant problem with organization? What problem are you willing to tackle? What is your intervention plan for this? Use goal-attainment scaling (Chapter 16) and develop a 5-point scale and a time frame for accomplishing your goal.
13. *Challenge activity:* With a classmate visit one or more stores that sell office equipment, supplies, and/or organizational aids. Locate items that you think would be helpful. Photograph them and present your ideas in class.

## REFERENCES

1. Allen AS, Cruickshank DR. Perceived problems of occupational therapists: A subset of the professional curriculum. Am J Occup Ther 1977;31:557–564.
2. American Occupational Therapy Association. Occupational therapy practice framework: Domain and process. Am J Occup Ther 2002;56:609–639.
3. Bachner JP, Cornelius E. Activities coordinator's guide: A handbook for activities coordinators in long-term care facilities. Washington, DC: U.S. Government Printing Office, 1978.
4. Gleeson K. The Personal Efficiency Program: How to Get Organized to Do More Work in Less Time. 3rd ed. Mississauga, ON: Wiley Canada, 2003.
5. Hafner K. You there, at the computer: Pay attention. New York Times, Feb 10, 2005.
6. Lakein A. How to Get Control of Your Time and Your Life. New York: Wyden, 1973, 1996.
7. Mann T. The Magic Mountain. New York: Knopf, 1927.
8. Ranke BEA. Documentation in the age of litigation. OT Practice 1998;3(3):20–24.

## SUGGESTED READINGS

Byofsky S. 500 Terrific Ideas for Organizing Everything. New York: Budget, 1997.

Covey, SR. The Seven Habits of Highly Effective People. New York: Simon & Shuster, 1991.

Jensen B. The Simplicity Survival Handbook: 32 Ways to Do Less and Accomplish More. Toronto: HarperCollins Canada, 2003.

Lakein A. How to Get Control of Your Time and Your Life. New York: Wyden, 1973, 1996.

Winston S. The Organized Executive: A Program for Productivity: New Ways to Manage Time, Paper, People, and the Electronic Office. New York: Warner, 1994.

APPENDIX A

# Case Examples

## CASE 1: A 21-YEAR-OLD WOMAN WITH DEPRESSION[1]

*H. Page* *Case #186302*

This 21-year-old single African-American woman with a *DSM-IV-TR* diagnosis of dysthymic disorder (300.4) on axis I and passive–aggressive personality disorder (negativistic personality disorder) on axis II (Table A-1) was admitted to the acute admissions ward of a state psychiatric hospital after a nearly fatal suicide attempt (pills) following several months of depression, withdrawal, and refusal to leave her mother's house. This is her first hospitalization. Patient is medicated with fluvoxamine (Luvox) 100 mg h.s.

Ms. Page is the oldest of three children, all living with their mother; the patient's father died when she was 13 years old. The patient states that she has no friends, her sole girlfriend having moved to Florida. She has dated some but has never had a serious relationship.

Ms. Page is a high school graduate and attended college for 2 years, majoring in psychology; she enrolled briefly in a nursing school but quit to move to Florida with her girlfriend. She stayed there only a few months and returned home, withdrawn and depressed. She subsequently refused to leave her mother's home, leading to this hospitalization.

Ms. Page has worked as a baby-sitter and a housekeeper in a private residence, most recently during her stay in Florida. At present, she has no income of her own, relying on her mother for economic support. She was referred to occupational therapy for general evaluation of task skills and work potential, leisure planning, and stress assessment.

The following evaluations were administered: *Comprehensive Occupational Therapy Evaluation (COTE)* scale, *Occupational Performance History Interview*, Interest Checklist, and Stress Assessment.[2]

### Interview

The interview revealed little new information. Most of Ms. Page's experience in occupational roles has been as a student. She said she enjoyed school and did well there. She expressed no interest in vocational activities, stating that she is not interested in going to school or getting a job. Patient appeared despondent throughout the interview. She was, however, clean, neat, and appropriately groomed.

### Comprehensive Occupational Therapy Evaluation

The *COTE* scale rating was based on a single performance of a simple mosaic tile task. The patient completed the task easily, requesting instruction from the therapist only twice. She did not interact with others, tended to isolate herself, and did not respond to casual conversation initiated by the therapist. She expressed indifference about the task, saying she didn't care whether she completed

[1] This case example is based on material contributed by Terry Brittell, COTA, ROH. Certain details have been altered for teaching purposes, but it is essentially a real case. The patient's name is fictitious.

[2] The Stress Assessment is a structured interview that collects data on situations that the person finds stressful and the way he or she typically reacts to stress.

**TABLE A-1. *DSM-IV-TR* DIAGNOSIS AT ADMISSION (CASE 1)**

| | |
|---|---|
| Axis I | 300.4 Dysthymic disorder |
| Axis II | Passive–aggressive personality disorder |
| Axis III | None |
| Axis IV | Severity 2, mild (best friend moved away) |
| Axis V | Current GAF: 50<br>Highest GAF past year: 60 |

*GAF,* global assessment of functioning.

it or not. No problems in cognition, memory, or coordination were noted.

Results of the Interest Checklist indicated a strong interest in social recreational activities (conversation, board games), athletic activities (volleyball, exercise, swimming), and manual activities (mending, sewing, manual arts). Patient reported a particular interest in rock collecting, a hobby she has pursued since childhood.

The Stress Assessment revealed that the patient frequently is subject to severe stress occasioned by frustration over situations such as fighting (especially among siblings), rules, financial worries, living conditions, and lack of activity. Ms. Page finds leisure time frustrating and feels she has no real accomplishments. She says living at home is too strict and cites her relationship with her mother as particularly stressful. She also reports a strong feeling of loss associated with the death of her father, her own graduation from school, and her separation from her friend who moved to Florida. In addition, Ms. Page has asthma, allergies, and acne and says she feels ugly. She feels that others do not understand her.

### Questions for Case 1

1. Assume that you are the OTA on the case. What additional assessment or assessments would you recommend to your supervisor? What additional information would you like to have, and how would you go about obtaining it?
2. Formulate an intervention plan. Assume Ms. Page can remain for 3 weeks more as an inpatient and can be discharged to a day treatment center within the state hospital center.

## CASE 2: A 72-YEAR-OLD WOMAN WITH ALZHEIMER'S DISEASE[3]

*J. Anderson* *Case #9801*

This 72-year-old married white woman was admitted to Green Manor Nursing Home, a skilled nursing facility, with a *DSM-IV-TR* diagnosis of dementia of the Alzheimer's type, late onset, with depressed mood (294.1) (Table A-2). Ms. Anderson, who also has axis III diagnosis of cerebral atherosclerosis and congestive heart failure, was first diagnosed with Alzheimer's disease 3 years ago. Until admission she was cared for at home by her husband of 45 years. However, Ms. Anderson has become weaker and incontinent, and Mr. Anderson, who is 74 years old, is not strong enough to help his wife transfer from bed to commode, so it was necessary to place her in a home.

**TABLE A-2. *DSM-IV-TR* DIAGNOSIS AT ADMISSION (CASE 2)**

| | |
|---|---|
| Axis I | 294.1 Dementia of the Alzheimer's type with late onset, with depressed mood |
| Axis II | None |
| Axis III | Cerebral atherosclerosis, congestive heart failure |
| Axis IV | Severity 3, moderate (recent move to nursing home) |
| Axis V | Current GAF: 22<br>Highest GAF past year: 25 |

*GAF,* global assessment of functioning.

[3] This case is based on actual clinical material, but names and other details have been changed to protect the resident's identity.

Ms. Anderson is of Norwegian ancestry; her religion is Lutheran. She was the fifth of nine children and is the only one still living. She has a high school diploma and was employed for 29 years as a bookkeeper in a local manufacturing business. The Andersons have one son, aged 51, who lives in another state. According to Mr. Anderson, his wife used to enjoy needlework, canasta, and gardening, activities that she abandoned as her illness became more severe. During the final 6 months Ms. Anderson remained at home, her husband took care of all of the cooking, cleaning, and household management. According to him, she complained constantly that he wasn't doing a good enough job, that she didn't like his cooking, and so on.

The following evaluations were attempted: structured interview and mental status examination, functional range of motion examination, functional daily living skills evaluation, and *Parachek Geriatric Rating Scale.*[4]

## Interview

At interview, Ms. Anderson was found seated in a wheelchair in her room. The wheelchair was the wrong size; it elevated her shoulders. Ms. Anderson was well groomed and neatly dressed; conference with the nursing staff revealed that her husband comes in early every morning to help. Ms. Anderson was able to state her name and knew she was in some sort of institution. She did not know the correct date, gave a month in a different season, and said the year was 1988 (19 years ago). When asked how she came to be in the home, she replied that she had come here for a job interview. ("They need someone to straighten out the books") She then said that she decided not to take the job. ("Who'd want to work in a place like this?") Resident incorrectly answered 7 of 10 questions on the mental status examination; recent memory and fund of general information seemed particularly impaired. She could follow a one-step command but not two steps. Her speech was clear and her hearing apparently unimpaired. Ms. Anderson wears glasses.

Functional range of motion examination revealed that Ms. Anderson could not walk, even with a walker, because of poor endurance and poor balance. She had full range in most motions of the upper extremities but was unable to elevate her arms above the level of her shoulders; range was more impaired on the right than on the left. Grasp was very weak. Range in the lower extremities was evaluated separately by a physical therapist, who noted limitations in all motions.

## Functional Daily Living Skills Evaluation

Functional daily living skills evaluation showed that resident had sufficient pinch and coordination to button and unbutton garments with front closures. She was unable to bathe or care for her teeth and hair without assistance but seemed aware of the need for help and asked for it. She could feed herself if the tray was prepared (e.g., meat cut up). Sitting balance was poor, and Ms. Anderson could not perform transfers unassisted.

Resident scored 28 on the *Parachek Geriatric Rating Scale.* Breakdown of the scores was as follows: physical condition, 10; general self-care, 11; social behaviors, 7.

## Questions for Case 2

1. Write an occupational therapy intervention plan, including goals and activities. *Hint:* The plan should focus on maintaining rather than improving function and should allow for deterioration in the resident's condition. State which activities are to be individual and which in a group.
2. Assuming the resident's condition deteriorates, at what point would you recommend that occupational therapy be discontinued? Identify specific behavioral and functional impairments that would indicate that the resident cannot

[4] A rating scale for physical capacities, self-care skills, and social interaction.

benefit from further treatment. Write a discharge plan (discontinuance from occupational therapy), including recommendations and directions for the nursing staff.

## CASE 3: A 54-YEAR-OLD WOMAN WITH SCHIZOPHRENIA, PARANOID TYPE[5]

*L. Lammermoor* *Case #082751*

This 54-year-old single white woman was admitted to the acute admissions ward on court certification following action by her neighbors. Commitment papers state that the patient has been complaining of people doing things against her; she is suspicious of her neighbors and has been breaking windows. Patient has had two previous psychiatric hospitalizations, in 1974 for 3 months and in 1977 for 6 months. Diagnosis is schizophrenia, paranoid type (295.30) (Table A-3). Patient also has chronic phlebitis in both legs. Prescribed medication includes olanzapine (Zyprexa) 10 mg h.s.; doxepin (Sinequan) 100 mg t.i.d.; docusate (Colace) 100 mg h.s., and prune juice 8 oz h.s.

At admission, Ms. Lammermoor was poorly groomed and dressed in dirty clothing. She appeared anxious, tense, and somewhat confused. Her speech was coherent but at times irrelevant. She denied hearing voices and denied having said that her food was poisoned. She said she had no idea why she was hospitalized other than the ill will of her neighbors.

**TABLE A-3. *DSM-IV-TR* DIAGNOSIS AT ADMISSION (CASE 3)**

| | |
|---|---|
| Axis I | 295.30 Schizophrenia, paranoid type |
| Axis II | None |
| Axis III | Phlebitis |
| Axis IV | Severity 2, mild (trouble with neighbors) |
| Axis V | Current GAF: 30<br>Highest GAF past year: 50 |

*GAF*, global assessment of functioning.

[5]This case example is based on material contributed by Terry Brittell, COTA, ROH. Certain details have been altered for teaching purposes, but it is essentially a real case. The patient's name is fictitious.

Patient is the third child in a family of eight and was raised in a rural section of northern New York State near the Canadian border. She has never married. She lives alone in an apartment with two cats. She has a 10th-grade education and has held numerous jobs as a domestic in private homes. She says she is now retired and living on Supplemental Security Income (SSI) and Social Security.

Patient was referred to occupational therapy 2 weeks after admission for evaluation of functional living skills and assessment of needs in relation to discharge planning. Evaluation instruments included a structured interview, the *Comprehensive Occupational Therapy Evaluation (COTE)* scale, and a functional living skills evaluation.

### Interview

Ms. Lammermoor arrived on time for the interview and each of the subsequent evaluation sessions. Though her hair was often slightly disheveled, she was otherwise clean and neat. She was cooperative in the interview and spoke at length about her apartment, the "things" (she refused to further define what she meant), and her two cats. She expressed sorrow over the death of her mother 5 years ago and seemed to have some unresolved feelings. She mentioned that she does not see her family; she feels positively about one of her brothers who lives in California but expressed hostility toward another brother who lives nearby. She spoke angrily of her neighbors, stating that she feels persecuted, that they pick on her, are stealing from her, and say bad things about her. She also mentioned that the neighborhood children harass her.

She said she neither has friends nor wants them. She said she is not interested in learning anything new to fill leisure hours, although she does enjoy solitary activities. The only group activity she expressed interest in was bingo. She was unaware of local resources and activity programs for retired people and said she wasn't interested in them.

## Comprehensive Occupational Therapy Evaluation

The *COTE* scale was used to rate the patient's performance of a simple craft activity (magazine picture collage). The patient worked at moderate speed and an acceptable level of activity. She appeared oriented to place, person, and time. She expressed concern about why certain other persons were not present or were late for the evaluation, which was administered in a group.

Patient was responsive and appropriate in her conversation, but most interactions were either dependent or impulsive. For example, she repeatedly asked for help, extra directions, and materials that she could obtain herself. Other patients appeared to view this as an attention-getting device, and several made negative remarks to the effect that she took needed attention from them. She also made comments that were unrelated to the conversation.

Patient needed no encouragement to engage in the activity; and after receiving repeated direction, which she requested, she was able to follow through and complete the task. She worked neatly, in an organized fashion; coordination and concentration were more than adequate for the task. She was able to make decisions and solve minor problems encountered in the activity despite her requests for assistance in other less difficult areas. She appeared highly motivated by the activity and expressed interest in other crafts displayed in the occupational therapy room.

## Functional Living Skills Evaluation

Ms. Lammermoor demonstrated an ability to function independently in the following areas: use of medication, use of her savings account, organization and cleaning of her home, selection of clothing and laundry and clothing maintenance, and single-serving cooking. She was unable to identify the correct response to several household emergencies, including what to do if the lights went out or if she smelled gas. She was able to use a telephone book to find emergency phone numbers, but she has limited reading and writing skills, which prevent her from writing simple messages or reading a bus schedule. She apparently relies on others to tell her when and where to take the bus, and she has a good knowledge of the public transportation system. She states that she does have a budget and could demonstrate how to break down her monthly income into weekly budgets. However, she was unable to demonstrate or explain how to make correct change from $5, and she could not figure the sales tax.

## Questions for Case 3

1. How do you interpret the patient's interest in bingo? Is this a good activity for developing social and interpersonal skills? Explain.
2. The physician wants to know whether Ms. Lammermoor can function well enough on her own to return to her own apartment or should be placed in a supervised living situation. Formulate a recommendation and justify it with evidence from the case history. Indicate any further evaluations or information that you think are needed or believe will help in making this determination. Document your recommendations in the form of a note suitable for the patient's chart.

# CASE 4: A 22-YEAR-OLD MAN WITH CHRONIC SCHIZOPHRENIA AND MILD MENTAL RETARDATION[6]

*J. Velasquez* *Case #085562*

This 22-year-old Hispanic man with an axis I diagnosis of chronic undifferentiated schizophrenia (295.90) and mild mental retardation (Table A-4)

[6] This case example is loosely based on an actual case. The names and certain other facts have been changed to protect the client's identity.

**TABLE A-4. *DSM-IV-TR* DIAGNOSIS AT ADMISSION (CASE 4)**

| | |
|---|---|
| Axis I | 295.90 Schizophrenia, undifferentiated type, chronic |
| Axis II | 317.00 Mild mental retardation |
| Axis III | None |
| Axis IV | Severity 1, none |
| Axis V | Current GAF: 20<br>Highest GAF past year: 20 |

*GAF,* global assessment of functioning.

was referred to a community day treatment center in a large East Coast city. The referral originated at another mental health clinic in a different part of the city. He had been attending that clinic for medication, and the staff there believed he could benefit from a structured day program and family therapy.

Mr. Velasquez was born in Colombia, South America. His parents were teenagers when he was born and have subsequently divorced (the father is reported to have been a drug addict and alcoholic). The client, who has four younger sisters and a younger brother, lived with his maternal grandparents in Colombia while his mother emigrated to the United States when he was 10. The rest of the family emigrated 6 years ago. Immediately after the move, the client became ill but was never hospitalized. He was followed at an outpatient clinic and stabilized on haloperidol (Haldol) and benztropine (Cogentin). Mr. Velasquez dropped out of school at age 16, without completing his high school education.

On admission, the social worker obtained the following information from the family. The mother is employed in a factory job. Mr. Velasquez, who speaks no English, stays home and masturbates all day. He sees no one but family members and has not been able to care for his own hygiene. His 14-year-old sister has been washing and dressing him. He appears to be hallucinating, says he is in the space shuttle, and has frequent loud outbursts of inappropriate laughter. Mr. Velasquez was also seen by the psychiatrist, who changed his medication to Risperdal.

The occupational therapy evaluation was performed 3 days later by an occupational therapy student under the supervision of the therapist. Evaluation instruments used were the *Occupational Role History Interview*[7] and the Allen Cognitive Level Screening test. Results were as follows:

## Interview

Mr. Velasquez appeared for the interview neatly dressed but with the back of his hair uncombed and his pants unzipped. He closed the zipper at the student's reminder to do so.

## Occupational Role History Interview

In the *Occupational Role History Interview*, Mr. Velasquez often gave tangential and irrelevant replies to questions asked by the student. He spoke of violent events, such as being beaten by a man with a club in school and having been accused by a classmate of killing her grandmother. When asked about school, he stated that he was good at drawing but bad at biology and physics. Mr. Velasquez said emphatically that he had no friends and could think of no one whom he had looked up to in the past as a role model.

Mr. Velasquez attended school in Colombia but has not attended since his family moved to this country when he was 16. He has never had a job. He has very limited understanding of English; the interview was conducted in Spanish.

## Allen Cognitive Level Screening Test

In the Allen Cognitive Level Screening test, the client was able to complete two running stitches and then two whip stitches. He was unable to complete the single cordovan stitch, and he recognized

[7] An abbreviated version of the *Occupational History Interview* (see Chapter 15).

that he had made errors but did not attempt to correct them. The student repeated the instructions (the client did not request this), but Mr. Velasquez was not able to complete the stitch on his second attempt. This performance was scored at cognitive level 4.

### Questions for Case 4

1. What additional information would you like to have about this client and his background?
2. What additional evaluations do you think might be useful?
3. From the available information, list the client's apparent assets (strengths) and deficits (problems). Include a discussion of the environment. Plan a schedule of daily activities at the treatment center. Choose one activity for each morning and afternoon except Wednesday morning, which is set aside for community meeting and medication groups. Give reasons for each activity choice. List two goals for one of these groups and explain what *specific* activity you would use and how you would structure and present it. These are the available activities:
   - Tools for living (daily living skills)
   - Art workshop
   - Music workshop
   - Sewing workshop
   - Woodworking
   - Boutique sales
   - Cooking school
   - Work preparation (prevocational)
   - Messenger training
   - Scrapbooking
   - Tai chi
   - Adult basic education
   - Social skills training
   - Assertiveness training
   - Anger management
   - Aerobic dancing
   - Drama workshop
   - Basic sensorimotor skills (parachute and ball play)
4. The client performed at level 4 on the Allen Cognitive Level Screening test. What additional information in the report supports this? Do you think this assessment is accurate or that a different result might be obtained at a different time? Explain your answer.

## CASE 5: A 30-YEAR-OLD MAN WITH BIPOLAR I DISORDER[8]

*D. Kennedy* *Case #291083*

This 30-year-old white man has an axis I diagnosis of bipolar I disorder (296.64), most recent episode mixed, severe with psychotic features (Table A-5). He was referred to occupational therapy for evaluation and development of skills needed to resume community living with his wife of 4 months. The patient was admitted to a general hospital following an incident on Valentine's Day 1 year ago in which he stabbed and enucleated his right eye. Mr. Kennedy cited a biblical passage as the reason for this self-mutilation.[9] Patient was subsequently

**TABLE A-5. *DSM-IV-TR* DIAGNOSIS AT ADMISSION (CASE 5)**

| | |
|---|---|
| Axis I | 296.64 Bipolar I disorder, most recent episode mixed, severe with psychotic features |
| Axis II | None |
| Axis III | Blind in right eye after self-inflicted enucleation |
| Axis IV | Severity 5, extreme (enucleation of eye, recent marriage) |
| Axis V | Current GAF: 10<br>Highest GAF past year: 30 |

*GAF,* global assessment of functioning.

[8] This case material was contributed by Beatrice White, COTA, OT Division, Springfield Hospital Center, Sykesville, MD. Certain details have been altered for teaching purposes, but it is essentially a real case. The patient's name is fictitious.

[9] Matthew 5:28–30.

transferred to an outpatient mental health clinic, but 3.5 years later he could not be maintained in the community and was admitted to a state hospital. This was his first psychiatric hospitalization, although he had a history of psychiatric consultations dating from adolescence; and since age 23, he has had had difficulty functioning at work because of emotional problems. Patient is medicated with lithium carbonate, although he has received thioridazine (Mellaril), haloperidol, and trihexyphenidyl (Artane) in the past (he was initially diagnosed as having schizophrenia, paranoid type). Patient has no history of drug or alcohol abuse.

Patient's family background is unclear; his parents separated when he was 6 years old, shortly after a sister, his only sibling, was born. He moved with his mother and sister from Virginia to Maryland and has had no contact with his father since. Patient's mother is described as rigid and controlling and very religious; church affiliation is Baptist. Patient's emotional problems were recognized during his school years; he was described as a "schizoid child" and received special education to compensate for his social isolation and difficulty with interpersonal relationships. Patient has a high school diploma. Mr. Kennedy worked for 7 years as a horse trainer and groomer at a race track and for 5 years at his mother's florist business.

Around his 24th birthday patient became ill and could no longer function at work. The precipitating incident occurred when a stranger knocked on the door of his home asking for a man with the same name as the patient; patient then became suspicious and concerned about men following him. He attended Bible class regularly with his mother, met his future wife there, and became engaged to her. Subsequently, he became anxious and indecisive about the pending marriage, and it was at this time that he mutilated his eye. After 4 months in acute care in a general hospital he was discharged and followed on weekly outpatient visits; at this point he was receiving thioridazine. He then married despite advice from the clinic not to do so. His medication was changed to haloperidol and trihexyphenidyl because of problems with rigidity and catatonic posturing. Patient was unable to consummate his marriage because of impotence, and he then became incontinent of urine and feces and was considered unmanageable at home; he was admitted to the state psychiatric hospital 4 months after his marriage. On admission, he was withdrawn and rigid, showed blunted affect, and exhibited festinating gait. He was delusional, expressing the idea that someone was gripping his mind and that Jesus was Satan. His medication was reviewed and changed to lithium, which seemed effective and has been continued since then.

Medical care of the right eye during the patient's tenure as an outpatient and during the first 2 months of his inpatient stay was extensive. Chronic infections, stretching of the eye socket, and poor hygiene and grooming due to carelessness and poor cooperation by the patient made it impossible for him to use a prosthesis. He has been wearing an eye patch.

The rehabilitation team in its initial treatment planning conference identified the primary goal as helping the patient make an effective adjustment to resume community living with his wife. Patient's wife was interested in a possible switching of roles: She would continue her work as a rental agent secretary in an apartment complex and he would take care of the home. It was not clear initially whether this was the best arrangement or whether patient should return to work at the race track and the florist's shop.

Occupational therapy evaluation included the *Kohlman Evaluation of Living Skills (KELS)*, a sensory-perceptual-motor assessment, and a street survival questionnaire. All of these were administered by the occupational therapist. A deficit in patient's standing balance was noted. In addition, patient was unable to perform basic household tasks; was unfamiliar with household situations; did not know proper first aid; was unable to identify household safety problems; had poor laundry skills; and was unfamiliar with budgeting, grocery shopping, paying bills, and banking. Patient was withdrawn and showed poor social skills. He was unable to identify leisure interests and showed no motivation for using leisure time productively. The occupational therapist established the following immediate goals:

- Improve standing balance
- Improve grooming, personal hygiene, and self-care
- Assess and develop work skills in preparation for return to full-time employment

The therapist began a series of one-to-one sensory integration sessions to improve standing balance and arranged for patient to attend daily occupational therapy self-care sessions and a work adjustment program for a 6-month work skills assessment and program in horticulture (the area was selected because of the patient's previous experience in a florist's shop). This vocational effort was coordinated by occupational therapy and the vocational rehabilitation counselor.

Patient's progress was reviewed prior to his completion of this program, at which time it seemed that patient would not be able to return to work because of overwhelming anxiety. Although Mr. Kennedy had participated actively in the work skills program, both patient and his wife agreed that it would be best for him to take over the household responsibilities rather than work full-time. Patient's wife rented a suburban efficiency apartment convenient to public transportation and shopping. Criteria for patient's release were based on his ability to maintain stability of mood and cooperate with daily treatment programs. Because the ultimate objective was to enable Mr. Kennedy to function as a homemaker in the community, he was referred to the home arts program[10] for evaluation and skills development.

[10] A home arts program is designed to help participants develop and improve homemaking skills in the following major areas: meal preparation, nutrition, housekeeping, self-care skills, play and leisure skills, sewing, social skills, and community trips. A protocol can be found in Fidler GS. Design of Rehabilitation Services in Psychiatric Hospital Settings. Laurel, MD: Ramsco, 1984.

The OTA in the home arts program used the *Comprehensive Evaluation of Basic Living Skills (CEBLS)*[11] to obtain more detailed information on patient's skills and needs. The following additional deficits were noted: unstable and unsafe posture; failure to compensate for loss of vision on the right; no knowledge of nutrition, menu planning, meal preparation, or grocery shopping; and a tendency to panic under stress. The following additional goals were established by the OTA and patient and approved by the OT:

- Increase sense of comfort and confidence in ability to carry out the home management role
- Improve ability to plan and execute basic household tasks
- Develop social skills in basic communication, ability to relate to others in small groups, and appropriate self-assertion
- Teach techniques to compensate for the visual defect
- Teach stress management techniques and establish a habit of using them
- Explore leisure interests and develop a habit of participating in leisure on a regular basis

Methods included attendance at the home arts program for 4 hours a day, four times a week for 10 weeks. Patient completed a course of instruction in all areas of home management. He became gradually more comfortable in social situations and showed appropriate curiosity and interest in the program and in other patients. He learned stress management techniques using music, progressive relaxation, and imagery, and he became less suspicious and more spontaneous in his interactions with others.

Patient was discharged from the hospital in the spring, a little more than 1 year after admission, following his successful completion of the home arts program. He consummated his marriage and now lives with his wife in the apartment she rented. He works part-time in a local greenhouse and

[11] Casanova JS, Ferber J. Comprehensive evaluation of basic living skills. Am J Occup Ther 1976;30:101–105.

nursery. He appears stable and is managing his role as homemaker and part-time worker very well. Maintenance checkups in the community mental health clinic in his neighborhood are continuing.

## CASE 6: A 22-YEAR-OLD WOMAN WITH POLYSUBSTANCE DEPENDENCE AND DEPENDENT PERSONALITY DISORDER[12]

*L. Balthasar* *Case # 112188*

This 22-year-old white woman, self-admitted to a detoxification unit, stated she sought treatment because she's pregnant and abusing drugs (Table A-6). Her father and maternal grandfather are alcoholics. Her parents were divorced when she was 13 years old, and she began using alcohol at that time. She has used pot since age 15, and over the past 6 months, crack cocaine. She stated she'd tried speed and acid once in her midteens. Ms. Balthasar's pattern of substance use is to drink more than a six-pack daily, one to two joints daily, and crack on weekends, anywhere from 10 rocks to two eight balls.[13] Client was transferred to rehabilitation after 5 days in detoxification.

**TABLE A-6. *DSM-IV-TR* DIAGNOSIS AT ADMISSION (CASE 6)**

| | |
|---|---|
| Axis I | 303.90 Alcohol dependence<br>304.30 Cannabis dependence<br>305.60 Cocaine abuse<br>304.90 Polysubstance dependence |
| Axis II | 301.6 Dependent personality disorder |
| Axis III | None |
| Axis IV | Severity 1, none |
| Axis V | Current GAF: 60<br>Highest GAF past year: 60 |

*GAF,* global assessment of functioning.

[12] Adapted from a case contributed by Susan Voorhies, COTA/CAO-DAC, of HCA Regional Hospital Rediscovery Unit, Jackson, TN, in consultation with Anne Brown, OTR, MS.

[13] An eight ball is equivalent to 10 to 12 rocks.

Client has a 10th-grade education, having dropped out of school during early years of drug use. She has been living with her mother, who works two jobs, and two younger sisters until this past week, when she went on a binge and stayed at various places. Client participates minimally in household chores (e.g., washes dishes and folds clothes).

### Interview

On interview by the occupational therapy assistant, she appeared sad, had poor eye contact, and said she has little self-confidence. She has no hobbies and no friends other than her drug-using peers. She stated she would like to get her general equivalency diploma (GED), have a job, live independently, and raise her baby. Client reported she's uncertain who is the father of her baby and so will be solely responsible for the child. She admitted that her life lacks structure and that she has no healthy leisure involvements. She stated that she values her family, sees her strengths in being a hard worker and straightforward and her weaknesses in using drugs and alcohol and allowing others to take advantage of her.

Goals, objectives, and treatment are shown in the treatment summary for this case (Table A-7).

### Occupational Therapy Discharge Summary (1 Month after Admission)

Ms. Balthasar was initially resistant to occupational therapy, but as she developed rapport with staff and interacted with peers, she began to participate and show motivation. She completed at least one project per week (e.g., painted sweatshirt, wooden carousel, stenciled teddy bear peg rack). In leisure education, she initially argued that she could not have fun without using chemicals. After several community out-trips and recreational activities (such as movies, cookouts, and swimming), she began identifying with fulfilling leisure activities such as playing recreational games with peers from Alcoholics Anonymous (AA) and

**TABLE A-7. OCCUPATIONAL THERAPY TREATMENT SUMMARY (CASE 6)**

| GOALS | OBJECTIVES | OT TREATMENT GIVEN |
|---|---|---|
| 1. To improve independent living skills (household, child care) | 1a. Client will identify areas of household skills she needs to learn (within 1 wk) | 1a. Individual OT 1 × wk |
| | 1b. Client will participate in independent living skills training, e.g., cooking a meal, planning a budget, 2 × wk. | 1b. Independent living skills training group 2 × wk |
| | 1c. Client will schedule parenting classes in the community (within 3 wk) | 1c. OT referral to Carl Perkins' parenting classes |
| 2. To identify leisure activities appropriate for a sober lifestyle | 2a. Client will identify leisure interests and hobbies (by 2 wk) | 2a. Leisure education 1 × wk; OT craft clinic 4 × wk; community out-trip 1 × wk |
| | 2b. Client will complete one craft project per wk while in treatment | 2b. OT craft clinic 4 × wk |
| | 2c. Client will identify specific leisure activities appropriate for herself and her baby (by 4 wk) | 2c. Leisure education 1 × wk; community out-trip 1 × wk |
| 3. To obtain a GED | 3. Client will schedule appointment with CARE about GED preparation classes (by 3 wk) | 3. Individual OT referral to CARE |
| 4. To improve assertiveness skills | 4a. Client will identify situations in which she could be more assertive (by 1 wk) | 4a. Assertiveness training group 2 × wk |
| | 4b. Client will role-play difficult situations using assertive techniques (by 3 wk) | 4b. Assertiveness training group 2 × wk |

*GED*, general equivalency diploma; *CARE*, Center for Adult Reading and Enrichment.

Narcotics Anonymous (NA). She identified sweatshirt painting as a possible hobby after discharge and plans to make clothing for herself and her baby using inexpensive paints, sale items, and clothing from thrift stores.

She continued to have difficulty demonstrating assertive behavior spontaneously. In structured role-playing, she was able to use assertive techniques effectively after they were modeled for her. OTA told client to continue working on assertive responses in daily interactions. Pt. scheduled three meetings a week at the Center for Adult Reading and Enrichment (CARE) program to prepare herself for her GED test. She will be discharged to a halfway house, where she will continue to receive treatment for the remainder of her pregnancy.

Ms. Balthasar has begun working on independent living skills, such as cooking from a recipe, planning and cooking a meal, developing a budget on her allowance from her mother, and general house cleaning. She will continue working on this at the halfway house. Ms. Balthasar will also be assigned part-time employment and will be referred to vocational rehabilitation for job training after she receives her GED. The halfway house will provide child care and a place for her to live while she continues her education and job training. She is scheduled to attend parenting classes two nights per week and will attend meetings of her 12-step programs nightly. This client has responded well to treatment, particularly to structure and support. OTA will follow up on referrals post discharge.

### Questions for Case 6

1. Identify the chief enabler in this client's situation.
2. What occupational roles is the client acquiring? What occupational roles can you foresee that she will need in the future?
3. What additional skills and social supports will the client need as her baby gets older?
4. The client's mother would like her to return home to live with her once the baby is born. What are the advantages and disadvantages in terms of Ms. Balthasar's maintaining and developing independent living skills and adult occupational roles?

## CASE 7: A 37-YEAR-OLD MAN WITH ALCOHOL DEPENDENCE DISORDER[14]

*B. Jebson* *Case #038947*

Mr. Jebson is a 37-year-old white married man admitted to detox unit after his employer confronted him about poor job performance and absenteeism owing to alcohol abuse (Table A-8). Client reported that his wife has been threatening to leave him over the past year. Client was transferred to rehabilitation after three days in detoxification.

**TABLE A-8. *DSM-IV-TR* DIAGNOSIS AT ADMISSION (CASE 7)**

| | |
|---|---|
| Axis I | 303.90 Alcohol dependence |
| Axis II | None |
| Axis III | None |
| Axis IV | Severity 2, mild (confrontation with employer) |
| Axis V | Current GAF: 70<br>Highest GAF past year: 80 |

*GAF,* global assessment of functioning.

Client began drinking alcohol at age 15 and stated that it has been a problem in his life for at least the past 5 years. He has been fired from two jobs during that time and is having difficulty at a local factory job in which he's been employed for almost 18 months. Client was able to maintain one job for 11 years, but that ended 5 years ago. He and his wife have been married for 10 years and have an 8-year-old daughter and 5-year-old son. Client denied any marital problems other than drinking.

Mr. Jebson has two brothers and one sister and was raised by his parents on a farm. He stated that he's the only one in his immediate family who drinks, but he's heard that his maternal great-grandfather was alcoholic. Client completed high school and vocational technical training, acquiring a welding certificate. He stated his pattern is to drink at least six to eight beers after work, and on weekends in excess of a case plus several half pints of whisky. Client says he has mainly drunk alone at home in his tool shop. He does very little individual or family leisure activity. He stated that he has difficulty expressing his feelings and drinks especially when he feels angry. Client admitted to being violent when drunk, throwing things and punching the wall on several occasions. He denies ever hitting his wife or children. Client said that he used to go to the local Baptist church with his family but quite because of his drinking. He had one DUI charge approximately 2 years ago and after that quit going to bars to drink.

[14] Adapted from a case contributed by Susan Voorhies, COTA/CAO-DAC, of HCA Regional Hospital Rediscovery Unit, Jackson TN, in consultation with Anne Brown, OTR, MS.

**TABLE A-9. OCCUPATIONAL THERAPY TREATMENT SUMMARY (CASE 7)**

| GOALS | OBJECTIVES | OT TREATMENT GIVEN |
|---|---|---|
| 1. To improve leisure and social involvement | 1a. Client will identify at least five leisure activities to provide socialization and support for his recovery (by 2 wk) | 1a. Leisure education 1 × wk; community out-trips 1 × wk |
| | 1b. Client will identify a variety of leisure activities to pursue with his family (by 2 wk) | 1b. Leisure education 1 × wk; community out-trips 1 × wk; family recreation night biweekly; OT clinic 4 × wk |
| | 1c. Client will introduce himself to at least one male peer at nightly 12-step meetings and will inquire about the group's recreational activities (by 3 wk) | 1c. 12-step meetings nightly; individual leisure assignment |
| 2. To improve assertive behavior and expression of feelings | 2a. Client will begin keeping a daily feeling log (within 3 d) | 2a. Individual OT assignment |
| | 2b. Client will identify situations in which he has withheld angry feelings (by 2 wk) | 2b. Assertiveness training 2 × wk |
| | 2c. Client will role-play specific situations in which he's been angry using assertive techniques to express his anger (by 3 wk) | 2c. Assertiveness Training 2 × wk |

Client identified his strengths as loving his family, being a skilled welder, and caring about people. He named his weaknesses as drinking and holding in his feelings. He identified his family and his job as most important to him. Client was verbal but tearful at times during the interview. He appears motivated to get sober because of pressure from employer and wife.

Goals, objectives, and treatment are shown in the treatment summary for this case (Table A-9).

## Occupational Therapy Discharge Summary (3 Weeks after Admission)

Mr. Jebson has been compliant throughout treatment. He made several projects in occupational therapy for his family and identified woodcraft as a hobby he could pursue and teach to his children. He named the following as family activities he would like to develop: cookouts, camping, movies, vacations, and community park excursions. He named as additional activities for himself hunting, fishing, boating, flea markets, and AA retreats. He has met several men from his community through AA and has asked two of them to be his sponsors in the program. Client had difficulty labeling his feelings in the log initially and was given a chart with facial expressions[15] to use as a guide. He began appropriately identifying feelings of anger

[15] Such a chart can be found as exercise 7, "Emotions," in Korb KL, Azok AD, Leutenberg EA. Life Management Skills: Reproducible Activity Handouts Created for Facilitators. Beachwood, OH: Wellness Reproductions, 1989.

and fear as dominant in his experience. In assertiveness group he identified himself as passive unless intoxicated, when he would become aggressive. He talked openly about things he's stuffed his anger over and role-played effective expression. He reported using assertion in a marital session with his wife with positive results. Client asked about becoming a volunteer after a year of sobriety. He identified this as a long-term goal for aftercare. Family and employer are expected to support and encourage client after discharge.

### Questions for Case 7

1. What are this client's occupational roles? How did his substance abuse affect his functioning in these roles?
2. Which aspects of this client's treatment as described fall specifically within the scope of occupational therapy? Which aspects could be managed equally well by another treatment discipline?
3. What are the elements of this client's preferred defensive structure (PDS) (see Chapter 6)?
4. Why was the emotions identification guide given to this client? What other activities could assist this client to develop knowledge in this area?

## CASE 8: A 21-YEAR-OLD WOMAN WITH COCAINE DEPENDENCE, POLYSUBSTANCE ABUSE, BULIMIA, AND BORDERLINE PERSONALITY DISORDER[16]

*T. Little* *Case #10391*

Ms. Little is a 21-year-old black woman who sought treatment after the Department of Social Services threatened to take her two children, a boy aged 6 and a girl aged 2. Client stated that her neighbor reported her for leaving her children alone. Client is unemployed and on welfare.

[16] Adapted from a case contributed by Susan Voorhies, COTA/CAO-DAC, of HCA Regional Hospital Rediscovery Unit, Jackson, TN, in consultation with Anne Brown, OTR, MS.

**TABLE A-10. *DSM-IV-TR* DIAGNOSIS AT ADMISSION (CASE 8)**

| | |
|---|---|
| Axis I | 304.20 Cocaine dependence<br>305.90 Polysubstance abuse (past)<br>307.51 Bulimia nervosa |
| Axis II | 301.83 Borderline personality disorder |
| Axix III | None |
| Axis IV | Severity 4, severe (poverty, unemployment, single parent status) |
| Axis V | Current GAF: 50<br>Highest GAF past year: 70 |

*GAF,* global assessment of functioning.

She said she can't make enough money working to pay bills and child care.

Client has drunk alcohol and used pot since age 11. She has tried speed and diazepam (Valium) and has used cocaine by snorting, injection, and smoking (Table A-10).

### Interview

Client stated she has used crack for the past 9 months and denies any other drugs since then except an occasional beer. Client admitted to using her welfare check for drugs and selling her food stamps to obtain money. She was never married and does not receive financial support from the fathers of her children. Client, who is slightly overweight, was observed purging food in the bathroom of the detoxification unit and admitted to episodic purging to control weight.

Ms. Little described herself as a good student in high school until her drug use became more important than studying. She has a high school diploma but did not attempt college, as she felt she could not afford it. Client's parents both drank and were physically abusive to one another. Ms. Little denies physical or sexual abuse of self or siblings by parents. Client reported she cooks, cleans, and

**TABLE A-11. OCCUPATIONAL THERAPY TREATMENT SUMMARY (CASE 8)**

| GOALS | OBJECTIVES | OT TREATMENT GIVEN |
|---|---|---|
| 1. To obtain a driver's license | 1. Client will spend 1 hr a day studying drivers manual and take her driver's test before discharge | 1. Individual OT as needed |
| 2. Destructive lifestyle | 2a. Client will identify for pursuit after discharge five leisure activities appropriate for a sober lifestyle (by 2 wk) | 2a. Leisure education 1 × wk; community out-trip 1 × wk |
| | 2b. Client will introduce herself to at least two women per night at 12-step meetings | 2b. Nightly 12-step meeting; leisure education assignment |
| | 2c. Client will identify at least five activities to pursue with children at home and five in the community (by 2 wk) | 2c. Leisure education 1 × wk; community out-trip 1 × wk |
| 3. To obtain job, educational training | 3a. Client will meet with vocational rehabilitation counselor (by 1 wk) | 3a. OT referral to vocational rehabilitation |
| | 3b. Client will identify job and educational training interests (by 1 wk) | 3b. Individual OT sessions |
| 4. To improve energy level and decrease craving for crack | 4a. Client will complete exercise assessment (by 3 d). | 4a. Individual OT assessment |
| | 4b. Client will participate in daily exercise program for 20 min initially (by 4 d, increasing to 45 min by 2 wk) | 4b. Daily structured exercise program |

takes care of all household chores independently. She stated she has been "out of control" since she took up crack 9 months ago, smoking approximately $200 worth 1 to 2 days per week at friends' homes or crack houses. She admitted to leaving the children alone twice over the last month and was appalled that she would do such a thing. She admitted to having slept with crack dealers to obtain drugs. Client stated that she knows she has to get clean or she will lose her children. She has never obtained a driver's license but does have a car of her mother's that she drives. She has no friends except other users, and other than drug use her only leisure activity is renting a movie for the children. Ms. Little stated that she feels depressed much of the time and has no energy.

Goals, objectives, and treatment are shown in the treatment summary for this case (Table A-11).

## Occupational Therapy Discharge Summary (3 Weeks after Admission)

Ms. Little has been alternately resistant and compliant with treatment throughout the 3 weeks. She argued that she didn't need a driver's license but became willing after this issue was addressed repeatedly by OTA, along with treatment team. Client was assigned specific study times and obtained her license 18 days after admission. She expressed pride at this accomplishment.

Client was resistant to identifying leisure activities for herself, but after several community outtrips began to identify enjoyable leisure interests such as putt-putt golf, swimming, movies, hiking, and eating out. Client selected as family interests board games, making cookies, and going to parks and McDonald's. She met with the vocational rehabilitation counselor and completed the application. OTA sent all records to the counselor, who has confirmed that client is eligible for assistance. One of her sisters has committed to keeping her children for her so that she can attend school when the time comes. Client appeared enthusiastic and stated that an opportunity for education and job preparation gives her hope. She identified a list of job interests and strengths, which was communicated to the counselor.

A goal to increase assertive behavior was added to treatment plan after client described how much difficulty she has saying no to peers. She role-played situations, was initially too aggressive, but after practice was able to express herself calmly but firmly. She introduced herself to other women at 12-step meetings, and spent time with two women volunteer alumnae who shared recovery experiences with her.

Client participated in the exercise program only after much encouragement from staff. Treatment team and OTA several times met with her to emphasize the importance of her following directions and increasing exercise participation. This client will continue to meet with OTA twice a week to work on leisure, assertiveness, and exercise compliance.

## Questions for Case 8

1. Compare this client with the client of similar age in case 6. What are the differences and what are the similarities?
2. What are this client's occupational roles now? What occupational roles might this client acquire for the future?
3. What additional community supports or aftercare strategies would be helpful for this client?

## CASE 9: A 12-YEAR-OLD BOY WITH ATTENTION DEFICIT-HYPERACTIVITY DISORDER AND OPPOSITIONAL DEFIANT DISORDER[17]

*Danny B.* *Case #38–499*

Danny is a 12-year-old boy who is in the fifth grade. He is being home-schooled by his father, who is a freelance illustrator; his parents feel that he is too distracted by peers to function in a school setting because of his behavioral problems (Table A-12). His school history shows below average academic achievement (he repeated fourth grade) despite average verbal and mathematical intelligence in testing with the *Wechsler Intelligence Scale for Children*, 3rd ed. (*WISC-III*). Since entering school he has had difficulty getting along with other children and has been picked on and ostracized. In kindergarten, he threw a chair across the classroom. Teachers in second and third grades restrained him several times when he struck out at classmates. He has been tested for learning disabilities but none were found. Danny is being

**TABLE A-12. *DSM-IV-TR* DIAGNOSIS AT ADMISSION (CASE 9)**

| | |
|---|---|
| Axis I | 314.01 Attention deficit–hyperactivity disorder, predominantly hyperactive-impulsive type<br>313.81 Oppositional defiant disorder |
| Axis II | None |
| Axis III | None |
| Axis IV | Severity moderate (conflicts in school, with siblings) |
| Axis V | Current GAF: 35<br>Highest GAF past year: 60 |

*GAF*, global assessment of functioning.

[17] Composite based on several clinical cases.

medicated with divalproex (Depakote), methylphenidate (Ritalin), and bupropion (Wellbutrin).

Danny is the oldest of four children, with a younger sister aged 9 and twin brothers aged 18 months. He was a full-term baby, delivered by cesarean section after unsuccessful attempts to move him from a breech presentation. Mother recalls that as an infant Danny was fussy and cried a lot in comparison with her other children. Developmental milestones were within normal limits (WNL). Since age 2 Danny has had intense temper tantrums and seemed easily frustrated. His parents assumed he would outgrow it, but the behavior continued. He would, for example, refuse to join in family activities, causing the entire family to miss planned events because he would kick anyone who attempted to drag him along. Parents and teachers have described Danny as absentminded and inattentive, demanding, argumentative, disruptive, loud, stubborn, withdrawn, suspicious, and moody.

Danny has no current peer friendships and no sustained peer relationships in the past. Teachers and parents describe his behavior with peers as bullying and unaware, insensitive to context, intense and needy, and in the words of one teacher "clueless about how to be a member of a group." Relationships with siblings are stormy, but Danny relies on his 9-year-old sister to be a friend and companion. He is jealous of his sister's friends; when friends visit his sister, Danny often disrupts their play, sometimes destroying toys and drawings.

Danny has few chores but does them if reminded several times. He enjoys taking in the mail and sorting it. He takes out the trash sometimes. His mother complains that he dawdles and takes forever to finish some chores, such as setting the table and taking out the trash. He feeds the two cats and the rabbits and likes to pet the animals. The cats have scratched him for being too rough. Danny's mother says she doesn't make him do too many chores because he is impatient and has broken too many things.

Danny has been home-schooled for the past year. On a typical day, he and his father work on the lessons for 2 hours, and then Danny has 4 to 6 hours of independent work. Danny's father says that Danny focuses well on his schoolwork and seems in particular to enjoy math and reading. However, Danny's father has to work longer hours to generate more income and would like to have Danny back in school.

Danny has had 3 years of psychotherapy with a psychologist; his parents say they see little change. They feel the medications have helped somewhat in curbing Danny's impulsivity and oppositional behaviors. The psychologist suggested occupational therapy for evaluation of social skills and for interventions to enable him to develop relationships with other children and to function in a public school classroom.

## Questions for Case 9

1. What challenges do you anticipate in forming a relationship with Danny?
2. Identify two major occupational roles appropriate to Danny's chronological age. For each, list the skills Danny already possesses. Then, based on the history, identify the specific skills Danny needs to develop to function in these roles.
3. The OT would like you to involve Danny in an activity to observe and assess his task skills and general approach to tasks. What activities would you consider? How would you present this to Danny? How would you try to engage him?
4. Write a long-term goal and two related short-term objectives corresponding to one of the problems you have identified. Explain why you think this goal and these objectives are a priority. Then describe *in detail* the methods you would use to work on the objectives.
5. What adaptations, compensations, and environmental supports would you suggest for the school setting? For the home? For social situations?
6. Looking ahead, 2 or 3 years from now, what developmental issues will be important for Danny? What risks do you predict? What preventive measures might help?

APPENDIX **B**

# Sample Group Protocols

## HOMEMAKER'S MANAGEMENT GROUP

### Description

A psychoeducation group for homemakers, focused on management and delegation of tasks and reduction of stress.

### Structure

Meets one afternoon per week for 1 hour. Written homework assignments assist members to practice concepts discussed in group. Group is limited to six members. Leader: OT or OTA who is also a homemaker.

### Goals

Through participation in this group, members will learn to:

1. Analyze and set priorities for their own household and caregiving tasks
2. Identify and report areas of difficulty for self in homemaker role
3. Learn and apply various problem-solving techniques to get household work done with less stress to self
4. Report results of problem-solving efforts to the group and receive feedback
5. Be able to state one's needs and request assistance from others

### Referral Criteria

Clients who are

- Homemakers
- Able to tolerate verbal group for 1 hour
- Able, with structure, to discuss their experience of homemaker role
- Willing to do homework assignments outside of group time

### Methodology

The group will be structured around a lesson or worksheet. After a brief introduction of members and of the group goals, leader will present the lesson or worksheet. Members will work on the lesson for approximately 20 minutes. A group discussion will follow. The meeting will end with an assignment to be done outside of group. The lesson or worksheet will vary with the needs of individuals and the group. Topics may include analysis of time use, time-management strategies, problem identification, generation of alternatives, assertiveness role-plays, finding social support, and so on.

### Role of the Leader

Leader will

- Structure and present group exercises
- Keep group on task and on time
- Facilitate discussion, feedback, and problem solving
- Contribute own experiences, serving as a role model
- Perform evaluations and outcomes assessment

### Evaluation

Clients will complete a forced-choice questionnaire on attitudes toward homemaker role as a pretest and posttest.

## Resources

Exercises on job stress, parenting, assertiveness, money management, role satisfaction, stress management, time management, values clarification, goal setting, coping skills, support systems, and so on are available from:

1. Korb KL, Azok SD, Leutenberg EA. Life Management Skills. Beachwood, OH: Wellness Reproductions, 1989.
2. Korb KL, Azok SD, Leutenberg EA. Life Management Skills: 2. Beachwood, OH: Wellness Reproductions, 1991.
3. Korb-Khalsa KL, Leutenberg EA, Azok SD. Life Management Skills: 3. Beachwood, OH: Wellness Reproductions, 1994.
4. Korb-Khalsa KL, Leutenberg EA. Life Management Skills: 4. Beachwood, OH: Wellness Reproductions, 1996.
5. Korb KL, Leutenberg EA, Brodsky AL. Life Management Skills: 5. Beachwood, OH: Wellness Reproductions, 2001.
6. Simmons PL, Mullins L. Acute Psychiatric Care. Thorofare, NJ: Slack, 1981.

# FAMILY RECREATION SKILLS[1]

## Description

A psychoeducation group for recovering substance abusers to assist the development or rediscovery of leisure activities in the context of the family.

## Structure

Group meets the first Monday of the month from 7:00 to 8:45 P.M. in the recreation room, OT workshop, or lounge, depending on activity, led by OTA or OT technician.

## Goals

Through participation in this group, the client will learn to:

1. Identify the effects of addiction and recovery on family leisure patterns
2. Interact pleasurably in a leisure situation with family members
3. Identify enjoyable leisure activities appropriate for families

## Referral Criteria

Clients who

- Are newly sober or drug free
- Have family members who can attend the group

## Methodology

Leader will assist those present to introduce themselves (10 minutes). Leader will lecture briefly on a leisure topic related to addiction, such as effects of addiction on family leisure; healing effects of fun and play; learning to enjoy each other again (10 to 15 minutes). Activities are then introduced, distributed. Session ends with a summary and comments from participants, facilitated by leader.

## Role of the Leader

Leader will

- Provide information and learning opportunities
- Facilitate pleasurable interaction in the group
- Assist participants to explore new recreational options

## Evaluation

Pretest, posttest: Clients asked to list recreational activities that they would like to do with their families.

[1] This protocol adapted with permission from one by Susan Voorhies, COTA, CSAC, and Anne Brown, OTR, MS, of ReDiscovery Unit, HCA Hospital, Jackson, TN.

## ADOLESCENT COOKING GROUP[2]

### Description

A role acquisition group for adolescents to develop more independence in meal preparation.

### Structure

Meets after school four afternoons per week for 2 hours. Each session includes a brief lesson followed by an activity such as shopping or cooking. Group makes meals two afternoons a week, shops two afternoons a week. Group meets in the kitchen.

### Goals

Through participation in this group, members will learn to:

1. Plan simple, nutritionally balanced dinners
2. Shop within a budget
3. Take advantages of sales, specials, and coupons
4. Prepare simple foods such as meat loaf, omelets, salads, puddings, and gelatin desserts

### Referral Criteria

Adolescent clients who

- Wish to assume greater responsibility for meal preparation
- Or are single parents and have this responsibility
- Or desire placement in supervised group apartments
- And do not already possess these skills

### Methodology

Each group session includes a lesson (e.g., food safety, nutrition, kitchen emergencies, stretching a budget) and an activity (either shopping or cooking). On cooking days, the members eat the meal and do the cleanup. Each session ends with discussion and planning for the next session.

### Role of the Leader

Leader will

- Provide structure and instruction
- Keep group oriented to task and time
- Encourage sharing among members
- Guide discussion and planning sessions
- Provide support to individuals to assist in skill development
- Perform outcomes assessment

### Evaluation

Members will complete a pretest before joining the group and a posttest after 12 weeks.

### Resources

Books and videos on cooking, nutrition, home management, and safety. Advertising circulars, newspapers, and coupons.

## DEMENTIA COOKING GROUP[3]

### Description

A group for persons with dementia for whom cooking was a major life activity, either as homemaker or as professional cook. Group is based on Allen's Cognitive Levels with accommodations for cognitive disabilities.

### Structure

Meets two mornings per week for 1 hour. Each session begins with sensory stimulation, followed by a highly structured food preparation activity. Participants eat the food at the end of the meeting and share their responses to the food and to the experience. Group meets in the kitchen. Group is limited to six participants at a time. Group is led by OTA with help from OT aides, students, and volunteers.

[2] The adolescent cooking group and the dementia cooking group use the same activity for different populations and for different goals.

[3] The adolescent cooking group and the dementia cooking group use the same activity for different populations and for different goals.

## Goals

Through participation in this group, members will

1. Identify specific scents, ingredients, and utensils
2. Recall pleasant experiences associated with cooking
3. Contribute to the completion of a task
4. Maintain awareness of environment
5. Watch and follow demonstrated directions

## Referral Criteria

Persons with dementia who

- Function at ACL levels 2.8 through 4.6
- Have previous experience of food preparation
- Are able to travel on foot or in wheelchair, with or without assistance
- Are not on dietary restrictions for sugar or salt

## Methodology

This is a highly structured group designed to permit maximum participation by persons with moderate to severe cognitive disabilities. Meeting will begin with sensory stimulation using food scents (e.g., vanilla, cinnamon, lime). Under leader's direction, members will prepare or assemble a food that requires no additional waiting time (i.e., does not require long baking or chilling before consumption). Members will then enjoy the food and participate in guided discussion of the experience and of any memories triggered by the experience.

## Role of the Leader

Leader or leaders will

- Provide structure, support, and environmental compensation commensurate with each member's task abilities
- Provide for safety of all participants
- Maintain appropriate hygiene of members during group (prevent contamination of food)
- Facilitate sharing by members of their responses to the experience

## Resources

Bottles, vials, bags of scented oils and spices. Adapted utensils to prevent injury.

# MANAGING WORK-RELATED STRESS[4]

## Description

A cognitive-behavioral group for persons with serious mental illness who are currently employed or placed in transitional work.

## Structure

Group meets in the conference room once a week on Wednesdays at noon for 1 hour. The duration of the program is 12 weeks. The OTA leads the group.

## Goals

Through participation in this group, the client will learn to

1. Monitor stress and stress-related symptoms
2. Recognize the effects of stress on work performance
3. Identify personal reactions to stress
4. Learn and practice alternative techniques for handling negative reactions and stress

## Referral Criteria

Clients who

- Are employed, are in supported employment, or are in some other work placement
- Identify work-related stress as a problem

## Methodology

Each session begins with a warmup to engage participation and increase motivation. This is followed by a lesson, which may include videos and demonstration. Clients then have the opportunity to discuss, analyze, and practice what they have

[4] This protocol based on ideas from Lee H, Tan HK, Ma H, Tsai C, Liu Y. Effectiveness of a work-related stress management program in patients with chronic schizophrenia. Am J Occup Ther 2006;60:435–441.

learned. Homework assignments for the week are distributed. Session ends with a summary and comments from participants, facilitated by leader. Topics included are stress and the stress reaction, communication strategies, assertiveness training, problem-solving strategies, mindfulness strategies, and stress reduction techniques.

### Role of the Leader

Leader will

- Present information about stress and the stress reaction in the workplace
- Assist clients to identify their own reactions to stress and to challenge the automatic thoughts that accompany stressful situations
- Assist to identify personal goals related to stress reduction
- Instruct and help clients practice techniques for stress management

### Evaluation

Pretest, post-test: Clients complete a quiz on stress and how they handle it as well as knowledge of stress management.

## THE GREEN TEAM (HORTICULTURE CLUBHOUSE GROUP)[5]

### Description

A horticulture group to give clubhouse members an experience of working with others, through the media of plants and floral objects.

### Structure

Group meets in a classroom or activity room once a week on Thursdays at 1 P.M. for 2 hours. During warm weather, the group also meets outside in the garden plot near the parking lot. The OTA leads the group.

[5] This protocol based on ideas from Perrins-Margalis NM, Rugletic J, Schepis NM, et al. The immediate effects of a group-based horticulture experience on the quality of life of persons with chronic mental illness. Occ Ther Ment Health 2000;16(1):15–32.

### Goals

Through participation in this group, members will learn to

1. Work together as a team, creating floral objects and planting and tending the garden
2. Learn to work with live and dried plant materials
3. Acquire work-related skills through plant culture and through making floral objects
4. Reflect on and explore feelings about the natural environment and plants

### Membership Criteria

Members must commit to staying with the group for 6 weeks.

### Methodology

This group has an object-relations orientation and also addresses task skills and project level group skills. Session content varies with time of year. During colder weather, indoor activities focus on using live and dried plant material to create objects such as terrariums, wreaths, pressed flowers, paper crafts with floral accents. During spring, seedling cultivation is introduced. In summer, garden planting and tending is the main activity. Members are encouraged to reflect on their experience of nature and their reactions to working with plants, and with each other. Exploration and sharing of feelings is encouraged through group discussion at the end of each session.

### Role of the Leader

- To select and introduce activities that will be meaningful to members
- To instruct members in techniques for working with plant materials
- To facilitate exploration and reflection on feelings
- To facilitate project-level group skills through short-term shared activities, as appropriate for individual members

# Index

## A

**B**

**H**

## S